REHABILITATION OF THE INJURED KNEE

EDITOR

Letha Y. Griffin

Staff, Peachtree Orthopaedic Clinic
Team Physician, Georgia State University
and Agnes Scott College
Atlanta, Georgia

SECOND EDITION

with *374* illustrations

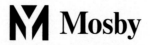 **Mosby**

St. Louis Baltimore Berlin Boston Carlsbad Chicago London Madrid
Naples New York Philadelphia Sydney Tokyo Toronto

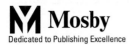
Mosby
Dedicated to Publishing Excellence

Editor: Robert Hurley
Developmental Editor: Leslie Neistadt
Associate Developmental Editor: Christine Pluta
Project Manager: Linda Clarke
Project Supervisor: Allan S. Kleinberg
Designer: Sheilah Barrett
Manufacturing Supervisor: John Babrick
Cover Artist: Diane Kay Davis

Printed in the United States of America
Composition by Graphic World
Printing/binding by Maple-Vail York

Mosby–Year Book, Inc.
11830 Westline Industrial Drive
St. Louis, Missouri 63146

Library of Congress Cataloging in Publication Data

Rehabilitation of the injured knee/editor, Letha Y. Griffin. —2nd
ed.
    p.   cm.
  Rev. ed. of: Rehabilitation of the injured knee/editors, Letha
Y. Hunter, F. James Funk, Jr. 1984.
  Includes bibliographical references and index.
  ISBN 0-8016-7556-1
  1. Knee—Wounds and injuries. 2. Knee—Wounds and injuries—
Patients—Rehabilitation.   I. Griffin, Letha Y.
  [DNLM: 1. Knee Injuries—rehabilitation. 2. Knee Joint—
  physiology.   WE 870 R345 1994]
RD561.R43 1994
617.5'82—dc20
DNLM/DLC   94-26852
for Library of Congress   CIP

95 96 97 98 99/9 8 7 6 5 4 3 2 1

Contributors

David F. Apple, Jr., M.D.
Associate Clinical Professor of Orthopaedic Surgery
Clinical Assistant Professor of Rehabilitation Medicine
Emory University
Clinical Professor of Orthopaedics
Georgia State University
Medical Director, Shepherd Spinal Center
Piedmont Hospital
Atlanta, Georgia

Elizabeth A. Arendt, M.D.
Assistant Professor, Department of Orthopaedic Surgery
University of Minnesota
Active Full-Time Staff
University of Minnesota Hospital
Minneapolis, Minnesota

Champ L. Baker, Jr., M.D.
The Hughston Clinic
Columbus, Georgia
Clinical Assistant Professor, Department of Orthopaedics
Tulane University
New Orleans, Louisiana

Robert M. Barnette, Jr., M.S., A.T.,C.
Instructor
Georgia State University
Coordinator of Sports Medicine
Peachtree Orthopaedic Clinic
Atlanta, Georgia

Dale F. Blair, M.S., A.T.,C., C.S.C.S.
Head Athletic Trainer
Wenatchee High School
Wenatchee, Washington

James E. Carpenter, M.D.
Assistant Professor of Surgery
University of Michigan Medical School
Orthopaedic Surgeon
University of Michigan Medical Center
Ann Arbor, Michigan

George N. Cernansky, Jr., M.S., A.T.,C.
Assistant Coordinator of Sports Medicine
Peachtree Orthopaedic Clinic
Atlanta, Georgia

T. Jeff Chandler, Ed.D., C.S.C.S., F.A.C.S.M.
Director of Sports Medicine Research and Education
Lexington Clinic Sports Medicine Center
Lexington, Kentucky

Mark S. De Carlo, M.S., P.T., A.T.,C.
Director of Physical Therapy
Methodist Sports Medicine Center
Indianapolis, Indiana

Peter J. Fowler, M.D., F.R.C.S.(C)
Professor of Orthopaedic Surgery
Head, Section of Sports Medicine
University of Western Ontario
University Hospital
London, Ontario, Canada

John P. Fulkerson, M.D.
Professor of Orthopaedic Surgery
The University of Connecticut School of Medicine
Farmington, Connecticut

William E. Garrett, Jr., M.D., Ph.D.
Associate Professor of Orthopaedic Surgery and Cell Biology
Duke University Medical Center
Durham, North Carolina

Brian P. Gastaldi, B.Sc. (P.T.), M.Sc., C.A.T.(C.)
Honorary Lecturer, Faculty of Kinesiology
University of Western Ontario
Clinical Specialist, Sports Physiotherapy
University Hospital
J. C. Kennedy Athletic Injuries Clinic
London, Ontario, Canada

Mark A. Gomez, Ph.D.
Assistant Adjunct Professor, Department of Orthopaedics
University of California, School of Medicine
San Diego, California

Daniel Gould, Ph.D.
Professor, Department of Exercise and Sport Science
University of North Carolina at Greensboro
Greensboro, North Carolina

Moya F. Hambridge, P.T., M.C.S.P. Dip PT
Physical Therapy Manager
Piedmont Hospital
Atlanta, Georgia

Jack Harvey, M.D.
Chief, Section of Sports Medicine
Orthopaedic Center of the Rockies
Fort Collins, Colorado

Stanley A. Herring, M.D.
Clinical Associate Professor
Department of Rehabilitation Medicine and Orthopaedics
University of Washington
Puget Sound Sports and Spine Physicians
Swedish Hospital
Seattle, Washington

Jack C. Hughston, M.D.
Clinical Professor Emeritus, Division of Orthopaedics
Tulane University School of Medicine
New Orleans, Louisiana
Professor Adjunct, School of Veterinary Medicine
Auburn University
Auburn, Alabama
Orthopaedic Surgeon
The Hughston Clinic
Chairman of the Board, The Hughston Sports Medicine
  Hospital
Orthopaedic Consultant, Martin Army Community Hospital
Columbus, Georgia

Mark R. Hutchinson, M.D.
Assistant Professor of Orthopaedics
Director of Sports Medicine Services
Orthopaedic Team Consultant
University of Illinois at Chicago
Chicago, Illinois

Mary Lloyd Ireland, M.D.
Assistant Professor, Department of Surgery (Orthopaedics)
University of Kentucky
Lexington, Kentucky

W. Ben Kibler, M.D., F.A.C.S.M.
Medical Director
Lexington Clinic Sports Medicine Center
Lexington, Kentucky

Thomas E. Klootwyk, M.D.
Clinical Instructor
Indiana University School of Medicine
Orthopaedic Surgeon, Department of Orthopaedics
Methodist Hospital of Indiana
Indianapolis, Indiana

Michael C. Koester, B.S., A.T.,C.
Student of Medicine
University of Nevada School of Medicine
Reno, Nevada

Mark G. Kowall, M.D.
Fellow
The Orthopaedic Specialty Hospital
Salt Lake City, Utah

Mark E. Longacre, M.P.T.
Sports Medicine Center
Omaha, Nebraska

Jerry A. Lubliner, M.D.
Assistant Attending Physician
Hospital for Joint Diseases
New York, New York

Gregory E. Lutz, M.D.
Instructor in Rehabilitation Medicine
Cornell University Medical College
Physiatrist
Hospital for Special Surgery
New York, New York

Terry R. Malone, Ed.D., P.T., A.T.,C.
Director and Associate Professor of Physical Therapy
University of Kentucky
Lexington, Kentucky

Frederic C. McDuffie, M.D.
Professor of Medicine
Emory University
Director, Arthritis Center
Piedmont Hospital
Atlanta, Georgia

Troy E. McIntosh, A.T.,C., C.S.C.S.
Graduate Assistant, Athletic Department
Georgia State University
Atlanta, Georgia

Lyle J. Micheli, M.D.
Associate Clinical Professor of Orthopaedic Surgery
Harvard Medical School
Director, Division of Sports Medicine
The Children's Hospital
Boston, Massachusetts

Thomas J. Moore, M.D.
Associate Professor
Emory University School of Medicine
Emory University Hospital
Crawford W. Long Memorial Hospital
Grady Memorial Hospital
Atlanta, Georgia

Lonnie E. Paulos, M.D.
Medical Director
Orthopaedic Biomechanics Institute
The Orthopaedic Specialty Hospital
Salt Lake City, Utah

Robert M. Poole, M.Ed., P.T., A.T.,C.
Director
The Human Performance and Rehabilitation Center
Atlanta, Georgia

James L. Sarni, M.D.
Assistant Professor
Departments of Orthopaedics and Rehabilitation Medicine
Tufts Medical School
Attending Physician
New England Medical Center
Boston, Massachusetts

Kevin P. Shea, M.D.
Assistant Professor of Orthopaedic Surgery
University of Connecticut School of Medicine
Assistant Clinical Chief of Orthopaedics
John Dempsey Hospital
Farmington, Connecticut

K. Donald Shelbourne, M.D.
Associate Clinical Professor
Indiana University School of Medicine
Orthopaedic Surgeon, Department of Orthopaedics
Methodist Hospital of Indiana
Indianapolis, Indiana

J. Andy Sullivan, M.D.
Professor and Chair
Department of Orthopaedic Surgery and Rehabilitation
University of Oklahoma College of Medicine
Children's Hospital of Oklahoma
Oklahoma City, Oklahoma

Suzanne M. Tanner, M.D.
Assistant Professor
Departments of Orthopaedics and Pediatrics
University of Colorado Health Sciences Center
Director, Adolescent Sports Medicine
Denver Children's Hospital
Denver, Colorado

Carol C. Teitz, M.D.
Associate Professor
Department of Orthopaedics
Division of Sports Medicine
University of Washington
Seattle, Washington

Laurie L. Tis, Ph.D., A.T.,C.
Assistant Professor
Director of Graduate Sports Medicine
Department of Kinesiology and Health
Georgia State University
Atlanta, Georgia

Eileen M. Udry, M.S.
University of North Carolina at Greensboro
Greensboro, North Carolina

Tim L. Uhl, M.S., P.T., A.T.,C.
Director of Physical Therapy
The Human Performance and Rehabilitation Center
Columbus, Georgia

W. Michael Walsh, M.D.
Adjunct Graduate Associate Professor
School of Health, Physical Education, and Recreation
University of Nebraska at Omaha
Clinical Associate Professor of Orthopaedic Surgery
University of Nebraska Medical Center
Active Staff
Nebraska Methodist Hospital and Children's Hospital
Omaha, Nebraska

Russell F. Warren, M.D.
Professor of Orthopaedic Surgery
Cornell Medical Center
Surgeon-in-Chief
Hospital for Special Surgery
New York, New York

Edward M. Wojtys, M.D.
Associate Professor
University of Michigan Medical School
University of Michigan Medical Center
MedSport
Ann Arbor, Michigan

Preface to Second Edition

This second edition of *Rehabilitation of the Injured Knee* comes a decade after the first edition was published. Not only does this edition incorporate new advances in rehabilitation techniques and equipment, but it gives greater emphasis to sport-specific functional rehabilitation programs as well as detailing rehabilitation schemes following specific injuries. It is hoped that the reader will find these more focused, practical applications helpful.

Letha Y. Griffin

Preface to First Edition

Much has been written regarding various surgical procedures of the knee, but very little has been written about the rehabilitation of this joint. Yet, in an athletic population, rehabilitation is the keystone to recovery. The best surgical efforts will not produce an adequate result unless coupled with such a program. In many cases surgery is not even required; a well-designed rehabilitation scheme is all that is needed to return the athlete's injured knee to its prior level of strength, endurance, and power. Such a program must take into consideration the condition of the athlete before injury, the type of injury sustained, the surgical procedures performed, and the level of competition to which the athlete must return. Not only must the anatomy of the knee and the physiology of ligament, cartilage, and muscle be understood in constructing this program, but the psychological profile of the athlete is also important.

Perhaps one reason so little has been written on knee rehabilitation is that the design of an adequate program takes the efforts of many health professionals—the physician, the physiologist, the biomechanics specialist, the therapist or trainer, and the psychologist. In this book we have tried, with the help of these health professionals, to describe the various facets of knee rehabilitation. The initial chapters deal with the basic knowledge of the knee. This basic knowledge is then used to build principles needed to design programs for regaining range of motion, muscle strength, power, and endurance following an injury. The remaining chapters present examples of rehabilitation schemes that may be useful to those designing their own programs.

To those of you reading this volume, we hope the information provided by the book's many authors will prove valuable in your efforts to achieve a rapid but safe return of your athletes to sport.

Letha Y. Griffin
F. James Funk, Jr.

Acknowledgments

A special thank you to all those who labored over the writing of the chapters enclosed within these covers . . . a thank you to the authors themselves and to their families who allowed them time away from home responsibilities to pursue this endeavor.

A thank you is also extended to all at Mosby for their attention to detail in final editing and production of this second edition, and to Jim Ryan, who is no longer with Mosby but who inspired all of us to develop the second edition of *Rehabilitation of the Injured Knee*.

To Leslie Neistadt, Developmental Editor, my grateful appreciation for the endless hours spent trying to keep all of us organized and focused until our task was completed.

To my family, Jim, Jordyn, and Ali, a special thank you for once again living on frozen dinners, doing your own laundry, and in general surviving without much help from this family member.

And to you, the readers, thank you for trusting us to provide you with a quality educational tool to help you better understand the complexities of rehabilitation of this truly intriguing joint, THE KNEE!

Letha Y. Griffin

Contents

Part I

INTRODUCTION AND HISTORICAL OVERVIEW

Chapter 1

INTRODUCTION AND HISTORICAL OVERVIEW

Jack C. Hughston

REHABILITATION

Rehabilitation is responsible for almost 100% of the recovery in patients with nonoperative knee disorders. Rehabilitation constitutes 50% of a good result in a surgically treated knee patient. Of course, successful rehabilitation requires a correct diagnosis and high-quality surgical achievement. Also, the prescribed rehabilitative exercises must be specific for the knee condition. Furthermore, the exercises must not be painful. Pain during exercise produces incomplete muscle contraction. The most frequent incorrect prescription I encounter is progressive resistance exercises from flexion to extension for patients with extensor mechanism disorders. The pain resulting from this exercise in this situation reduces muscle contraction and prevents patient compliance.

In addition to prescribing specific quadriceps and hamstrings exercises to strengthen the knee, we on the knee rehabilitation team must see to it that the whole of the lower extremity is rehabilitated. This requires exercises for the gastrocnemius and soleus and the hip adductors and abductors. So, all of the muscles of the lower extremity must be rehabilitated. Occasionally I see functional disability of the knee that is a result solely of weakness of one of these muscle groups. For instance, if the hip abductor is weak, a patient places the affected lower limb more centrally under the pelvis for balance during weightbearing. The result is medial joint line pain at the knee. Again, weak hip abductors may cause the patient to overuse the iliac muscle and iliotibial band, with the result being anterolateral knee pain. The knee itself in these instances is normal.

To achieve successful rehabilitation, endurance exercises must accompany muscle-strengthening exercises. Last, we cannot forget to make patients attain joint mobility through stretching exercises.

Now that we know the requirements of knee rehabilitation, how do we achieve them? Success requires the efforts of the entire rehabilitation team: the doctor, the therapist, the trainer, the coach, and the patient's family members and friends. Motivation is the key. Rehabilitation is organized boredom. Persistence requires constant encouragement and stimulation of the patient. It is human nature to begin letting up (slacking off) once the goal is in sight. This is the critical time for motivation. Only with motivation can the goal of strength and endurance be met.

I think frequency of exercise is most important. It is illogical to think that exercising only once in every 24-hour period will be sufficient. The prescribed exercises should be performed every 8 hours, or more frequently, during a day. To accomplish this, the exercises must be adaptable to various physical locations and must fit into the patient's lifestyle without too much interruption of the routines of daily life.

I like to have patients demonstrate their routine exercises to me on their first return clinic visit. Not infrequently the demonstration reveals that the patient has forgotten or misunderstood some of the finer points of the prescribed rehabilitation. The incorrect performance can then be corrected. Patients need to demonstrate how they perform the exercises, not merely tell you how they are performing them.

Once the patient is approaching a functional level in the rehabilitation program, the exercise prescription must be adjusted toward the requirements of the sport or activity level anticipated by the patient.

The use of a knee brace upon return to sports participation

may be an aid to further rehabilitation, according to some. I have never prescribed a brace. I think the muscles protect the knee, and thus I send the athlete back to action when the muscles are rehabilitated. Over my 40 years of experience, the rate of reinjury is minimal, almost zero. Rehabilitation is the true answer, not knee braces. Once knee stability, motion, function, and bony congruity are obtained and rehabilitation is complete, there is no subsequent ligamentous loosening or joint deterioration in the long-term follow-up.

HISTORICAL PERSPECTIVE

The World War II era was the beginning of rehabilitation as we know it today. During that time, I was on an orthopedic service in the Army Medical Corps and thus present for some important developments in the field of rehabilitation. Howard Rusk had developed the Rehabilitation Centers for Neurological Illness and Injury. I happened to be working in one of these neurologic centers, which was also combined with an amputation center. We quickly learned the importance of rehabilitation for the whole body, including the knee.

At this same time in history, Marcus Stewart was serving as an orthopedic consultant in the armed forces stationed in England. He championed rehabilitation of extremities in general, but the knee in particular. DeLorme reported the techniques and benefits of repetitive quadriceps exercises in knee rehabilitation toward the close of the war (1946). Immediately after the war, Phelps was utilizing rehabilitation to great advantage in cerebral palsy patients. Then Sister Kenny added her stimulus to rehabilitation of the polio patient.

In the years 1950 through 1955, I saw just about all of the patients with acute polio in southern Georgia. Orthopedists, especially those interested in children's disorders and acute polio, were relatively scarce in the Southeast at that time. Each summer I would have about 50 patients with acute polio in the local hospital. My physical therapist, Celia Craig, and I worked about 18 hours a day so that we could implement our rehabilitation routine in these patients. Warm Springs was just 20 miles up the road; however, Irvin and Bennett were primarily concentrating on the residuals of polio. They did give us considerable consultation when we requested it.

During the 1950s, sports medicine was emerging, although not recognized by name as it is today. It was, however, beginning to make its presence known in the orthopedic treatment and rehabilitation of the athlete, and at that time this was mostly concentrated toward the knee. This attention to the knee and to sports medicine grew significantly during the 1960s through the educational activities of the American Medical Association Committee on the Medical Aspects of Sports and as a result of the annual postgraduate courses produced by the Sports Medicine Committee of the American Academy of Orthopaedic Surgeons. Rehabilitation became much more sophisticated. Great strides in progress have continued since then.

With the outstanding faculty of this book covering each aspect of knee rehabilitation, conditioning, and physiologic muscle response in detail, I feel it would be improper for me to consume time and space by expounding on these specific areas in this introduction. These authors furnish us with the fine details and the latest advances related to rehabilitation of the knee.

Part II

GENERAL CONSIDERATIONS

Chapter 2

FUNCTIONAL ANATOMY AND BIOMECHANICS OF THE KNEE JOINT

Peter J. Fowler
Jerry Lubliner

The accurate diagnosis and optimum treatment of knee problems depend on the knowledge and understanding of the anatomy and biomechanics involved in both normal and abnormal function. In the knee, stability is not a function of the bony architecture to the same extent that it is in joints such as the hip and ankle. Performance at maximal efficiency is the result of the coordinated effort of all components: ligamentous, muscular, osseous, and cartilaginous. In this chapter the complex interplay of structure and function is presented by categorizing the structures of the knee as five separate units: (1) bony architecture, (2) cruciate-meniscus complex, (3) semimembranosus posteromedial-medial complex, (4) biceps femoris posterolateral-lateral complex, and (5) quadriceps anteromedial-anterolateral complex.

In the knee, motion occurs between the tibia and femur and between the articulating surfaces of the patella and femur. The knee is capable of six independent motions or "degrees of freedom": three rotational and three translational.[1] These occur on three axes and can occur in combination (Fig. 2-1; Table 2-1). All components interact to limit more than one motion. Injury to any component results in increased laxity. During clinical examination, specific structures are assessed individually by positioning the knee so that other structures do not resist motion. The three primary forces that act on the knee are described by Frankel and Nordin as ground reaction force, patellar tendon force, and joint reaction force.[2] In ground reaction, the major load is transmitted through the tibia during heel strike. At the knee the reaction takes place as forces transmitted by ligaments, muscles, and tendons and by the contact between the bony surfaces.

The knee is inherently unstable, particularly in flexion. It is characterized by features of both a ginglymoid (hinged) and a trochoid (pivot) articulation. Normal movement involves flexion and extension but very little action in any other direction. The bulk of the posterior soft tissues limits extreme flexion; the bony configuration and the tension created in the capsular and ligamentous structures limit extension. Rotation can be variable but is usually less than 10 degrees, with the greatest amount passively obtained at 90 degrees of flexion. As the knee comes into extension during weightbearing, the femur internally rotates on the tibia. In complete extension, no rotation is possible, and the knee is most stable.

Flexion and extension are a combination of rolling and gliding movements,[3] with rolling occurring during the first 20 degrees of flexion, and gliding during the rest of the motion. During normal flexion a combination of these two motions results in a typical posterior shift of contact points of both articular surfaces so that the femur does not impinge on the posterior tibial plateau (Fig. 2-2). Abnormal motion of the knee caused by trauma or internal derangement alters normal mechanics and results in pathology. Frankel and Burstein[4] have used instant center analysis (first described by Reuleaux[5]) to prove that an internal derangement of the knee causes a displaced instant center and interferes with the screw-home mechanism. The knee may counteract by stretching soft tissue support structures or by exerting increased or abnormally directed forces on articular cartilage.[6]

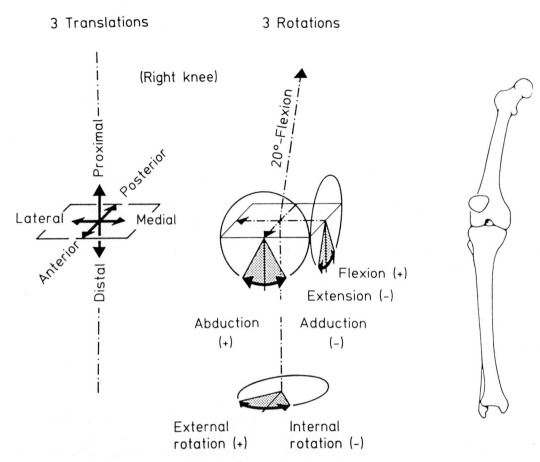

Fig. 2-1. The six degrees of freedom of knee motion: three translations and three rotations, right knee. (From Jakob RP, Staübli HU: *The knee and cruciate ligaments,* 1990, Fig. 1, p. 3.)

Table 2-1. Independent motions of the knee: degrees of freedom

Joint rotations and axes		Knee translations and axes	
Flexion-extension	Medial-lateral located in femur	Medial-lateral	Flexion-extension
Internal-external	Parallel to tibial shaft	Anterior-posterior	Abduction-adduction
Abduction	Parallel to femoral sagittal and tibial transverse planes	Compression-distraction	Internal-external rotation

BONY ARCHITECTURE

In extension there is a high degree of tibiofemoral congruency, which helps to stabilize the joint[7] (Fig. 2-3). Viewed from the lateral side, the **femoral condyles** are cam-shaped with a flatter distal end and a highly curved posterior margin.[8] The **lateral femoral condyle** is broader in both the anteroposterior and transverse planes than in the medial plane (Fig. 2-3, *A*). Distally, the **medial femoral condyle** projects to a slightly lower level than the lateral condyle[9] (Fig. 2-3, *B*). The lateral condyle has a more flattened curve and a characteristic notch by which it can be identified on a lateral radiograph[10] (Fig. 2-3, *C*). The disparate shape of the condyles facilitates the screw-home mechanism or terminal rotation of the femur at final extension (Fig. 2-4).

The articular surface of the medial femoral condyle is prolonged anteriorly, and as the knee comes into full extension, the femur internally rotates until the anterior articular surface of the medial condyle is in contact with the tibial plateau. In this position the knee is locked.

The femoral condyles have a smaller radius of curvature than the tibial plateaus.[7] During rotational movements, the medial condyle describes a smaller arc than the lateral condyle.[9] This potentially unstable condition is improved by the menisci, which increase tibiofemoral congruency. Aberrations in the anatomy of the femoral condyles can lead to unstable conditions. A subluxating patella may result from a hypoplastic lateral femoral condyle. The trochlear groove, the patellofemoral articulation, is formed by the

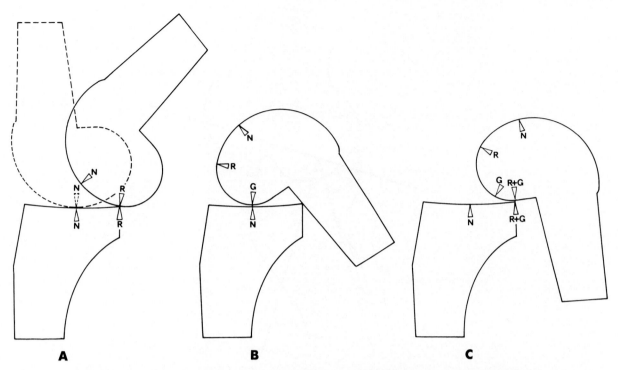

Fig. 2-2. Combination of rolling and gliding during knee flexion allows the femur to flex without impinging on the posterior tibial plateau. **A,** Movement of the femur relative to the tibia if only rolling occurred. **B,** Movement of the femur relative to the tibia if only gliding occurred. **C,** True knee flexion as combination of rolling and gliding. (From Parisien JS: *Arthroscopic surgery*, McGraw-Hill, New York, 1988.)

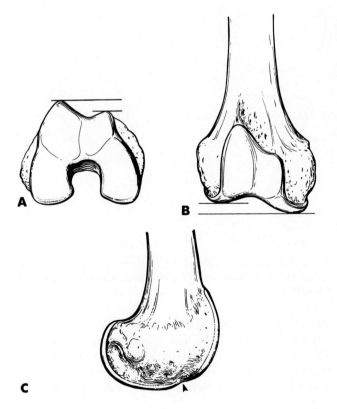

Fig. 2-3. A, The lateral femoral condyle is broader than the medial femoral condyle. **B,** The medial femoral condyle projects distally to a level slightly lower than the lateral condyle. **C,** The characteristic notch of the lateral femoral condyle assists in x-ray identification in the lateral view. (From Parisien JS: *Arthroscopic surgery*, McGraw-Hill, New York, 1988.)

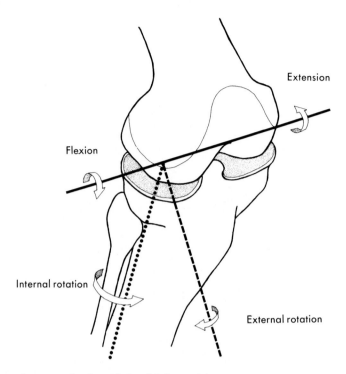

Fig. 2-4. Screw-home mechanism of the tibiofemoral joint. During extension, the tibia rotates externally; during flexion, the motion is reversed.

channel between the femoral condyles and is usually 130 degrees when viewed from superior to inferior. An angle greater than 130 degrees may lead to a subluxating patella.

The *tibial plateaus* provide reciprocal articular surfaces for the femoral condyles. In the sagittal plane the medial tibial plateau is slightly concave, whereas the lateral plateau has a slight convexity[8] (Fig. 2-5). This convexity matching the flattened lateral femoral condyle increases the stability of the knee when it is loaded and aids in identification of the lateral tibial plateau on radiograph.

The contact areas of the medial tibial plateau are up to 50% larger than those of the lateral tibial plateau.[11] The articular cartilage of the medial tibial plateau is thicker than the articular cartilage of the lateral tibial plateau, which allows it to sustain the high forces to which it is subjected.

THE CRUCIATE MENISCUS COMPLEX

The formation of a meniscoligamentous complex is apparent at the seventh week of embryonic development. The intimate relationship between the menisci and the cruciate ligaments is established as they develop from this common structure[12,13] (Fig. 2-6). The importance of the menisci to knee stability has only recently been appreciated by many investigators.[14-17]

The role of the menisci as stabilizers and weight transmitters is a function of their structure.[18] In the extended knee, the menisci resemble crescents that are triangular when cross-sectioned. The menisci work to reduce peak loads between femur and tibia, help maintain knee congru-

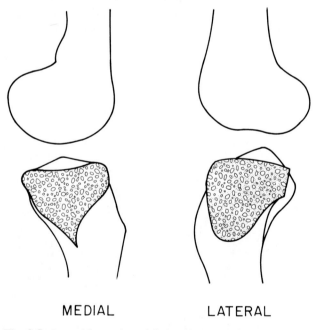

MEDIAL   LATERAL

Fig. 2-5. Lateral femoral condyle has characteristic notch. Lateral tibial condyle is slightly convex with a more squared-off posterior projection.

ity, resist capsular and synovial impingement, and aid the screw-home mechanism. The lateral meniscus transmits 75% and the medial meniscus 50% of the load in their respective compartments.[19] Scanning electron microscope studies of the normal meniscus demonstrate that the fiber

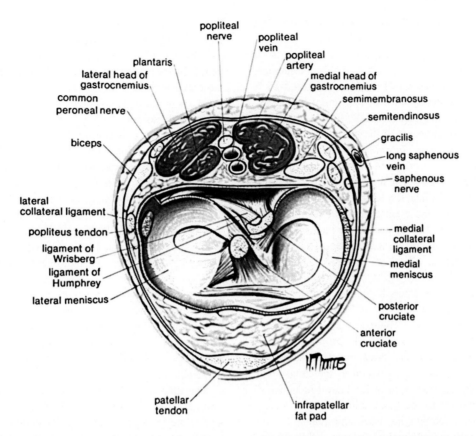

Fig. 2-6. Transverse section of the knee joint demonstrating the interrelationships of the cruciate-meniscus complex. (From Parisien JS: *Arthroscopic surgery,* McGraw-Hill, New York, 1988.)

orientation is predominantly in the long axis, with a few fibers running in other directions.[20] The shape of the meniscus helps dissipate tensile stresses loaded on the long axis of the knee. Meniscectomy causes a reduction in the tibiofemoral contact area and an increase in the magnitude of stresses on the articular cartilage.[6] As a result, fibrillation of the articular cartilage of the tibial plateau and the femoral condyle occurs more readily when a meniscus is absent. This supports the view that the menisci absorb significant loads in the knee joint.[16,17]

During flexion the menisci move backward and follow the contact points of the femur. This action is facilitated by the pull from the attachments of the semimembranosus posteromedially and the popliteus posterolaterally. The anterior and posterior horns of both menisci are anchored to the intercondylar area of the tibia by the meniscotibial ligaments. The cartilaginous substance of the meniscus is nourished through (1) the synovial fluid at the inner free meniscal border, (2) the blood vessels in the peripheral third of the menisci, and (3) the diffusion to the inferior and superior surfaces from vessels and synovia that pass within the meniscofemoral and meniscotibial ligaments.[3] Because the central portion of the meniscus has the most precarious source of nutrition, it is the area most at risk for injury.

The *medial meniscus* is longer than the lateral in the anteroposterior plane and is more firmly attached to the capsular structures. Anteromedially, it is attached to the femur by capsule and is reinforced with the medial retinaculum. Centrally, it is attached to capsule by the medial capsular ligament, and the wider posterior horn is attached to the posteromedial capsular complex. Its attachment to the posterior oblique ligament component is particularly firm, which limits its mobility relative to the lateral. As a result, because the ability of the medial meniscus to move out of harm's way during rapid acceleration and deceleration is decreased, tears to it tend to occur in the area of the posterior oblique ligament attachment.[3] The midportion of the meniscus is attached to the femur and tibia through a thickened joint capsule, the deep medial ligament.[21] Posteromedially, through the capsular complex, the medial meniscus is attached to the very strong semimembranosus muscle. This attachment helps move the medial meniscus posteriorly during knee flexion.

The more spherical *lateral meniscus* covers up to two thirds of the articular surface of the tibial plateau. Its capsular attachments are similar to those of the medial meniscus except for a defect through which the popliteus traverses to attach to the femur. Because of this popliteal hiatus, the lateral meniscus has increased mobility, which may explain why in the presence of anterior cruciate ligament stability, it is torn less frequently.[3] The posterolateral attachment of the lateral meniscus is to the popliteus, which anchors it to both tibia and femur and aids its backward movement during knee flexion.

The *meniscofemoral ligaments* are important accessory structures (Fig. 2-6). The anterior meniscofemoral ligament, also known as the *ligament of Humphry,* is formed by a continuation of the posterior horn of the lateral meniscus, runs anterior to the posterior cruciate ligament (PCL), and inserts on the lateral aspect of the medial femoral condyle. The posterior meniscofemoral ligament, the *ligament of Wrisberg,* has the same origin but runs behind the PCL to its insertion.[22] These two structures emphasize the relationship between the PCL and the lateral meniscus. Flexion and extension occur in this meniscofemoral compartment (Fig. 2-7). With flexion, the menisci move backward; with extension, they move forward through capsular expansions to the quadriceps muscle. Also with extension, the meniscotibial or coronary ligaments facilitate external rotation of the tibia on the femur (the screw-home mechanism).

The *anterior cruciate ligament (ACL)* and the menisci originate as a condensation of blastoma at 6½ weeks of gestation.[23] The ACL, although entirely intra-articular, is extrasynovial within its synovial envelope. It attaches to a depression in the tibia just anterolateral to the tibial spine and blends with the anterior horn of the lateral meniscus.[24] There is no attachment to the tibial spine itself. The ACL spirals through the intercondylar notch and attaches to the lateral femoral condyle in an arched fashion. It has no discrete bundles;[25] however, at 90 degrees of flexion it is twisted 90 degrees, so that the most anterior portion of the tibial attachment inserts on the most medial and proximal portions of the femoral attachment. The fibers arising from the posterior part of the tibial attachment insert on the most lateral and distal parts of the femoral attachment. The anteromedial fibers are taut in 90 degrees of flexion, and the posterolateral fibers are taut in extension. The tension in the ACL is increased with internal rotation and decreased with external rotation.[3] This anatomic configuration helps the ACL prevent forward movement of the tibia on the femur throughout the entire arc of motion.[7,9] The average length of the ACL is 31 ± 3 mm, the average width 10 ± 2 mm, and the average thickness is 5 ± 1 mm. It remains isometric throughout its arc of motion and creates an angle of 26 ± 7 degrees with the long axis of the femur.[25] Kennedy found the strength of the cadaveric ACL of a median age of 62 years to be 640 N.[26] Trent et al reported the average stiffness to be 141 N and ultimate load to be 633 N.[27] Noyes and Grood demonstrated the linear stiffness to be 182 ± 56 N and the ultimate load 1730 ± 660 N.[28] More recently, Woo et al. have found that linear stiffness, ultimate load, and energy absorbed decrease significantly with the specimen's age.[29]

In twisting deceleration injuries of the lower extremity, the ACL is damaged more than any other support structure of the knee. Chronic instability, specifically anterior tibial subluxation, can result from such disruptions.[30] Progressive instability of the ACL-deficient knee may contribute to meniscal tears and osteoarthritis.[31,32]

The main blood supply of the ACL is derived from the middle geniculate artery and from branches of the inferior geniculate arteries.[33] These richly endow the synovial fold covering both cruciates. This fold originates from the posterior inlet of the intercondylar notch and extends to the anterior tibial insertion of the ligament, where it joins the synovial tissue of the joint capsule distal to the infrapatellar fat pad, a structure important to preserve during ACL reconstructive procedures. Minimal blood supply is derived from the ligamentous osseous junctions.

Histologic studies have identified mechanoreceptors on

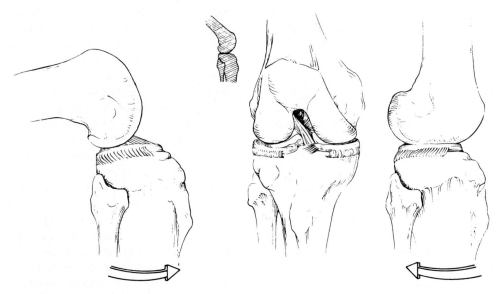

Fig. 2-7. Flexion and extension occur in the meniscofemoral compartment; rotation occurs in the meniscotibial compartment.

the surface of the ACL. These play an important role as the proprioceptive reflex arcs that serve to protect the knee structures from deformation beyond the anatomic limit.[34] The preservation of these mechanoreceptors in ACL surgery may facilitate rehabilitation.

The *posterior cruciate ligament (PCL)*, an intrasynovial and extra-articular structure, is a main stabilizer of the knee.[35] It averages 38 mm in length and 13 mm in width.[35] This ligament is a composite structure consisting of superficial and deep tibiofemoral and meniscofemoral fibers. The PCL is directed vertically in the sagittal plane from its broad tibial attachment approximately 1 cm inferior to the joint (Fig. 2-8). The semicircular femoral attachment is on the lateral aspect of the medial femoral condyle. The PCL is medial to the center of the joint and does not cross the ACL alignment.[35] Anteriorly, it attaches in the femoral notch on the medial femoral condyle. The tibial attachment is in a depression in the posterior tibia between the two tibial plateaus approximately 1 cm below the tibial surface.[36] It is thicker, less oblique than the ACL, and requires more force to tear.[26,37] The PCL is taut in all degrees of flexion and extension, but the tension is increased in internal rotation as it wraps around the ACL.[3] It prevents hyperextension and posterior subluxation and is responsible for 90% to 95% of restraint to posterior displacement of the tibia on the femur.[38,39]

The major blood supply is provided by the supreme genicular artery, the medial and lateral geniculate arteries, and the anterior and posterior tibial recurrent arteries, with some additional contribution by the synovial tissue.[40] Mechanoreceptors are found primarily on the femoral portion of the ligament.[34] The most common mechanisms of injury to the PCL are hyperextension (common in football), hyperflexion, and violent posterior displacement of the tibia with the knee flexed (dashboard injury).[37] When the PCL has been torn, complete dislocation of the knee must be ruled out.[41]

Unlike tears of the ACL, which affect knee function in the stance phase of gait, tears of the PCL may result in a limitation of knee function in the swing phase of gait. The knee may be affected during descent when the heel strike occurs before full extension and reduction of the tibia.

THE SEMIMEMBRANOSUS POSTEROMEDIAL-MEDIAL COMPLEX

The structures of the medial and posteromedial aspect of the knee help resist abduction and external rotatory forces. Various investigators have described the interplay of these structures.[42-44]

The *semimembranosus muscle* is the main structure of the posteromedial corner and provides much of the stability to this area. Of its five insertions, two are tendinous and the others are fibrous extensions of the tendon sheath[44] (Fig. 2-9). A direct tendinous branch attaches to the posteromedial aspect of the tibia (infraglenoidal tubercle).[43] A portion of this tendon then continues around the medial side of the

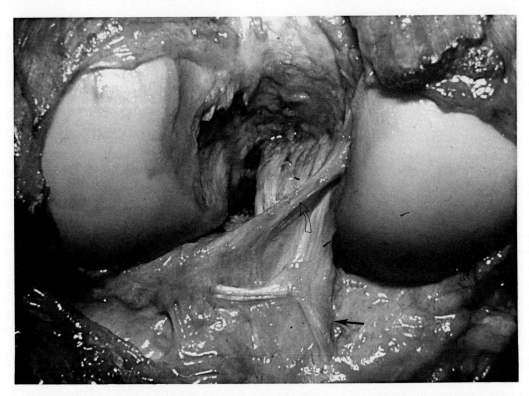

Fig. 2-8. The posterior cruciate ligament is strong and broad. The tibial attachment is 1 cm inferior to the joint *(solid arrow)*. Note the meniscofemoral ligament rising from the lateral meniscus *(open arrow)*.

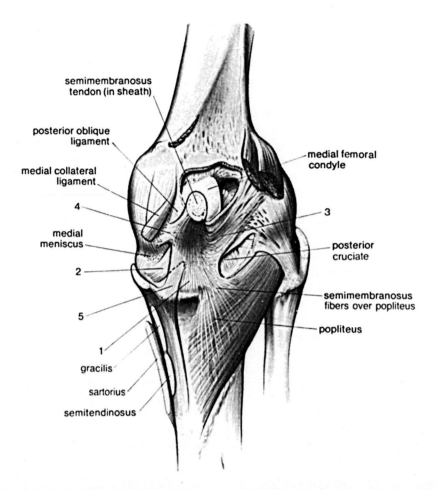

Fig. 2-9. The insertions of the semimembranosus muscle into the posteromedial corner of the knee: *(1)* the direct tendinous insertion; *(2)* the tendinous continuation of the direct insertion deep to the superficial medial ligament; *(3)* the oblique popliteal ligament formed by the posterior capsule and a fibrous tract of the semimembranosus; *(4)* the fibrous insertion of the semimembranosus into the posterior oblique ligament; and *(5)* the fibrous insertion of the semimembranosus into the superficial medial ligament inferiorly. (From Parisien JS: *Arthroscopic surgery,* McGraw-Hill, New York, 1988.)

tibia deep to the superficial medial ligament. From these two tendinous insertions, the semimembranosus sends three main fibrous tracts into the posteromedial corner. The most clearly defined of these tracts are the ones that blend with the capsule posteriorly and form the *oblique popliteal ligament*.[44] A second fibrous insertion extends into the *posterior oblique ligament,* and a third distribution of fibers blends into the *superficial medial ligament* inferiorly. Above the direct insertion, the tendon of the semimembranosus is attached to the medial meniscus and is responsible for posterior displacement of the medial meniscus in knee flexion.[41]

The *posterior oblique ligament,* a thickening of the capsular ligament, is attached proximally to the adductor tubercle of the femur and distally to the tibia and posterior capsule. This ligament is also attached to the medial meniscus, although one third to one half of its fibers pass uninterrupted from the femur to the tibia. It is a true femorotibial ligament in which there exist fibers in the deep portion that form femoromeniscal and meniscotibial fibers

(coronary ligament). The distal attachment of the posterior oblique ligament has three arms.[43] The most prominent of these attachments is the central arm, which attaches to the edge of the posterior surface of the tibia close to the margin of the articular cartilage. Second, there is a superior or capsular arm that is continuous with the posterior capsule and the proximal portion of the oblique popliteal ligament. Last, there is a poorly defined distal arm attached to the sheath of the semimembranosus and to the tibia distal to the direct insertion of the semimembranosus. The posterior oblique ligament is relaxed at 60 degrees of flexion. It is responsible for a great deal of the stability of the posteromedial aspect of the knee, and attention must be paid to its integrity at the time of surgery.

The *deep medial ligament,* also known as the *medial capsular ligament,* originates distal to the medial epicondyle and attaches to the center of the medial meniscus. The meniscotibial portion of this ligament contributes to the coronary ligament and limits excessive movement of the anterior horn of the medial meniscus.[44] The deep medial ligament is of primary importance to the stability of the medial side of the knee; it is the first ligament to tear when the flexed knee is subjected to forced external rotation and abduction.[10]

The *superficial medial ligament* or *medial collateral ligament* originates from the medial epicondyle of the femur and then passes anteriorly to attach to the tibia approximately 7 cm below the joint. Its anterior fibers first lengthen and then shorten as the knee is flexed,[45] whereas its posterior fibers shorten as the knee is flexed. These fibers are joined by those of the deep medial ligament to form the anterior fibers of the posterior oblique ligament.

The *pes anserine* is composed of the combined tendons of the *sartorius*, the *gracilis*, and the more posterior *semitendinosus* fused with the local fascia. It inserts not more than 1 cm anterior to the medial collateral ligament. By functioning as a flexor and internal rotator of the knee, it provides dynamic stability. In extension, the tendons of the pes are parallel to the medial capsular ligament and closely overly it. Because of their accessibility, these tendons are used in various repairs and reconstructions of the knee.[46] The semitendinosus attaches to the medial gastrocnemius muscle approximately 7 cm proximal to its insertion of the tibia by way of a crural fascia that at times resembles a tendon-like band. Noteworthy is the anatomical relationship of the saphenous nerve. This lies deep to the sartorius and pierces the fascia between the sartorius and gracilis tendons to become subcutaneous. The infrapatellar branch of this nerve also penetrates the sartorius fascia more anteriorly.

The *gastrocnemius* overlies the posterior knee capsule and consists of two large and powerful muscle bellies that originate from the posterior and superior aspects of the femoral condyles. The medial head has a variable thick tendinous origin above the medial femoral condyle, which interdigitates extensively with a muscular origin. The tendon becomes fully replaced by muscular fibers 4 to 6 cm distal to the origin.

The most posterior border of the posteromedial-medial complex is formed by the *oblique popliteal ligament*, which is an important posterior stabilizing structure and receives portions of the tendon of the semimembranosus and of its sheath. It transverses the back of the knee and inserts onto the lateral femoral condyle.

THE BICEPS FEMORIS POSTEROLATERAL-LATERAL COMPLEX

The structures on the lateral side of the knee resist excessive adduction and internal rotatory forces. The muscular and ligamentous structures also combine to help prevent anterior and posterior translation of the lateral tibial condyle (Fig. 2-10).

The *biceps femoris muscle* is the main motor unit on the lateral side of the knee and exerts a stabilizing influence akin to the semimembranosus on the medial side. It consists of short and long heads that fuse to become a thick tendon at the level of the fibular head, which then separates into three layers: superficial, middle, and deep. The superficial layer of the biceps forms three expansions: (1) a very strong anterior expansion that blends with the anterior crural fascia (the orientation of these fibers is similar to that of the pes anserine on the lateral side), (2) a middle expansion that spreads to the lowest part of the lateral collateral ligament and the head of the fibula and blends with the fascia over the peroneal muscles, and (3) a posterior expansion that extends inferiorly to blend with the fascia over the calf muscles.

The middle expansion is a thin layer that encircles the distal attachment of the lateral collateral ligament. Through this attachment, the biceps muscle can transmit tension to the lateral collateral ligament. The deep layer of the biceps is bifurcated. One layer inserts on Gerdy's tubercle. The other sweeps around the posterolateral corner and sends fibers to the anterolateral tibia, the tibiofibular syndesmosis, the fibula, and the posterolateral capsular structures.

Through its capsular attachments, the biceps muscle helps to stabilize the lateral collateral ligament, the posterolateral capsule, and the lateral meniscus. It also exerts an influence on the iliotibial band, especially at 10 to 30 degrees of flexion, and is a strong flexor and external rotator of the knee. These functions must be considered before modification of the biceps is undertaken to reconstruct other structures of the knee.[4,19]

The *lateral collateral ligament* originates on the flare of the lateral epicondyle of the femur just anterior to the origin of the gastrocnemius and inserts into the head of the fibula distally, with some fibers coursing more anteriorly to insert on the proximal tibia anterior to the fibular head. The tendon of biceps femoris blends with the lateral collateral ligament.[48] The lateral collateral ligament is taut in extension and external rotation and lax in flexion and internal rotation.[3] In this latter position the biceps transmits tension to the lateral collateral ligament.

The *oblique popliteal ligament* blends with the semimembranosus tendon medially to form a three-dimensional triangle linking the medial proximal femur, posteromedial tibia, and the posterolateral femur. Laterally, it attaches with the lateral head of the gastrocnemius, the arcuate ligament, and the fabellofibular ligament (if present) on the femur. The oblique popliteal ligament reinforces the posterior capsule. The anatomy of this ligament establishes the intricate balance between the medial and lateral stabilizing structures.

The *popliteus muscle*, tripartite in origin, is the only muscle that has a rotatory effect when the knee is hyperextended.[49] The main tendon attaches to the lateral condyle of the femur just anterior to the lateral collateral ligament. It proceeds distally through an aperture in the lateral capsule and is joined by its attachment to the posterior horn of the lateral meniscus and its attachment to the fibular head. It crosses and reinforces the lateral side of the knee, and its

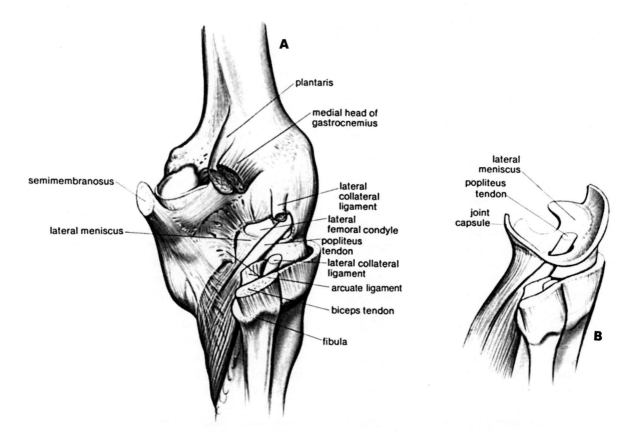

Fig. 2-10. The posterolateral corner of the knee. **A,** The arcuate ligament and a small portion of the lateral capsule have been removed to expose the popliteus muscle and tendon and the lateral meniscus. Note the intimate relationship of the structures of the posterolateral corner. During knee flexion the popliteus pulls the lateral meniscus backward. **B,** The popliteal hiatus and penetration of the popliteal tendon into the joint are shown. (From Parisien JS: *Arthroscopic surgery,* McGraw-Hill, New York, 1988.)

insertion on the tibia is fleshy. The popliteus muscle helps to initiate and maintain internal rotation of the tibia on the femur and to stabilize the posterolateral ligaments and the posterior horn of the lateral meniscus.[50,51] It pulls the lateral meniscus backward during flexion and internal rotation and is a synergist to the PCL.[49] The popliteus plays an important role in restraining excessive hyperextension and abduction rotation.[52] In anterior cruciate–deficient knees, the incidence of structural lesions of the popliteus system exceeds 85%. This explains the posterolateral tenderness in this group of patients.[52]

The *arcuate ligament* and the *fabellofibular ligaments* are variable structures on the lateral side of the knee. The arcuate ligament consists of a condensation of fibers of the origin of the popliteus, including those fibers from the fibula. This Y-shaped ligament transverses the posterior capsule and joins the oblique popliteal ligament at its femoral insertion. It is variable in thickness and thus variable in potential contribution to knee stability. When the fabella is present, the fabellofibular ligament, described as the "short lateral collateral ligament" by Kaplan,[42] is present as well (15% of the population).[53] It originates on the fabella in

conjunction with the fleshy lateral head of the gastrocnemius and oblique popliteal ligament and inserts on the fibula. This triangular structure acts as a rotatory stabilizer of the knee.[3]

The *lateral head of gastrocnemius* originates on the posterolateral aspect of the lateral femoral condyle as it fuses with the origins of the oblique popliteal ligament, the fabellofibular ligament, and the arcuate ligament. This strong plantar flexor of the ankle covers the posterolateral knee capsule and must be relaxed for knee ligamentous disruptions to be correctly assessed.

The *lateral capsular ligament* is triangular in shape and variable in thickness. It is located in the midlateral part of the capsule and has both a vertical component and a horizontal component.[54] This strong thickening of the lateral capsule may cause an avulsion of the tibial metaphyseal bone when stressed.[55] Radiologically, this has been termed the lateral capsular sign.[56]

The *iliotibial band (ITB),* a thick dynamic stabilizer of the lateral aspect of the knee, is formed proximally from the tensor fascia lata anteriorly and the gluteus maximus posteriorly. As it courses along the thigh, the ITB attaches to the linea aspera of the femur by blending with the intermuscular septum. The distal portion of this attachment consists of the strong transverse fibers described by Kaplan.[57] Further distally, this structure sends fibers to the lateral patellar retinaculum and eventually inserts on Gerdy's tubercle.

The ITB is an extensor when the knee is in 0 to 30 degrees of flexion and a flexor when the knee is flexed from 40 to 145 degrees. Passage of this axis is between 30 and 40 degrees of flexion. The pivot shift phenomenon in ACL insufficiency is intimately dependent on this normal function of the ITB.[58] Detachment of the ITB at its bony insertion results in immediate and pronounced varus laxity of the joint.[3] This may be present following substitution of the ACL using strips of ITB. The ITB acts a femorotibial ligament. Abnormal biomechanical factors across the knee joint can cause a friction syndrome of the ITB. It is especially common in runners with rotatory deformities of the forefoot.

THE QUADRICEPS ANTEROMEDIAL-ANTEROLATERAL COMPLEX

Whereas the quadriceps muscle is an important component of overall knee function, many clinicians have felt it to be the key to normal knee function. Consequently, rehabilitation of knee joint dysfunction has all too frequently been exclusively synonymous with quadriceps muscle strengthening.[59] Other muscle groups are now recognized as equally important to the proper maintenance of knee function and stability. In this discussion we have emphasized the critical role of other motor structures, particularly the semimembranosus and biceps femoris muscles. Attention should be paid to them in total rehabilitation, and in specific clinical situations their rehabilitation may be even more important.

Nonetheless, the *quadriceps-patellar mechanism,* along with its medial and lateral expansions, is essential to normal knee function. In its healthy state, this is a powerful muscle that works to counteract gravity and allow us to assume the upright position. The quadriceps muscle comprises different extensors that show a combined axial deviation of about 10 to 15 degrees in their course to the patella. The fiber direction is the superior component of the quadriceps-patellar tendon angle, commonly called the *Q-angle*.[60] The common quadriceps tendon receives its contributions from the *vastus intermedius, vastus lateralis,* and *vastus medialis muscles,* as well as from the *rectus femoris muscles*. The rectus femoris is also a hip flexor. During athletic activity, the extensor mechanism must stabilize the knee joint. Weakness of the extensor mechanism is caused by generalized quadriceps dysfunction and may cause buckling and pain.

The selective function of each component of the quadriceps tendon has been studied extensively from an anatomic, biomechanical, and electrodiagnostic standpoint by Lieb and Perry.[61,62] These authors queried earlier beliefs that the vastus medialis muscle had a selective function that was more important during 15 degrees of terminal knee extension. All components are important, and in the normal setting each makes a contribution.

The *vastus medialis* has a very thin fascial covering and is separated into two muscles distinguished by fiber orientation. The *vastus medialis longus* is the larger division, and it has vertically oriented fibers that deviate approximately 15 to 18 degrees from the longitudinal axis of the femur. The *vastus medialis obliquus* fibers, located in the distal quarter of the vastus medialis, are more horizontal, deviating an average of 50 to 55 degrees from the femoral axis. The primary function of the vastus medialis is to maintain patellar alignment. Without the pull of this component, the patella would dislocate laterally from the unopposed pull of the vastus lateralis muscle, which is directed 12 to 15 degrees laterally in the frontal plane. Both the rectus femoris, which assumes a central and superficial position in the quadriceps complex, and the vastus intermedius, which lies deep to it, rotate the tibia internally on the femur.[3]

All four muscle bellies of the quadriceps complex become aponeurotic at the anterior aspect of the knee.[63] Loss of the bulk of the quadriceps is common in patients with knee lesions.[61,62]

Encased in the common quadriceps tendon is the patella, the body's largest sesamoid bone. The main function of the patella is to increase the efficiency of the quadriceps muscle by shifting its line of pull anteriorly. The main distal insertion of the quadriceps-patellar mechanism is through the patellar ligament (tendon) to the tibial tubercle. More knee complaints are associated with the patellofemoral articulation than with any other area within or immediately surrounding the knee.

The *patella* is the guard on the anterior surface of the femoral condyles lying deep to the fascia lata and the fibers of the rectus femoris. Its main function is to increase the biomechanical efficiency of the quadriceps complex in knee extension. It also allows a better distribution of compressive stresses on the femur by increasing the area of contact between the patellar tendon and the femur.[64] Patellofemoral joint forces increase with flexion of the knee in the presence of a constant quadriceps muscle force.[4] During stair climbing and descent, peak patellofemoral joint reactive force is 3.3 times the body weight.[65]

The height of the patellar articular surface is 3.5 cm ± 4 mm, the height of the anterior surface is 4.5 cm ± 7 mm, the width is 4.7 cm ± 7 mm, and the thickness is 2.3 cm ± 4 mm.[63] The shape of the patella helps determine the congruity of the trochlear groove: The smaller the medial facet, the more likely are instability and articular cartilage damage.[66] The patella is divided into two facets separated by vertical ridges. The lateral facet is concave in both planes and accommodates the lateral femoral condyle well. The medial facet is convex and touches the medial femoral condyle (MFC) over only a small part of its surface. A vertical ridge near the medial border isolates a narrow strip known as the *odd facet*. Recently, a distal nonarticulating pole of the patella has been described.[67] It is important to recognize this variant as this long distal pole can normalize the Insall Salvati index and give the impression of normal patellar height in cases of patella alta.[68,69]

The *patellar ligament* and *retinaculum* are the distal extensions of the quadriceps complex. Anatomically, the patellar ligament is a tendon, but because it attaches bone to bone, it is called a ligament. The patellar ligament is composed mostly of fibers of the rectus femoris with an occasional contribution from the vastus lateralis. The *medial patellar retinaculum* (medial quadriceps expansion) arises mainly from the vastus medialis obliquus, the medial edge of the quadriceps tendon, and the adjacent medial patellar border. The fibers then proceed with the superficial medial ligament to a combined insertion on the tibia.[70] There is a negative correlation between the length of the patellar ligament and that of the medial patellar retinaculum.[63] The medial patellar retinaculum is an important stabilizer of the knee. In patients with patella alta, it is flimsy and weak and contributes to patellar dislocation.

The *lateral patellar retinaculum* is formed by an aponeurotic expansion of the vastus lateralis and the ITB; it has a superficial layer and a deep layer. The superficial layer originates from the ITB interdigitating with the fibers of the vastus lateralis and patellar tendon and inserts on the anterior aspect of the patella and patellar tendon. The deep layer forms the lateral patellofemoral ligament, which extends from the patella to the epicondyle of the femur. This is a static guide for the patella, and variations in its length and thickness are related to the shape and thickness of the patella.[63] At the lower border of the deep retinacular layer is a distinct patellotibial ligament whose fibers insert on the lateral meniscus and the tibia. Lateral retinacular release is a procedure commonly performed to relieve patellar tracking abnormalities. This may be carried out through the superficial layer only or through both layers.[48]

The broad tibial insertion of the quadriceps muscle not only provides active extension to the knee but also controls stability and rotation. With powerful contractions of the quadriceps mechanism during rapid deceleration and direction change, acute tears of the ACL can occur as the tibia subluxates anteriorly. Also, there may be anterior tibial subluxation in the nonweight bearing situation. In chronic ACL insufficiency, when there is deceleration through the quadriceps mechanism, such subluxations may occur with minimum provocation. Grafts for ACL reconstruction are frequently fashioned from the central third of the patellar ligament and adjacent quadriceps tendon.

SUMMARY

To achieve maximal rehabilitation, the knee joint must be considered in the light of total body function. Similarly, as rehabilitation of one injured knee structure is planned, the whole knee as a synchronized functional unit must be kept in mind. No structure or complex works in isolation.

For example, we describe the menisci as part of the cruciate-meniscus complex, yet they modify the bony architecture and, because of their connections, are inseparable from all other complexes. Following meniscectomy, each unit has lost a component. In the same way, rehabilitation of an ACL-injured knee must take into account the adverse effect of quadriceps muscle strengthening alone, when in fact a balanced strength ratio with the hamstring muscles must be maintained.

Rehabilitation must be prescribed with regard for the interplay of the five anatomic units, their biomechanical function, and the demands to be ultimately placed on the knee.

REFERENCES

1. Noyes FR, Grood ES: *Diagnosis of knee ligament injuries: biomechanical precepts.* In Feagin JA Jr, editor: *The crucial ligaments,* New York, 1988, Churchill Livingstone.
2. Frankel VH, Nordin M: *Biomechanics of the knee.* In Hunter LY, Funk FJ Jr, editors: *Rehabilitation of the injured knee,* St Louis, 1984, Mosby–Year Book.
3. Müller W: *The knee: form, function and ligament reconstruction,* Berlin, 1983, Springer Verlag.
4. Frankel VH, Burstein AH: *Orthopaedic biomechanics,* Philadelphia, 1970, Lea & Febiger.
5. Reuleaux F: *The kinematics of machinery: outline of a theory of machines,* London, 1876, Macmillan.
6. Frankel VH, Nordin M: *Basic biomechanics of the musculoskeletal system,* ed 2, Philadelphia, 1989, Lea & Febiger.
7. Shoemaker S, Markolf K: Effects of joint load on the stiffness and laxity of ligament deficient knees. *J Bone Joint Surg [Am]* 67:136, 1985.
8. Welsh RP: Knee joint structure and function, *Clin Orthop* 7:147, 1980.
9. Campbell's operative orthopaedics, ed 6, St Louis, 1980, Mosby–Year Book.
10. Kennedy JC, Fowler PJ: Medial and anterior instability of the knee, *J Bone Joint Surg [Am]* 7:349, 1971.
11. Kettlecamp DB, Jacobs AW: Tibiofemoral contact area: determination and implications, *J Bone Joint Surg [Am]* 54:349, 1972.
12. Gray DJ, Gardner E: Prenatal development of the human knee and superior tibiofibular joints, *Am J Anat* 86:235, 1950.
13. Kaplan EB: The embryology of the menisci of the knee, *Orthop Clin North Am* 4:647, 1973.
14. Nicholas JA: Injuries to the menisci of the knee, *Orthop Clin North Am* 4:647, 1973.
15. Helfet AJ: Mechanism of derangements of the medial semilunar cartilage and their management, *J Bone Joint Surg [Br]* 41:319, 1959.
16. Noble J, Alexander K: Studies of tibial subchondral bone density and its significance, *J Bone Joint Surg [Am]* 67:295, 1985.
17. Bourne RB, et al: The effect of medial meniscectomy on strain distribution in the proximal part of the tibia, *J Bone Joint Surg [Am]* 66:1431, 1984.
18. Fowler PJ: *Meniscal lesions: the role of arthroscopy in the management of adolescent knee problems.* In: Kennedy JC, editor: *The injured adolescent knee,* Baltimore, 1979, Williams & Wilkins.
19. Walker PS, Erkman MJ: The role of the menisci in force transmission across the knee, *Clin Orthop* 109:184–192, 1975.
20. Cameron HU, Macnab I: The structure of the meniscus of the human knee joint, *Clin Orthop* 89:215, 1972.
21. Arnoczky S, et al: *Injury and repair of the musculoskeletal soft tissues,* Chicago, 1987, American Academy of Orthopaedic Surgeons.
22. Heller L, Langman J: The menisco-femoral ligaments of the human knee, *J Bone Joint Surg [Br]* 46:307, 1964.

23. Ellison AE, Berg EE: Embryology, anatomy and function of the anterior cruciate ligament, *Orthop Clin North Am* 16:3, 1985.
24. Marshall JL, Girgis FG, Zelko RR: The biceps femoris tendon and its functional significance, *J Bone Joint Surg [Am]* 54:1444, 1972.
25. Odentsten M, Gilquist J: Functional anatomy of the anterior cruciate ligament and a rationale for reconstruction, *J Bone Joint Surg [Am]* 67:257, 1985.
26. Kennedy JC, et al: Tension studies of human knee ligaments, *J Bone Joint Surg [Am]* 58:350, 1976.
27. Trent PS, Walker PS, Wolf B: Ligament length patterns, strength and rotational axis of the knee joint, *Clin Orthop* 117:263, 1976.
28. Noyes FR, Grood ES: The strength of the anterior cruciate ligament in humans and rhesus monkeys: age related and species related changes, *J Bone Joint Surg [Am]* 58:1074, 1976.
29. Woo SL, et al: Tensile properties of the human femur–anterior cruciate ligament–tibia complex, *Am J Sports Med* 19:217, 1991.
30. Kennedy JC, Weinberg HW, Wilson AS: Anatomy and function of the anterior cruciate ligament, *J Bone Joint Surg [Am]* 56:223, 1974.
31. Fetto JF, Marshall JL: The natural history and diagnosis of anterior cruciate ligament insufficiency, *Clin Orthop* 147:29, 1980.
32. Noyes FR, et al: The symptomatic anterior cruciate–deficient knee, *J Bone Joint Surg [Am]* 65:154, 1983.
33. Arnoczky SP: Blood supply to the anterior cruciate ligament and supporting structures, *Clin Orthop* 16:15, 1985.
34. Schuttz PA, Miller DC, Kerr CS, Michel L: Mechanoreceptors in human cruciate ligaments, *J Bone Joint Surg [Am]* 66:1072, 1984.
35. Hughston J: The posterior cruciate ligament in knee joint stability, *J Bone Joint Surg [Am]* 51:1045, 1969.
36. Van Dommelon BA, Fowler PJ: Anatomy of the posterior cruciate ligament: a review, *Am J Sports Med* 17:24, 1989.
37. Kennedy JC, Grainger RW: The posterior cruciate ligament, *J Trauma* 7:367, 1967.
38. Butler DL, Noyes FR, Grood ES: Ligamentous restraints to anterior-posterior drawer in the human knee: a biomechanical study, *J Bone Joint Surg [Am]* 62:259, 1980.
39. Kennedy JC, Roth JR, Walker DM: Posterior cruciate ligament injuries, *Orthop Digest* 7:19, 1979.
40. Scapinelli R: Studies on the vasculature of the human knee joint, *Acta Anat (Basel)* 70:305, 1968.
41. Fowler PJ: Classification and early diagnosis of knee joint instability, *Clin Orthop* 147:15, 1980.
42. Kaplan EB: Some aspects of functional anatomy of the human knee, *Clin Orthop* 23:18, 1962.
43. Hughston J, Eilers AF: The role of the posterior oblique ligament in repairs of acute medial (collateral) ligament tears of the knee, *J Bone Joint Surg [Am]* 55:923, 1973.
44. Warren LF, Marshall JL: The supporting structures and layers on the medial side of the knee, *J Bone Joint Surg [Am]* 61:56, 1979.
45. Bartel ME, et al: Surgical repositioning of the medial collateral ligament, *J Bone Joint Surg [Am]* 59:107, 1977.
46. Slocum DB, Larson RL: Pes anserinus transplantation: a surgical procedure for control of rotatory instability of the knee, *J Bone Joint Surg [Am]* 50:226, 1968.
47. Kennedy JC, Galpin RD: The use of the medial head of the gastrocnemius muscle in the posterior cruciate ligament–deficient knee, *Am J Sports Med* 10:63, 1982.
48. Fulkerson JP, Gossling HR: Anatomy of the knee joint lateral retinaculum, *Clin Orthop* 153:183, 1980.
49. Basuajian JV, Lovejoy JF: Functions of the popliteus in man, *J Bone Joint Surg [Am]* 53:557, 1971.
50. Mann RA, Hagy HL: The popliteus muscle, *J Bone Joint Surg [Am]* 59:924, 1977.
51. Last RJ: The popliteus muscle and lateral meniscus, *J Bone Joint Surg [Br]* 32:93, 1950.
52. Staübli HU, Birrer S: The popliteus tendon and its fascicles at the popliteal hiatus: gross anatomy and functional arthroscopic evaluation with and without anterior cruciate ligament deficiency, *J Arthro Rel Surg* 6:209, 1990.
53. Pritchett JW: The incidence of fabellae in osteoarthritis of the knee, *J Bone Joint Surg [Am]* 66:1379, 1979.
54. Johnson LL: Lateral capsular ligament complex: anatomical and surgical considerations, *Am J Sports Med* 7:156, 1979.
55. Seebacher JR, et al: The structure of the posterolateral aspect of the knee, *J Bone Joint Surg [Am]* 64:536, 1982.
56. Woods GW, Stanley RF, Tullos HS: Lateral capsular sign: x-ray clue to significant knee instability, *Am J Sports Med* 7:27, 1979.
57. Kaplan EB: The iliotibial tract, *J Bone Joint Surg [Am]* 40:817, 1958.
58. Jakob RP, Hassler H, Staübli HU: Observations on rotatory instability of the lateral compartment of the knee: experimental studies on the functional anatomy and the pathomechanism of the true and reversed pivot shift sign, *Acta Orthop Scand* 52:1, 1981.
59. Smillie IS: *Injuries of the knee joint,* rev ed, London, 1962, E & S Livingstone.
60. Insall J, Falvo KA, Wise DW: Chondromalacia patellae, *J Bone Joint Surg [Am]* 58:1, 1976.
61. Lieb FJ, Perry J: Quadriceps function: an electromyographic study under isometric conditions, *J Bone Joint Surg [Am]* 53:749, 1971.
62. Lieb FJ, Perry J: Quadriceps function: an anatomical and mechanical study using amputated limbs, *J Bone Joint Surg [Am]* 50:1535, 1968.
63. Reider B, Marshall JL, Koslin B: The anterior aspect of the knee joint, *J Bone Joint Surg [Am]* 63:351, 1981.
64. Frankel VH, Nordin M: *Basic biomechanics of the skeletal system,* Philadephia, 1980, Lea & Febiger.
65. Reilly DT, Martens M: Experimental analysis of the quadriceps muscle force and patello-femoral joint reaction force for various activities, *Acta Orthop Scand* 43:126, 1972.
66. Grana WA, Krieghauser LA: Scientific basis of extensor mechanism disorders, *Clin Sports Med* 4:247, 1985.
67. Grelsamer RP: Patellar morphology in the sagittal plane: clinical correlation, *Am J Sports Med* 17:725, 1989.
68. Insall J, Salvati E: Patella position in the normal knee joint, *Radiology* 101:101, 1971.
69. Grelsamer RP, Meadows S: The modified Insall-Salvati ratio for assessment of patellar height, *Clin Orthop* 282:170, 1992.
70. Greenhill BJ: The importance of the medial quadriceps expansion in medial ligament injury, *Can J Surg* 10:312, 1967.

Chapter 3

ASSESSMENT OF THE ATHLETE WITH AN ACUTELY INJURED KNEE

Elizabeth A. Arendt

The foundation of injury diagnosis is combining knowledge of anatomy and biomechanics with clinical correlates, including history, physical exam, tests, and their interpretation. There has been an explosion of knowledge in the past decade concerning the dynamic and static stabilizers of knee joint motion and how that knowledge correlates to clinical diagnosis, treatment plan, and treatment outcomes. This knowledge, combined with the clinical correlates of history, physical exam, and select clinical tests, gives the clinician an approach to the acutely injured knee.

CLINICAL ASSESSMENT
History

As with many other physical conditions, an accurate history can be extremely useful in guiding your clinical assessment and ultimate diagnosis. Certain features in the history are particularly useful in evaluating an acute knee.

An accurate description of the mechanism of injury, when possible, is important to elicit from the injured patient. In contact injuries one should elicit the point of application of the contact force. This helps analyze what potential structures might have been damaged by an application of a force in a given direction. For instance, in a clipping injury from the lateral side of the knee, one might expect contact discomfort on the lateral side of the knee, with potential injury to the supporting structures on the medial side of the knee, due to the medially directed force placed on the joint. If a straight anterior force is applied to the proximal aspect of the tibia, one might expect a contact bruise or abrasion on the anterior surface of the leg, with a suspicion for a posterior cruciate ligament injury (Fig. 3-1). Noncontact injuries can also be associated with significant force, as a result of internally generated energy created by body momentum. If a body in motion suddenly changes direction, the foot-leg complex can become momentarily trapped or caught as the body continues to pivot, resulting in significant rotatory torque being absorbed by the knee.

The degree of pain or disability cannot be used as a reliable indicator of the seriousness of an injury. Pain can be felt at the time of the injury but quickly subside, especially in complete ligament disruptions when capsular tears are common. Frequently the degree of discomfort is related to a tense joint effusion, which is diminished when a capsular tear is present and the fluid is able to escape to the surrounding tissues. In a study of 50 severe injuries to the medial side of the knee, 76% of patients were able to walk off the playing field and into the doctor's office unaided and without crutches.[1] Instability of the knee joint can be masked in the early stages by muscle spasm, patient guarding secondary to pain and apprehension, or tightness of the knee joint due to a tense effusion.

Perhaps most useful to elicit in the history of an acute knee injury is presence or absence of swelling in the early postinjury period. Joint swelling up to the first 12 hours from an injury indicates hemorrhage into the joint. Effusion that occurs after 12 to 24 hours is suggestive of synovial fluid accumulation that can be caused by irritation to an intra-articular structure such as an in-substance meniscal injury. In two separate studies, traumatic hemarthrosis of the knee signified "significant intra-articular injury"[2] and "lesions of surgical significance"[3] in 90% of cases reviewed. The differential diagnosis of acute knee hemarthrosis is:

1. Ligament injury: The cruciate ligaments are intra-articular/extra-synovial structures that when torn can bleed into the joint. The lateral collateral ligament and the superficial medial collateral ligament are extra-articular structures that by themselves do not cause hemarthrosis (Fig. 3-2).

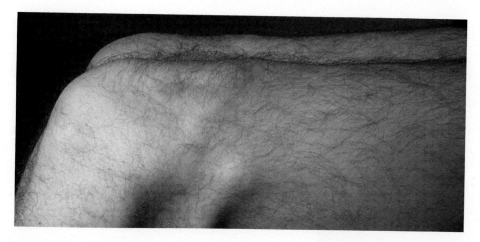

Fig. 3-1. Skin abrasion on the anterior surface of the proximal tibia, sustained by an athlete who fell on a bent knee, making contact with artificial turf. The athlete's physical exam was consistent with a posterior cruciate ligament disruption.

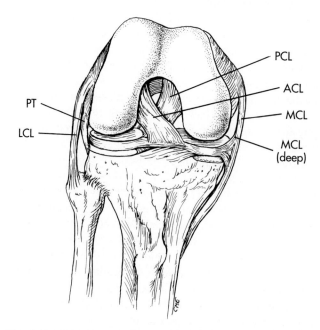

Fig. 3-2. PCL (posterior cruciate ligament); ACL (anterior cruciate ligament); MCL (medial collateral ligament); LCL (lateral collateral ligament); PT (popliteus tendon).

2. Peripheral meniscus tear: The outer or peripheral third of the meniscus is vascular, and a tear of the meniscus in this region can be a source of hemarthrosis. Meniscus tears in the vascular zone have potential for healing and can be repaired (Fig. 3-3).

3. Fractures: In addition to obvious condylar fractures, occult fractures can be a cause of hemarthrosis. These include ligament avulsions of the intra-articular ligaments (ACL/PCL) (Fig. 3-4), osteochondral fractures secondary to a patella dislocation, or blunt trauma to the knee resulting in a shear injury, which can produce an osteochondral fracture.

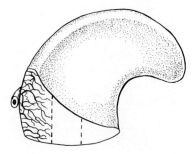

Fig. 3-3. The outer or peripheral third of the meniscus is vascular and has the potential for healing.

4. Synovial/capsular tears: Patella dislocations, even in the absence of an osteochondral fracture, are a source of hemarthrosis. This category also includes other disruptions of the extensor mechanism including quadriceps ruptures and infrapatellar tendon ruptures.

The most frequent cause of an acute hemarthrosis of the knee is a tear of the anterior cruciate ligament.[2,3]

The patient's report of a pop frequently signifies the tearing of a ligament, most commonly the anterior cruciate ligament.[2]

It is also important to ask the patient if this joint has been previously injured. Frequently this uncovers an acute-on-chronic injury. This is common with a secondary subluxation event in a chronic anterior cruciate deficient knee, or an acute-on-chronic patella dislocation. Injury analysis and treatment options may differ, depending on this knowledge.

Physical exam

The physical exam components should be systematically organized and performed in every patient, making each step a part of a consistent routine. A general impression of the patient's appearance, level of distress, and comfort level with the physician or exam environment is helpful to assess before proceeding with the physical exam. An ideal exam

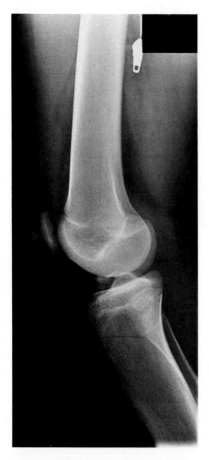

Fig. 3-4. Lateral radiograph of a knee in a 14-year-old female soccer player who sustained an acute knee injury. Surgical findings at the time of knee arthroscopy revealed a bony avulsion of the tibial origin of the anterior cruciate ligament.

environment contains a relaxed patient, a calm and confident physician, and a methodical manual exam void of sudden limb movements or extremes of force. The more ideal the exam environment, the more accurate the physical exam.

The physical exam can be divided into four parts: inspection, palpation, range of motion, and stability testing.

Inspection. Identifying joint effusion within the first 12 hours from injury is helpful in the differential diagnosis, as discussed previously. The absence of intra-articular swelling does not rule out ligament rupture. A severe ligament tear can have associated large capsular disruption, fluid can escape into the surrounding soft tissue, and swelling may not be readily apparent. The absence of swelling in an acute knee injury may indicate an extra-articular source of pain or disability.

Color, deformity, and previous scars are noted. Localized bruises and abrasions can be useful to identify the point of application of a force, helping you to surmise structures involved in the injury.

Muscle atrophy is assessed by inspecting muscle shape and tone and by comparing it to the contralateral limb. This raises concern that the limb has been injured before and one

could be dealing with an acute-on-chronic injury. This can also suggest muscle weakness or imbalance as a possible predisposing factor in the cause of the injury.

Palpation. Direct palpation of the injured area in regions corresponding to the origin and insertion of anatomic structures can be very useful in distinguishing pathology in menisci, patellofemoral joint, and collateral ligaments. Because the cruciate ligaments do not have a direct insertion point corresponding to a palpable area on the external knee, direct palpation is not as helpful in distinguishing a cruciate ligament injury. However, the anterolateral joint line can be tender after an anterolateral subluxation event. This can be seen in an acute anterior cruciate ligament disruption or a chronic subluxation event. One must bear in mind, however, that diffuse tenderness is common in extensive ligament disruptions. If the knee exam is not performed in the immediate postinjury period, palpable discomfort and ecchymosis may be more indicative of the most dependent portion of the limb, rather than reflecting an injured structure.

If one elicits discomfort to palpation in an area that corresponds to more than one anatomic structure, one must further refine the elements of the physical exam to isolate the different pathologies. Palpable discomfort along the mid-medial joint line can correspond to both meniscus and medial collateral ligament pathology. Further refinement in the physical exam is necessary. Stress on an injured ligament elicits pain, whereas pain with compression of a joint may indicate meniscal pathology.

Range of motion. Range of motion should be assessed both actively and passively. A locked knee is a knee unable to obtain full passive motion of the joint secondary to a mechanical block. A displaced meniscus tear classically presents as an acutely locked knee. An osteochondral fracture can impose a mechanical block to motion. Loose bodies may be secondary to a patella dislocation or a displaced osteochondritis dissecans fragment. Rarely, a loose body may represent a foreign substance such as a staple or screw from a previous surgical procedure.

A pseudo-locked knee is when full range of motion cannot be obtained secondary to pain (hamstring spasm) or swelling. A swollen joint rests in the position where there is maximum capsular space. For the knee this is approximately 30 degrees of flexion.

Active range of motion assesses the integrity of the motor units surrounding the knee.

Stability testing. Stability testing of the knee establishes whether there has been ligamentous injury to the joint. The sine qua non of a ligament disruption is the presence of pathologic motion. When a knee is examined by a qualified clinician immediately after an injury, the presence or absence of joint laxity can be reliably determined. The evaluation becomes increasingly difficult when pain, swelling, or muscle spasm is present.

The Standard Nomenclature of Athletic Injuries defines three degrees of ligament sprains.[4] Grade I is a mild injury, with mild point tenderness, little local swelling and hemorrhage, and no abnormal motion of the joint when the ligament is stressed. A grade II sprain is a moderate injury with increased pain and swelling and with abnormal joint motion elicited when the ligament is stressed. There is an end point to the limits of motion when force is applied, implying a partial tearing or stretching of the ligamentous structures. Concerning straight plane instabilities, a grade II injury implies abnormal motion between 5 and 10 mm greater than the opposite side. A grade III sprain implies a complete disruption of the ligament. Abnormal motion is increased, and a soft end point is felt when the limits of joint motion are tested.

Examiners appear to be better able to detect end point differences than displacement differences.[5] Experience in appreciating the quality of the end point will give the examiner a higher degree of accuracy in making the diagnosis of a complete anterior cruciate ligament tear.[6]

The method of joint testing is important, and a consistent and organized approach is essential. In order to compare exams between two limbs or to compare serial exams, the examination conditions (i.e., the position of the limb, the force applied, the point of application of that force, and the point of detection of the joint displacement) must be constant. Frequently the uninjured knee is tested first, both for patient relaxation and to assess the degree of physiologic laxity in the patient's ligaments. Joint motion varies within the normal population, but there is little right-left variation in a normal subject.[7]

Tests to determine pathologic knee motion are numerous. Much of our knowledge concerning ligament disruptions are based on the correlation of the physical exam with known surgical pathology and on laboratory sectioning studies. Disruption of a ligament alters the limits of knee motion in predictable ways. Commonality between tests is to measure the displacement of the tibia in relation to the femur. Primary tests to measure the limits of knee motion examine straight plane instabilities (medial, lateral, anterior, posterior) as well as axial rotation displacements (Fig. 3-5). In addition to defining knee laxity in straight and rotatory directions, the concept of estimating the rotation and translation of the medial and lateral tibial plateaus has been recently advanced.[8,9] The clinical assessment of compartment motion has not been established in regard to accuracy, reproducibility, and applicability.

The concept of primary and secondary ligamentous restraints to joint motion was introduced by Butler[10] in 1980. A primary restraint is that structure that accounts for the majority of the restraining force to an externally applied load in a given direction. A secondary restraint provides a lesser contribution to the same externally applied force. However, when the primary restraint is disrupted, the secondary structures are then responsible for limiting motion to the applied force. This concept has proven useful to understanding the interrelationship of the ligaments in re-

straining joint motion. Using this concept, the roles of the various primary knee ligaments can be addressed.

The anterior cruciate ligament (ACL) functions as the primary stabilizer to limit anterior tibial displacement[11,12] and as a secondary restraint to tibial rotation.[12] The posterior cruciate ligament (PCL) acts primarily to restrain posterior tibial displacement and secondarily to restrain external tibial rotation.[12] The medial collateral ligament's (MCL) primary function is to limit medial or valgus angulation of the knee and internal rotation,[12,13] best appreciated at 20 degrees of flexion. Its secondary role is in restraining anterior tibial motion.[12,14] The lateral collateral ligament (LCL), together with the deep posterior lateral structures, acts as a primary stabilizer to lateral or varus angulation of the knee, as well as a primary restraint to limit external rotation.[12,15,16] Secondary function is to limit anterior and posterior tibial motion.[15,16]

The manual exam for the stability testing of the knee assesses both straight plane instabilities and rotatory instabilities. With the patient supine, abduction and adduction forces are placed alternately on the knee, both at 0 and 20 degrees of flexion. Varus and valgus opening of the knee joint at 20 degrees indicates injury to the lateral and medial ligament complexes, respectively. If opening persists at 0 degrees, injury to posterior structures is involved as well.

The drawer test is performed by flexing the knee to 90 degrees, securing the foot in a neutral position, and attempting to translate the tibia in an anterior and posterior direction. If posterior translation is present, and it increases with the foot externally rotated and decreases with the foot internally rotated, injury to the posterolateral structures is present. The drawer test is most useful for evaluating PCL injuries. In the awake patient, the quadriceps neutral position should be established before testing for the PCL. This is done by asking the patient to actively contract the quadricep muscle while the examiner holds the leg at more than 70 degrees of flexion. This actively translates the tibia anteriorly to the anatomic position (Fig. 3-6). This maneuver is critical when assessing ACL and PCL instabilities. The posterior sag sign indicates PCL insufficiency. The tibial tubercle becomes less prominent on the involved side when the knees and hips are flexed to 90 degrees.

The Lachman's test is a manual test for evaluating ACL integrity. It is performed with the knee held in slight flexion (20 degrees), with anterior translation of the tibia attempted against a fixed femur (Fig. 3-7). According to Torg et al.,[17] this negates hamstring spasm, is more comfortable for the patient, and removes the "door-stopper" effect of the medial meniscus.

Tests to determine rotatory laxity are complex and best described elsewhere. The tests for anterolateral instability include the lateral pivot shift test as advocated by Galway and MacIntosh,[18] the Losee test,[19] and the Noyes flexion rotation drawer test.[20]

Tests to examine for posterolateral instability include the

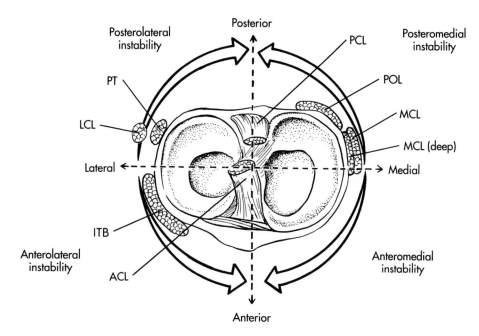

Fig. 3-5. PCL (posterior cruciate ligament); POL (posterior oblique ligament); MCL (medial collateral ligament); ACL (anterior cruciate ligament); ITB (iliotibial band); LCL (lateral collateral ligament); PT (popliteal tendon).

reverse pivot shift as described by Jakob et al[21] and the external rotation recurvatum test.[22]

Despite the ubiquitous use of manual exams to determine pathologic joint laxity, the accuracy and reproducibility of these exams needs to be more thoroughly assessed. This is necessary to help us better develop treatment programs for given knee injuries, to help clinicians communicate more effectively with each other, and to report and compare the results of surgical and conservative intervention more accurately. In one recent study 10 patients were examined by 11 experienced surgeons and 3 arthrometers. There was appreciable difference between measurements recorded by different examiners, particularly anterior-posterior measurements in combined ACL-PCL injuries.[23] A second study looked at knee motion limits and subluxations by recording actual right-left values in instrumented cadaver knees. These were compared to the clinical assessment of 11 experienced knee surgeons. There was wide variability between examiners in the starting position of knee flexion and tibial rotation and wide variation in the loads applied by examiners to the knee joints during the tests. The most frequent misdiagnosis was the interpretation of increased external rotation (ER) of the tibia to represent PCL injury when in fact the injury was to the MCL and ACL. The researchers felt the diagnosis of rotatory subluxations was highly subject to diagnostic error, especially the interpretation of increased ER of the tibia as a posterior subluxation of the tibia.[24]

There exists an unmet need for reliable measurements of pathologic knee motion under specific loading conditions, especially rotatory subluxations. When examining the in-

jured knee, the clinician performs a given motion test, defines the magnitude and direction of abnormal motion, and then determines the structures injured and the degree of that injury. Each step is a source of potential error. Despite the current concern for the accuracy and reproducibility of standard manual exams for ligament instability, these exams continue to be central to the assessment of acute knee injuries. Concern for error is greatest when multiple ligaments have been injured and when assessing the integrity of the posterolateral corner. Physical exam tests continue to have a high specificity in diagnosing injuries to the anterior cruciate ligament.[6,25]

Stability testing of the extensor mechanism is an important and frequently overlooked part of the examination of the acutely injured knee. The extensor mechanism should be examined in a superior-to-inferior direction for completeness and consistency. The patient should be asked to perform a straight leg-raising effort. (One should look carefully for the presence of an extensor lag in this maneuver.) This establishes the integrity of the extensor mechanism. Quadriceps ruptures are frequently misdiagnosed in the evaluation of the injured knee. If the patient's knee is quite swollen, it will likely be resting in a slightly flexed position for comfort. The patient must still demonstrate the ability to raise the leg without an extensor lag greater than that of the resting position of the knee. Frequently, in a quadricep rupture, the patient may be able to elevate the leg off the table, but a significant lag is present, and the patient is not able to hold the leg against gravity or any minor resistance. If you have the advantage of examining the knee immedi-

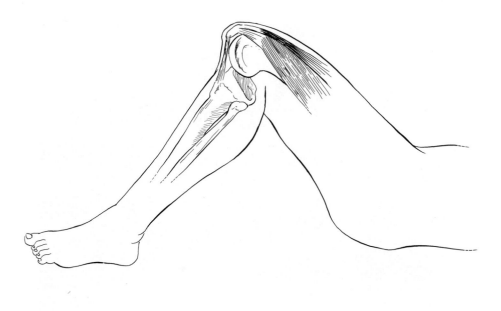

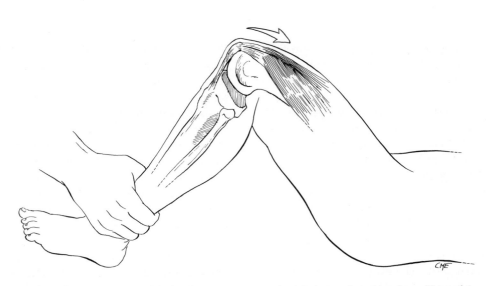

Fig. 3-6. With the knee held at 90 degrees, an active quadricep muscle contraction will translate the tibia forward to the neutral position. At this point in the physical exam the degree of anterior and posterior translation of the tibia should be assessed.

ately after injury, a palpable defect should be present in the quadricep mechanism. However, this can quickly fill with blood, and the presence of swelling and blood can eliminate the palpable defect.

A second source of misdiagnosis is tearing of the infrapatella tendon. This is associated with patella alta when compared to the contralateral knee, and patella height should be assessed and compared. A palpable defect can frequently be palpated. Other injuries compromising the integrity of the extensor mechanism are transverse patella fractures and avulsions of the patella tendon origin.

In addition to examining the integrity of the extensor mechanism, medial-lateral stability of the patella must be assessed. One first establishes the position of the patella. A complete dislocation of the patella is clinically apparent in most cases (Fig. 3-8). Frequently the patella reduces spontaneously soon after the injury. Signs that an acute lateral dislocation has occurred should be sought. Swelling is usually present; frequently it is quite dramatic. Palpable pain along the medial restraining structures is present. Passive lateral movement of the patella may cause pain or apprehension. Increased motion in the lateral direction may be

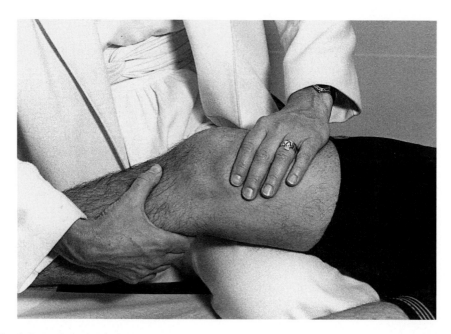

Fig. 3-7. Lachman's hand exam: one way to stabilize the leg, particularly with the larger thigh, is to place the patient's distal femur over the examiner's bent knee. The femur is then stabilized between the examiner's hand and thigh, providing a stable post by which to judge anterior translation of the tibia.

present but is usually guarded against secondary to pain. Straight leg raising is possible but this frequently causes pain and may be associated with an extensor lag.

Patella dislocation occurring without acute swelling of the joint implies constitutional features in the patella-femoral articulation that allows the kneecap to be highly mobile without tearing of the soft tissue restraints. These features include increased tissue laxity, atrophic or underdeveloped musculature, and hypoplastic bony anatomy.

Instrumented testing devices. Concern about the accuracy of the clinical exam and its reproducibility, both between examiners and in serial exams, has led researchers to create instrumented measurement systems designed for objective documentation of knee motions. A second driving force in the development of such instruments is to document and measure the success of ligament surgery in regard to the reestablishment of normal motion limits.

Motion measurements consist of three parameters. The limb is positioned in a set manner. A force applied in a set manner, preferably quantified. The resultant joint displacement is measured. A testing device may perform one, two, or all of these tasks.

The earliest reports of instrumented testing devices consisted of applying a standard displacement force and documenting the resultant joint position change by comparing photographs[26] or radiographs.[27,28] These were taken of the knee both stressed and unstressed. Perhaps the first instrumented knee laxity machine was the pneumatic stress machine, introduced by Kennedy and Fowler in 1971.[29]

Stress radiographic techniques are widely known to the

clinician and have a long history. However, they have not been widely used as an instrumented testing device by clinicians, possibly because of the expense, radiation exposure, and vigorous parameters that need to be followed to obtain reproducible results.

The use of an instrumented measurement machine has been popularized by some to add to clinical acumen in the evaluation of acute knee injuries. In 1985 Daniels et al. published a study of 138 patients with acute knee injuries. In 53 patients whose ACL tears were confirmed by arthroscopy, the anterior laxity measurements performed in the clinic were suggestive or diagnostic of pathologic anterior laxity in 50 patients.[7]

Anderson and Lipscomb in 1989 examined 50 patients with suspected cruciate ligament tears with a clinical exam, exam under anesthesia (EUA), and an instrumented test with KT-1000 (MED-metric, San Diego), Stryker (Stryker, Kalamazoo, Michigan), and Genucom (Faro Medical Technologies, Champlain, New York).[30] The findings were then confirmed by arthroscopy and/or arthrotomy. Thirty had acute (within 2 weeks) knee injuries. The KT-1000 can be used to identify the quadriceps neutral position and therefore is more accurate in assessing PCL instability. However, this must be done in the awake patient. The accuracy in correctly predicting injured cruciates was 92% with the clinical exam, 98% with the EUA, 75% using KT-1000, 75% using Stryker, and 70% using Genucom. The authors felt that this study suggested that the clinical exam by an experienced examiner is the most accurate way to determine cruciate ligament integrity, but in many cases the confidence in clinical di-

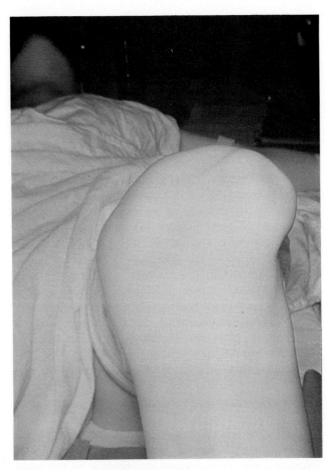

Fig. 3-8. A young female presents in the emergency room with an acute knee injury. An obvious deformity of lateral dislocation of the patella is noted on gross knee exam.

agnosis was improved with instrumented machine confirmation. Performing a max manual improves the accuracy of these testing devices.[31]

Clearly, there is a cost difference among the devices. The Stryker device sells for approximately $900; KT-1000, approximately $3000; and Genucom, $50,000. The Genucom certainly has increased versatility. It is a complex computerized system that allows a full battery of knee laxity tests for analysis of knee ligament stability, including varus-valgus, pivot shift, and recurvatum. It has a computer capacity that allows storage of patient data for subsequent comparison.[32] However, with increased versatility also comes increased complexity. The Genucom results can vary from day to day, and care must be taken in interpreting the meaning of a single measurement. Meticulous care in the digitization process must be adhered to, with diligence in assuring patient relaxation.[33]

In summary, instrument testing devices are not meant to substitute for a thorough history and physical exam, but rather supplement and substantiate them.[34] Due to differences in device sensitivities and functional design, numer-

ical results from one device cannot be generalized to another.[32]

The KT-1000 is perhaps the most popular portable instrumented knee machine clinically used. It has been widely researched and popularized by Dale Daniels. In a classic 1985 study,[7] he and co-authors noted a wide range of laxity within the normal population. However, there was a small right-to-left knee difference. Of his normal population 88% had a right-to-left difference less than 3 mm. This has been confirmed by others.[28] When using a KT-1000, a side-to-side difference of 3 mm or more is suggestive of anterior laxity.

Another parameter that instrumented measurements can record is stiffness or end point. The inverse of stiffness or compliance can be measured on KT-1000 and Stryker. A measurement of compliance increases the diagnostic accuracy of these machines. Compliance index as measured by the KT-1000 is the difference between values at 15 and 20 pounds of force. A compliance index greater than 1 is suggestive of pathologic anterior laxity.[35]

Dale Daniels in his clinics routinely performed KT-1000 measurements on patients with acute knee injuries with suspected ACL disruptions. To allow better stabilization of the patella and perhaps to increase patient comfort, an aspiration of the knee prior to testing is performed, if one estimates the effusion as greater than 50 cc. Patients who have received an injury to the patella may not tolerate the pressure needed to stabilize the patella sensor. Performing four displacement tests (20 pound, 30 pound, max manual, and quadriceps active) is the manufacturer's suggested routine. If any of these four tests has an injured minus normal knee displacement value of 3 mm or more, the likelihood of a cruciate ligament disruption is greater than 95%.[35]

In all instrumented machines that measure anterior-posterior motion as diagnostic of an ACL injury, careful assessment of PCL integrity must be ruled out or accounted for in performing the instrumented measurements.

Clearly, to gain diagnostic accuracy, the patient must be relaxed, and the instrument must be appropriately utilized per the manufacturer's instructions. There is a learning curve with regards to the use of these machines. Clinicians who routinely utilize instrumented testing should document their own test-retest reproducibility on different patients and on different days for the highest accuracy.

TESTS AND THEIR INTERPRETATION
Conventional radiography

The assessment of an acutely injured knee is incomplete without radiographic evaluation, and this continues to be a requirement of a complete work-up of the acutely injured knee. The radiographic examination of the knee should contain, at a minimum, three views: an anterior-posterior (A/P) view, a lateral view, and an axial view of the patellofemoral joint. A tunnel or notch view is frequently helpful in certain conditions.

The A/P views of the acutely swollen knee are often done in a nonstanding position. If the patient has any degree of a flexion contracture secondary to trauma or spasm, a standing radiograph shows overlap of the femur and tibia and is less useful for examination of the articular surface. Therefore, in a knee that cannot obtain full extension, or if standing may be painful for the patient, a nonstanding view is ordered. However, a standing A/P radiograph offers the additional advantage of assessing tibial-femoral alignment in the weightbearing position.

The A/P view's primary usefulness is to rule out pertinent negatives in regard to bony pathology, as well as to search for occult fractures.

The lateral view of the knee evaluates the superior-inferior position of the kneecap. With regard to the acutely injured knee, patella alta should raise the suspicion of an infrapatella tendon injury. This may need to be compared to a view of the other side, either by x-ray or by physical exam, to confirm the diagnosis. Additionally, avulsion fractures of the posterior cruciate ligament (Fig. 3-9), which frequently arise from the tibia, are best seen on lateral view.

Axial views of the patellofemoral joint should be a routine part of all acute knee injuries. One primarily assesses the position of the kneecap in a medial-lateral plane, in relationship to the trochlear groove. Patella tilt can also be evaluated. Search for occult fractures is necessary. Acute swelling is easily visualized in this view.

There have been many conventions established for axial or tangential viewing of the patellofemoral joint.[36] Popular axial views of the kneecap are those of Laurin et al.[37] and Merchant et al.[38] Important to remember is that each view has its own established criteria based on population studies done by the given researchers, in establishing normal and abnormal values for given views. Therefore, one could question the validity of drawing Merchant lines on a Laurin view and the like. One should become familiar with an individual convention and use that routinely, as this will increase the diagnostic assistance that axial views can provide.

In a suspected patellar dislocation, the axial view should be carefully analyzed for the presence of an osteochondral fracture. In an acute patellar dislocation, the kneecap is dislocated laterally. Fractures are most common as a result of the relocation of the patella, as a forceful quadricep contraction pulls the kneecap back in alignment. As the laterally displaced kneecap relocates into the trochlear groove, osteochondral fractures can occur by the contact of the medial patella facet against the lateral femoral condyle. Therefore, fractures should be sought along the medial patellar facet and the lateral femoral condyle (Fig. 3-10). The fragment may consist of a thin flake of osseous bone, appearing tangentially on x-ray as a thin eggshell fragment (Fig. 3-11). However, a fairly large cartilaginous fragment may be associated with these osseous fragments. The radiographic picture cannot estimate the size or importance of the fragment. In addition to searching for osteochondral fragments, one should assess the position of the patella within the trochlear groove and the presence of any translation or tilt in the kneecap (Fig. 3-12). The Laurin view is particularly helpful in this regard.

The notch view has the most applicability for better assessment of an osteochondritis dissecans lesion and for searching for loose bodies. In anterior cruciate ligament injuries, an intercondylar notch view has some application

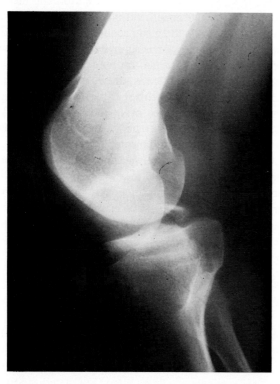

Fig. 3-9. A lateral radiograph of the knee reveals a fracture of the posterior aspect of the tibia. Surgical exploration revealed an avulsion fracture of the tibial insertion of the posterior cruciate ligament.

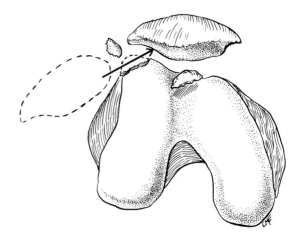

Fig. 3-10. Osteochondral fractures occurring at the time of patella dislocation usually occur when the patella relocates and the medial patella facet can make contact with the lateral aspect of the femoral condyle, at which time osteochondral fragmentation can result.

in assessing the shape and the width of the intercondylar notch.[39,40] Frequently, avulsion injuries of the tibial insertion of the cruciate ligaments, as well as tibial spine fractures, are best seen in the notch view.

Manual stress films occasionally are employed to identify ligament damage. Stress x-rays are most useful to rule out epiphyseal injury (Salter type I) versus ligamentous pathology in an adolescent[41] (Fig. 3-13). Anterior and posterior stress films can evaluate the integrity of the cruciates, and angular deformity of the knee can be documented with varus and valgus stress views. Stress views used to evaluate angular deformity are most frequently performed at 20 to 30 degrees of flexion, comparable to the degree of flexion used in the physical exam.

Stress radiography can also be used to diagnose and document the pathologic knee motion. This technique enjoys more popularity in central Europe. In this capacity, stress radiography utilizes a machine to hold and control the limb and provides a known force application to the tibia. Stress radiography and instrumented arthrometer testing are both useful in substantiating the clinical diagnosis of an anterior cruciate ligament injury.[42] Stress radiography in this setting is most helpful in establishing known force levels and in providing a retrievable record to document the exact tibial position in relation to the femur. It also has the advantage of being able to provide varus and valgus stressing of the knee to document angular deformity of the knee. Current portable instrumented knee machines are limited to evaluation of anterior-posterior motion alone. The disadvantages of stress radiography are obvious. It is an exacting technique and requires special equipment. It is expensive and offers radiation exposure to the patient.

Routine radiographs by themselves do not allow direct visualization of injured ligaments. Their primary importance is to rule out the presence of condylar fractures as well as other occult fractures. They also play an important role in ruling out pertinent negative pathologies of the bony knee. Extensive fractures about the knee are readily demonstrated by standard radiography, but careful analysis is necessary to detect avulsion injuries at the attachment sites of ligaments and tendons. This is especially true among children in whom cruciate ligament injuries are commonly of the avulsion type.[43] One should examine ligament origin and insertion, including the collaterals, for possible small avulsion fractures that might give radiographic support to the clinical exam in diagnosing a ligament injury. This is particularly true of an avulsed fragment of the fibular head at the site of the biceps femoris insertion or fibular collateral ligament insertion, suggesting an injury to the lateral ligamentous complex of the knee. A small fracture along the anterolateral portion of the knee, frequently referred to as a Segond fracture,[44] is considered an indirect sign of an anterior cruciate ligament injury. It represents tension on the lateral capsular ligament of the knee associated with anterolateral instability. The Segond fracture is referred to as a lateral capsular sign.

A bloody effusion is detected as a soft tissue density in the suprapatellar pouch primarily on axial or lateral projections. The presence of fat in the effusion or a lipohemarthrosis suggests an osseous injury and can be seen as a fat-fluid line on a cross-table lateral projection. The accumulation of fat is greatest in the cases of acute trauma.[45]

Because routine radiographs by themselves do not allow direct visualization of injured ligaments and soft tissue structures, other forms of diagnostic imaging have evolved to help analyze these structures. From a historical perspective, arthrography has been a valuable adjunctive tool in evaluating acute knee injuries,[46,47] most used to diagnose meniscal lesions. Its value in defining cruciate ligaments is more limited. However, it is technique dependent, and its accuracy for meniscal and ligament injuries is in part dependent on the frequency of its use at an individual institution.

Arthrograms have the most application in the evaluation of the menisci in the acute and chronic knee injury. However, this standard use of the arthrogram has been largely replaced at the current time by use of magnetic resonance

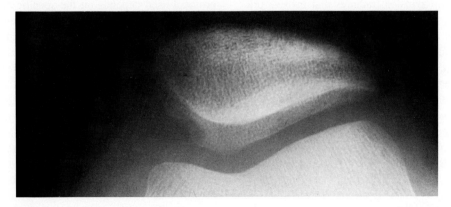

Fig. 3-11. Axial radiograph of a patient who sustained an acute patella dislocation. Radiographic findings reveal a disruption in the normally smooth margins of the medial patella facet, which correlates to an acute fracture fragmentation.

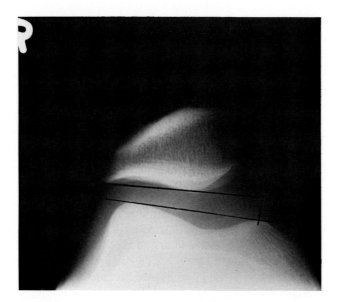

Fig. 3-12. Twenty-degree axial view (Laurin's view) of a patient who sustained an acute patella dislocation. Radiographic lines drawn along the lateral patella facet and across the highest point of the medial and lateral femoral condyles reveal converging lines, which represent continued tilt of this kneecap. A perpendicular line drawn from the highest point of the medial femoral condyle reveals more than 3 mm lateral displacement of the patella from this perpendicular line, indicating continued subluxation of this kneecap.

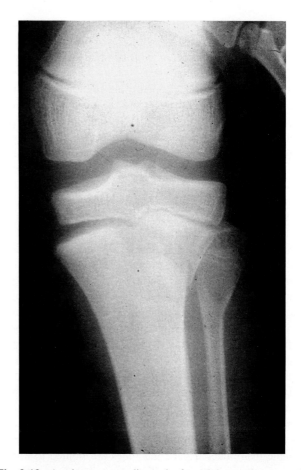

Fig. 3-13. A valgus stress radiograph of an adolescent knee reveals a Salter I injury of the proximal tibial epiphysis.

imaging (MRI) studies. Arthrograms continue to be useful, particularly when combined with tomograms for the evaluation of the stability of osteochondral lesions, in particular, osteochondritis dissecans defects. The leakage of dye in and around an osteochondral fragment clearly represents instability of that lesion.

Computed tomography (CT) is a reliable diagnostic tool for a number of musculoskeletal conditions but has never found specific application for routine imaging of acute knee injuries. It continues to have application in evaluating complex fractures around the knee, particularly those involving cortical surfaces, in evaluating the integrity of the cortical surfaces, in picking up avulsion fractures that involve primarily cortical bone, and, combined with contrast, in evaluating osteochondral defects.

CT has also found application in the analysis of patellofemoral malalignment. To date, however, there has been a paucity of published studies,[48,49] involving small numbers of normals, with little correlation of the CT findings with the clinical exam. The role that CT scan plays in the clinical work-up and management of patellofemoral alignment has yet to be clearly defined.

Bone scans have their best application for evaluation of a suspected stress fracture or infection in bone. Their value in diagnosing reflex sympathetic dystrophy is variable.

MRI clearly has revealed the most useful diagnostic applicability for evaluation of the musculoskeletal system, particularly in the acute knee injury. It is able to image sup-

porting soft tissue structures, acute and chronic bone marrow changes, and, to a lesser degree, articular surface cartilage changes. It is currently the test of choice to evaluate meniscal and ligamentous injuries to the knee.

MRI is based on the concept of magnetization of soft tissue ions. Multiple pulse sequences and imaging planes can be used in evaluation in MRI of tissues. The precise protocol used depends on the specific clinical situation. In general, T1-weighted images best view subcutaneous fat and bone marrow, which have the brightest signal intensity. Hyaline cartilage is of intermediate signal density, and muscle has even less density. On T2-weighted images, effusions have the brightest signals, followed in decreasing order by subcutaneous fat, bone marrow, and muscle. Ligaments, tendons, and cortical bone remain low in signal intensity.

For the knee, MRI has its greatest application in evaluation of meniscus (Fig. 3-14) and, secondarily, cruciate ligaments. MRI has an overall accuracy rate for detection of meniscal abnormalities at 93% (sensitivity, 95%; specificity, 91%). It has a false negative rate of 4.8%.[50] It has the advantage of evaluating extra-articular structures and therefore may pick up pathology that is masquerading as meniscal pathology. The accuracy of MRI in imaging an-

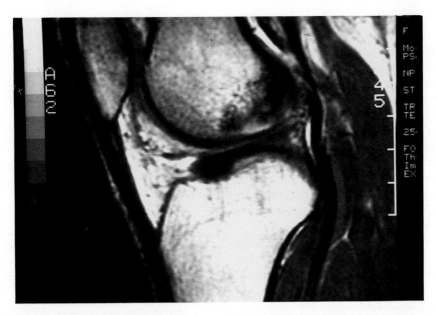

Fig. 3-14. T1-weighted sagittal MRI of an acutely injured knee, revealing a tear in the posterior aspect of the medial meniscus.

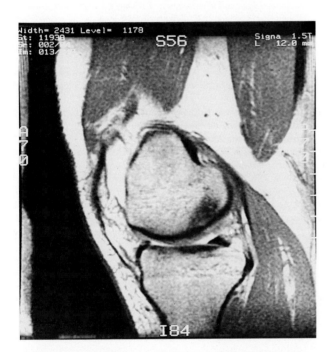

Fig. 3-15. T1-weighted sagittal MRI of an acutely injured knee. Although conventional radiographs were normal, MRI reveals an area of decreased signal intensity in the subchondral bone of the posterior aspect of the medial femoral condyle.

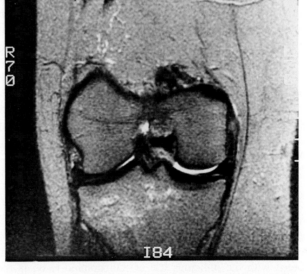

Fig. 3-16. T2-weighted coronal MRI of an acutely injured knee. Although conventional radiographs were normal, MRI reveals an area of increased signal intensity in the subchondral bone of the lateral tibial condyle.

terior cruciate ligament injuries has also proved helpful, with a 95% accuracy rate in one recent study.[50] The MRI is showing increasing accuracy as a modality to evaluate the integrity of the PCL.[51]

MRI offers increased detail in detecting and defining the partial cruciate ligament injury. It can detect edema, swell-

ing, and partial-thickness tearing within the cruciate ligament bundle that may be difficult to assess on physical exam or arthroscopic visualization and probing. One consideration in reviewing current studies that assess MRI accuracy is the use of arthroscopy as the gold standard. Arthroscopy has its own limitations, making it imperfect as a gold standard.

MRI of the collateral structures is useful to assess ligament continuity as well as surrounding edema and local hemorrhage. A complete tear (grade III) of the collateral ligament is diagnosed on the basis of discontinuity of the ligament. However, the differentiation between grade I and grade II injuries of the collateral ligament depends on the clinical diagnosis rather than on MRI findings. Isolated injuries of the lateral collateral ligament structures are rare. The preceding discussion has more application for medial collateral ligament structures. However, MRI has the advantage of evaluating acute edema in the region of the lateral and posterolateral complex and of evaluating the possibility of associated PCL-ACL injuries in these complex and often severe injuries to the knee.[52]

An additional advantage of MRI over other forms of diagnostic imaging is that one is able to make a statement about the age of the injury. The presence of acute swelling, tissue edema, or early hematoma formation signifies that the injury is of recent onset. As a result of MRI of acutely injured knees, subchondral bone changes have been identified that occur in the absence of conventional radiographic changes (Figs. 3-15 and 3-16).[53-55] There is some suggestion that these MRI changes may lead to subsequent cartilage degeneration.[54] Their role in the development of post-traumatic arthritis continues to be investigated.[56]

The advantages of MRI are numerous. It has the advantage of evaluating intra-articular as well as extra-articular structures with excellent soft tissue discrimination. It has multiplane imaging capacity. When appropriate, it has the ability to identify right-to-left differences. It uses no ionizing radiation.

MRI continues to be costly and should be used only as an adjunct in an acutely injured knee if it will alter the treatment protocol. It should never be used in the absence of a thorough history and physical exam. As with many clinical situations, its usefulness is as an adjunctive test. When it is combined with the physical exam and other clinical studies, the most accurate diagnosis can be achieved.

SUMMARY

A correct diagnosis is central to the institution of appropriate treatment for the injured knee. A careful evaluation using the foundation of history and physical exam, combined with the judicious use of radiographic tests, is the essential basis from which subsequent management schemes are laid.

REFERENCES

1. Hughston JC: *Surgical repair of acute ligamentous tears of the knee.* Presented at AAOS postgraduate course, *The injured knee in sport: special reference to the surgical knee,* Eugene, Oregon, July 23–25, 1973.
2. Paulos L, Noyes F, Malek M: A practical guide to the initial evaluation and treatment of knee ligament injuries, *J Trauma* 20:498, 1980.
3. DeHaven K: Diagnosis of acute knee injuries with hemarthrosis, *Am J Sports Med* 8:9, 1980.
4. American Medical Association: *Standard nomenclature of athletic injuries,* Chicago, 1966, American Medical Association.
5. Daniel D: *Diagnosis of a ligament injury.* In Daniel D, O'Connor J, Akeson W, editors: *Knee ligaments: structure, function, injury and repair,* New York, 1990, Raven Press.
6. Donaldson W, Warren R, Wickiewicz T: A comparison of acute anterior cruciate ligament examinations, *Am J Sports Med* 13:5–10, 1985.
7. Daniel D, et al: Instrumented measurement of anterior knee laxity in patients with acute anterior cruciate ligament disruption, *Am J Sports Med* 13:401–407, 1985.
8. Miller W, et al: Oak knee evaluation: a new way to assess knee ligament injuries, *Clin Orthop* 232:37–50, 1988.
9. Noyes FR, Grood ES: *Diagnosis of knee ligament injuries: clinical concepts.* In Feagin J, editor: *The crucial ligaments,* vol I, New York, 1988, Churchill Livingstone.
10. Butler D, Noyes F, Grood E: Ligamentous restraints to anterior-posterior drawer in the human knee: a biomechanical study, *J Bone Joint Surg [Am]* 62:259–270, 1980.
11. Fukubayashi T, et al: An *in vitro* biomechanical evaluation of anterior-posterior motion of the knee: tibial displacement, rotation, torque, *J Bone Joint Surg [Am]* 64:258–269, 1982.
12. Markolf K, Mensch J, Amstatz H: Stiffness and laxity of the knee—the contributions of the supporting structures: a quantitative *in vitro* study, *J Bone Joint Surg [Am]* 58:583–594, 1976.
13. Seering W, et al: The function of the primary ligaments of the knee in varus-valgus and axial rotation, *J Biomech* 13:785–799, 1980.
14. Shoemaker S, Markolf K: Effects of joint load on the stiffness and laxity of ligament-deficient knees: an *in vitro* study of the anterior cruciate and medial collateral ligaments, *J Bone Joint Surg [Am]* 67:136–146, 1985.
15. Gollehon D, Torzilli P, Warren R: The role of the posterolateral and cruciate ligaments in the stability of the human knee: a biomechanical study, *J Bone Joint Surg [Am]* 69:234–242, 1987.
16. Grood E, Stowers S, Noyes F: Limits of motion in the human knee: effect of sectioning the posterior cruciate ligament and posterolateral structures, *J Bone Joint Surg [Am]* 70:88–97, 1988.
17. Torg JS, Conrad W, Kalen V: Clinical diagnosis of anterior cruciate ligament instability in the athlete, *Am J Sports Med* 4:84, 1976.
18. Galway HR, MacIntosh DL: The lateral pivot shift: a symptom and sign of anterior cruciate ligament insufficiency, *CORR* 147:45, 1980.
19. Losee RE, Ennis TR, Southwick WO: Anterior subluxation of the lateral tibial plateau, *J Bone Joint Surg [Am]* 60:1015–1030, 1978.
20. Noyes FR, et al: Clinical laxity tests and functional stability of the knee: biomechanical concepts, *CORR* 146:84, 1980.
21. Jakob RP, Hassler H, Staeubli H: The reversed pivot shift sign: a new diagnostic aid for posterolateral rotatory instability of the knee, *Acta Orthop Scand* Suppl 52:18, 1981.
22. Hughston JC, Norwood LA: The posterolateral drawer test and external rotational recurvatum test for posterolateral rotatory instability of the knee, *CORR* 147:82, 1980.
23. Daniel D: Assessing the limits of knee motion, *Am J Sports Med* 19:139–147, 1991.
24. Noyes FR, et al: The diagnosis of knee motion limits, subluxations, and ligament injury, *Am J Sports Med* 19:163–171, 1991.
25. Katz J, Fingeroth R: The diagnostic accuracy of ruptures of the anterior cruciate ligament comparing the Lachman test, the anterior drawer sign, and the pivot shift test in acute and chronic knee injuries, *Am J Sports Med* 14:88–91, 1986.
26. Sprague RB, Asprez GM: Photographic method for measuring knee stability: a preliminary report, *Phys Ther* 4:1055–1058, 1965.
27. Torzilli PA, Greenberg RL, Insall JN: An *in vivo* biomechanical evaluation of A-P motion of the knee: roentgenographic measurement technique, stress machine, and stable population, *J Bone Joint Surg [Am]* 63:960–968, 1981.

28. Jacobson K: Stress radiographical measurement of the anteroposterior, medial and lateral stability of the knee, *Acta Orthop Scand* 47:335–344, 1976.

29. Kennedy JC, Fowler PJ: Medial and anterior instability of the knee: an anatomical and clinical study using stress machines, *J Bone Joint Surg [Am]* 53:1257–1270, 1971.

30. Anderson AF, Lipscomb AB: Preoperative instrumented testing of anterior and posterior knee laxity, *Am J Sports Med* 17:387–392, 1989.

31. Anderson AF, et al: Instrumented evaluation of knee laxity: a comparison of five arthrometers, *Am J Sports Med* 20:135–140, 1992.

32. Highgenboten CL, Jackson A, Meske NB: Genucom, KT-1000, and Stryker knee laxity measuring device comparisons: device reproducibility and interdevice comparison in asymptomatic subjects, *Am J Sports Med* 17:743–746, 1989.

33. Wroble RR, et al: Reproducibility of Genucom knee analysis system testing, *Am J Sports Med* 18:387–395, 1990.

34. Sherman OH, Markolf KL, Ferkel RD: Measurements of anterior laxity in normal and anterior cruciate absent knees with 2 instrumental test devices, *Clin Orthop* 215:156–161, 1987.

35. Daniel DM, Stone ML: *KT-1000 anterior-posterior displacement measurements.* In Daniel D, O'Connor J, Akeson W, editors: *Knee ligaments: structure, function, injury, and repair,* New York, 1990, Raven Press.

36. Carson WG, et al: Patellofemoral disorders—physical and radiographic examination: part II, radiographic examination, *Clin Orthop* 185:178–186, 1984.

37. Laurin CA, Dussault R, Levesque HP: The tangential x-ray investigation of the patellofemoral joint: x-ray technique, diagnostic criteria and their interpretation, *Clin Orthop* 144:16, 1979.

38. Merchant AC, et al: Roentgenographic analysis of patellofemoral congruence, *J Bone Joint Surg [Am]* 56:1391–1396, 1974.

39. Souryal TO: Bilaterality in anterior cruciate ligament injuries: associated intercondylar notch stenosis, *Am J Sports Med* 16:449–454, 1988.

40. Anderson AF, Lipscomb AB: Analysis of the intercondylar notch by computed tomography, *Am J Sports Med* 15:547–552, 1983.

41. Bright RW: *Physeal injuries.* In Rockwood CA, Wilkins KE, King RE, editors: *Fractures in children,* vol 3, Philadelphia, 1984, JB Lippincott.

42. Staubli H, Jakob RP: Anterior knee motion analysis: measurement and simultaneous radiography, *Am J Sports Med* 19:172–177, 1991.

43. Bradley GW, Shives TC, Samuelson KM: Ligament injuries in the knees of children, *J Bone Joint Surg [Am]* 61:588–591, 1979.

44. Wood GW, Stanley RF, Tullos HS: Lateral capsular sign: x-ray clue of significant knee instability, *Am J Sports Med* 7:27–33, 1979.

45. Resnick D, Goergen TG, Niwayama G: *Physical injury.* In Resnick D, Niwayama G, editors: *Diagnosis of bone and joint disorders,* ed 2, Philadelphia, 1988, WB Saunders.

46. Tongue JR, Larson RL: Limited arthrography in acute knee injuries, *Am J Sports Med* 8:19–23, 1980.

47. Wang J, Marshal J: Acute ligamentous injuries of the knee: single contrast arthrography, a diagnostic aid, *J Trauma* 15:40–43, 1975.

48. Schutzer SF, Ramsby GR, Fulkerson JP: The evaluation of patellofemoral pain using computerized tomography: a preliminary study, *Clin Orthop* 204:286–293, 1986.

49. Inoue M, et al: Subluxation of the patella, *J Bone Joint Surg [Am]* 70:1331–1337, 1988.

50. Mink JH, Levy T, Crues JH: Tears of the anterior cruciate ligament and menisci of the knee: MR evaluation, *Radiology* 167:769–774, 1988.

51. Gross ML, et al: Magnetic resonance imaging of the posterior cruciate ligament: clinical use to improve diagnostic accuracy, *Am J Sports Med* 20:732–737, 1992.

52. Mink JH: *The ligaments of the knee.* In Mink JH, editor: *Magnetic resonance imaging of the knee,* New York, 1987, Raven Press.

53. Mink JH, Deutsch AL: Occult cartilage and bone injuries of the knee: detection, classification and assessment with MR imaging, *Radiology* 170:823–829, 1989.

54. Vellet AD, et al: Occult posttraumatic lesions of the knee: prevalence, classification, and short-term sequelae evaluated with MR imaging, *Radiology* 178:271–276, 1991.

55. Yao L, Lee JK: Occult intraosseous fracture: detection with MR imaging, *Radiology* 167:749–751, 1988.

56. Vener MJ, et al: Subchondral damage after acute transarticular loading: an in vitro model of joint injury, *J Ortho Res* 10:759–765, 1992.

Chapter 4

THE PHYSIOLOGY AND BIOCHEMISTRY OF SOFT TISSUE HEALING

Mark A. Gomez

Successful rehabilitation of an injured knee demands an understanding of the physiology of healing within the wounded soft tissues. Therefore, the goal of this chapter is to provide knowledge of the progression of biochemical and physiologic events that occur as a result of an injury to particular soft tissues in the knee. First, each of the primary biochemical constituents of normal tissues and their physiologic function is described. Next, how these constituents are affected subsequent to tissue injury is presented. Finally, factors that augment or diminish the material properties of these damaged tissues during the healing process are described.

NORMAL SOFT TISSUE: BIOCHEMISTRY AND PHYSIOLOGY

Soft tissues about the knee, such as ligament, meniscus, and articular cartilage, consist of components that are the products of particular synthetic (or anabolic) mechanisms. These extracellular matrix components include collagen, proteoglycans, elastin, and glycoproteins such as fibronectin. Descriptions of these principal biochemical constituents follow.

Collagen

Collagen typically constitutes 65% to 80% of the dry weight of the aforementioned connective tissues (Fig. 4-1). It is synthesized by fibroblasts within the soft tissue in a sequence of intracellular and extracellular enzymatic steps (Fig. 4-2). Within the cell, the amino acids proline and lysine of a single alpha helical polypeptide chain are first hydroxylated (i.e., OH groups are added using propyl and lysyl hydroxylase; note that iron and ascorbate are also necessary for this reaction to take place). Next, three of these chains combine to form a triple helix called *procol-*

lagen. This procollagen molecule is then exocytosed from the cell, where the enzyme procollagen peptidase cleaves the registration peptides off each end of the structure. The removal of these peptides, which augmented the assembly of the triple helix, produces tropocollagen, a molecule approximately 2800 angstroms long. It is this molecule that is used to produce the collagen fibril. A quarter-length stagger describes how these "building blocks" then fit together. If one envisions two tropocollagen molecules side by side, the second one is shifted longitudinally by an amount equal to a quarter of the length of the first molecule. A third tropocollagen would be shifted relative to the second molecule by a quarter length, and so on. Finally, the enzyme lysyl oxidase causes the formation of aldehydes on the peptide-bound lysines and hydroxylysines of the tropocollagen molecules. These aldehydes permit the formation of both intramolecular and intermolecular crosslinks between the tropocollagen molecules. These crosslinks in turn play a key role in defining the mechanical characteristics of the soft tissue.

Different collagenous structures are composed of different types of collagen. As represented in Figure 4-1, the total collagen dry weight of ligament consists of both type I and type III collagen in a ratio of about 9:1.

In articular cartilage, collagen represents about 50% of the tissue's dry weight. Type II collagen accounts for 90% to 95% of this total collagen, with the remainder defined by the minor type V, VI, IX, and XI collagens. It should be noted that the high hydroxylysine and/or glycosylated hydroxylysine content of type II collagen is typically associated with high proteoglycan and/or water content. This association helps maintain a very hydrated matrix, which is necessary for normal articular cartilage function. Preliminary work on the minor collagens indicates that they are

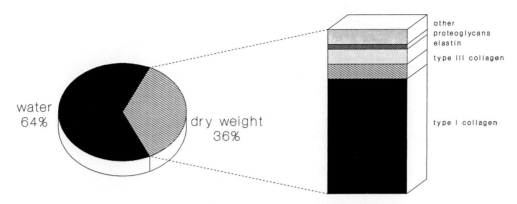

Fig. 4-1. Biochemical composition of normal ligament tissue.

probably involved in the formation as well as the structural stability of the type II collagen mesh.

Finally, meniscus contains mostly type I collagen (90% of the total collagen dry weight), with the remainder made up of types II, V, and VI in approximately similar amounts. What is unusual about the type I collagen found in meniscus is that it too has a high hydroxylysine and/or glycosylated hydroxylysine content, which is usually low in the type I collagens found in other tissues.

As mentioned before, there is a balance of synthesis and degradation of collagen in soft tissues. It has been estimated that the half-life of collagen in tendon is between 300 and 500 days. However, detailed descriptions of the complete mechanism of collagen turnover and the factors that contribute to it are still needed. An example of one of these factors would be a mediator that activates collagenase (i.e., the enzyme that breaks down collagen) initially bound to an inhibitor and secreted in toto by a fibroblast.

Proteoglycans

Proteoglycans comprise only 1% of the dry weight of tendon, but up to 30% of the dry weight of articular cartilage. A proteoglycan subunit consists of a core protein on which glycosaminoglycan (GAG) side chains are covalently bound (Fig. 4-3). These subunits are typically found in both ligament and tendon structures, but in tissues such as articular cartilage, they can aggregate with hyaluronic acid to form large hydrophilic molecules. Physically, these molecules are negatively charged with a large number of hydroxyl groups. These groups in turn attract water through hydrogen binding to form a gel-like extracellular matrix. This matrix helps maintain the spatial relationship between other proteoglycan monomers and the type II collagen fibrils as well as provide a means to regulate the flow of water through the entire matrix, particularly during loading of the tissue.

Elastin and fibronectin

Elastin contributes less than 5% of the dry weight of ligaments, and it is believed to contribute to the tissue's ability to recover to its original length after the application of a load or strain. In normal human meniscus, it has been determined that this protein makes up only 0.6% of the dry weight, and little is known about its functional significance.

The glycoprotein fibronectin is normally involved in the interaction of the fibroblasts with the surrounding matrix. This includes the cell's ability to adhere to other cells as well as any substratum. Further, there is a heterogeneity among various soft tissues regarding the amount of this protein. For example, cruciate ligaments have approximately 2 μg of fibronectin for every milligram of dry tissue, which is twice that contained in the collateral ligament or the patellar tendon. A study by Banes et al., however, demonstrates that if the surface synovial cells from avian tendons are removed with collagenase, no positive reaction with antifibronectin antibody can be detected within the cells internal to the tendon. If the external surface was allowed to remain intact, the flexor tendon surface stained positively with antibody to cellular fibronectin. Based on these results, it was hypothesized that the fibronectin may help prevent cell removal by frictional forces normally experienced by the tendon. Also, because this protein has binding sites for hyaluronic acid and collagen, it may contribute to lubrication at the tendon surface boundary.

HEALING SOFT TISSUE: BIOCHEMISTRY AND PHYSIOLOGY

The overall process of scar formation follows a series of cellular and biochemical events that are to a large degree similar in different soft tissues. In this next section, four phases of the soft tissue response to injury are discussed using a ligament healing model. These sequential phases embody traumatic inflammation and destruction, matrix and cellular proliferation, remodeling, and maturation of the injured tissue.

Phase I: inflammation and destruction

This first phase begins within a few minutes after injury. Blood vessels are disrupted, causing the gap between the ligamentous ends to fill with blood to form a hematoma (Fig. 4-4). The release of histamines from mast cells and

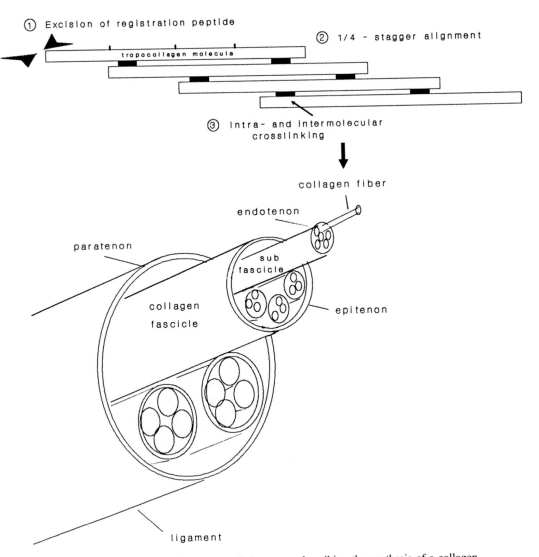

alpha-helical collagen body

Glycine

Hydroxyproline
HO

Proline

Precursor registration peptide

Hydroxylation of certain proline and lysine residues

Glycosylation of certain hydroxylysine residues

OH   OH
Triple helix or procollagen
OH

Cell membrane

① Excision of registration peptide

② 1/4 - stagger alignment

tropocollagen molecule

③ Intra- and intermolecular crosslinking

collagen fiber

endotenon

paratenon

sub fascicle

collagen fascicle

epitenon

ligament

Fig. 4-2. Sequence of intracellular and extracellular events describing the synthesis of a collagen fiber.

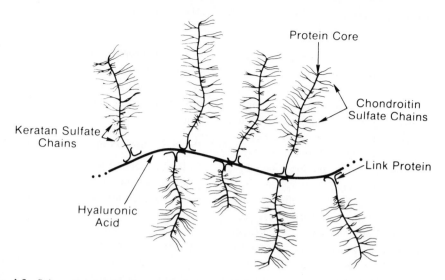

Fig. 4-3. Schematic showing how proteoglycans noncovalently associate with link proteins and a central hyaluronic acid filament to form an aggregate.

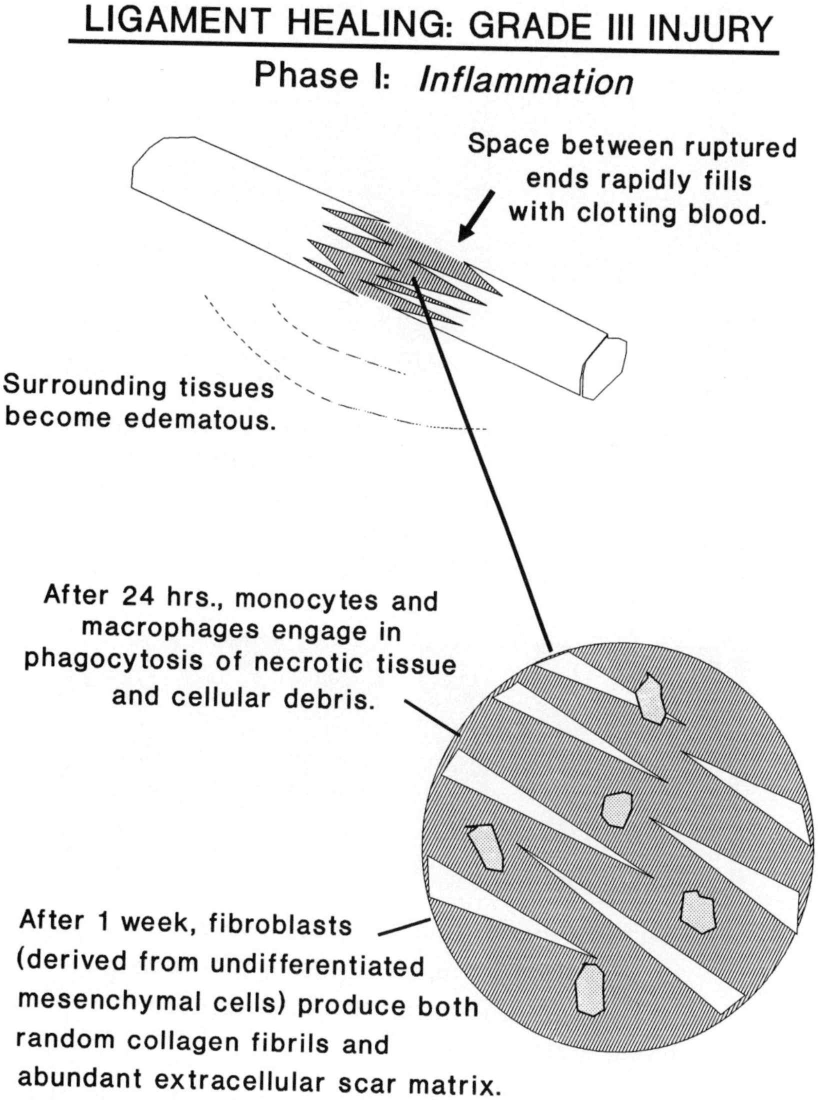

Keratan Sulfate Chains

Protein Core

Chondroitin Sulfate Chains

Link Protein

Hyaluronic Acid

LIGAMENT HEALING: GRADE III INJURY

Phase I: *Inflammation*

Space between ruptured ends rapidly fills with clotting blood.

Surrounding tissues become edematous.

After 24 hrs., monocytes and macrophages engage in phagocytosis of necrotic tissue and cellular debris.

After 1 week, fibroblasts (derived from undifferentiated mesenchymal cells) produce both random collagen fibrils and abundant extracellular scar matrix.

Fig. 4-4. Drawing of the events occurring in phase I of ligament healing.

serotonin from platelets causes vasodilation and increased permeability of precapillary arterioles. The subsequent edematous or vasodilatory state of the tissue is augmented by mediators such as bradykinins, which cause the capillaries to be more permeable. Further, an increased concentration of smaller proteins produced by enzymatic degradation increases the water volume through osmosis. After about 24 hours, complement activation produces anaphylatoxin, which chemotactically attracts polymorphonucleocytes, monocytes, and macrophages. These inflammatory cells then actively engage in phagocytosis of necrotic tissue, cellular debris, and blood clot in the wound site. The function of these cells, however, can be negatively affected by disease or even steroid use. After several days, these macrophages help recruit new fibroblasts and also release factors that initiate the growth of capillary buds into the wound.

Water, glycosaminoglycan, fibronectin, and DNA content all increase during this phase. Collagen synthesis, particularly of type III collagen, is also increased in order to provide for early stabilization of the nascent extracellular matrix.

Phase II: matrix and cellular proliferation

By the second week after injury, vascular albeit disorganized granulation tissue is visible to the naked eye. Fibroblasts predominate in number, although macrophages and mast cells are still in evidence (Fig. 4-5). The endoplasmic reticulum of the fibroblasts is pronounced under transmission electron microscopy, which indicates that matrix is being actively synthesized. Again, the collagen fibrils are still somewhat random in their organization and are surrounded by an indeterminate fibrous material or ground

LIGAMENT HEALING: GRADE III INJURY
Phase II: *Matrix and Cellular Proliferation*

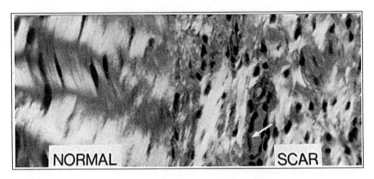

NORMAL   SCAR

Two weeks subsequent to a partial ligament injury, vascular granulation tissue fills the gap between the ligament ends (arrow denotes vessel in scar tissue). Fibroblasts predominate and actively synthesize extracellular matrix.

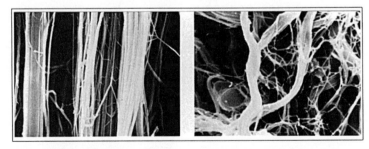

Scanning electron microscopy demonstrates disorganized collagen fibrils in the healing scar (right) compared to those of normal tissue (left).

Fig. 4-5. The microscopic appearance of healing ligament during phase II, in which matrix and cellular proliferation occurs.

substance. Within this matrix, water and glycosaminoglycan concentrations remain elevated, and both the DNA concentration (which reflects the increased cellularity) and the concentration of type III collagen reach their maximum amounts for the entire reparative process (i.e., phases I through IV) (Fig. 4-6). Type I collagen begins to become the principal matrix component. Finally, optimization of collagen synthesis in this phase is provided by a slightly acid environment and the presence of vitamin C.

Phase III/IV: remodeling and maturation

After approximately 3 weeks, the reddish scar becomes pinkish and translucent and bridges the gap between the dense white ligament ends (Fig. 4-7). Histologically, fibroblasts have shrunk in size and are synthetically less active. Further, the collagen fibers have begun to orient themselves longitudinally (i.e., in the direction loads are normally experienced by the ligament).

As the scar material "matures," the ratio of type III to type I collagen approaches normal, the numbers and types of reducible collagen crosslinks reflect those of normal ligament tissue, and water and DNA contents return to normal. The disappointing fact is that, despite these positive changes, animal studies have shown that the ligament scar can undergo a stress (i.e., force/area) that is only two thirds

that of a normal ligament for a given strain (i.e., new length − original length/original length).

FACTORS AFFECTING THE HEALING OF SOFT TISSUE

Many clinical and basic science studies have been performed to augment the properties of healing soft tissues about the knee. Although much success has been achieved toward our understanding of optimal treatment regimens, there is still considerable work to be done. In the following sections, factors that have been determined to either improve or prevent healing are presented.

Positive factors that affect healing

Ligament. Examples of factors that can improve the material properties of healing ligament are the application of increased stress and increased motion (e.g., the use of a locking-hinge rehabilitative brace for grade III tears as opposed to a plaster cast) during the healing process. Basic science studies have demonstrated that when increased stress is applied to a healing medial collateral ligament, there is improved alignment of the collagen fibers (Fig. 4-8, *A* and *B*). This improved structural organization gives the scar the ability to resist a higher stress for a given strain (Fig. 4-8, *C*). However, further knowledge of the proper level of stress

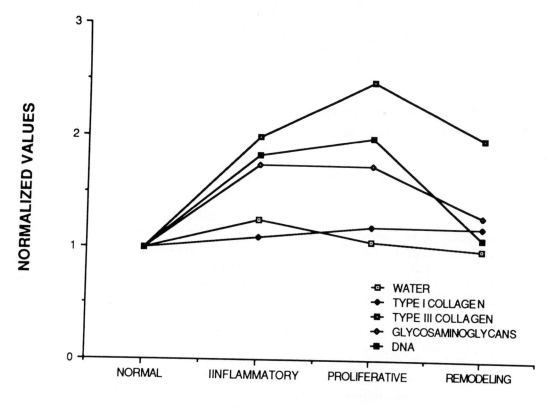

Fig. 4-6. Normalized changes in biochemical constituents of injured rabbit medial collateral ligament as a function of the different stages of healing.

LIGAMENT HEALING: GRADE III INJURY

Phase III: *Remodelling*

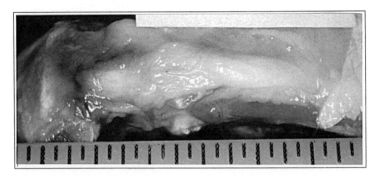

After several weeks, the ligament ends are bridged
with a translucent scar.

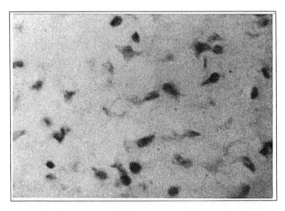

The number of fibroblasts is still increased,
but are less active based on their ultrastructure.
They appear to have a lower ratio of cytoplasm
to nucleus volume and less endoplasmic reticulum.

Fig. 4-7. Gross and microscopic appearance of healing ligament during the remodeling phase.

and the timing of its application is required to optimize particular therapeutic exercise programs. Once this information is acquired, the appropriate rehabilitative regimen would enhance the mechanical or material properties of the ligament and thus allow for a quicker and possibly complete return of normal joint function.

Clinically, physical modalities such as cryotherapy (e.g., the application of ice packs) and ultrasound can decrease the edema during the inflammatory phase. Further, it is believed that more rapid regeneration of the injured ligament may be achieved because of increased vascular ingrowth into the wound site. The proposed mechanism for this increase while using ultrasound is that low-intensity sound waves increase the flow or transport of calcium ions within mast cells. This in turn allows for the release of chemotactic

agents that attract macrophages and other cellular components active in the healing process.

Meniscus. Surgical repair of a tear in the outer third or vascular region of the meniscus promotes healing. This is true as long as the lesion is in contact with the meniscal blood supply in the periphery of the meniscus. The healing response follows that described previously and is considered extrinsic in origin. The contribution of meniscal cells or the intrinsic response is unknown at this time.

Articular cartilage. Much work has been performed to augment healing of full-thickness defects in articular cartilage. For example, perforation of the subchondral bone permits the initiation of the aforementioned phases of the innate repair response. However, despite histologic and biochemical evidence that the healing tissue exhibits charac-

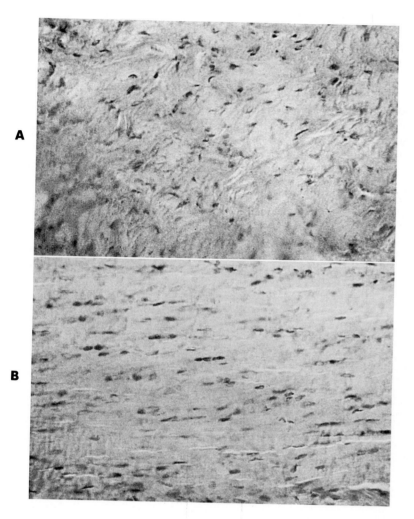

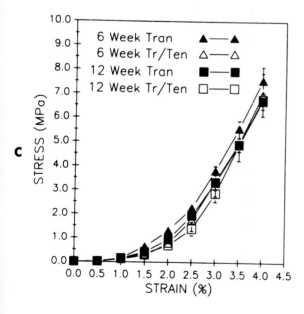

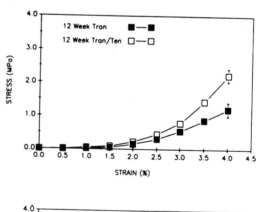

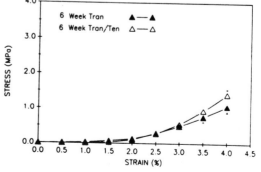

Fig. 4-8. A, Transected/healing ligament at 12 weeks after injury. **B,** Transected/healing ligament after 4 weeks of healing and 8 weeks of added tension. Note in the latter that many cells are spindle-shaped and that there is improved fiber orientation. **C,** The stress-strain curves for control ligaments *(left)* and for transected/healing ligaments with and without added tension at 6 and 12 weeks after injury *(right)*.

teristics not unlike that of normal hyaline cartilage, it is still not clear if the biomechanical properties of the newly formed tissue can provide for normal joint function in a long-term clinical setting.

This repair of damaged cartilage is also found in patients' knees that undergo an alteration of the loads across the joint. Much clinical success has been achieved, for example, by performing a high tibial osteotomy in patients with extreme varus of the knee and radiographic indications of osteoarthritis in the medial compartment. This act of load redistribution frequently relieves symptomatic pain and may prevent the need for total knee arthroplasty.

Negative factors that affect healing

Ligament. Injury can be thought of as the disruption of the normal homeostatic environment in which a tissue functions. This environment is defined by the biochemical mi-

lieu, mechanical factors, and vascular anatomy, among other things. If a particular component is removed from the environment, then the native healing response is not optimal. For example, immobilization (i.e., prevention of normal motion and stresses) of the knee joint by casting has been found to have a negative impact on the properties of healing ligament tissues. Typical effects include reduced matrix organization, lowered total collagen levels, and a reduction in the mechanical properties (i.e., the quality of the ligament material) (Fig. 4-9). Depending on the length of time immobilization is utilized, however, these effects can be reversible.

In the case of anterior cruciate ligament (ACL) healing, it would appear that many components necessary for the healing sequence to begin are disrupted at the time of injury. Nutrition is supplied to the ACL by means of a synovial layer that covers the entire ACL, originating from the in-

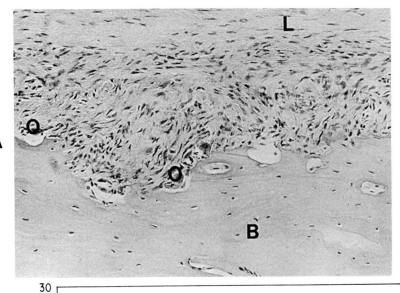

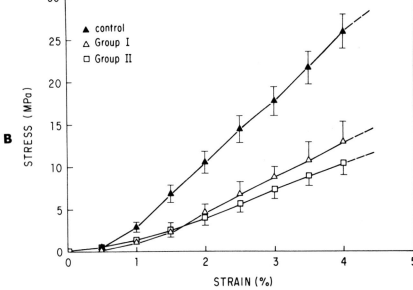

Fig. 4-9. A, Photomicrograph of a tibial insertion after 12 weeks of immobilization. Note the juxtaposition of osteoclasts *(O)* with the scalloped edges of bone *(B)*. Disorganization of the ligament *(L)* near the insertion is also in evidence. **B,** Stress-strain curves of control ligaments and those with 9 (group I) and 12 (group II) weeks of immobilization.

tercondylar notch and extending anteriorly to the tibial insertion site of the ligament. This synovium is supplied with blood from the fat pad via the inferior medial and lateral geniculate arteries. It is because of this layer that the ACL is considered extrasynovial. Simultaneous rupture of the synovium and the ACL would in turn cause several things: disruption of the blood supply, exposure of the ACL's fibroblasts to the synovial fluid, and a cessation of the normal in situ stress normally experienced by the ligament. Thus, not only are the cells not getting proper nutrition but also they cannot proliferate as well because of their exposure to the synovial fluid. Further, the injury causes the ACL fibroblasts to release collagenase, which causes the breakdown of the matrix. Clinical attempts to suture the ACL have failed for these reasons and for the fact that it is very difficult to maintain reduced stress on the surgically repaired tissue. Normal knee function causes very high load demands on the sutured tissue and prevents the ends from keeping close proximity to one another. In fact, in animal studies it has been shown that if there is a substantial gap initially between ruptured ends of a collateral ligament that *can* heal, the healing scar remodels at a slower rate.

Meniscus and articular cartilage. Injuries to the inner two thirds of the meniscus or to partial-thickness articular cartilage defects typically lack any sort of inflammatory healing response. This is attributed to the fact that these tissues have an avascular, alymphatic, and aneural composition. Investigators have attempted to provide a vascular supply to a longitudinal tear of the inner meniscus by using a channel bored into the inner meniscus from the outer vascular periphery. This channel permits the migration of fibroblasts into the avascular tear region, with the eventual formation of fibrous connective tissue. Although a response is elicited with this type of technique, it is not clear if the newly formed scar tissue is capable of withstanding the stresses typically experienced by a normal meniscus.

CONCLUDING REMARKS

The overall process by which soft tissues renew both their cell population and their extracellular matrix is termed *morphostasis*. In mature tissues, this renewal of the matrix involves the balance between synthesis of matrix components and their degradation through catabolic processes. The proper balance defines normal homeostasis. However, in an injury situation, this normal balance changes dramatically and quickly and places many demands on the host's resources to "fix" the wound and restore joint function.

As one of the primary goals of the body is to restore function, it is interesting that in the first phase of the ensuing inflammatory repair process, collagenase is released. In other words, the disrupted extracellular matrix has to be removed *first* before the wound repair and remodeling processes can begin. The tissue fibroblasts make up for this in the proliferative phase by actively synthesizing more collagen. The problem here is that the collagens being synthesized include type III collagen, which has inferior material properties compared to those of the normal type I collagen. Moreover, all the collagen is initially laid down in a very disorganized fashion (Fig. 4-5). Again, the tissue compensates for what appears to be yet another backward

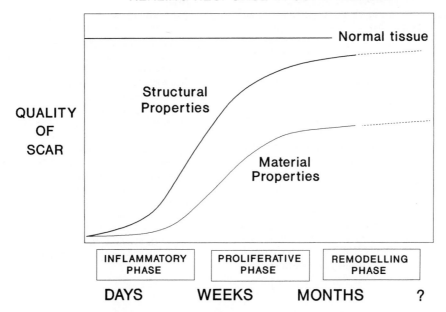

Fig. 4-10. Conceptual changes in the structural properties (i.e., those properties dictated by the size and shape of the tissue) and the material properties (i.e., those properties dictated by the quality of the tissue) as a function of healing time.

step by producing great amounts of this extracellular matrix material. This effectively causes an increase in the cross-sectional area of, for example, an injured or healing collateral ligament. By having a lot of "inferior" material, the healing structure can behave more like a normal ligament (i.e., a structure with a smaller amount of "normal," albeit better material).

The conceptual difference between the quality of the healing scar as a structure and as a material is graphically shown in Figure 4-10. Again, it shows a singular preference by the host to establish the return of function as indicated by a return in the structural properties (e.g., the load capability) of the tissue after a few months. The quality of the scar in terms of its material properties (e.g., load capability divided by cross-sectional area) does not always return to normal even after 1 year. Again, from a rehabilitative point of view, optimal joint function will more than likely be expedited through the proper timing and use of treatment regimens that optimize the material properties of the injured or healing tissue.

REFERENCES

1. Amiel D, et al: Tendons and ligaments: a morphological and biochemical comparison, *J Orthop Res* 1:257–265, 1984.

2. Arnoczky SP, et al: Meniscal repair using an exogenous fibrin clot: an experimental study in the dog, *Trans Orthop Res Soc* 11:452, 1986.

3. Arnoczky SP, Warren RF: Microvasculature of the human meniscus, *Am J Sports Med* 10:90–95, 1982.

4. Arnoczky SP, Warren RF: The microvasculature of the meniscus and its response to injury: an experimental study in the dog, *Am J Sports Med* 11:131–141, 1983.

5. Bailey AJ, Bazin S, Delaunay A: Changes in the nature of the collagen during development and resorption of granulation tissue, *Biochim Biophys Acta* 328:383–390, 1973.

6. Bailey AJ, Robins SP, Balian G: Biological significance of the intermolecular cross-links of collagen, *Nature* 251:105, 1974.

7. Banes AJ, et al: Tendon synovial cells secrete fibronectin in vivo and in vitro, *J Orthop Res* 6:73–82, 1988.

8. Cabaud HE, Rodkey WG, Fitzwater JE: Medial meniscus repairs: an experimental and morphologic study, *Am J Sports Med* 9:129–134, 1981.

9. Chimich D, et al: The effects of initial end contact on medial collateral ligament healing: a morphological and biomechanical study in a rabbit model, *J Orthop Res* 9:37–47, 1991.

10. Daniel DM, Akeson WH, O'Connor JJ, editors: *Knee ligaments: structure, function, injury, and repair,* New York, 1990, Raven Press.

11. Donohue JM, et al: The effects of indirect blunt trauma on adult canine articular cartilage, *J Bone Joint Surg [Am]* 65:948–957, 1983.

12. Eyre DR, Paz MA, Gallop PM: Cross-linking in collagen and elastin, *Annu Rev Biochem* 53:717–748, 1984.

13. Frank CB, et al: Medial collateral ligament healing: a multidisciplinary assessment in rabbits, *Am J Sports Med* 11:379–389, 1983.

14. Frank C, Schachar N, Dittrich D: Natural history of healing of the repaired medial collateral ligament, *J Orthop Res* 1:179–188, 1983.

15. Furukawa T, et al: Biochemical studies on repair cartilage resurfacing experimental defects in the rabbit knee, *J Bone Joint Surg [Am]* 62:79–89, 1980.

16. Gamble JG, Edwards CC, Max SR: Enzymatic adaptation in ligament during immobilization, *Am J Sports Med* 12(3):221–228, 1984.

17. Gomez MA, et al: The effects of increased tension on healing medial collateral ligaments, *Am J Sports Med* 19:347–354, 1991.

18. Grinnell F: Fibronectin and wound healing, *J Cell Biochem* 26:107–116, 1984.

19. Heatley FW: The meniscus: can it be repaired? An experimental study in the rabbit, *J Bone Joint Surg [Br]* 62:397–402, 1980.

20. Kastelic J, Galeski A, Baer E: The multicomposite structure of tendon, *Connect Tissue Res* 6:11–23, 1978.

21. Levene CI: Diseases of the collagen molecule, *J Clin Pathol* 12:82, 1978.

22. Mankin HJ: The response of articular cartilage to mechanical injury, *J Bone Joint Surgery [Am]* 64:460–466, 1982.

23. Mayne R, Irwin MH: *Collagen types in cartilage.* In Kuettner KE, Schleyerbach R, and Hascall VC, editors: *Articular cartilage biochemistry,* New York, 1986, Raven Press.

24. Miller EJ: *The collagen of the extracellular matrix.* In Lash JW and Berger MM, editors: *Cell and tissue interactions,* New York, 1977, Raven Press.

25. Mosher DF: Physiology of fibronectin, *Annu Rev Med* 35:561–575, 1984.

26. Mow VC, Ratcliffe A, Woo SLY, editors: *Biomechanics of diarthrodial joints,* New York, 1990, Springer Verlag.

27. Neuberger A, Slack HGB: Metabolism of collagen from liver, bone, skin and tendon in normal rat, *Biochem J* 53:47–52, 1953.

28. Nimni ME: Collagen: structure, function and metabolism in normal and fibrotic tissues, *Semin Arthritis Rheum* 13:1–86, 1983.

29. Ogston AG: *The biological functions of the glycosaminoglycans.* In Balasz EA, editor: *Chemistry and molecular biology of the intercellular matrix,* vol 3, London, 1970, Academic Press.

30. Peters TJ, Smillie IS: Studies on the chemical composition of the menisci of the knee joint with special reference to the horizontal cleavage lesion, *Clin Orthop* 86:245–252, 1972.

31. Polverini PJ, et al: Activated macrophages induce vascular proliferation, *Nature* 269:804–806, 1977.

32. Salter RB, et al: The biological effect of continuous passive motion on healing of full-thickness defects in articular cartilage: an experimental study in the rabbit, *J Bone Joint Surg [Am]* 62:1232–1251, 1980.

33. Tanzer ML: Crosslinking of collagen, *Science* 180:561, 1973.

34. Vailas AC, et al: Physical activity and its influence on the repair process of medial collateral ligaments, *Connect Tissue Res* 9:25–31, 1981.

35. Williams IF, McCullagh KG, Silver IA: The distribution of types I and III collagen and fibronectin in the healing equine tendon, *Connect Tissue Res* 12:211–227, 1984.

36. Woo SLY: The biomechanical and morphological changes in the medial collateral ligament of the rabbit after immobilization and remobilization, *J Bone Joint Surg [Am]* 69:1200–1211, 1987.

37. Woo SLY, et al: Treatment of the medial collateral ligament injury: II. Structure and function of canine knees in response to differing treatment regimens, *Am J Sports Med* 15:22–29, 1987.

38. Woo SLY, Buckwalter JA, editors: *Injury and repair of the musculoskeletal soft tissues,* Park Ridge, Ill, 1988, American Academy of Orthopaedic Surgeons.

39. Woo SLY, Gomez MA, Akeson WH: *Mechanical behavior of soft tissues: measurements, modifications, injuries and treatment.* In Nahum AM, Melvin J, editors: *The biomechanics of trauma,* Norwalk, Conn, 1985, Appleton-Century-Crofts.

Chapter 5

THE PHARMACOLOGY OF REHABILITATION: THEORETICAL AND PRACTICAL CONSIDERATIONS

Michael C. Koester

Electrical modalities, ice, heat, and therapeutic exercise all have an accepted and valued role in the rehabilitation of musculoskeletal injuries. The effect of each is well understood, and the indications and contraindications are precise and often inherent. However, the role of anti-inflammatory and analgesic drugs in the rehabilitation process is the subject of controversy. The exact actions of many of these agents are still unknown, and treatment regimens are debated. Despite these uncertainties, prescription and over-the-counter nonsteroidal anti-inflammatory drugs (NSAIDs), corticosteroids, and analgesics have become an integral part of the treatment of most musculoskeletal injuries.

The use of NSAIDs and aspirin in the treatment of sports-related injuries has increased in conjunction with the growing popularity of sports and exercise.[1] In fact, there were 70.3 million NSAID prescriptions filled across the United States in 1991.[2] Past studies have shown that NSAIDs and aspirin, when included with traditional acute injury therapy, can decrease pain and swelling and hasten an athlete's return to competition.[1] Chronic injury research indicates that certain NSAIDs have positive analgesic and significant anti-inflammatory properties.[3] However, recent research suggests that some NSAIDs may actually slow the mechanism of tissue repair.[4-7] (As a note of clarification, aspirin is technically an NSAID but is not included in the generic term, which describes the newer agents.) Corticosteroid use in the treatment of chronic injuries has decreased in recent years, following several decades of what some believed was ex-

cessive use; their popularity, though, does now appear to be again on the rise.

THE INFLAMMATORY RESPONSE

To set our discussion in the proper perspective, a brief review of the inflammatory response is necessary. Inflammation is the response of vascular tissue to physiologic damage. The response prevents the extensive spread of injury-causing agents to nearby tissues, disposes of cellular debris, and sets the stage for the repair process.[8] The process begins with the initial tissue trauma (Fig. 5-1). Following a short period of vasoconstriction, the cellular injury signals the release of chemical mediators such as histamine and bradykinin from mast cells and thromboxane, leukotrienes, and prostaglandins from cell membranes.[9] These chemical mediators increase cellular and capillary permeability and stimulate capillary vasodilation. The changes in vascular permeability directly result in edema because of the flow of fluid out of the vasculature and into the interstitial space.[10] The increased blood flow and vascular permeability allow for white blood cells to migrate toward the injury site, infiltrate the site, and initiate the healing process.[11] Within 48 hours of the initial insult, fibroblasts begin the process of wound repair and collagen synthesis.[10]

By definition, the inflammatory response is essential to the resolution of the injury. However, excessive edema, coupled with vascular dilation and damage that result in vascular stasis, disrupts the flow of oxygen to the healthy tissue surrounding the injury site. The resultant hypoxia can lead to further tissue damage, appropriately referred to as *secondary hypoxic injury*.[12]

If the inflammatory condition persists without resolution, it is termed *chronic inflammation*. This condition arises

Adapted with permission from Koester MC: An overview of the physiology and pharmacology of aspirin and the nonsteroidal anti-inflammatory drugs, *J Ath Training* 28:252–259, 1993.

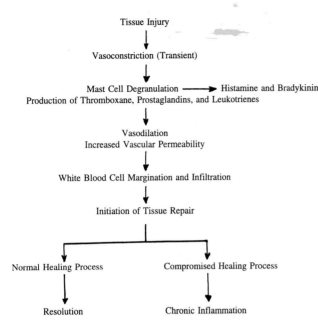

Fig. 5-1. The inflammatory response.

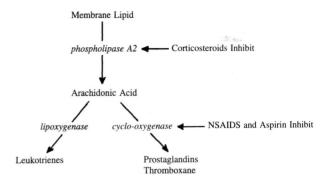

Fig. 5-2. The stepwise synthesis of the eicosanoids. Italics denote the enzymes involved in the pathway.

because for some reason the normal healing process is compromised. This can often result from decreased vascular perfusion caused by an accumulation of inflammatory products (vasodilators), cellular debris, and scar tissue. Thus, the process of inflammation must often be interfered with for the healing process to begin. The reestablishment of vascular perfusion is also accomplished through careful mobilization.

The implementation of cryotherapy and other modalities in an effort to decrease pain and inflammation has been well understood by sports medicine professionals for several years. The following discussion sheds light on the specific roles played by the various chemical mediators in the inflammatory response, which can be influenced through the use of NSAIDs and corticosteroids.

THE EICOSANOID FAMILY

As noted earlier, the prostaglandins, thromboxane, and the leukotrienes all play a role in the inflammatory response. They are all members of the eicosanoid family, derivatives of the 20-carbon–fatty acid molecule arachidonic acid (Fig. 5-2). Arachidonic acid is a component of cell membranes and must be released from the membrane by phospholipase A_2, prior to being synthesized to an eicosanoid. Once free, arachidonic acid can be converted to either an initial leukotriene or to a common prostaglandin and thromboxane precursor via two separate pathways. Aspirin and NSAIDs exert their effects by blocking the production of prostaglandins and thromboxanes, whereas corticosteroids have been implicated in blocking the activity of phospholipase A_2. Most of the NSAIDs have little or no effect upon leukotriene synthesis.

Leukotrienes are synthesized from arachidonic acid by the action of the enzyme lipoxygenase. The leukotrienes consist of a family of chemicals that function to mediate chemotaxis, increase vascular permeability, and activate leukocytes.[13] The leukotrienes are also believed to play an important role in asthma. A lipoxygenase inhibitor would be of enormous therapeutic value, but most pharmacologic agents that block leukotriene production have so far been too unspecific or too toxic to use therapeutically.[13]

Effects of prostaglandins and thromboxane

The prostaglandins represent a variety of very important chemicals that are produced by almost every tissue in the body. Different prostaglandins play various roles in many physiologic processes. Those roles are examined in the following discussion and outlined in Table 5-1.

Mediation of inflammatory process. The term *mediation* is important in describing the activities of prostaglandins. On their own prostaglandins do not appear to be capable of inducing either pain or edema.[14] They are capable of directly causing vasodilation, but are dependent upon histamine and bradykinin to increase the permeability of the blood vessels. In addition, prostaglandins act synergistically with other chemicals to sensitize pain receptors to mechanical and chemical stimulation.[15]

Fever mediation. Prostaglandins have been implicated in the role of fever mediation through their release into the hypothalamus. The hypothalamus acts as the thermoregulatory control center of the body. Although the exact mechanism remains unknown, animal studies have shown that the injection of specific prostaglandins into the cerebral ventricles causes an increase in body temperature.[16]

Gastrointestinal system. Prostaglandins interact in a number of ways to protect the delicate lining of the gastrointestinal system. They appear to inhibit gastric acid secretion and may have an antiulcer effect.[17] Prostaglandins also appear to have the property of *cytoprotection*, defined as the ability to protect the gastric mucosa from exposure to harmful substances. Although the mechanism is unknown,

Table 5-1. A summary of the major effects of the eicosanoids

Eicosanoid	Major effects
Leukotrienes	Chemotaxis
	Leukocyte activation
	Increase in vascular permeability
Thromboxane	Platelet aggregation
Prostaglandins	Mediation of inflammation
	Increase in vascular permeability*
	Sensitization of pain receptors*
	Mediation of fever
	Induction of uterine contractions
	Inhibition of gastric secretion
	"Cytoprotection" of gastric mucosa
	Systemic and renal vasodilation
	Inhibition of platelet aggregation

*Synergistic actions.

cytoprotection may result from a specific prostaglandin that stimulates mucus formation.[17]

Reproductive system. In the uterus, prostaglandins act to stimulate the contraction of the smooth muscle layer, known as the *myometrium*. This smooth muscle contraction serves two important purposes. During childbirth the prostaglandin-stimulated contractions of the myometrium aid in delivering the baby through the birth canal. They are also released at the end of the menstrual cycle to facilitate the shedding of the uterine lining by stimulating muscular contractions.[18] These continuous contractions can result in ischemic pain, referred to as *cramping* or *primary dysmenorrhea*.

Renal blood flow. During exercise the autonomic nervous system releases chemicals into the bloodstream that act as potent vasoconstrictors in many peripheral tissues, including the kidneys. Prostaglandins can serve to dilate renal blood vessels, counteracting those chemicals and thus maintaining a constant flow of blood to the kidneys.[19] This action of the prostaglandins appears to be more significant if the kidneys are functioning abnormally and is usually not a concern in young, healthy patients.[20]

Other effects. A specific prostaglandin, prostacyclin, is released by the internal lining of the blood vessels. This substance appears to inhibit the aggregation of blood platelets on blood vessel walls. Also highlighting the importance of prostaglandins, a recent study suggests they may promote the repair of cartilage by inhibiting the action of interleukin-1.[21] This discovery could be of major importance for people suffering from rheumatoid arthritis.

Thromboxane, produced in blood platelets, functions as a powerful inducer of blood platelet aggregation to aid in the clotting mechanism.[13] Therefore, thromboxane and prostacyclin have an antagonistic relationship. This stands as a good example of how prostaglandins attenuate the actions of other chemicals in a variety of tissues.

Table 5-2. Conditions of the knee for which corticosteroid therapy may be indicated

Prepatellar bursitis
Pes anserine bursitis
Medial collateral ligament bursitis
Semimembranous bursitis
Iliotibial band friction syndrome
Medial patellar plica
Tendonitis
Joint disorders

Adapted from Kerlan RK, Glousman RE: Injections and techniques in athletic medicine, *Clin Sports Med* 8:541–560, 1989.

Actions of corticosteroids

Inhibition of phospholipase A_2
Decrease in cytokine production
Induction of T-lymphocyte death
Reduction of the number of basophils
Prevention of mast cell degranulation
Overall inhibition of chemotactic agents
Inhibition of protein synthesis
Inhibition of fibroblast proliferation
Inhibition of collagen synthesis

Given this basic understanding of the inflammatory response and the properties of the arachidonic acid derivatives, the following discussion centers upon how different pharmacologic agents can affect these processes.

Corticosteroids

With the wide use and accessibility of NSAIDs and the past history of overuse, corticosteroid injection therapy is currently limited.[22] If used properly, however, corticosteroids can play an important role in the rehabilitation and resolution of certain chronic inflammatory conditions (Table 5-2). Corticosteroids act to subvert the inflammatory response, allowing the body to reinitiate the healing process by increasing overall vascular perfusion to the area and thus clearing the site of debris and additional inflammatory products so that the reparative process may begin.

The complete mechanism of action of corticosteroids is not completely understood (see box above). It is known that the activities include the inhibition of phospholipase A_2, which then directly limits the production of thromboxane, leukotrienes, and prostaglandins. In addition, corticosteroids limit the migration of neutrophils and monocytes to the inflamed area, prevent the degranulation of mast cells, and induce the death of certain lymphocytes.[24]

Corticosteroids should be used only when frontline therapy fails and infection has been ruled out.[25] Because of the potentially adverse effects of corticosteroids on collagen and protein synthesis, direct tendon injection should be avoided, as it has been associated with tendon rupture.[22] Instead, peritendinous injections are recommended for tendonitis. Some physicians consider even peritendinous injections of the patellar tendon too much of a risk.[26] It is also advised that a single weightbearing joint be injected no more than three times in a year and that the injected joint be rested for a time following each treatment.[22]

ASPIRIN

Aspirin (acetylsalicylic acid) is a derivative of salicylic acid. Found in the bark of willow trees, salicylic acid's medicinal benefits and side effects have been known for more than 2000 years. Aspirin was first synthesized by a Bayer Company chemist in the late nineteenth century. It proved to be far less of a gastric irritant than salicylic acid and was introduced to the marketplace in the spring of 1899. Heralded as a wonder drug, it quickly became one of the most widely used pharmaceutical products in the world. Annual aspirin consumption in the United States now ranges between 26 and 74 million pounds.[15]

Surprisingly, aspirin's mechanism of action has been known only since 1971. John Vane discovered that the aspirin molecule transfers a functional group onto the cyclo-oxygenase enzyme.[27] As a result, the enzyme is irreversibly inhibited and unable to bind arachidonic acid; therefore, the enzyme can no longer convert arachidonic acid to prostaglandins and thromboxane.

Effects of aspirin

Following the ingestion of aspirin (3000 to 6000 mg per day for anti-inflammatory action), a series of chemical events results from the blockage of cyclo-oxygenase. The decrease in prostaglandin production leads to a corresponding reduction in inflammation and edema.[20] The inhibition of prostaglandin and thromboxane synthesis may not be the only effect that aspirin exerts upon the tissues. In some systems aspirin may impinge upon the formation of 12-HETE, a leukotriene derivative that acts as a chemotactic agent.[20] Aspirin may also reduce inflammation and pain by influencing the migration of chemical potentiators such as neutrophils and monocytes, and activate neutrophils as well.[20]

Negative consequences may also result from aspirin use. In the gastrointestinal tract, aspirin can cause gastric upset, bleeding, and even ulcers. Various studies have shown an incidence of anywhere from 2% to 40%, depending upon the parameters of the investigation.[20] It does not appear that the gastrointestinal side effects are due to the inhibition of prostaglandin synthesis alone, although this area is subject to debate.[20,28]

The mechanism of gastric irritation does, however, appear to be related to the direct effect of aspirin upon the lining of the stomach.[29] Unbuffered aspirin lowers the electrical potential of the gastric membrane, which then affects the flow of hydrogen ions. Davenport's theory contends that this disruption of hydrogen ions triggers a series of events

Table 5-3. Stages of Reye's syndrome

Stage	Signs and symptoms
1	Vomiting, lethargy, indifference
2	Delirium, hyperventilation, combativeness
3	Light coma, hypoventilation, intact pupillary response, decorticate posturing
4	Deep coma, loss of spontaneous ventilation, decerebrate posturing, fixed and dilated pupils
5	Flaccidity, seizures

Adapted from Lovejoy FH, et al: Clinical staging in Reye's syndrome, *Am J Dis Child* 128:36–41, 1974.

that lead to gastric erosion and bleeding.[20] Studies have shown that enteric-coated aspirin does not cause as many abnormalities in the stomach lining because of its buffering action.[20] Mild gastrointestinal upset can often be avoided if aspirin is taken with a meal because of the "buffering" action of the food.

Aspirin use can also result in complications such as prolonged bleeding time and tinnitus. Prolonged bleeding time results from the inhibition of thromboxane. In that aspirin irreversibly binds to cyclo-oxygenase, the decreased platelet function lasts from 4 to 6 days (the platelet life-span) following aspirin intake.[28] In addition, many people taking high doses of aspirin may develop tinnitus. It is probably due to an effect on the inner ear, not the central nervous system, and it often results from a dosage that is too high.

Reye's syndrome. A presentation of aspirin would be incomplete without a brief discussion of Reye's syndrome. First described in 1963, Reye's syndrome is a rare and potentially devastating acute illness that usually strikes children following a viral infection. For several years epidemiologic data suggested a relationship between Reye's syndrome and aspirin use by children infected with either the influenza or chicken pox virus. Those early reports were highly criticized. More recently, a study conducted by the Center for Disease Control linked the occurrence of Reye's syndrome to aspirin and other salicylates administered in the management of viral illnesses.[30] Based on current knowledge, it would appear prudent to disallow the use of aspirin and other salicylates by anyone under the age of 18 who may have a viral infection.

The exact cause of Reye's syndrome remains a mystery. It is known that the illness impairs mitochondrial function, resulting in liver and neurologic damage.[31] In 1974, Lovejoy et al.[32] proposed a five-stage system on which to chart the symptoms of Reye's syndrome (Table 5-3). Reye's syndrome is potentially fatal, and the symptoms must be treated as a medical emergency; however, a diagnosis can be made only through laboratory tests.

THE NSAIDS

In the latter half of this century, chemists have used aspirin as a prototype to develop the NSAIDs. The main

NSAIDs available in the United States

Carprofen
Diclofenac sodium
Diflunisal
Etodolac
Fenbufen
Fenoprofen
Flurbiprofen
Ibuprofen
Indomethacin
Ketoprofen
Ketorolac tromethamine
Meclofenamate sodium
Nabumetone
Naproxen
Naproxen sodium
Oxaprozin
Phenylbutazone
Piroxicam
Suldinac
Tolmetin

Chemical classes of NSAIDs

Carboxylic acids

PYRANOCARBOXYLIC
Etodolac
PROPIONIC
Naproxen
Ibuprofen
Fenoprofen
Oxaprozin
ACETIC
Tolmetin
Diclofenac
Indomethacin
SALICYLIC
Aspirin

Enolic acids

OXICAMS
Piroxicam
PYRAZOLONES
Phenylbutazone
PYRROLOPYRROLE
Ketorolac tromethamine

goal of this research has been to produce agents that do not present aspirin's sometimes severe side effects. Although there are differences in potency, specificity, and specific mechanisms of action, all NSAIDs inhibit the activity of cyclo-oxygenase in some manner.[14] The inhibition is not an irreversible reaction like aspirin but, instead, dependent upon concentration.[28]

Along with blocking cyclo-oxygenase, NSAIDs are thought to have additional properties. Possible activities include modulation of T-cell function, inhibition of inflammatory cell chemotaxis, lysosomal membrane stabilization, and free radical scavenging, as well as an effect on the activation of neutrophils.[28,33,34] The beneficial activities of the different NSAIDs seem to be quite similar, although there are some differences in specific action and side effects.

There are many different chemical classes and brands of NSAIDs currently available (see box above). New NSAIDs are introduced to the market at a surprising rate. The following discussion represents a clinical overview of frequently used chemical classes of NSAIDs (see box at top of next column), as well as those agents with special clinical significance and their standard prescription dosages. The doses listed are for anti-inflammatory action unless otherwise noted. Analgesic doses tend to be 50% to 75% of those for anti-inflammatory activity.

Ibuprofen (Advil, Motrin, Nuprin)

A propionic acid derivative, ibuprofen is the most frequently prescribed NSAID.[2] It boosts aspirin's potency for analgesic and anti-inflammatory action, but has a lower incidence of side effects. This reduced incidence may be linked to ibuprofen's decreased inhibition of platelet aggre-

gation, lessening possible gastric bleeding.[16] In addition, it appears that ibuprofen may be the most beneficial NSAID in easing the pain of primary dysmenorrhea. A prescription regimen consists of 2200 to 2400 mg per day, taken in three separate doses.[30,35,36] Such a schedule enables it to be taken at mealtimes, lessening the likelihood of gastric irritation, as mentioned previously, and perhaps improving compliance. Daily dosage should not exceed 3200 mg.[33]

Naproxen (Naprosyn) and naproxen sodium (Anaprox)

The second most prescribed NSAID, naproxen is chemically similar to ibuprofen.[2] Naproxen is 20% more potent than aspirin, with side effects much like ibuprofen.[16] In comparison studies with ibuprofen, naproxen was found to be marginally superior in decreasing joint inflammation.[36] Because of naproxen's long half-life, the daily recommended dosage of 750 to 1000 mg can be taken on a twice-daily schedule, reducing gastric upset with only two exposures.[30,33] Naproxen is eliminated from the body mainly by way of the kidneys; therefore, it should be used with caution in persons with renal complications.[33] Naproxen can also cross the placenta and should not be prescribed during any stage of pregnancy.[37] The sodium salt of naproxen (Anaprox) is more quickly absorbed than naproxen and more readily concentrates in the synovium.[37] For this reason, sodium naproxen is often indicated for joint pain and inflammation.

Oxaprozin (Daypro)

Oxaprozin is a recently introduced propionic acid derivative. Unlike the other propionic acids, oxaprozin offers the convenience and advantages of once-a-day dosing. This schedule is credited to the agent's long half-life. Studies of patients with rheumatoid arthritis and osteoarthritis found 1200 mg of oxaprozin to have similar efficacy to naproxen (250 mg t.i.d.), piroxicam (20 mg once per day), and ibuprofen (300 to 400 mg q.i.d.).[38] The usual NSAID-related adverse effects were found to be less than aspirin, but comparable to ibuprofen.[39] Dosage should not exceed 1800 mg per day. In short, oxaprozin offers the advantages of once-a-day dosing with efficacy and side effects similar to other NSAIDs.

Fenoprofen (Nalfon)

This agent deserves special mention because it appears to be more damaging to the kidneys than other NSAIDs of the propionic class.[28] The reason for this apparent relationship is unknown. However, in a study of people suffering from rheumatoid arthritis, fenoprofen was found to have fewer gastrointestinal side effects than the other NSAIDs to which it was compared.[28] Usual dosage consists of 300 to 600 mg three or four times daily, with total dosage not exceeding 3200 mg.[33] Because of the increased incidence of renal damage, fenoprofen should be used cautiously in patients who may be at risk for renal complications.

Piroxicam (Feldene)

Although derived from a different chemical group, piroxicam has properties similar to ibuprofen, naproxen, and fenoprofen. Its most important asset lies in that it was the first NSAID to offer a once-a-day dosage schedule of 20 mg.[30,33] The single daily dose greatly benefits compliance and gastrointestinal irritation can be decreased even more if the drug is taken with the largest meal of the day.[3] Piroxicam has been found to increase the percentage of suppressor T-cells in peripheral blood and inhibit neutrophil migration.[28,33] Such research suggests that a person with a cold or other infection may want to avoid the drug. Piroxicam is cleared from the plasma mainly by the liver; hence, it can be administered to people with renal deficiency.[20]

Tolmetin (Tolectin)

Tolectin is chemically different than the previously discussed NSAIDs but has similar effects. The most frequently reported side effect is gastrointestinal disturbance.[33] When given in conjunction with acetaminophen, the analgesic properties of tolmetin are enhanced.[33] Tolmetin is administered in three or four doses of 200 to 400 mg. A daily dose of 1200 to 1500 mg roughly approximates 2400 mg of ibuprofen.[28]

Diclofenac sodium (Voltaren)

As with other NSAIDs, diclofenac sodium inhibits the synthesis of prostaglandins and thromboxane. However, it also reduces the amount of arachidonic acid made available from the cell membrane, thereby decreasing the amount of leukotrienes produced as well.[33] Standard dosage is 50 mg three times per day or 75 mg twice a day.[33] In addition, renal damage may be associated with diclofenac less frequently, but this difference is yet to be verified.[33] Diclofenac sodium is similar to naproxen sodium in that it accumulates in the inflamed synovium; thus it is also indicated for joint pain and inflammation.

Indomethacin (Indocin and Indocin-SR)

Indomethacin, introduced in 1963, was one of the first NSAIDs developed and continues to be among the most powerful inhibitors of cyclo-oxygenase.[1] Although particularly effective in maladies such as rheumatoid arthritis, ankylosing spondylitis, and gout arthritis, indomethacin is not recommended for use as a simple analgesic or antipyretic because of its potentially severe side effects, such as gastrointestinal disturbances and headaches.[33] Daily dosage ranges from 75 to 100 mg taken in three or four doses.[33] Prolonged-release formulas are available (75 mg one to two times per day); however, gastrointestinal and other adverse effects appear to be similar to the regular formula.[33]

Ketorolac tromethamine (Toradol)

Recently introduced, ketorolac tromethamine is the first NSAID to be available for intramuscular injection as well as oral administration. Although it also has anti-inflammatory and antipyretic properties, it is currently being marketed primarily as an analgesic, particularly in postoperative patients.[33] Studies have shown ketorolac to be equal to, or more effective than, morphine.[40,41] Although administered intramuscularly, damage to the gastrointestinal mucosa may still occur. However, doses of 10 to 30 mg given four to five times per day produced less mucosal injury than 650 mg of aspirin using the same dosage schedule.[33] The maximum recommended daily dose is 150 mg for the first day, followed by no more than 120 mg per day for the remainder of the regimen.[33] Ketorolac represents an exciting step in NSAID development, an agent with the analgesic efficacy of morphine, easily delivered, and nonaddictive.

Etodolac (Lodine)

Etodolac is a pyranocarboxylic, unique among the NSAIDs. This agent offers a flexible daily dosing schedule of 600 to 1200 mg divided into two or four doses.[42] Maximum dosage should not exceed 1200 mg per day. In two separate studies etodolac was found to be as effective as piroxicam in treating osteoarthritis[43] and to have an efficacy comparable to diclofenac sodium in the treatment of rheumatoid arthritis.[23] Endoscopic studies have indicated that etodolac is better tolerated in the gastrointestinal tract than naproxen and similar to placebo.[28] However, etodolac is a newly introduced agent in the United States, so wide experience has not yet been gained.

Nabumetone (Relafen)

Nabumetone is a unique NSAID in that the ingested compound is a relatively weak inhibitor of cyclo-oxygenase.[28] In the liver, nabumetone is metabolized to 6-methoxy-2-naphthylacetic acid (6-MNA), a strong cyclo-oxygenase inhibitor.[28] Theoretically, this method of metabolism should limit gastrointestinal side effects because the active metabolite is not absorbed in the gut and hence local prostaglandin concentrations should not be affected. Endoscopic studies show fewer new occurrences of gastric damage in patients taking nabumetone (1000 mg per day for 12 weeks) than those taking naproxen (500 to 750 mg per day for 12 weeks) or indomethacin (150 mg per day for 3 weeks).[44] However, postmarketing results in the United Kingdom have indicated similar peptic ulcer rates to other NSAIDs.[44] Nabumetone is a nonacidic naphalalkylone that is structurally similar to naproxen.[28] Dosing varies from 1000 mg once per day to 2000 mg in two doses.

Phenylbutazone (Butazolidin)

Introduced in 1949, phenylbutazone has decreased in popularity with the development of less toxic NSAIDs. Its use is recommended only after other NSAID therapies have failed, and then only if the physician and patient decide that the benefits outweigh the risks of therapy.[33] The long-term use of phenylbutazone can result in various blood dyscrasias including aplastic anemia (destruction of the bone marrow) and severe hepatic reactions.[28] At the present time, phenylbutazone's significance is more historical than clinical.

Choosing an NSAID

The main considerations in the design of an NSAID or aspirin therapy regimen are efficacy of the agent, patient compliance, adverse side effects, and cost of treatment. Incidence and severity of side effects weigh heavily upon compliance and treatment cost. Compliance is more easily attained if the drug causes minimal discomfort and the dosage requirements easily fit into the patient's schedule. The cost of treatment can be difficult to determine because there are factors other than the price of the drug to consider. An inexpensive option such as aspirin can become quite expensive if an ulcer or other gastrointestinal pathology develops, requiring more medication or even hospitalization.[3] It must also be remembered that patients respond differently to drugs. A drug that works well on one patient may have no efficacy in another. Because of this, patients are often moved from one drug to another in an attempt to find the most effective agent. Other factors are listed in the box on this page.

Effects on the healing process

An additional factor to consider in designing an NSAID program has recently been discovered. Several studies have shown that NSAIDs may affect the healing process through direct action upon specific tissue components. In a study conducted by culturing rabbit articular cartilage chondrocytes in the presence of NSAIDs, diclofenac sodium and indomethacin—and piroxicam to a lesser degree—inhibited the secretion of proteoglycans.[5] Proteoglycans are extracellular molecules involved in the formation of cartilage, tendons, and ligaments. They are vital to the process of tissue repair. Other studies have shown that indomethacin and aspirin can interfere with the synthesis or transport of such connective tissue components.[4,6,7]

In contrast to these findings, a recent study indicated that indomethacin, diclofenac, and piroxicam are capable of suppressing enzymes responsible for the degradation of collagen and cartilage.[45] Such results indicate that NSAIDs may actually diminish the process of osteoarthritis. Numerous other studies have found different NSAIDs to have either positive or detrimental effects upon articular cartilage in either animal models or in vitro.[46-49] As of yet, no study has proven that NSAIDs cause damage to articular cartilage in humans. All studies concerning the effects of NSAIDs must be carefully critiqued, considering the method of investigation, the agents studied, and whether clinically significant concentrations of the agent were used. These areas of NSAID activity are certain to be the focus of intensive investigation and controversy for the next several years.

Acute injuries

Controversy also exists over when—or if—an NSAID regimen should begin following an acute injury. Some feel drug therapy should be initiated immediately along with rest, ice, compression, and elevation (RICE) in an attempt to arrest the inflammatory process. Others believe that NSAID therapy should begin no sooner than 48 to 72 hours following the injury and implementation of RICE, the idea being that blockage of thromboxane synthesis will promote additional bleeding as well as diminishing the inflammatory process, perhaps slowing the initiation of healing. Evidence on either side of the argument is largely anecdotal, most coming from the clinical setting. The number of well-done studies conducted in this area are few. One cannot draw any definite conclusions from such studies because of the variability of the selected populations, treatment regimens, injuries, and rehabilitation programs.[50] None of the studies, however, indicates that NSAIDs hinder the recovery process. To the contrary, some of the studies showed a slightly quickened recovery time in the patients taking NSAIDs following acute injury.[51-55] Much more research needs to be conducted in this area.

Risk factors to consider when prescribing NSAIDs

Age
Gender
Pregnancy
History of peptic ulcer disease
Gastritis
Gastrointestinal hemorrhage
Renal disease
Acute infection

Table 5-4. Drugs that may interact with NSAIDs and their common clinical uses

Drug	Common use
Angiotensin-converting enzyme (ACE) inhibitor (Capoten, others)	Treatment of hypertension
Anticoagulants (Coumadin, Panwarfin)	Prophylaxis and treatment of pulmonary embolism and venous thrombosis
Beta-blockers (Inderal, others)	Decrease cardiac output and peripheral vascular resistance
Diuretics (Lasix, others)	Promote the excretion of urine
Lithium	Treatment of manic depression
Methotrexate	Treatment of cancer
Metoclopramide (Reglan)	Antiemetic
Phenytoin sodium (Dilantin)	Treatment of seizure disorders
Probenecid (Benemid)	Treatment of gout, maintenance of serum levels of cephalosporins or penicillins
Sulfonylureas (Glucotrol, others)	Treatment of non-insulin-dependent diabetes

Drug interactions

NSAIDs bind strongly to plasma proteins, thus competing for binding sites with other agents. Usually, such interactions are of little clinical significance, except for instances when NSAIDs are administered in conjunction with other highly bound drugs (Table 5-4). Therefore, caution should be taken before combining NSAID therapy with drugs such as methotrexate, phenytoin sodium (Dilantin), warfarin sodium (Coumadin, Panwarfin), captopril (Capoten), and ionically bound oral hypoglycemics.[37] Concomitant use of NSAIDs and lithium has resulted in lithium toxicity due to a decrease in the renal clearance of lithium.[37] In addition, different NSAIDs should not be used simultaneously because of potential toxicity. Owing to the variability of possible interactions and the large number of potentially reactive agents, I recommend that the prescribing physician be aware of all drugs the patient is taking prior to the initiation of NSAID therapy.

ACETAMINOPHEN

Although not an anti-inflammatory agent, acetaminophen (Tylenol, Anacin 3) is an important drug that deserves our attention for its clinical uses. Acetaminophen, discovered in 1877, has analgesic and antipyretic properties through its actions upon the central nervous system. Acetaminophen has no anti-inflammatory properties because it cannot inhibit cyclo-oxygenase in the peripheral tissues.[56] Therefore, it also does not present complications such as gastrointestinal disturbance and prolonged bleeding time, and so acetaminophen is indicated for mild pain and fever in those who are contraindicated for aspirin use due to Reye's syndrome risk (as discussed previously) or who cannot tolerate aspirin or NSAIDs. Usual dosage of acetaminophen is 325 to 650 mg at 4-hour intervals.[33]

Acetaminophen, like all drugs, can be a toxic substance if used in excess. The minimum toxic dose in adults is 5 to 15 g.[57] Overdoses or prolonged overuse (5 to 8 g per day for several days) may result in severe hepatic damage or death.[33] The liver damage appears to be produced by a metabolite of acetaminophen. In therapeutic doses, the toxic metabolite is detoxified by glutathione; however, with extreme intake, if the glutathione drops below 30% of normal values, tissue necrosis occurs.[57]

CONCLUSION

Anti-inflammatory and analgesic agents currently play an important role in the treatment of musculoskeletal injuries and other disease processes. In many instances they may be as important in the rehabilitation program as the traditional modalities. As new agents are marketed and new methods of delivery are introduced, NSAIDs will likely assume an even larger role in rehabilitation and treatment. For example, topical NSAIDs are currently available in Europe and are being tested in the United States. They allow for local application while presenting decreased risks and side effects.[50] As these new drugs and formulations are introduced and discoveries concerning the action and effects of these agents are made, practitioners must keep a watchful eye on the literature, balancing the results of each new study with their knowledge of the pharmacology of these agents as well as past clinical experience.

REFERENCES

1. Knych ET: *Anti-inflammatory agents.* In Thomas JA, editor: *Drugs, athletes, and physical performance,* New York, 1988, Plenum.
2. Anti-arthritic medication usage: United States, 1991, *Stat Bull Metrop Insur Co* 73:25–34, 1992.
3. Calabrese LH, Rooney TW: The use of nonsteroidal anti-inflammatory drugs in sports, *Phys Sportsmed* 14:89–97, 1986.
4. Bassleer C, Henrotin Y, Franchimont P: Effects of sodium naproxen on differentiated human chondrocytes cultivated in clusters, *Clin Rheumatol* 11:60–65, 1992.
5. Collier S, Ghosh P: Comparison of the effects of NSAIDs on proteoglycan synthesis by articular cartilage explant and chondrocyte monolayer cultures, *Biochem Pharmacol* 41:1375–1384, 1991.
6. David MJ, et al: Effect of NSAIDs on glycosyltransferase activity from human osteoarthritic cartilage, *Br J Rheumatol* (suppl 1):13–17, 1992.
7. Henrotin Y, Bassleer C, Franchimont P: In vitro effects of etodolac and acetylsalicylic acid on human chondrocyte metabolism, *Agents Actions* 36:317–323, 1992.

8. Marieb EN: *Human anatomy and physiology,* Redwood City, Calif, 1989, Benjamin/Cummings.
9. Teitz CC: *Scientific foundations of sports medicine,* Philadelphia, 1989, BC Decker.
10. Ryan GB, Majno G: *Inflammation,* Kalamazoo, Mich, 1977, Upjohn.
11. Booher JM, Thibodeau GA: *Athletic injury assessment,* St Louis, 1989, Mosby–Year Book.
12. Knight KL: *Cold as a modifier of sports induced inflammation.* In Leadbetter WB, Buckwalter JA, Gordon SC, editors: *Sports induced inflammation: clinical and basic science concepts,* 1990, American Academy of Orthopaedic Surgeons.
13. Glew RH: *Lipid metabolism II: pathways of metabolism of special lipids.* In Devlin TM, editor: *Textbook of biochemistry with clinical correlations,* New York, 1992, Wiley-Liss.
14. Goldstein IM: *Agents that interfere with arachidonic acid metabolism.* In Gallin JI, Goldstein IM, Snyderman R, editors: *Inflammation: basic principles and clinical correlates,* New York, 1988, Raven.
15. Miller RL, Insel PA, Melmon KL: *Inflammatory disorders.* In Melmon KL, Morrelli HF, editors: *Clinical pharmacology: basic principles in therapeutics,* New York, 1978, Macmillan.
16. Shires TK: *Anti-inflammatory drugs.* In Conn PM, Gebhart GF, editors: *Essentials of pharmacology,* Philadelphia, 1989, FA Davis.
17. Robert A, Ruwart MJ: *Effects of prostaglandins on the digestive system.* In Lee JB, editor: *Prostaglandins,* New York, 1982, Elsevier.
18. Guyton AC: *Medical physiology,* Philadelphia, 1991, WB Saunders.
19. Oates JA, et al: Clinical implications of prostaglandin and thromboxane A2 formation, *N Engl J Med* 319:761–767, 1988.
20. Kimberly RP, Plotz PH: *Salicylates including aspirin and sulfasalazine.* In Kelley WN, et al, editors: *Textbook of rheumatology,* Philadelphia, 1989, WB Saunders.
21. Dajani EZ, Wilson DE, Agrawal NM: Prostaglandins: an overview of the worldwide clinical experience, *J Assoc Acad Minor Phys* 2:23, 27–35, 1991.
22. Pfenninger JL: Injections of joints and soft tissue: (part I) general guidelines, *Am Fam Physician* 44:1196–1202, 1991.
23. Khan FM, Williams PI: Double-blind comparison of etodolac SR and diclofenac SR in the treatment of patients with degenerative joint disease of the knee, *Curr Med Res Opin* 13:1–12, 1992.
24. Sternberg EM, Wilder RL: *Corticosteroids.* In McCarty DJ, Koopman WJ, editors: *Arthritis and allied conditions: a textbook of rheumatology,* Philadelphia, 1993, Lea & Febiger.
25. Birrer RB: Aspiration and corticosteroid injection, *Phys Sportsmed* 20:57–71, 1992.
26. Kerlan RK, Glousman RE: Injections and techniques in athletic medicine, *Clin Sports Med* 8:541–560, 1989.
27. Vane JR: Inhibition of prostaglandin synthesis as a mechanism for aspirin-like drugs, *Nature* 231:232–234, 1971.
28. Furst DE, Paulus HE: *Aspirin and other nonsteroidal anti-inflammatory drugs.* In McCarty DJ, Koopman WJ, editors: *Arthritis and allied conditions: a textbook of rheumatology,* Philadelphia, 1993, Lea & Febiger.
29. Lehne RA, et al: *Pharmacology for nursing care,* Philadelphia, 1990, WB Saunders.
30. Clark WG, Brater DC, Johnson AR: *Goth's medical pharmacology,* St Louis, 1988, Mosby–Year Book.
31. Weil ML: *Infections of the nervous system.* In Menkes JH, editor: *Textbook of child neurology,* Philadelphia, 1990, Lea & Febiger.
32. Lovejoy FH, et al: Clinical staging in Reye's syndrome, *Am J Dis Child* 128:36–41, 1974.
33. *Antiarthritic drugs.* In: *Drug evaluations annual,* Chicago, 1993, American Medical Association.
34. Lindsley CB: Uses of nonsteroidal anti-inflammatory drugs in pediatrics, *Am J Dis Child* 147:229–236, 1993.
35. Meyers FH, Jawetz E, Goldfien A: *Review of medical pharmacology,* Los Altos, Calif, 1980, Lange.
36. Nuki G: Nonsteroidal analgesic and anti-inflammatory agents, *Br Med J* 287:39–43, 1983.
37. Amadio P, Cummings DM, Amadio P: Nonsteroidal anti-inflammatory drugs: tailoring therapy to achieve results and avoid toxicity, *Postgrad Med* 93:73–78, 93–97, 1993.
38. Al-Faks MA, Pugh MC: Oxaprozin: a new NSAID, *Orthop Rev* 21:558, 560–563, 1992.
39. Oxaprozin for arthritis, *Med Lett Drugs Ther* 35:15–16, 1993.
40. O'Hara DA, et al: Ketorolac tromethamine as compared with morphine sulfate for treatment of postoperative pain, *Clin Pharmacol Ther* 41:556–561, 1987.
41. Yee JT, et al: Analgesia from intramuscular ketorolac tromethamine compared to morphine in severe pain following major surgery, *Pharmacotherapy* 6:253–261, 1986.
42. Etodolac, *Med Lett Drugs Ther* 33:79–80, 1991.
43. Paulsen AP, et al: Efficacy and tolerability comparison of etodolac and piroxicam in the treatment of patients with osteoarthritis of the knee, *Curr Med Res Opin* 12:401–412, 1991.
44. Nabumetone—a new NSAID, *Med Lett Drugs Ther* 34:38–40, 1992.
45. Vignon E, et al: In vitro effect of nonsteroidal anti-inflammatory drugs on proteoglycanase and collagenase activity in human osteoarthritic cartilage, *Arthritis Rheum* 10:1332–1335, 1991.
46. Bjelle A, Eronen I: The in vitro effect of six NSAIDs on the glycosaminoglycan metabolism of rabbit chondrocytes, *Clin Exp Rheum* 9:369–374, 1991.
47. Brandt KD, Albrecht M: Effect of naproxen sodium on the net synthesis of glycosaminoglycans and protein by normal canine articular cartilage in-vitro, *J Pharm Pharmacol* 42:738–740, 1990.
48. Glazer PA, Rosenwasser MP, Ratcliffe A: The effect of naproxen and interleukin-1 on proteoglycan catabolism and on neutral metalloproteinase activity in normal articular cartilage in vitro, *J Clin Pharmacol* 33:109–114, 1993.
49. Obeid G, Zhang X, Wang X: Effect of ibuprofen on the healing and remodeling of bone and articular cartilage in the rabbit temporomandibular joint, *J Oral Maxillofac Surg* 50:843–849, 1992.
50. Weiler JM: Medical modifiers of sports injury: the use of nonsteroidal anti-inflammatory drugs (NSAIDs) in sports soft-tissue injury, *Clin Sports Med* 11:625–644, 1992.
51. Blazina ME: Oxyphenbutazone as an adjunct to the conventional treatment of athletic injuries, *Clin Med* 76:19–22, 1969.
52. Fredberg U, Hansen PA, Skinhoj A: Ibuprofen in the treatment of acute ankle joint injuries: a double-blind study, *Am J Sports Med* 16:641–646, 1988.
53. Lereim P, Gabor I: Piroxicam and naproxen in acute sports injury, *Am J Med* 84(suppl 5A):45–49, 1988.
54. McLatchie GR, et al: Variable schedules of ibuprofen for ankle sprains, *Br J Sports Med* 19:203–206, 1985.
55. Van Marion WF: Indomethacin in the treatment of soft tissue lesions: a double blind trial against placebo, *J Int Med Res* 1:151–158, 1973.
56. Rang HP, Dale MM: *Pharmacology,* New York, 1987, Churchill Livingstone.
57. Ellenhorn MJ, Barceloux DG: *Medical toxicology: diagnosis and treatment of human poisoning,* New York, 1988, Elsevier.
58. White S: Topical non-steroidal anti-inflammatory drugs (NSAIDs) in the treatment of inflammatory musculoskeletal disorders, *Prostaglandins Leukot Essent Fatty Acids* 43:209–222, 1991.

THE ROLE OF PHYSICAL MODALITIES: PART I— ELECTRICAL MODALITIES IN SPORTS MEDICINE

Edward M. Wojtys
James E. Carpenter

The clinical use of electrical modalities in the rehabilitation of musculoskeletal injuries has flourished in the past decade. Unfortunately, most of this practice is based on anecdote and experimentation rather than controlled scientific investigation. It is unfortunate that the wealth of basic science information available in some of these areas has not been applied to clinical practice.

HISTORY

The use of electricity in an attempt to heal injured, painful, or weakened body parts is not a new idea. Scribonius Largus, who practiced medicine in ancient Rome, employed torpedo fish, rays, and electric eels to treat difficult patients with gout or headaches.[1] Apparently, these painful areas were submerged in water, allowing contact with the stimulus-emitting creature. Statistics on patient and physician satisfaction for those services, unfortunately, are not available.

Very little is written in the medical literature about the use of electricity as a therapeutic agent until the 1800s, when sporadic reports on hand-cranked devices for the treatment of everything from acne to constipation to lumbago began to appear. Not until the 1960s, when Melzack proposed the "gate theory" of pain, were scientific investigations focused on the effects of electricity on pain, bone and soft tissue healing, scoliosis and muscle function.[2] In 1971, a review of 234 physical therapy practices nationally showed that 89% used electrical stimulation (ES) as a therapeutic regimen.[3] Unfortunately, very little was known about their success rates from controlled studies. Typical uses included neuromuscular reeducation in patients with peripheral nerve lesions, hemiplegia, paralysis, attempts at prevention of disuse muscle atrophy, and reduction of spasticity.

INTRODUCTION

Electrical modalities are therapeutic techniques in which electrical potentials are applied across a biologic tissue to produce a desired physiologic effect. When an electrical potential is applied across tissues, an electric current flows. The amount of current that flows is dependent upon the magnitude of the potential and the tissue resistance. As these currents pass through biologic tissue, they can produce physiologic effects, such as thermal changes, and psychologic benefits, all of which need to be considered when deciding the usefulness of a device.

All biologic tissues contain positively and negatively charged ions. These particles with electrical charges have the ability to move, usually from a higher concentration to a lower concentration, but also with respect to electrical signals. Positively charged ions tend to move toward negatively charged electrodes and vice versa, creating current flow. The concentration of ions in part establishes the electrical resistance of a tissue. As the ion concentration of a tissue increases, so does the ability to transmit electrical energy. All of these phenomena affect the response of a tissue to ES.

Applied electrical energy can mimic the natural flow present in normal tissue or can be designed to produce a desired effect (e.g., fracture healing) by changing amplitude, pulse duration, frequency, wave form, rate of rise, signal decay time, and other factors.

TECHNIQUES OF ELECTRICAL CURRENT APPLICATION

The path an electrical current follows reflects, in part, the direction of the least resistance offered. Those tissues offering low resistance to ion flow are called *good conductors*. Also, those tissues with the highest ion concentration are usually the best conductors of electricity. Consequently, biologic tissues that have a high water content, such as blood, are very good conductors.

Skin, because of its layered structure, is considered an insulator; it generally resists electrical current flow. Therefore, when currents are applied through skin, solutions of low resistance are applied to the skin's surface to improve electric signal penetration and increase the area of contact.

ES can be applied to musculoskeletal tissues by several different techniques: direct stimulation, capacitive stimulation, or inductive stimulation.[4] In addition to the differing methods of application of ES, there are differences in the stimulation signals that can be delivered. The magnitude (or amplitude), polarity, waveform, frequency, and duration of signals can all be varied independently. These have been referred to in the past by a variety of names, which can be confusing and frequently misleading to the clinician. Some of the more common terms are explained further in this chapter.

Direct current

Direct current (DC) describes a constant electrical potential between two electrodes. It is also referred to as *galvanic* or *faradic* stimulation. The frequency, amplitude, waveform, and polarity can all be varied independently. Battery-powered devices usually produce DC at low voltage, and the current can be interrupted or uninterrupted. Electrodes can be implanted in tissue or applied to the overlying skin surface. Implanted electrodes offer the most efficient and accurate stimulation method but require invasive procedures to place the electrodes. Alternatively, surface stimulation, which does not require invasive electrode placement, must traverse tissues other than those specifically targeted to produce a deep effect. In particular, skin, which is an electrical insulator, must be overcome by the electrical potential. Care must be taken to protect the tissues between the target area and the electrical source, especially when dissimilar layers of tissue are present.

Charged particles that flow in an electrical field can accumulate at the electrodes when a constant field is applied (DC-ES). These charged particles may cause local tissue inflammation or skin irritation at the electrodes. Beneficial effects may also be produced, such as increased local blood flow. The area surrounding the negative electrode tends to become relatively alkaline and may be of help in the treatment of infected tissues by inhibiting bacterial growth.[5] Conversely, the region surrounding the positive electrode can become acidic, which can increase cell migration.[5] The amount of current used in DC stimulation depends on the individual's pain tolerance and the desired effect of the stimulation. Fracture healing, for instance, may require invasive placement of electrodes in order to obtain the desired level of stimulation.[6-10]

Indirect current

Capacitive. Capacitive stimulation is achieved by placing electrodes on opposite sides of the limb and applying an electrical potential that cycles with time. The external potential created by the electrodes generates an internal electrical field across the tissues. A stimulating current then flows in this electrical field. This technique is felt to be less selective than direct stimulation. Attaining the desired effect (interval, amplitude, etc.) in a deep target region can be clinically challenging. The thickness and insulating capacity of the overlying tissues need to be considered.

Inductive. Inductive stimulation employs a pair of wire coils on a common axis placed on opposite sides of the limb. Varying currents are applied through these coils, which generate a time-dependent magnetic field and, consequently, a secondary electrical field. It is this secondary electrical field that causes current flow in the tissues between the coils. The location of the electrical field can be used to target specific tissues; however, the placement of the coils needs to be precise.

Neither the capacitive nor the inductive stimulation technique generates electrode by-products as direct stimulation can. Unfortunately, the differences in the biologic effects at the cellular level of these three techniques of ES are not known.

Alternating current

In order to avoid the potential problems caused by the accumulation of electrolytic by-products during DC-ES, alternating or pulsed electrical currents are more commonly used today in clinical practice. This group of stimulators includes galvanic, faradic, high-voltage, inferential, and Russian current types. In alternating current (AC) ES, polarity is reversed constantly by the changing direction of the electrical field. Sometimes these pulses of stimulation are called *biphasic* because of their changing direction. Charged particles continue to flow between the electrodes, but the polarity or direction is constantly changing, producing little to no net movement. If ion accumulation is desired, as in the case of an infected nonunion, then AC-ES would not be appropriate. However, if ion accumulation is not needed to produce the desired clinical effect, AC is preferred. Most therapeutic ES utilizes AC or pulsed current.

Pulsed current. *Pulsed current* ES refers to the pattern in which electrical signals are delivered over time. If rest periods (no stimulation) are utilized between periods of stimulation, the current is described as *pulsed*. These patterns can be symmetric (balanced) or asymmetric (unbalanced), depending on the signal intensity and tolerance of the patient. Pulses can also be monophasic or biphasic, depending on the desired tissue effect. When the stimulation period is shorter than the rest period, the active phase is called a *burst*. Many currently popular electric stimulators deliver pulsed stimulation with the burst capacity.

Inferential current. Inferential current combines the effects of two separate sets of electrodes, producing a biplanar, direct pattern of ES. These sets of electrodes are placed in different planes but are centered over the same focal area. Stimulator signals can be adjusted for each set of electrodes. It is hypothesized that where the two electrical fields produced by these pairs of electrodes intersect, electrical interference is produced. Ideally, the electrical interference occurs in the targeted tissue. If the two signals that are applied via the two sets of electrodes are in phase (same polarity), their effect is additive in the region of current overlap. If these signals are out of phase, their opposite polarities cancel out. These combination electrical waves are called *heterodynes*.

It is further hypothesized that a greater stimulus can be delivered to the tissues of interest with inferential current because it produces lower levels of stimulation in the non-target tissues, such as the skin. This stimulation technique is frequently used to decrease pain and/or swelling in a well-localized area. However, because the body is not homogeneous in its tissue make-up (i.e., bone, fat, muscle), it is sometimes difficult to predict the desired route of application or the exact pattern of effect produced by two simultaneous currents. Understandably, well-localized, superficial pain and swelling is easier to target. When three sets of electrodes are used, the technique is called *stereodynamic inferential current*, which can complicate these considerations.[11,12]

Russian current. Russian current was popularized when reports of exceptional results with muscle training and conditioning were presented at a Canadian Symposium in 1977.[13] This method does not represent a different technique of applying ES, only a different type of stimulation signal. Specifically, the typical Russian stimulator generates a time-modulated AC, typically using direct stimulation. Interestingly, the fantastic results reported by Kots have never been reproduced.[13]

Iontophoresis. Iontophoresis is a technique that employs DC-ES to drive ions through the insulating superficial layers of the body (skin, subcutaneous fat) to deeper targets (tendon, muscle). Using knowledge of ion polarity and pharmacokinetics, positively charged ions of medications can be driven away from a positively charged electrode, whereas negatively charged ions may require the use of a negative electrode. Frequently medications, such as corticosteroids, are applied to the skin in the hope that, as charged substances, they can be driven through the skin and subcutaneous tissues to the target sites. Deep delivery of these substances could, in theory, reduce local tissue inflammation while minimizing the undesirable systemic effects of many medications. Unfortunately, this has not been well substantiated scientifically.

USES OF ELECTRICAL SOFT TISSUE STIMULATION

Biologic tissues exhibit many electrical phenomena. Bone and collagen have been extensively studied.[14,15] Both soft and hard biologic tissues demonstrate electrical potentials when strained, representing, in part, a piezoelectric phenomenon.[16] This activity occurs because of a change in the relative position of the charged particles when deformation of the structure occurs with applied forces. Moistened collagen in tendon has been shown to develop electrical potentials along its fiber axis when subjected to axial loads.[17] These potentials occur as a result of fluid flow and ion movement through tissue, producing streaming potentials as well as piezoelectric effects. Entire tendons also demonstrate electrical potentials along their functional axis. Kappel et al. found, in dogs, "a consistent resting potential difference in the intact tendon with definite polarity, positive proximally."[18] This potential increased when the tendon was stretched, averaging 7.5 mV across a 2-cm length of tendon. This potential dropped toward zero if the tendon was interrupted by an incision, and the potential did not return to normal with repair. Thus, it is clear that the tendon and probably ligamentous soft tissue, as well as bone, have normal bioelectric activity, which is determined by mechanical stress and can be significantly altered by injury. The exact role that these potentials play in tissue maintenance remains unclear, but their presence and importance are clear. These electric charges probably act as key signals for response or repair at the cellular level, but their exact role is not yet agreed upon.

The discovery of electrical phenomena in musculoskeletal tissue has generated interest in attempting to manipulate the biology of these tissues through externally applied electrical potentials. Nessler and Mass demonstrated that this can be done with tendons in vitro.[19] They found increased cellular activity and subsequent increases in collagen production in whole tendons in culture in response to continuous DC. Most other in vivo soft tissue studies have focused on the effect of ES on tendon or ligament repair following injury.

Soft tissue healing

Clinicians from multiple disciplines have shown great interest in the effect that ES may have on soft tissue healing. Most recent studies have attempted to enhance or speed tissue repair with ES. In 1983, Frank et al. reported on an experimental model for medial collateral ligament (MCL) healing in rabbits.[20] After transection and repair, the experimental group underwent ES with U-shaped electromagnets 7 hours per day, 5 days per week, for 21 or 42 days. The experimental group demonstrated a higher hydroxyproline content in the repaired ligaments, with increased stiffness and strength noted at 21 days. The differences were not significant between the control and experimental groups at earlier points in time.

In the patellar tendon of rabbits, Akai et al. created 4- by 4-mm defects and followed their healing. Using constant DC-ES generated by implanted electrodes, they found increased stiffness and a decrease in type III:type I collagen ratio compared to controls.[21] Similar positive effects on ligament healing have been seen with ES in rabbits and rats after ligament transection.[22-24] Unfortunately, most animal studies have utilized implanted electrodes with direct, constant, or alternating current, whereas most clinical studies utilize noninvasive surface electrodes, making direct correlations between animal and human studies difficult at best. Other than the surface coils used in the work by Frank[20] none of the techniques for delivering ES studied in animals is directly comparable to the techniques available for human use.

The polarity of a current, which dictates the direction of ion flow through soft tissue, appears to be a significant factor in determining the response of soft tissue to ES. In a rat MCL model, Kenney and Dahners found significantly improved healing when the electrical field was colinear with the axis of the ligament.[23] When the electric field was perpendicular to the axis of the ligament, no effect was seen. Interestingly, Tart and Dahners found ES to be protective against joint contracture when the field was applied transversely to the limb in a rat model.[25]

In contrast to the in vitro studies, there have been very few clinical studies on the effectiveness of ES in the healing process of injured ligaments or tendons. Wilson studied a group of 40 patients with grade I and II ankle sprains randomly divided into two groups.[26] He found improved subjective scores of pain and disability after 3 days of treatment with high-frequency ES for 1 hour per day. However, no objective measurement of ankle function was statistically significant between the two groups. Michlovitz et al. also studied the effect of ES on ankle sprains.[27] They randomly divided 30 patients into three groups: ice, ice plus ES (28 pulses per second), and ice plus ES (80 pulses per second). Each patient received one 30-minute treatment per day for 3 days. There was no statistically significant difference between the groups in edema reduction measured volumetrically or in ankle range of motion on day 1 or day 3. These limited studies do not provide compelling evidence for using ES to enhance healing of soft tissue injuries. More in-depth investigation may prove differently.

The lack of objective support for the clinical use of ES for the enhancement of ligament or tendon healing is reflective of the major gaps in our basic science understanding of ES. Also, it must be emphasized that most existing experimental studies differ from the clinical setting in very fundamental ways. The majority of the experimental studies have employed electrodes directly implanted in the soft tissue, whereas surface electrodes are generally used clinically.

Although the signal being delivered at the skin may be well defined in terms of amplitude, duration, and frequency, what signal reaches the target area remains unknown. The effects of the insulating layers of skin and subcutaneous tissue and the dampening effect of different soft tissue depths remain a mystery in need of further investigation. In addition, many experimental studies use continuous ES, yet clinically, short, infrequent periods of stimulation are more commonly used due to practical considerations of medical treatment duration as well as the negative effects of continuous DC discussed earlier in this chapter.

Because of the difficulty and costs of treating chronic dermal wounds, there has been much interest in techniques to enhance healing. Animal models of wound healing utilizing incisions[28,29] and skin grafts[30] have consistently demonstrated an increased healing rate with ES over the control. Unlike the clinical studies on ligament healing, the studies on chronic dermal wound healing agree with the experimental reports. The best available study is a blinded, randomized, multicenter study of chronic dermal wounds.[31] The authors found healing rates to nearly double in patients treated with pulsed ES. A sponge electrode was used directly in the open wound. These findings are in general agreement with other studies of chronic wound healing.[32-35]

Despite some success with the use of ES in the clinical treatment of dermal wounds and experimental ligament injuries, the mechanism is unclear. Electrical fields have been shown to inhibit the rate of bacterial growth, especially in regions closest to electrodes, and this may play a role in the healing of open wounds.[36] Enhanced circulation through vascular proliferation in response to pulsed electromagnetic fields has been demonstrated in the rabbit.[37] Increased tissue perfusion from this phenomenon could improve the healing response in the affected soft tissues. There may, as well, be a direct stimulation of the soft tissue repair response at the cellular level through ion manipulation.

Unfortunately, adequate corresponding clinical studies evaluating the efficacy of ES in promoting healing of ligament and tendon injuries are not available to support its use for these conditions. No clinical studies exist on the effects of ES on the difficult problems of chronic, refractory soft tissue injuries such as tendonitis. Controlled clinical studies in this area are necessary before these techniques should be routinely used to treat patients with these conditions. In contrast, ES has been shown to improve chronic dermal wound healing under certain conditions. Whether the cost in terms of equipment, personnel, and time justify its use has not been addressed. It will likely depend on the individual clinical situation.

Pain control

ES has been promoted by some as a treatment modality for pain control. Despite years of investigation into the area of pain control, however, agreement is lacking on the mechanism of action of electricity on pain-stimulus propagation and perception. It is unclear whether electricity primarily affects β-endorphin release in the pituitary, affects enkephalin release in the spinal cord, or simply acts as an impulse between the periphery and the brain capable of blocking painful afferent input. When electrical stimuli reach the slow, small, unmyelinated nerve fibers in the periphery, pain impulses traveling to the cortex along larger myelinated fibers can be blocked if the electrical impulse is of the correct amplitude, frequency, and duration.[2] This effect can be powerful and should not be overlooked when considering the positive effects of ES on soft tissue. During rehabilitation after operation or injury, a decrease in pain may very well be the key to a quicker return to normal function. However, because pain control is not the primary focus of this review, suffice it to say that clinical questions remain concerning the positive effects seen and reported on pain control.

Muscle inhibition

Reflex inhibition of muscles can be a major problem for athlete and nonathlete alike after injury or surgery on limbs or around joints. Overriding this negative effect by directly stimulating nerve or muscle through the use of ES can be quite helpful clinically. The lower extremity muscles in this posttrauma scenario may benefit significantly from ES-assisted attempts at muscle contraction. Fortunately, ES is not always needed, but when voluntary muscle contractions cannot be generated, ES can be very beneficial. Even when pain is not present, joint effusion can make limb control difficult for patients.[38] This is frequently due to lower motor neuron reflex inhibition. Stokes and Young[39] and de Andrade et al.[40] reported that this reflex mechanism occurs when afferent stimuli from pain and pressure receptors in and around the injured joint prevent activation of α-motor neurons in the anterior horn of the spinal cord, which are responsible for muscle activation. Stokes and Young have shown that in patients undergoing arthrotomy and meniscectomy, there was significant inhibition of the quadriceps muscle on the operated side.[39] During the first few hours after surgery, the inhibition was usually significant but incomplete (50% to 70%), with partial muscle control possible. It became more pronounced later during the first 24 hours (80%) and could continue at high levels (70% to 80%) for days after surgery. Lesser degrees of inhibition can persist for even weeks after surgery (35% to 40%). Young et al. attempted to eliminate the efferent block on skeletal muscle caused by painful afferent input by injecting a local anesthetic into the involved joint.[41] Unfortunately, this inhibition continues if an effusion persists even when painful stimuli are blocked by anesthetic agents. Joint aspiration can decrease intra-articular pressure and may improve attempts at muscle rehabilitation. In fact, de Andrade et al.[40] and Jayson and Dixon[42] showed that the inhibition of the quadriceps could be significantly reduced by aspiration of the knee joint effusion.

Recurrent effusions in athletes or laborers who want to be physically active as soon as possible following injury or surgery should be treated with caution. The inhibition produced by an effusion may be a protective mechanism necessary to allow a synovial joint to rest in the early injury or postoperative period, when joint loading might be deleterious. Routine, repeated aspiration solely to improve muscle performance may in fact produce hazardous joint loading.

Tourniquets commonly used in the operating room are frequently blamed for postoperative quadriceps muscle dysfunction.[43,44] Stokes and Young studied the quadriceps of four normal subjects before and after the maximum tolerable periods of unilateral tourniquet ischemia.[45] The tourniquets were used exactly as they would have been in the operating room. Quadriceps function did not change with the induced ischemia, leading the authors to conclude that this was not a factor in postoperative inhibition.

Extra-articular pain can also have a negative effect on quadriceps muscle function.[46] Ekholm et al. showed that pinching the anterior aspect of the knee joint capsule inhibited the quadriceps stretch reflex and quadriceps activity in decerebrate cats.[47] Interestingly, blocking afferent spinal cord input by dorsal root section prevents muscle atrophy secondary to experimental arthritis.[48,49] Therefore, the mechanism of the positive effects seen with ES needs to be considered. It is possible in the posttrauma scenario that the positive effects seen with ES on muscle may be in part due to a pain-relieving action caused by the stimulation of nociceptive afferent nerve fibers. Interestingly, the quadriceps inhibition resulting from an experimental knee effusion can be partially prevented by intra-articular injection of a local anesthetic.[40] All of these studies indicate a lower motor neuron reflex loop (H reflex) that modulates muscle performance based on afferent input from pain or pressure receptors (effusions) and provides a target for ES. In fact, in the lower extremity, ES of IA afferents of the femoral nerve reduces excitability of the α-motorneuron pool and consequently inhibits the quadriceps and hamstrings.

Wolf[50] has shown that certain sensory stimulation patterns can block other afferent sensory input to the spinal cord, whereas Delwaide et al.[51] have demonstrated that cutaneous sensory nerve stimulation can also increase motorneuron excitability in humans. The precise mechanism of action for ES is unclear. ES may reduce quadriceps inhibition by blocking painful afferent input or by simply increasing the excitability of anterior horn cells.

Immobilization. The direct effects of joint immobilization on neuromuscular excitability are difficult to isolate because immobilization is frequently utilized when other neuromuscular inhibitors are present (joint pain and swelling). Consequently, it is unclear how ES can best be utilized when immobilization becomes necessary. Voluntary muscle contractions should first be encouraged. If a muscle contraction is not attainable, ES should then be considered. Mayer has shown that IA excitatory post-synaptic potentials were reduced in gastrocnemius motorneurons of cats whose knee and ankle joints were immobilized by pinning.[52] Unfortunately, pinning these joints probably induced some discomfort, so again the relevant factors are difficult to decipher. Fuglsang-Frederiksen and Scheel showed that voluntary activation of motor units in the human quadriceps was reduced after knee immobilization for treatment of collateral ligament injuries.[53] Unfortunately, we do not know if knee effusions were present or the level of discomfort experienced by the patient. The best indication that limb immobilization does have a negative effect on motor neuron excitability was reported by Sale et al.,[54] who demonstrated in the upper extremity that immobilization of human thenar muscles alone produced a reduction in reflex potentiation (the enhancement of reflex responses by voluntary effort, a function of motor neuron excitability).

Further work by Gould et al. compared three groups of normal volunteers in long leg casts.[55] One group performed isometric exercises, another used ES, and a third group remained sedentary. Protein intake was controlled. Isokinetic testing after 2 weeks of immobilization showed ES to be helpful in maintaining voluntary power and in decreasing muscle bulk loss.

Overcoming muscle inhibition and atrophy. Significant muscle inhibition and partial denervation are good indications for ES until voluntary muscle contractions are possible. ES can be very useful in reactivating and conditioning skeletal muscle that has been inhibited or atrophied by injury, surgery, immobilization, or partial denervation. Whether the affected muscles are the external rotators of the shoulder after glenohumeral dislocation, the peroneals at the ankle following a sprain, or the abdominal muscles in the postpartum period, ES appears to be helpful in overcoming inhibition and regaining active muscle control. ES appears to be most effective when muscle inhibition is profound and voluntary muscle contractions cannot be generated. Near-maximal muscle contractions produced by ES can improve strength, and submaximal levels of stimuli appear to reeducate or "turn on" dysfunctional muscles after injury or surgery. The challenge to the clinician remains the identification of the correct stimulus for the muscle problem in terms of pulse, intensity, duration, and frequency. Unfortunately, the positive effects may be of short duration and do not appear to outweigh those produced by voluntary muscle activity.

An anterior cruciate ligament (ACL) reconstruction rehabilitation protocol designed by Eriksson and Haggmark produced better results with ES and exercise than exercise alone, in terms of muscle performance.[56] Several studies have shown that ES can retard the deleterious biochemical changes that occur in the muscles of immobilized limbs as they atrophy.[57-59] However, if immobilization after injury or surgery is avoided and active muscle contractions can be performed, the indications for the use of ES are less clear. ES appears to lose its benefits when active resistance exercise is possible. Unfortunately, most investigations have

focused only on isometric training. What effect ES will add to isotonic, isokinetic, concentric, or eccentric modes of training is not known.

Morrissey et al. also studied the effects of ES on the immobilized extremity after ACL surgery.[60] They used two groups of patients: quadriceps isometrics with and without ES. All strength testing was done in the isometric mode on 15 male volunteers. The group that did not use muscle stimulation lost 80% of its preoperative quadriceps torque in 6 weeks of immobilization. ES did decrease the strength loss during cast immobilization; however, the benefit was short-lived, being undetectable 6 weeks after immobilization was discontinued (12 weeks after surgery). In this study, ES could not prevent loss of thigh girth in the immobilized limb and had no effect on pain.

Wigerstad-Lossing et al. also investigated the use of ES in the immobilized limb.[59] After ACL surgery, 23 patients used ES during voluntary muscle contractions. Four 10-minute sets of quadriceps stimulation were used three times a week at a frequency of 30 Hz in addition to the standard program of quadriceps isometric contractions performed by the control group for 6 weeks. ES decreased muscle strength loss, muscle wasting (computed tomography scan measurements), and losses in oxidative and glycolytic muscle enzyme activity (assessed by muscle biopsy). In the control group (no ES), muscle biopsies showed a significant decrease in the area occupied by type I muscle fibers compared with the stimulated group. Unfortunately, only isometric muscle strength at 30 degrees was measured postoperatively.

Gould et al. compared the effects of ES alone to isometric exercise training in two groups of 10 patients undergoing open meniscectomy.[61] A protocol consisting of "tetanizing" 5-second muscle contractions was used 400 times a day for 2 weeks. At 4 weeks after surgery, the stimulated group showed better muscle volume and strength and less knee swelling, discarded crutches earlier, had an improved range of motion, and experienced less pain than the nonstimulated group.

Jensen et al. demonstrated the positive effects of postoperative ES in 90 arthroscopic knee surgery patients.[62] Less muscle inhibition and pain were expected in this group, compared with the Gould study,[61] because of the arthroscopic, closed technique. Use of postoperative pain medication and isokinetic strength at 1, 3 and 7 weeks after surgery was evaluated. Isokinetic strength (60 degrees and 180 degrees per second) and endurance (at 50% fatigue) were measured. ES was effective in decreasing the amount of pain medication used in 93% of patients. The ES group regained preoperative isokinetic strength in flexion and extension, range of motion, and leg volume an average of 1 month sooner than the nonstimulated group.

In order to evaluate adequately the use of ES in these postoperative studies, it would be useful to know how many patients had true muscle inhibition and needed ES to generate a contraction in their quadriceps or hamstrings. Postoperative inhibition of the quadriceps and hamstrings muscles after injury or surgery is a known phenomenon, usually due to knee joint swelling and pain.[38] When the thigh musculature is not functioning after an injury or operation, the stage is set for complications.[63] Although problems do not always occur with induced muscle dysfunction, when they do, the consequences can be devastating.[63] Therefore, aggressive treatment of muscle dysfunction after injuries or surgery to the lower extremity is warranted. There is no doubt that the added cost of ES is well worth the investment if significant complications can be avoided. However, the added cost of ES probably cannot be justified in routine situations where voluntary muscle contractions can be generated.

ELECTRICAL STIMULATION FOR NORMAL MUSCLE TRAINING

The dream of muscle strength, tone, and endurance enhancement through the use of ES is appealing to today's physique-conscious society. The fascination of plugging in a device to obtain a body beautiful, strong, and fit without hard physical effort is understandable. The physiology that makes this scenario believable stems from the understanding that muscles need only vigorous contractions to improve strength, tone, and endurance. The key question becomes, Can an externally initiated contraction (ES) be as productive as an internally generated one? After all, Kernell et al. have shown that absolute muscle tension is the critical factor in determining a muscle's response to functional ES.[64] Secondary factors in the development of muscle tension include the training mode involved (muscle length, resistance applied, speed). Muscle tension can be produced in one of three basic modes: isometric, in which the muscle length remains the same while the load may vary; isotonic, in which the length of the muscle changes while the load remains the same; and isokinetic, in which the speed of contraction remains the same as the resistance varies. During isotonic or isokinetic activities, muscles can shorten (concentric activity) or lengthen (eccentric activity) while under tension. Activities of daily living frequently require slow, concentric muscle activity at low load levels, whereas athletic activities frequently utilize the eccentric mode, producing high loads in the muscle-tendon complex.

Eccentric activity is capable of generating very large loads in the muscle-tendon unit. They are essential in activities such as running and throwing and need to be emphasized in training for sports. Unfortunately, strength gains in each particular mode do not necessarily carry over to other modes of activity. Strength gained through isometric exercises does not necessarily mean improvements in isokinetic performance. Therefore, all three training modes are needed in a balanced muscle-training program.

Because the eccentric mode stresses the muscle-tendon units to the highest degree, it closely resembles the injury situation and demands caution when used in training. Un-fortunately, most research on combination programs of ES and muscle training have utilized the isometric mode only. Very little is known about the use of ES with eccentric contractions. The role of ES in isotonics and isokinetics with either concentric or eccentric mechanisms of muscle training remains open to debate.

Incorporation of ES into a training program requires an understanding of its mechanism of action. When used with exercise, electricity may enhance the contractile force of a given set of muscle fibers by simply augmenting the propagation of an impulse through those fibers that would have been stimulated voluntarily, or the electric stimulus may allow additional fibers to be recruited beyond those recruited by normal voluntary activity.[65] It is unclear whether this is purely a muscle phenomenon, a combined effect on nerve and muscle, or the effect of "neural conditioning" alone.

The goal of any ES conditioning program for strength should be tetanic or near-tetanic contractions of the involved muscle. Most investigators agree that increasing the stimulation frequency beyond that necessary to achieve tetanic contraction is not helpful and may be quite painful, resulting in further muscle inhibition.[66-69] Painful ES, especially in the injury situation, should be avoided.

The quality of a muscle contraction produced by ES depends directly upon the parameters of the electric signal. Intensity, frequency, pulse amplitude, and shape, as well as electrode placement and soft tissue resistance, are important details that need to be considered. Because muscle stimulation is usually generated with surface electrodes, it may be difficult to tell what signal is reaching the target muscle. The success of this modality is determined by how well the stimulus reproduces the desired clinical effect. For the quadriceps femoris muscle, the following frequencies have been examined: 25 Hz,[70] 30 to 35 Hz,[71] 45 Hz,[72] 50 Hz,[73-75] 60 Hz,[75,76] 65 Hz,[77] 75 Hz,[75,78] 100 Hz,[72,76,79,80] 2000 Hz,[81] 2200 Hz,[75,82] and 2500 Hz.[83,84] This range of frequencies indicates the many possibilities that deserve investigation.

Interest in the sports world was stirred in 1977 by Kots at a Canadian symposium on athletic conditioning.[13] His reports of ES-improved muscle strength in the range of 30% in normal muscle over a 3-week period were previously unheard of. Kots used a program of 2500 cycles per second in 10-msec intervals coupled with 10 msec of rest. This type of electric protocol is now referred to as *Russian current*. Morphometric changes, including increased muscle girth and decreases in limb fat content, were also reported. Since that report 16 years ago, despite numerous attempts in various centers, the same promising results have not been duplicated. ES has not replaced traditional conditioning programs in athletics. However, some well-known anecdotal stories are impressive enough to warrant interest by strength coaches and athletic trainers.

More research is definitely needed to define the role of ES in athletic training. Only a small portion of our current training regimens have been investigated with ES augmentation.[74,85-87] Continued investigation at the clinical level does seem appropriate. ES may provide the cellular stress necessary to provoke muscle remodeling and strengthening. If the generation of tension is linearly related to stress at the cellular level, then the parameters needed to improve strength should be a solvable problem. The torque generated by a maximal voluntary contraction (MVC) is the benchmark that should be used for comparison of ES programs. Walmsley et al. compared the maximum torque generated by voluntary isometric contractions, low- and medium-frequency ES, and combinations of these factors.[75] No single method or combination was able to generate more torque than an MVC. In each case, the torque generated by the electrical devices was significantly less than that produced by an MVC; the effect of ES combined with maximum voluntary activity was not additive at either low or medium frequency.

The lack of an augmentation effect by ES on MVC was further substantiated by Kramer,[88] whose results were similar to those of Walmsley et al.[75] He used asymmetrical, bidirectional waveforms of 1-msec pulse duration at frequencies of 20 Hz, 50 Hz, and 100 Hz delivered over the femoral nerve and superficial quadriceps femoris muscle at their maximum tolerated intensities. Kramer concluded that superimposing ES on MVC produced no additional benefit.

Other reports vary on muscle torque gains produced by exercise augmented with ES in male subjects.[76,78,81-83,89]

Most ES-augmented exercise investigated has focused on the lower extremity. In the upper extremity, Ikai has reported ES-induced contractions producing 30% more torque than those produced by MVC in the adductor pollicis muscle only.[90]

Electrical stimulation training without exercise

Kramer showed that ES-induced contractions at 100 Hz generated 87% of the maximal voluntary torque (MVT) produced on voluntary isometric contractions (50 Hz, 84%).[72] ES-only training contraction intensities of 33%,[83] 67%,[89] 80%,[78] and 87%[76] of the MVT have been reported to be as effective as an MVT program in producing knee extension torque increases. Intuitively, there are problems with these reports: A contraction producing 33% the MVT possible should not produce the same effect as one that generates 87% of the MVT.

A recurring question in ES research has been, Can the electrical signal provide as powerful a stimulus as one generated from the CNS? Selkowitz was able to achieve an ES-only training intensity of 91% of the pretraining MVC.[82] In this group, he reported strength gains of 44% after nine treatments, an improvement acceptable to most. Training intensity has been strongly correlated to net strength gains.[91,92] However, this is primarily based on voluntary contraction data. It is not known if voluntary and ES-induced

contractions vary in their effect on muscle tissue; fiber type response (I versus II) may vary with the stimulus. Delitto et al. have reported a reversal of the motor unit recruitment order during electrically elicited contractions.[93]

The target level of ES is dependent upon the desired muscle effect, training mode, and the prestimulation condition of the muscle. If increasing the peak torque (strength) is the main objective, short, high-intensity stimulation is preferable. However, if improved endurance is the goal, lower-intensity stimulation over longer periods may be better. This is an area of confusion in the current ES literature. There are literally hundreds of protocols varying in intensity, frequency, pulse duration, and rest time for each muscle parameter: tone, power, and endurance.

The amount of rest between bursts of activity in the stimulation pattern is an important aspect to consider when addressing muscle endurance. Kelly and Lieber studied the effect of functional ES in 90 healthy male and female subjects at 10-, 30-, and 50-Hz frequencies at 50% (5 seconds on, 5 seconds off) or 70% (5 seconds on, 2 seconds off) duty cycle.[94] Treatment sessions were 30 minutes in duration and focused on the quadriceps femoris muscle torque attained during the 30 minutes of functional ES. Kelly and Lieber concluded that the average torque produced when stimulating at 50% duty cycle was always greater than the average torque achieved using a 70% duty cycle. The 70% duty cycle always resulted in earlier fatigue for all three frequencies tested, indicating it may be best for endurance training; torque declined by 50% or more within the first 5 minutes of the 30-minute treatment session. The absolute torque produced by the 50-Hz, 50% duty cycle group was greatest throughout the 30-minute treatment period, suggesting that the 50-Hz, 50% duty cycle may be the preferred setting for muscle strengthening.

Soo et al. investigated ES at 2500-Hz sine waves, interrupted for 50 pulsed bursts per second, to improve the lower extremity muscle torque of young, healthy subjects.[95] The target of the stimulation pattern was isometric torques equivalent to 50% of MVC, 8 contractions per session for 10 sessions. The strength increases using ES in knee extensor muscle torque for women and knee flexor muscle torque for men and women were not significant. However, there was a mean quadriceps torque gain of 4.8% per week in knee extensors of men. This rate of improvement is comparable to the studies published by Atha, who showed that standard isometric exercise could produce a 1.8% to 12% per week strength increase.[96] However, the difference between men and women, although not large, is of interest. Numerous explanations exist, but the fact that the difference was seen in knee extensors but not flexors is surprising.

Selkowitz showed that after 12 sessions of ES training most of his subjects were producing electrically stimulated contraction torques that were higher than the MVC torques produced prior to the ES training program.[82] These strength increases are consistent with Fahey et al.[96] (2% increase per week), Currier and Mann[89] (2.8% increase per week), and Laughman et al.[83] (4.4% increase per week), all in knee extensor muscles of men.

Endurance training

It is usually easier to generate a single contraction than multiple repetitions at maximal effort. Also work performance over time is a more difficult factor to quantify than peak torque. Therefore, in vivo endurance evaluations must consider both psychological and physiologic parameters. Endurance (work per unit time) is an important parameter in muscle performance. The duration a force can be produced can be as important as the amount of the force itself. Studies on young adult upper extremities by Ikai and Yabe suggest that endurance could be improved up to 130% over a 13-week training period.[97] The physiologic improvements in endurance were explained by increases in blood flow and oxygen intake in the muscle, based on capillarization; the psychologic gains were attributed to increased discharge of the neuromuscular unit.[97]

The effectiveness and indications for comfortable, low-intensity ES training programs need to be defined. Because high-intensity stimulation targets type II muscle fibers preferentially, low-intensity stimulation (20 Hz) may be the preferred signal for type I fibers. Some clinical problems (patellofemoral pain) would benefit more from less aggressive, less intense programs targeting type I fibers. These individuals often do not tolerate the very powerful, near-maximal contractions produced by higher-intensity stimulation that targets type II muscle fibers.

For muscle endurance, Selkowitz recommends regimens consisting of short intervals between ES-induced contractions with contraction durations approximately equal to the rest period (4 to 15 seconds on and off, for a total of 6 to 15 minutes in each session) using lower frequencies, usually between 50 and 200 Hz.[98] The more typical muscle strength training regimen has longer rest intervals and shorter muscle stimulation times and usually depends upon higher frequencies (2500 Hz).

Electrical stimulation effect on nonstimulated muscles

Cocontraction of knee flexor muscles while the extensors are being stimulated may be a possible explanation for the small gains in the hamstring torque reported in the study of Soo et al.[95] In muscles even more distant from the site of stimulation, Laughman et al. have described the cross-education effects of ES in the nonstimulated extremity.[83] Strength improvements in the opposite limb suggest a mechanism that reaches beyond the local area of muscle stimulation, possibly through retrograde as well as anterograde conduction along the nerve fiber. Singer has found alterations in voluntary motor unit activation patterns after strengthening atrophic muscles with ES, indicative of a profound neural change.[99] These changes were suggestive of increased neural drive synchronization to the contractile ap-

paratus. This effect also was seen in the opposite, uninjured, untrained limb. This change seems to indicate that the signal must be getting back at least to the spinal cord level, if not higher in the central nervous system.

Ultrastructural muscle changes with electrical stimulation

Sinacore et al. biopsied quadriceps femoris muscles before and after ES workouts at 80% of maximum isometric torque.[100] After training with a 2500-Hz sinusoidal carrier wave with interruptions at 50 pulses per second, muscle biopsies showed glycogen depletion in the type II muscle fibers, primarily type IIA fibers. The authors concluded that this profile of ES activates type II skeletal muscle fibers more than type I. Even though type IIA fibers have greater oxidative potential and fatigue-resistant characteristics, they appear to be readily activated by this pattern of ES and depleted of glycogen more completely than type IIB fibers.

Gender effect

Clinically, ES appears to be used more often in women after injury or surgery due to significant muscle inhibition. However, ES is thought to have the same effect in males and females, according to the work done by Kramer et al.[72] When the torques generated by ES were expressed as a percentage of the MVC of the individual, the percentages obtained for both males and females were comparable. Unfortunately, MVC is a subjective measurement and, therefore, is suspect as a control.

Fahey et al. found no difference between the torque gains of knee extensor muscles of men and women in their 6-week ES program.[96]

Recent work by Arvidsson noted more positive effects with ES in females, possibly because of a decreased concentration of anabolic testosterone that allows more profound muscle wasting after injury or surgery.[101]

GENERAL GUIDELINES

A thorough literature review by Selkowitz[98] in 1989 reached several conclusions about ES, and several of those conclusions still appear to be valid, based on the most recent medical literature.

1. Training isometrically with ES significantly increases isometric quadriceps femoris strength in certain positions.
2. The increase in isometric strength for a group training with ES alone is significantly and positively correlated with the mean training contraction intensity.
3. The increase in isometric strength for a group using ES alone may be dependent upon mean training contraction duration.
4. There may be upper limits to training contraction intensity and duration (and, therefore, strength increases) with ES. These limitations appear to be affected by neuromuscular and muscle fiber fatigue factors.

5. Neuromuscular education may also mediate increases in isometric strength due to training with ES.

REFERENCES

1. Kane K, Taub A: A history of local electrical analgesia, *Pain* 1:125–138, 1975.
2. Melzack R: *The puzzle of pain,* New York, 1973, Basic Books.
3. Amrein L, Garrett TR, Martin GM: Use of low-voltage electrotherapy and electromyography in physical therapy, *Phys Ther* 51:1283–1287, 1971.
4. Black J: Electrical stimulation of hard and soft tissues in animal models, *Clin Plast Surg* 12:243–251, 1985.
5. Gault WR, Gatens PF: Use of low intensity direct current in management of ischemic skin ulcers, *Phys Ther* 56:265–269, 1976.
6. Becker RO, Selden G: *The body electric,* New York, 1985, William Morrow.
7. Brighton CT: Bioelectric effects on bone and cartilage, *Clin Orthop* 124:2–4, 1977.
8. Connolly JF, Hahn H, Jardon OM: The electrical enhancement of periosteal proliferation in normal and delayed fracture healing, *Clin Orthop* 124:97–105, 1977.
9. Marino A, Becker RO: Biologic effects of extremely low frequency electric and magnetic fields: a review, *Phys Chem Physics* 9:131–143, 1977.
10. Wolf SL: *Electrotherapy,* New York, 1981, Churchill Livingstone.
11. Nelson RL, Currier DP: *Clinical electrotherapy,* Norwalk, Conn, 1987, Appleton and Lange.
12. Nikolova L: *Treatment with interferential current,* New York, 1987, Churchill Livingstone.
13. Kots YM: Notes from lectures and laboratory periods, Canadian-Soviet exchange symposium on electro-stimulation of skeletal muscles, Concordia University, December 6–15, 1977.
14. Bassett CAL, Pawluk EJ: Electrical behavior of cartilage during loading, *Science* 178:982–983, 1972.
15. Brighton CT, Black J, Pollack S: *Electrical properties of bone and cartilage: experimental effects and clinical applications,* New York, 1979, Grune & Stratton.
16. Fukada E, Yasuda I: Piezoelectric effects in collagen, *Jpn J App Physics* 3:117–121, 1964.
17. Anderson JC, Eriksson C: Electrical properties of wet collagen, *Nature* 218:166–168, 1968.
18. Kappel DA, Zilber S, Ketchum LD: *Biological and clinical effects of low-frequency magnetic and electric fields,* Springfield, Ill, 1974, Thomas.
19. Nessler JP, Mass DP: Direct-current electrical stimulation of tendon healing in vitro, *Clin Orthop* 217:303–312, 1987.
20. Frank C, et al: Electromagnetic stimulation of ligament healing in rabbits, *Clin Orthop* 175:263–272, 1983.
21. Akai M, et al: Electrical stimulation of ligament healing, *Clin Orthop* 235:297–301, 1988.
22. Adams EL, Bradford DS, Oegema TR: Early histological and biomechanical change in ligament healing under electrical stimulation, *Trans ORS* 13:106, 1988.
23. Kenney TG, Dahners LE: The effect of electrical stimulation on ligament healing in a rat model, *Trans ORS* 13:107, 1988.
24. Litke DS, Dahners LE: The effects of low level direct current electrical stimulation on ligament healing in a rat model—with a dosage study, *Trans ORS* 13:669, 1988.
25. Tart RP, Dahners LE: Effects of electrical stimulation on joint contracture in a rat model, *J Orthop Res* 7:538–542, 1989.
26. Wilson DJ: Treatment of soft-tissue injuries by pulsed electrical energy, *Br Med J* 2:269–270, 1972.
27. Michlovitz S, Smith W, Watkins M: Ice and high voltage pulsed stimulation in treatment of acute lateral ankle sprains, *J Orthop Sports Phys Ther* 9:301–304, 1988.

28. Brown M, McDonnell MK, Menton DN: Electrical stimulation effects on cutaneous wound healing in rabbits, *Phys Ther* 68:955–960, 1988.
29. Konikoff JJ: Electrical promotion of soft tissue repairs, *Ann Biomed Eng* 4:1–5, 1976.
30. Politis MJ, Zanakis MF, Miller JE: Enhanced survival of full-thickness skin grafts following the application of DC electrical fields, *Plast Reconstr Surg* 84:267–272, 1989.
31. Feedar JA, Kloth LC, Gentzkow GD: Chronic dermal ulcer healing enhanced with monophasic pulsed electrical stimulation, *Phys Ther* 71:639–649, 1991.
32. Carley PJ, Wainapel SF: Electrotherapy for acceleration of wound healing: low intensity direct current, *Arch Phys Med Rehabil* 55:443–446, 1985.
33. Gentzkow GD, Miller KH: Electrical stimulation for dermal wound healing, *Clin Podiatr Med Surg* 8:827–841, 1991.
34. Kloth LC, Feddar JA: Acceleration of wound healing with high voltage, monophasic, pulsed current, *Phys Ther* 68:503–508, 1988.
35. Weiss DS, Kirsner R, Eaglstein WH: Electrical stimulation and wound healing, *Arch Dermatol* 126:222–225, 1990.
36. Kincaid CB, Lavoie KH: Inhibition of bacterial growth in vitro following stimulation with high voltage monophasic, pulsed current, *Phys Ther* 69:651–655, 1989.
37. Greenough CG: The effects of pulsed electromagnetic fields on blood vessel growth in the rabbit ear chamber, *J Orthop Res* 10:252–262, 1992.
38. Jensen KA, Graf BK: *The effects of knee effusion on quadriceps strength and intra-articular pressure of the knee during isokinetic exercise.* In *AANA Book of Abstracts, Instructional Courses & Symposia,* 1992.
39. *Stokes M, Young A: Investigations of quadriceps inhibition: implications for clinical practice, Physiotherapy 70:425–428, 1984.*
40. de Andrade JR, Grant C, Dixon A: Joint distension and reflex muscle inhibition in the knee, *J Bone Joint Surg [Am]* 47:313–322, 1965.
41. Young A, et al: The effect of intra-articular bupivacaine on quadriceps inhibition after meniscectomy, *Med Sci Sports Exerc* 15:154, 1983.
42. Jayson MIV, Dixon A: Pressure changes during passive joint distension, *Ann Rheum Dis* 29:261–265, 1970.
43. Dobner JJ, Nitz AJ: Post-meniscectomy tourniquet palsy and functional sequelae, *Am J Sports Med* 10:211–214, 1982.
44. Saunders KC, et al: Effect of tourniquet time on post-operative quadriceps function, *Clin Orthop* 143:194–199, 1979.
45. Stokes M, Young A: The contribution of reflex inhibition to arthrogenous muscle weakness, *Clin Sci* 67:7–14, 1984.
46. Stener B: Reflex inhibition of the quadriceps elicited from a subperiosteal tumour of the femur, *Acta Orthop Scand* 40:86–91, 1969.
47. Ekholm J, Eklund G, Skoglund S: On the reflex effects from the knee joint of the cat, *Acta Phys Scand* 50:167–174, 1960.
48. Harding B: An investigation into the cause of arthritic muscular atrophy, *Lancet* 1:433–434, 1929.
49. Raymond: Recherches experimentales sur la pathogenie des atrophies musculaires consecutive aux arthrites traumatiques, *Rev Med* 10:374–392, 1890.
50. Wolf SL: Perspectives on central nervous system responsiveness to transcutaneous electrical nerve stimulation, *Phys Ther* 58:1443–1449, 1978.
51. Delwaide PJ, Crenna P, Fleron MH: Cutaneous nerve stimulation and motoneuronal excitability: I, soleus and tibialis anterior excitability after ipsilateral and contralateral sural nerve stimulation, *J Neurol Neurosurg Psychiatry* 44:699–707, 1981.
52. Mayer RF, et al: The effect of long-term immobilization on the motor unit population of the cat medial gastrocnemius muscle, *Neuroscience* 6:725–739, 1981.
53. Fuglsang-Frederiksen A, Scheel U: Transient decrease in number of motor units after immobilization in man, *J Neurol Neurosurg Psychiatry* 41:924–929, 1978.

54. Sale DG, et al: Effect of strength training upon motoneuron excitability in man, *Med Sci Sports Exerc* 15:57–62, 1983.

55. Gould N, et al: Transcutaneous muscle stimulation as a method to retard disuse atrophy, *Clin Orthop* 164:215–220, 1982.

56. Eriksson E, Haggmark T: Comparison of isometric muscle training and electrical stimulation supplementing isometric muscle training in the recovery after major knee ligament surgery, *Am J Sports Med* 7:169–171, 1979.

57. Eriksson E, et al: Effects of electrical stimulation on human skeletal muscle, *Int J Sports Med* 2:18–22, 1981.

58. Standish WD, et al: The effects of immobilization and of electrical stimulation on muscle glycogen and myofibrillar ATPase, *Can J Appl Sports Sci* 7:267–271, 1982.

59. Wigerstad-Lossing I, et al: Effects of electrical muscle stimulation combined with voluntary contractions after knee ligament surgery, *Med Sci Sports Exerc* 20:93–98, 1988.

60. Morrissey MC, et al: The effects of electrical stimulation on the quadriceps during postoperative knee immobilization, *Am J Sports Med* 13:40–45, 1985.

61. Gould N, et al: Transcutaneous muscle stimulation to retard disuse atrophy after open meniscectomy, *Clin Orthop* 178:190–197, 1983.

62. Jensen JE, et al: The use of transcutaneous neural stimulation and isokinetic testing in arthroscopic knee surgery, *Am J Sports Med* 13:27–33, 1985.

63. Noyes FR, Wojtys EM, Marshall MT: The early diagnosis and treatment of developmental patella infera syndrome, *Clin Orthop* 265:241–252, 1991.

64. Kernell D, et al: Effects of physiologic amounts of high- and low-rate chronic stimulation on fast-twitch muscle of the cat hindlimb, *J Neurophysiol* 58:598–613, 1987.

65. Nowakowska A: Influence of experimental training by electric current stimulation on skeletal muscles, *Acta Physiol Pol* 13:37–44, 1962.

66. Edwards RHT, et al: Human skeletal muscle function: description of tests and normal values, *Clin Sci Mol Med* 52:283–290, 1977.

67. Freund HJ: Motor unit and muscle activity in voluntary motor control, *Physiol Rev* 63:387–436, 1983.

68. Petrofsky JS: *Isometric exercise and its clinical implications,* Springfield, Ill, 1982, Charles C Thomas.

69. Sugai N, Worsley R, Payne JP: Tetanic force development of adductor pollicis muscle in anesthetized man, *J Appl Physiol* 39:714–717, 1975.

70. Currier DP, Lehman J, Lightfoot P: Electrical Stimulation in exercise of the quadriceps femoris muscle, *Phys Ther* 59:1508-1512, 1979.

71. Bohannon RW: Effect of electrical stimulation to the vastus medialis muscle in a patient with chronically dislocating patellae: a case report, *Phys Ther* 63:1445–1447, 1983.

72. Kramer JF, et al: Comparison of voluntary and electrical stimulation contraction torques, *J Orthop Sports Phys Ther* 5:324–331, 1984.

73. Edwards RHT, Hill DK, Jones DA: Heat production and chemical changes during isometric contraction of the human quadriceps muscle, *J Physiol (Lond)* 251:303–315, 1975.

74. Halbach JW, Straus D: Comparison of electro-myo-stimulation to isokinetic training in increasing power of the knee extensor mechanism, *J Orthop Sports Phys Ther* 2:20–24, 1980.

75. Walmsley RP, Letts G, Vooys J: A comparison of torque generated by knee extension with maximal voluntary muscle contraction vis-à-vis electrical stimulation, *J Orthop Sports Phys Ther* 6:10–17, 1984.

76. Kramer JF, Semple JE: Comparison of selected strengthening techniques for normal quadriceps, *Physiother Can* 35:300–304, 1983.

77. Johnson DH, Thurston P, Ashcroft PJ: The Russian technique of faradism in the treatment of chondromalacia patellae, *Physiother Can* 29:266–268, 1977.

78. McMiken DF, Todd-Smith M, Thompson C: Strengthening of human quadriceps muscles by cutaneous electrical stimulation, *Scand J Rehabil Med* 15:25–28, 1983.

79. Cox AM, et al: Effect of electrode placement and rest interval between contractions on isometric knee extension torques induced by electrical stimulation at 100 Hz, *Physiother Can* 38:20–27, 1986.

80. Lainey CG, Walmsley RP, Andrew GM: Effectiveness of exercise alone versus exercise plus electrical stimulation in strengthening the quadriceps muscle, *Physiother Can* 35:5–11, 1983.

81. Romero JA, et al: The effects of electrical stimulation of normal quadriceps on strength and girth, *Med Sci Sports Exerc* 14:194–197, 1982.

82. Selkowitz DM: Improvement in isometric strength of the quadriceps femoris muscle after training with electrical stimulation, *Phys Ther* 65:186–196, 1985.

83. Laughman RK, et al: Strength changes in the normal quadriceps femoris muscle as a result of electrical stimulation, *Phys Ther* 63:494–499, 1983.

84. Owens J, Malone T: Treatment parameters of high frequency electrical stimulation as established on the Electro-Stim 180, *J Orthop Sports Phys Ther* 4:162–168, 1983.

85. Hartsell HD: Electrical muscle stimulation and isometric exercise effects on selected quadriceps parameters, *J Orthop Sports Phys Ther* 8:203–209, 1986.

86. Nobbs LA, Rhodes EC: The effect of electrical stimulation and isokinetic exercise on muscular power of the quadriceps femoris, *J Orthop Sports Phys Ther* 8:260–268, 1986.

87. Wolf SL, et al: The effect of muscle stimulation during resistive training on performance parameters, *Am J Sports Med* 14:18–23, 1986.

88. Kramer JF: Effect of electrical stimulation current frequencies on isometric knee extension torque, *Phys Ther* 67:31–38, 1987.

89. Currier DP, Mann P: Muscular strength development by electrical stimulation in healthy individuals, *Phys Ther* 63:915–921, 1983.

90. Ikai M: Training of muscle strength and power in athletes, *Br J Sports Med* 7:43–47, 1973.

91. Berger RA, Hardage B: Effect of maximum loads for each of ten repetitions on strength improvement, *Res Quarterly* 38:715–718, 1967.

92. Knuttgen HG: *Development of muscular strength and endurance.* In Knuttgen HG, editor: *Neuromuscular mechanisms for therapeutic and conditioning exercise,* Baltimore, 1976, University Park Press.

93. Delitto A, et al: Electrical stimulation versus voluntary exercise in strengthening thigh musculature after anterior cruciate ligament surgery, *Phys Ther* 68:660–663, 1988.

94. Kelly MJ, Lieber RL: Human quadriceps muscle fatigue at three frequencies and two duty cycles using electrical stimulation, *Trans ORS* 16:41, 1991.

95. Soo CL, Currier DP, Threlkeld AJ: Augmenting voluntary torque of healthy muscle by optimization of electrical stimulation, *Phys Ther* 68:333–337, 1988.

96. Atha J: *Strengthening muscles.* In Hutton RS, Miller DI, editors: *Exercise and sport sciences review,* Philadelphia, 1981, Franklin Institute.

97. Ikai M, Yabe K: Training effect of muscular endurance by means of voluntary and electrical stimulation, *Int Z Angew Physiol* 28:55–60, 1969.

98. Selkowitz DM: High frequency electrical stimulation in muscle strengthening, *Am J Sports Med* 17:103–111, 1989.

99. Singer KP: The influence of unilateral electrical muscle stimulation on motor unit activity patterns in atrophic human quadriceps, *Aust J Physiotherapy* 33:31–37, 1986.

100. Sinacore DR, et al: Type II fiber activation with electrical stimulation: a preliminary report, *Phys Ther* 70:416–422, 1990.

101. Arvidsson I: *A study of rehabilitation after knee surgery with special emphasis on pain inhibition on voluntary muscle activation,* PhD thesis, Karolinska Institutet, Stockholm, 1985.

THE ROLE OF PHYSICAL MODALITIES: PART II— THERMAL MODALITIES

Laurie L. Tis

Thermal modalities consist of superficial and deep heating modalities and cryotherapy. These modalities are the most frequently utilized modalities in the clinical setting. Superficial heating modalities include hot packs, warm whirlpool baths, paraffin baths, and fluidotherapy. Hot packs and warm whirlpool baths are the modalities most commonly employed in knee rehabilitation. Practical discussion is limited to those modalities, but physiologic effects apply to any of the superficial heating modalities. Deep heating modalities include ultrasound and the diathermies. Diathermies are rarely utilized, so all discussion of the deep heating modalities is limited to ultrasound. *Cryotherapy* is an umbrella term that refers to any modality capable of tissue cooling. This includes superficial tissue ice packs, ice massage, and cold whirlpools.

SUPERFICIAL HEATING MODALITIES

Superficial heating modalities, such as hot packs and warm whirlpool baths, heat superficial tissue layers, with a depth of penetration limited to 1 to 2 cm. The maximum depth of penetration is dependent upon variables such as the type of heat applied, duration of treatment, area to be treated, and size of the area to be treated.[1,2] The use of hot packs and warm whirlpool baths is common because this modality is convenient, inexpensive, and very soothing to the patient.

Physiologic effects

Effects of superficial heating modalities include metabolic changes, neuromuscular changes, vascular changes, and connective tissue changes. Metabolic changes occur in any tissue with a change in tissue temperature. This change is due to the "Q_{10} effect," where an elevation in tissue temperature of 10°C results in a doubling of the rate of metabolic activity, within physiologic limits.[3] Small changes in tissue temperature with the use of hot packs or warm whirlpool baths result in local temperature elevation and increase local metabolism. In order to elicit the physiologic effects discussed, local tissue temperature must be elevated to 40 to 45°C.[4]

Vascular changes occur with the application of heat in the form of vasodilation. Vasodilation occurs both at the skin and skeletal muscle tissue layers.[1] The responses of the two tissues must be addressed individually because the changes are due to different mechanisms and vary in terms of the degree of effect. Increased blood flow in the skin occurs because of a local axon reflex,[5] chemical mediator release (bradykinin, prostaglandin, and histamine) due to a mild inflammatory response, and local spinal cord reflexes that relax smooth muscle tissue.[6] Additionally, heating of a large area, such as the quadriceps, results in indirect vasodilation of distal areas through this spinal cord reflex.[7,8] Superficial heat produces little change in skeletal muscle blood flow.[5]

The application of superficial heating modalities induces neuromuscular changes, including the alteration of the pain threshold, nerve conduction velocity, and muscle spindle activity. It has been observed that heat increases the pain threshold.[9] Although the mechanism for this response is not well documented, it is hypothesized that this response is related to the gate control theory of pain modification.[10] Similarly, an increase in tissue temperature also results in an increase in nerve conduction velocity. The advantages or disadvantages of an increase in nerve conduction velocity have not been established, but may be related to the increased pain threshold observed with the application of superficial heat.[11,12] Changes in muscle spindle activity have also been documented with the application of superficial heat. Heating has been established to alter the firing rate of the γ-efferent fibers,[13] which would decrease the stretch on the muscle spindle. This indirectly results in a decrease in the firing rate of the α-motoneuron. This may account for the typically observed relaxation of a muscle spasm with the application of a hot pack or warm whirlpool.[13-15]

Connective tissue changes may also be elicited with tissue temperature increases. A complication associated with injury requiring prolonged immobilization is connective tissue shortening (joint contracture). This, in addition to the formation of adhesions and scar tissue, can result in significant loss of range of motion. When connective tissue temperature is elevated to between 40 and 45°C, in conjunction with a gradual stretch, elongation occurs.[15-17] This effect on connective tissue may also be beneficial in the symptomatic treatment of joint stiffness in patients with arthritis.

Indications for the use of superficial heat

Superficial heat is an appropriate modality for any subacute or chronic condition or any situation that the desired effects would be to increase range of motion, increase tissue healing, decrease pain, or decrease muscular spasm.

Methods of application

Hot packs are kept in a water cabinet, which is maintained at a temperature of 71.1°C. The hot packs are removed and wrapped in several layers of toweling or placed in a hot pack cover and then placed on the area to be treated. It is important that the hot pack be placed on the patient, rather than the patient on the hot pack, in order to avoid excessive heating. A hot pack size should be chosen appropriate to the size of the area being treated. Typically, a hot pack maintains its heat for the duration of the desired treatment (20 to 30 minutes). The hot pack is then returned to the water cabinet and reheats in approximately 30 minutes.

It is important to position the patient properly in order to maximize the effects of hot packs. When a muscle group is the target tissue, this group should be put on a gentle stretch during the time the heat pack is applied. Similarly, when heating the anterior knee (i.e., patellar tendon, infrapatellar bursae, or patellar fat pad), the knee should be flexed slightly (15 to 30 degrees) to increase the amount of exposed target tissue (Fig. 6-1). Likewise, when targeting the popliteal space, the patient should be in the prone position, with the knee in extension.

Warm whirlpools are often considered the superficial heat agent of choice because, in addition to the warmth effects, the whirlpool agitation creates a mechanical massaging effect, stimulating skin receptors and potentially decreasing pain more effectively than hot packs. Additionally, range-of-motion exercises can be performed while in the whirlpool, potentially enhancing the therapeutic effects of the tissue temperature increase and the exercises. The recommended temperature range for a warm whirlpool is 36.5 to

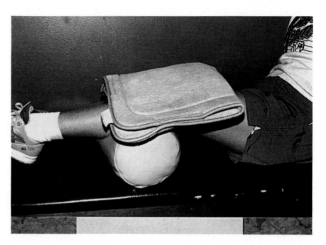

Fig. 6-1. Knee flexed to 15 to 30 degrees during hot pack application.

40.5°C when the body is not fully immersed. The patient should perceive a sensation of moderate warmth, but not burning or excessive heating.

Contraindications and precautions

Contraindications to the use of superficial heat include areas of malignancy and areas of uncontrolled bleeding and hemorrhaging. Similarly, if a patient is taking medication that may affect vascular wall strength, superficial heat is not the modality of choice. Precautions should be taken when making the decision to utilize superficial heating modalities in areas of impaired sensation or impaired vascular circulation.

THERAPEUTIC ULTRASOUND

The effects and indications for ultrasound are very similar to those of the superficial heating agents, but ultrasound has the advantage of heating tissue at depths of 3 to 5 cm. Clinical ultrasound units produce soundwaves at frequencies of 1, 2, or 3 mHz. These soundwaves are generated from a solid crystal, located in the head of the ultrasound applicator. The application of electricity to the crystal results in the production of soundwaves via the reverse piezoelectric effect. Most ultrasound units are capable of producing ultrasonic energy in a continuous or pulsed mode, with an intensity range of 0 to 2 watts per square centimeter (w/cm²).

Physiologic effects

Ultrasound is capable of producing both thermal and nonthermal physiologic effects. When ultrasound is used in a continuous mode, both thermal and nonthermal effects are elicited, whereas pulsed ultrasound elicits only nonthermal effects.

Thermal. The thermal effects of ultrasound are the same as those of the superficial heating modalities, including:
1. Increased collagen tissue extensibility[15,16]

2. Increased local blood flow[17,18]
3. Increased nerve conduction velocity[19-21]
4. Decreased sensation of pain[9,12,13]
5. Increased local metabolism[3,4]
6. Change in the contractile activity of skeletal muscle[13,14]

The physiologic changes elicited by continuous ultrasound are temperature-dependent, with changes occurring with tissue temperature increased to 40 to 45°C.[4] These physiologic alterations depend on the frequency, duration, and intensity at which ultrasound is applied and on the structures involved. At a frequency of 3 mHz, ultrasound penetrates to a depth of 1 to 2 cm, whereas at a frequency of 1 mHz, penetration can achieve depths up to 5 cm. Duration of ultrasound application is also a factor in tissue temperature increases. A direct relationship exists between the duration application and degree of tissue temperature increase, with prolonged exposure potentially leading to excessive tissue temperature elevation. The intensity of ultrasound application is also directly related to the degree of heating that occurs in any given structure. Absorption of ultrasonic energy is related to the amount of collagen present in a tissue. The higher the collagen content, the greater the absorption of ultrasonic energy. Hence, ultrasound is absorbed by blood, fat, muscle, blood vessels, skin, tendon, cartilage, and bone in least to greatest amounts, respectively. Ultrasound is best utilized to heat periarticular structures and muscle-bone junctions.[22-24]

Nonthermal. The primary nonthermal effects of ultrasound are cavitation and acoustical streaming. *Cavitation* is the vibration of gas bubbles by the ultrasonic waves. Cell function can be altered by the expansion and compression, within physiologic limits, of the gas bubbles that result from this vibration. However, research has not established which, if any, of the nonthermal effects of ultrasound are due to cavitation.[20,22]

Acoustical streaming is defined as the movement of fluid along cell membranes due to the force of the ultrasound beam creating a "wave" effect. This acoustical streaming has been credited with increasing cell and vessel wall permeability.[25] Increased protein synthesis, calcium ion flux, decreased nerve conduction velocity, and increased blood flow have also been documented. Although pulsed ultrasound is nonthermal in nature, the aforementioned effects are intensity-dependent.[26-28] The intensity of pulsed ultrasound should remain below 1.5 w/cm[2] to avoid adverse effects.

Indications for the use of ultrasound

A variety of conditions respond favorably to the adjunctive use of therapeutic ultrasound. Ultrasound is an appropriate modality for any subacute or chronic condition.

Contraindications and precautions

Contraindications for the use of ultrasound include administration over the eyes, heart, pregnant uterus, and genitals. Ultrasound should not be administered to malignant tissue or to an individual who has thrombophlebitis. Ultrasound should be only cautiously administered to areas of impaired pain and temperature sensation, areas of reduced or impaired circulation, and epiphyseal plates. Caution must also be used when administering ultrasound to an artificial joint.

Method of application

When utilizing ultrasound as an adjunctive therapy, several decisions must be made in regard to proper application. These decisions include selection of a conductive medium, selection of the size of the ultrasound head, and selection of the treatment time, frequency, and intensity. Ultrasonic energy waves do not travel well in air and therefore require a conductive medium. This conductive medium (coupling agent) is typically either a gel or water. Gel is spread evenly and moderately in the area to be treated. Although ultrasound can also be administered in water, this would not be an appropriate technique for treatment of the knee. The submersion technique is best utilized in areas such as the feet and hands.

Ultrasound units have heads in the sizes of 1, 5, and 10 cm[2]. The size of head selected is dependent upon the area to be treated. A general rule is that the area to be treated should not be more than four times the size of the ultrasound head. For example, the quadriceps musculature is large, and a 10-cm[2] head would be ideal, whereas the distal patellar tendon region may be best treated with the 1-cm[2] head.

After the size of the head has been selected, the frequency, intensity, and duration of the treatment application must be determined. As has been previously noted, frequency selection would be determined by the depth of penetration desired. For example, the quadriceps musculature would be treated at a frequency of 1 mHz. The intensity is adjusted to the desired level (0.5 to 1.5 w/cm[2]). Intensity is proportionately determined by the amount of tissue heating desired and the amount and depth of tissue being treated. The patient should never feel more than a mild warming effect in the area to be treated. More than a gentle warming is indicative of excessive tissue heating. The ultrasound treatment time is set, with the general guidelines for duration being 5 minutes per 3- by 5-inch area or an area 3-4 times the size of the ultrasound head.

The position of the patient is also an important consideration when utilizing ultrasound. The effect of ultrasound can be maximized if the target tissue is maximally exposed. For example, when treating an anterior patellar structure, the knee should be slightly flexed. If one of the desired effects of ultrasound is the elongation of muscle or connective tissue, this tissue should be gently stretched during the application of the ultrasound treatment (Fig. 6-2). It is imperative that proper positioning techniques be used when applying any modality; otherwise, the effects of the modality will not be optimal.

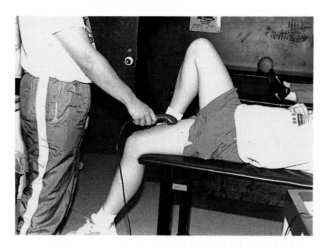

Fig. 6-2. Rectus femoris on a gentle stretch during ultrasound application.

CRYOTHERAPY

Cryotherapy refers to any physical agent capable of cooling superficial or articular structures. It includes ice packs, cold packs, cold immersion, and ice massage. Cryotherapy is commonly employed in acute injury situations. During the normal course of injury repair and tissue healing, cryotherapy is also employed as an adjunct therapy to therapeutic exercise. The use of ice, in so many situations, is based upon the physiologic effects of cryotherapy and tissue cooling.

Physiologic effects

The effects of cold can largely be summarized as the opposite of the effects of tissue temperature increases as induced by superficial and deep heating modalities. Cold decreases local tissue and joint temperatures. Decreased local tissue temperature leads to local vasoconstriction, decreased metabolism, and decreased sensation of pain.

Short-duration cold exposure results in the vasoconstriction of arterioles and venules. This response is due to several interrelated factors. Cold directly causes a contraction of smooth muscle. Cold also causes a reflex vasoconstriction of cutaneous blood vessels, a physiologic "heat conservation" response. It is due to numerous local reflex mechanisms and a hypothalamic response to cooled blood in general circulation.[6,29,30] It should also be noted that extreme cold or prolonged exposure to cold results in vasodilation. This vasodilation may or may not by cyclical in nature. Cyclical vasodilation is also referred to as the *hunting response*. Cyclic vasodilation and vasoconstriction has been observed to follow cooling in excess of 15 minutes.[31,32]

The application of cold also induces neural adaptations. Cold decreases nerve conduction velocity in small-diameter, unmyelinated nerve fibers. This decreased nerve conduction velocity results in decreased pain sensation. This decreased

sensation of pain may effectively break into the pain-spasm-pain cycle that is typically observed in any injury.[33-35]

Indications

A variety of conditions may positively respond to the application of ice. Conditions specific to the knee include
1. Any acute injury to the knee
2. Any situation that has caused a resumption in the inflammatory response or local swelling
3. Knee extensor and flexor musculature strains and spasms
4. Bursitis (prepatellar, pes anserine, suprapatellar, infrapatellar)
5. Tendonitis (patellar, pes anserine)
6. Contusions

This list is merely a suggested group of injuries that often respond well to cryotherapy. Cryotherapy is the modality of choice in an acute injury and an appropriate adjunctive modality for any subacute or chronic condition.

In an acute injury, ice helps to *prevent* the formation and accumulation of edema. Following any acute trauma due to tissue damage at the cellular level, excess free proteins are present in the extracellular space. This change in the concentration of proteins in the extracellular space, in turn, causes more fluid to leave the capillaries than is resorbed, leading to an accumulation of excess edema at the injury site.[6] Some edema formation is inevitable and is the result of the primary tissue damage. However, excess edema limits the amount of oxygen in the area, potentially leading to secondary tissue damage from hypoxia. This tissue damage in turn leads to an increase in the number of free proteins in the extracellular space, continuing the destructive cycle related to edema formation. Ice application has the potential to limit the amount of secondary tissue trauma related to hypoxia because cooling of local tissue decreases local cellular metabolism, which decreases the oxygen requirement of the local cells and limits the amount of cell death related to hypoxia.

Contraindications and precautions

As with any modality, there are conditions that would contraindicate the use of cryotherapy, and there are conditions that would warrant caution when using any form of ice application. Contraindications to the use of cryotherapy include peripheral vascular disease and areas of decreased sensation or circulation. Ice should not be applied over open wounds.

Care must be taken when using cryotherapy with a person with cold sensitivity, cold allergies, or Raynaud's phenomenon. Some individuals with these conditions can tolerate ice application and others cannot. Elevated blood pressure is also a precaution to treating with cryotherapy. Prolonged cold exposure should also be avoided in areas of superficial peripheral nerves. In the knee, this would specifically involve the common peroneal nerve as it crosses the head of the fibula. Unfortunately, there are several reported case studies where common peroneal nerve palsy has been the result of inappropriate ice application to the lateral aspect of the knee joint.[36-38] To avoid damage to the skin or underlying tissue from cold therapy, ice or cold packs should be used intermittently for no longer than 10 to 15 minutes at a time and the area to be cooled should be padded with a towel or dressing. Avoid placing a cold pack directly on the skin.

Methods of application

Several common methods of cryotherapy are available and easily employed. Cold packs are the most common method of cold application. Cold packs come in the commercially prepared and reusable form, ice packs, and instant cold packs. Commercial cold packs are stored in a freezer and kept at −15°C. Ice packs are easily made with crushed or cubed ice and a plastic bag. Fill the bag approximately half full with ice, evacuate the air from the bag, and tie a knot at the open end of the bag. A small to moderate amount of water can also be added to the ice (enough to create a slush), particularly to cubes, to increase the ease at which the ice bag will form with the contours of the body. Chemical instant cold packs are also available. These packs are single use, and a blow to the bag will mix the chemicals, causing a cooling mixture to form. These packs do not get very cold or maintain their temperature for very long. Because of the thermal limitations, the fact that the packs often break and cause chemical burns, and the expense, these packs are not ideal. However, if no other form of ice is available, they are better than nothing.

When using any of the three types of cold packs, it is important to position the patient properly in order to maximize the cooling effects. When treating an acute injury, it is important to elevate the knee. When treating an acute muscle injury it is often helpful to put the muscle on a gentle stretch during the time the cold pack is applied. When cooling the patellar tendon, infrapatellar bursae, or patellar fat pad, the knee can be flexed slightly (15 to 30 degrees) to increase the amount of exposed target tissue (Fig. 6-3). Likewise, to target the popliteal space, the patient should be in the prone position, with the knee in extension. When using commercial cold packs, place several layers of toweling between the skin and the cold pack because the temperature of the commercial cold pack is well below the freezing point.

Cold immersion is another form of cryotherapy that is commonly seen in the clinical setting. The whirlpool is filled with cold water and cooled to approximately 13 to 18°C. This temperature is just a suggested range as the tolerance to cold varies greatly among individuals. The patient should feel a moderate cooling effect, achieving analgesia within several minutes. In addition to the cooling effect, the whirlpool agitation creates a mechanical massaging effect, stimulating skin receptors and potentially decreasing pain. Because of the decreased pain, muscle spasms may relax, facilitating range-of-motion exercises that can be performed in the whirlpool.

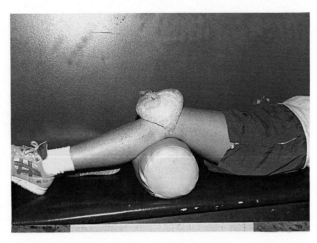

Fig. 6-3. Knee flexed to 15 to 30 degrees during ice pack application.

Because the patient in a cold whirlpool is in the dependent position, this form of cryotherapy may not be the method of choice in an acute knee injury where edema formation is expected. The cold whirlpool may be an appropriate choice for a subacute or chronic injury with minimal edema formation or when minimal edema formation is expected with the acute injury. The primary advantage of cold immersion is that it provides consistent, circumferential tissue cooling of the entire region, whereas the area of application is limited when using cold packs.

Treatment time for cold packs or cold immersion is the typical 15 to 20 minutes. During the cryotherapy process, the individual experiences four sensations: intense cold, burning, aching, and analgesia. Analgesia is achieved after several minutes, but moderate discomfort prior to analgesia is typical.

Ice massage is another common form of cryotherapy that is frequently utilized in the clinical setting. A medium-sized paper or styrofoam cup is filled with water and frozen. When needed, the cup is taken out of the freezer, and the paper or styrofoam is peeled away, exposing approximately 1 cm of ice. This is then massaged in a circular motion over the involved area (Fig. 6-4). As the ice melts, continue to peel away the paper or styrofoam. Analgesia is achieved in several minutes. The ice massage treatment should be performed for a minimum of 10 minutes. Typical patient positioning guidelines, as have been previously discussed, should be carefully followed.

Because cryotherapy is the modality of choice in any acute injury, it is often used in conjunction with compression. The use of compression is very effective in both preventing and reducing edema formation and hence can effectively be utilized in the treatment of both acute and subacute injuries. The use of compression in the prevention of edema formation and in the reduction of edema already present is the result of increasing the lymphatic and venous flow through mechanical increases in pressure, forcing the

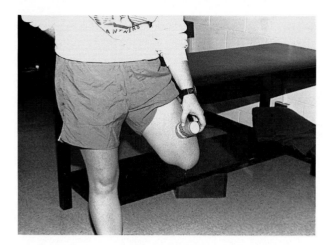

Fig. 6-4. Ice massage application to the quadriceps.

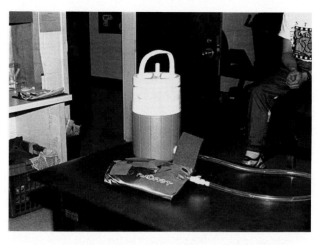

Fig. 6-5. Cryo/Cuff unit with knee attachment.

edema out of the area.[39-41] Compression can be applied through an elastic wrap applied around the cold pack, or several commercial compression devices are currently on the market. Pneumatic compression devices utilize a sleeve attached to a hose that will apply intermittent pressure, using either air or cold water. The devices using air are placed on the limb, with cold packs placed between the skin and the compression sleeve. Another simple commercial device, the Cryo/Cuff, has recently come into wide use in many settings. This device uses a thermal container filled with ice water that is elevated above the limb. The bottom spout is attached to a hose that runs to a compression sleeve. The sleeve is placed around the knee, and the water runs into the sleeve, resulting in even, circumferential cooling and compression (Figs. 6-5 and 6-6). This device is simple to use and inexpensive and provides very effective compression and cooling.

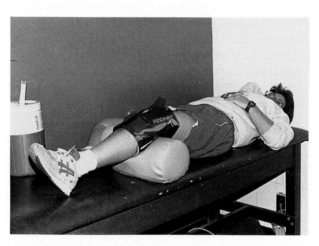

Fig. 6-6. Cryo/Cuff unit applied to an acutely injured knee.

SUMMARY

The thermal modalities have physiologic effects including a change in local tissue metabolism, vascular adaptations to temperature changes, changes in neuromuscular responses, and changes in connective tissue pliability. The superficial and deep heating modalities have similar physiologic responses related to an increase in tissue temperature. However, these changes occur at different tissue levels because of the depth of penetration of the two types of physical heating agents. When selecting a modality, the physiologic effects and desired treatment outcomes must be determined prior to initiation of any modality of use.

When using these modalities, it is imperative to understand the nature of the injury and the physiologic effects of the modalities. Then the modality choice is based upon the desired therapeutic outcomes and treatment goals. When physical agents are used randomly, without regard to physiology or treatment goals, optimal treatment effects are not elicited. Likewise, proper application and patient position-

ing guidelines must be observed in order to maximize the effects of the modality. It is also important to remember that any physical agent is to be used as an adjunct to a total rehabilitation program. All too often, the modality is viewed as the rehabilitation program.

REFERENCES

1. Abramson DI, et al: Changes in blood flow, oxygen uptake and tissue temperature produced by the topical application of wet heat, *Arch Phys Med Rehabil* 42:305, 1961.
2. Lehmann JF, et al: Temperature distributions in the human thigh produced by infrared, hot pack and microwave applications, *Arch Phys Med Rehabil* 47:291, 1966.
3. Brooks GA, and Foley TD: *Exercise physiology: human bioenergetics and its applications,* New York, 1985, Macmillan.
4. Lehmann JF, Delateur BJ: *Therapeutic heat.* In Lehmann JF, editor: *Therapeutic heat and cold,* ed 4, Baltimore, 1990, Williams & Wilkins.
5. Crockford GW, Hellon RF: Vascular responses of human skin to infrared radiation, *J Physiol* 149:424, 1959.
6. Guyton AC: *Textbook of medical physiology,* ed 7, Philadelphia, 1986, WB Saunders.

7. Abramson DI, et al: Indirect vasodilation in thermotherapy, *Arch Phys Med Rehabil* 46:412, 1965.

8. Wessman MS, Kottke FJ: The effect of indirect heating or peripheral blood flow, pulse rate, blood pressure and temperature, *Arch Phys Med Rehabil* 48:567, 1967.

9. Lehmann JF, Brunner GD, Stow RW: Pain threshold measurements after therapeutic application of ultra sound, microwaves, and infrared, *Arch Phys Med Rehabil* 39:560, 1958.

10. Prentice WE: *Therapeutic modalities in sports medicine*, ed 2, St Louis, 1990, Mosby–Year Book.

11. Abramson DI, et al: Effect of temperatures and blood flow on motor nerve conduction velocity, *JAMA* 198:1082, 1966.

12. Halle JS, Scoville CR, Greathouse DG: Ultrasound's effect on the conduction latency of the superficial radial nerve in man, *Phys Ther* 61:345, 1981.

13. Fisher E, Solomon S: *Physiological responses to heat and cold.* In Licht S, editor: *Therapeutic heat and cold,* ed 2, Baltimore, 1965, Waverly.

14. Michlovitz SL: *Thermal agents: rehabilitation,* ed 2, Philadelphia, 1990, FA Davis.

15. Lehmann JF: Effect of therapeutic temperatures on tendon extensibility, *Arch Phys Med Rehabil* 51:481, 1970.

16. Warren GC, Lehmann JF, Koblanski JN: Heat and stretch procedures: an evaluation using rat tail tendon, *Arch Phys Med Rehabil* 57:122, 1976.

17. Paul ED, Imig CJ: Temperature and blood flow studies after ultrasonic irradiation, *Am J Phys Med* 34:370, 1955.

18. Abramson DI, et al: Changes in blood flow, oxygen uptake and tissue temperatures produced by therapeutic physical agents, I: effect of ultrasound, *Am J Phys Med* 39:51, 1960.

19. Currier DP, Greathouse D, Swift T: Sensory nerve conduction: effect of ultrasound, *Arch Phys Med Rehabil* 59:181, 1978.

20. Halle JS, Scoville CR, Greathouse DG: Ultrasound's effect on the conduction latency of superficial radial nerve in man, *Phys Ther* 61:345, 1981.

21. Kramer JF: Ultrasound: evaluation of its mechanical and thermal effects, *Arch Phys Med Rehabil* 65:223, 1984.

22. Lehmann JF, et al: Heating of joint structures by ultrasound, *Arch Phys Med Rehabil* 49:28, 1968.

23. Lehmann JF, et al: Heating produced by ultrasound in bone and soft tissue, *Arch Phys Med Rehabil* 48:397, 1968.

24. Lehmann JF, et al: Therapeutic temperature distribution produced by ultrasound as modified by dosage and release of tissue exposed, *Arch Phys Med Rehabil* 48:662, 1967.

25. Lota MJ, Darling RC: Change in permeability of the red blood cell membrane in a homogeneous ultrasonic field, *Arch Phys Med Rehabil* 36:282, 1955.

26. Harvey W, et al: The simulation of protein synthesis in human fibroblasts by therapeutic ultrasound, *Rheumatol Rehabil* 14:237, 1975.

27. Lehmann JF, Biegler R: Changes of potentials and temperature gradients in membranes caused by ultrasound, *Arch Phys Med Rehabil* 35:287, 1954.

28. Hogan RD, Burke KM, Franklin TD: The effect of ultrasound on microvascular hemodynamics in skeletal muscle: effects during ischemia, *Microvasc Res* 23:370, 1982.

29. Perkins J, et al: Cooling and contraction of smooth muscle, *Am J Physiol* 163:14, 1950.

30. Cobbold AF, Lewis OJ: Blood flow to the knee joint of the dog: effect of heating, cooling, and adrenaline, *J Physiol (Lond)* 132:379, 1956.

31. Fox RH, Wyatt HT: Cold induced vasodilation in various areas of the body surface in man, *J Physiol (Lond)* 162:289, 1962.

32. Lewis T: Observation upon the reactions of the vessels of the human skin to cold, *Heart* 15:177, 1930.

33. Douglas WW, Malcolm JL: The effect of localized cooling on conduction in cat nerves, *J Physiol (Lond)* 130:53, 1955.

34. Zankel HT: Effect of physical agents on motor conduction velocity of the ulnar nerve, *Arch Phys Med Rehabil* 47:787, 1966.

35. Li C-L: Effect of cooling on neuromuscular transmission in the rat, *Am J Physiol* 194:200, 1958.

36. Collins KI, Storey M, Peterson K: Peroneal nerve palsy of cryotherapy, *Physician Sports Med* 14:105, 1986.

37. Basset FH, et al: Cryotherapy-induced nerve injury, *Am J Sports Med* 20:516–518, 1992.

38. Malone TR, et al: Nerve injury in athletes caused by cryotherapy, *J Athletic Training* 27:235–237, 1992.

39. Starkey J: Treatment of ankle sprain by simultaneous use of intermittent compression and ice pack, *Am J Sport Med* 4:142, 1976.

40. Quillen WS, Rouillier LH: Initial management of acute ankle sprains with rapid pulsed pneumatic compression and cold, *JOSPT* 4:39, 1982.

41. Sloan J, Giddings P, Hain R: Effects of cold and compression on edema, *Physician Sports Med* 8:116, 1988.

Chapter 7

EXERCISE AND ASSESSMENT EQUIPMENT FOR THE KNEE: APPROPRIATE USE AND FUNCTION

Terry R. Malone
William E. Garrett, Jr

This chapter is designed to provide a "framework of evaluation" for clinicians to review exercise and assessment equipment that may be used in rehabilitation of the patient afflicted with a knee disorder. It is important to recognize the actual impact of knee pathology on lower extremity function. Unfortunately, many of the traditional concepts of strength and function are not as specific and synonymous as we would like to believe. In fact, strength assessment is often not the measurement of muscular ability but rather a level of neurologic drive or inhibition. We frequently discuss function but recognize the limitations presented by multiple joint actions (closed kinetic chain patterns) versus single joint actions (open kinetic chain) as being more appropriate for assessment. Thus, in this chapter we present basic exercise concepts and information regarding the proper application of exercise equipment and its integrated applications involving assessment and relationship to dysfunction.

BASIC CONCEPTS

Muscle performance is a difficult entity to evaluate, requiring operational definitions of specific parameters if appropriate communication is to be accomplished. The muscle-tendon unit is composed of active (contractile element) and passive (noncontractile connective tissue) structures. A definition of strength is typically based on the maximal level of output an individual can generate through the contractile element. Although this first appears relatively simplistic, the measurement occurs secondarily (through the skeletal system) rather than primarily (tension generated within the muscle tendon unit) and as such allows alteration of tension within muscle versus measured output to be the product. (Although muscle may function optimally when slightly stretched, the maximal torque seen occurs in the middle of the available range of motion because skeletal leverage and length tension ratios interact.) Different muscles vary greatly in their capacity to produce force and thus to shorten, with a basic rule of cross-sectional area of muscle fiber being directly related to force generation capacity.[14,15] Also related to maximal output is the orientation or architectural arrangement of the muscle fibers within the specific muscle assessed. Alterations in architecture produce a unique characteristic for a specific muscle, as it may increase the given number of fibers in a cross-sectional area but may decrease the length of the tissue, thus providing greater force but lessening the range of motion in which the muscle may be functional.[6,22]

Unfortunately, clinicians frequently do not recognize the importance of neural control of the muscle when they attempt to assess maximal output (strength) or functional ability. The central nervous system (CNS) drive may be tremendously limited by pain, apprehension, swelling, effusion, or other factors. Thus clinicians are not assessing a fully activated muscular component but one inhibited through a lack of neural drive.[18,25]

Three basic forms of muscle activation occur and can be measured through clinical means. We recommend the terminology *muscle activation,* and the action or response is isometric (maintenance of position, stabilizer), concentric (shortening with a resultant movement), or eccentric (lengthening or controlled lowering). Thus the resultant action is a balance between what is applied to the system and what the system applies in return. Assessment of these actions can be accomplished through a variety of means, ranging from manual techniques to mechanical dynamometers. Each system or technique has specific strengths and weaknesses.

ISOMETRIC ASSESSMENT

Most commonly applied clinical assessments are through manual muscle testing (MMT), which is used to provide a screen of the patient presenting with musculoskeletal dysfunction. It involves an isometric contraction typically performed in the middle of the available range of motion at a specific joint. It requires a skillful practitioner and attention to detail to allow replication. Because it is isometric, an obvious limitation involves lack of dynamic action, which requires the synchronous action of multiple muscle groups to provide movement as well as proximal stabilization. It also is somewhat range-specific (only one position in the length-tension ratio) and does not assess how quickly or how often (endurance). Also, the interrater reliability is relatively low, particularly for assessing maximal efforts of large muscle groups.[20]

Handheld dynamometry has been developed in an attempt to add objectivity to the existing manual techniques. Reliability and quantification of these devices are quite acceptable for most clinical settings, and this technique does minimize some of the limitations previously described.[2] If clinicians are utilizing handheld dynamometers, we recommend multiple test positions, thus allowing capabilities to be assessed at different points of the range of motion, as well as in different functional positions.

ISOTONIC ASSESSMENT

Frequently referred to as *weightlifting,* isotonic assessment involves a controlled movement of a weight through a range of motion. Limiting factors for this activity include a person's ability to recruit and coordinate muscle activity via neural action, appropriate integrity of the ligamentous supports for a specific joint, and stabilization allowing controlled actions over a fixed extremity or trunk during action. As in isometric assessment, it is imperative to recognize the importance of skeletal leverage in the assessment procedure (in that the distance the weight is placed distal to the axis of rotation is responsible for the effect of loading as it multiplies the weight applied). Biomechanically weak positions within the specific range of motion limit the load that can be placed on the extremity and force the concentric lifting action to be maximally stressful only at the specific point. This forces the remainder of the range of motion to be submaximal in activation and demand. It must be recognized that concentric action (the lifting of the weight) provides information concerning the contractile element but does not provide a maximal assessment of the other soft tissue structures involved with eccentric action. To do a

maximal assessment of the isotonic capabilities of the muscle tendon unit thus requires a concentric assessment of the maximal ability to raise the weight through a range of motion, whereas the eccentric involves a higher amount of weight being controllably lowered. Clinicians must also be mindful of always placing the weight the same distance from the axis of rotation and attempting to have the movement occurring at a similar rate of speed. The majority of isotonic assessment occurs at approximately 60 degrees per second, which is one of the limitations in attempting to correlate this assessment to functional movements. Unfortunately, functional patterns are not isolated activities, and the isotonic assessment lacks the integrated activation demands involving a variety of demands, such as isometric stabilization, concentric-generation capacity, and eccentric absorbing-dissipating function.

ISOKINETIC ASSESSMENT

Whereas isotonic movements involve a fixed amount of weight placed on the extremity, isokinetic movements can best be described as a mechanism of controlling the speed of movement as the patient attempts to accelerate the extremity, which is interfaced to a controlling device. Rather than the output of muscle being limited by the provided resistance (weight multiplied by lever arm length), the maximal speed is controlled by a dynamometer; the torque output of the muscle tendon unit varies through the range of motion, with the maximal level dictated by the effort provided through the patient. Dynamometers control the maximal velocity through a variety of techniques with the newer devices allowing both concentric and eccentric evaluation. It is interesting to note that the eccentric activation pattern used through dynamometry assessment might be presenting the central nervous system with unique demands of a different sort than those seen with the typical muscle function in eccentric activation (i.e., the in vivo stretch-shortening cycle; the muscle typically undergoes an eccentric stretch prior to a concentric activation).

Major advantages of isokinetic assessment include the ability to control the function of a specific muscle group through a particular range of motion and joint axis, specific recruitment and speed demands, and the provision of isolated reproducible assessment patterns.[5,13] Data collected through dynamometry should be reviewed on a machine-specific format, as differing manufacturers use specific techniques for gravity correction, point-to-point assessment, and other reliability factors.[22,24] The dynamic assessment provided through isokinetics allows us to assess reliably the ability of the individual to drive (neural activation) maximally a specific muscle group to provide action at a particular joint and exercise pattern. Any direct comparison of this performance and that which occurs during functional activities should be cautious. Interestingly, the aforementioned strength of isokinetics (determination of maximal output at a specific joint) is also the major limitation to applying it to functional activities that involve multiple joints in a variety of sequenced actions. Clinicians are urged not to dismiss the importance of isokinetic assessment in that functional performance may allow a weakened structure to be "substituted for" by a secondary muscle pattern that may be less efficient but readily adapted by the individual.

One of the interesting areas of isokinetic assessment involves the relationship of what is known as the *force-velocity curve*. In concentric actions the maximal torque decreases as the maximal speed of performance increases. There is a significant decrease in torque production at very high speeds, particularly when the movement requires a fairly large body mass to be accelerated to a predetermined maximal speed, thus presenting a steep decrease in peak torque from 60 to 300 degrees per second. The relationship in peak torque and speed is not as inverse in eccentric muscle action. It should be noted that eccentric peak values are always larger than concentric peak torques, but that the slope (decrease in torque related to increasing speed of movement) in peak values is not nearly as steep; thus, eccentric torque-velocity relationships are much more stable over speeds.

SPECIAL EXERCISE MODALITIES

Clinicians have realized that rehabilitation involves much more than pure strengthening and have recently become more functionally oriented.[9,17,21] As this functional approach is utilized, clinicians have increasingly provided a varied demand for muscular action, requiring the patient's neural system to activate and synchronize a broad spectrum of muscular actions. An interesting array of exercise devices has emerged that include combining activities (Fig. 7-1) to facilitate the training of these responses. Although these devices provide different stimuli, their use as testing devices is somewhat questionable. In addition, it should be recog-

nized that the ability of these devices to provide carryover to other functional tasks remains to be proven.

BALANCE TRAINING

Proprioceptive exercise sequences (balance training for the lower extremity) have become an accepted part of most lower extremity rehabilitation programs. Their use is frequently viewed as originating with the work of Freeman and Wyke,[8] who reported on the loss of functional stability to a small group of patients who had experienced ankle sprains. From this original work, many authors have examined a variety of exercise sequences to enhance what is frequently termed *proprioceptive ability*. This term may be unfortunate as the aforementioned proprioception may be only one portion of the total problem for many individuals. We recommend the use of the terms *balance* or *kinesiologic activities*. It is recognized that such exercise activities may lack desired scientific specificity. An advantage to their use, however, is that they are fairly easily accepted by patient and clinician alike.

Several balance devices are used, including single-axis boards (fore and aft, anterior to posterior, and side to side) (Fitter-Slide unit, Fig. 7-2) and multiaxial devices such as the BAPS board (Biomechanical Ankle Platform System, Fig. 7-3), the circular balance board (18- to 20-inch, ¾-inch-thick plywood circle with a hemispheric object centered under the inferior aspect), and the Kinesthetic Awareness Trainer. The KAT system has a multiaxial pivot point similar to the other disks (BAPS and circular balance boards), but also has adjustable pneumatic pressure to alter the stiffness, thus allowing balance activities as well as strengthening activities to be performed. The clinical efficacy of these devices has been shown.[7] Although these devices were initially designed for ankle problems, clinicians

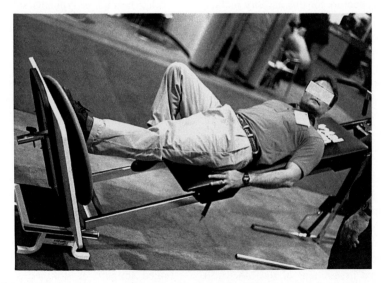

Fig. 7-1. Balance work in a partial weightbearing "closed kinetic chain" exercise pattern.

were quick to realize that patients who have hip and knee injuries can have alterations in balance abilities. Thus, these patients may benefit from such training programs. In fact, balance training has become an accepted part of the majority of protocols for all lower extremity patients.

PLYOMETRICS

Somewhat related to the recent emphasis on balance activities has been the growing use of closed kinetic chain rehabilitation of the lower extremity (Fig. 7-4). Balance and closed kinetic chain movements are synonymous with most functional activities. Komi et al.[11,12] emphasized the importance of eccentric activity with functional patterns and described the stretch-shortening cycle, which allows a potentiated concentric movement preceded by an eccentric stretch.[10] This exercise sequence has become known as *plyometric training* and is often incorporated in rehabilitation programs for athletes involved in jumping activities. As recognition of the worth of plyometrics in lower extremity rehabilitation increased, this exercise technique began to be used in upper extremity rehabilitation as well.

Lower-quarter plyometric programs typically involve depth jumping and normally begin with an emphasis on lower-intensity activities and progress to higher-intensity movements. The depth jumping often begins with jumping from a standing position, followed by performing a rebound jump on landing, and then progresses to jumping from a box to the floor, followed by reciprocal rebound action. Athletes are urged to perform this rebound jump as quickly as possible and the athletes must learn to emphasize quality of movement rather than performing large numbers of repetitions. It is our recommendation that before depth jumping is initiated, in-place jumping into a rebound pattern should be performed with skill and comfort. Often the incorporation of these activities in a preseason sequence can be very beneficial and can decrease some of the early-season acclimatization that may be seen in the less-trained participants in volleyball, basketball, or football. The effectiveness of plyometric activities appears similar to or superior to other training techniques.[3,4]

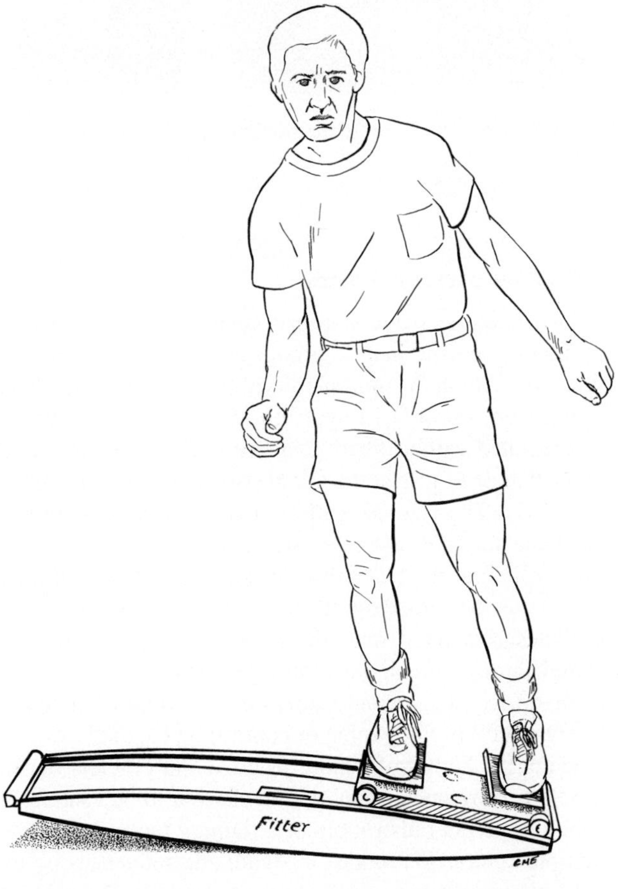

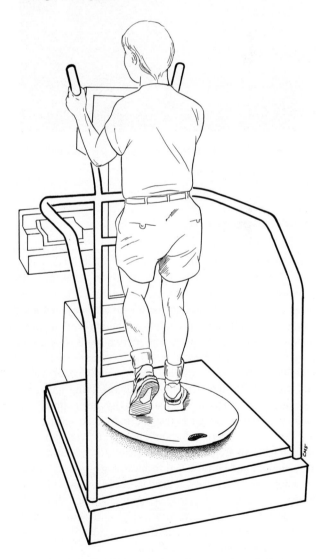

Fig. 7-2. The Fitter exercise unit allowing fore and aft and side-to-side movement patterns in a closed-chain, weightbearing position.

Fig. 7-3. BAPS board adapted to a testing platform.

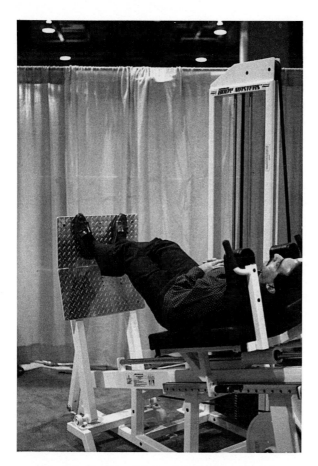

Fig. 7-4. Traditional "closed-chain" leg press unit.

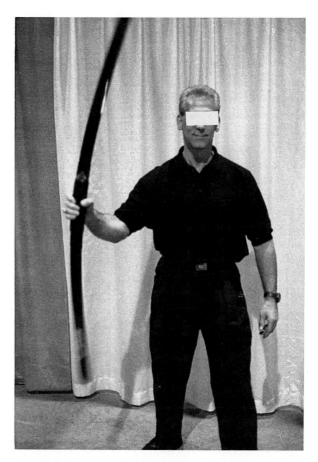

Fig. 7-5. The Body Blade oscillatory exercise device.

INERTIAL TRAINING

The clinical device for training involving inertial loading was developed and introduced to the rehabilitation community as the IMPULSE (EMA, Newnan, Georgia). The impulse simulates the functional momentum activities seen in general activities through the use of a trolley that slides along a horizontal track providing a minimal level of friction but an opportunity for adjustable inertial loads. Contrary to progressive resistance exercise, the progression for the individual using inertial training begins with heavier weights and proceeds to lighter weights, thus involving greater acceleration and shorter times of activity but a higher frequency. The one caveat is that the individual must control the movement pattern and should not be allowed to increase the intensity of training until the pattern is performed in a very smooth and coordinated fashion. Early results of studies using this device show it to be useful as a neural muscular trainer rather than primarily a "strengthening" device.[1] It may be that this device is also useful as a pain modulator when used in oscillatory sequence in a fairly low demand pattern through neural mechanisms.[1]

Oscillatory exercise devices

Two exercise devices utilize oscillatory sequences for training of specific muscle groups as well as requiring stabilization actions of multiple body parts. The Body Blade (Hymanson, Playa Del Ray, California) is a training device of integrated carbon fibers approximately 5 feet in length with a handle or grip at the middle of the length of the blade (Fig. 7-5). The exercise pattern involves the oscillation of the blade forward and rearward in a coordinated pattern. The oscillation is predetermined, and the effort of the exerciser can be varied quite markedly. Because the blade oscillates at a fixed rate, the intensity of the workout is altered through the application rather than by the demand of the device. The manufacturers of the Body Blade claim it to be useful in fine-tuning or controlling oscillations, thus allowing the body to be more reactive and efficient during muscle performance. They do not claim it to be a strengthening device but rather more of a training tool that requires multiple contraction modes in stabilizing influences by the body, allowing it to be a very versatile and effective training device. They also feel that it might be quite useful in pain modulation through the oscillatory pattern provided by the blade.

The B.O.I.N.G. (Body Oscillation Integrates Neuromuscular Gain) (OKPT, Minneapolis) is a unique oscillating exercise unit that provides a grip on the end of the device rather than in the middle, as seen with the Body Blade. The action is to allow a deflection or bending in an oscillatory pattern involving muscular activation similar to that previously described with the Body Blade. The manufacturers claim that this device is extremely useful for enhancing the rehabilitation sequence in a variety of patients and also effective in pain modulation.

It is interesting to note that the people evaluating these devices have not seen a carryover from these devices to isokinetic testing but have seen changes in functional sequence and decreases in pain. Although most of these reports are anecdotal, the recognition of neural integration to the overall exercise sequence during rehabilitation is obvious. These devices, although typically applied through the upper extremity, can be useful in the stabilization and positioning aspects of the lower extremity during the performance of these oscillatory techniques.

Shuttle 2000

The Shuttle 2000 (Contemporary Design, Glacier, Washington) is a closed kinetic chain device that allows an individual to perform a horizontal or supine squat. Resistance is applied through rubber tubing, which is adjusted by the number of tubes against which the individual exerts. The feet are placed on a platform and a horizontal sled is thus driven from the platform through the action of the lower extremities. Training with this type of device has demonstrated an increase in vertical leap and a carryover to isokinetic assessment.[19]

Many individuals utilize the Shuttle and similar types of functional weight-shifting patterns in a progression culminating in plyometric movements. Thus the individual extends off the platform, moving the sled rapidly from the starting position and allowing the feet to move from the platform but then requiring "them" (the lower extremity) to absorb the energy as the sled is pulled back to the platform via the rubber tubing.

ISOINERTIAL EXERCISES

Several companies manufacture devices that mix control (Isotechnologies, Hillsborough, North Carolina; Hydra-Fitness Industries, Belton, Texas) of some portion of resistance or some portion of speed, thus not being purely isokinetic or isotonic. These devices typically work on the application of a hydraulic principle or pneumatic device that either prioritizes resistance and requests the individual to accelerate a fixed resistance or uses some other type of regulating pattern. As these devices provide a different requirement of neural activity, their relationship or correlation to other ex-

ercise modes has not been well delineated. One of the authors has observed that some individuals who perform well on isotonic or isokinetic assessment have a similar response on these devices.

TO TEST OR NOT TO TEST?

One of the most difficult questions to be asked and thus answered by the rehabilitation specialist is when and how to "test" the musculoskeletal "output" of an individual patient. As stated previously, we frequently are assessing the level of neural inhibition rather than the level of muscular performance that is available. To avoid this aberrant pattern, clinicians are urged to use testing in a more appropriate fashion that is cognizant of its inherent limitations.

RECOMMENDATION OF TESTING FORMATS

If maximal effort of a specific agonist or movement pattern is desired, isokinetic dynamic assessment is very apropos. This should include multiple speeds and be conducted on a quiet joint (no effusion or inflammatory condition) that possesses inherent stability (no ligamentous incompetence) while the patient is able and willing to provide uninhibited maximal efforts. When these conditions are present, reliable testing may be performed. The normal sequence in testing includes generalized exercise warm-up, beginning with submaximal efforts and then moving to the specific dynamic movement expected at submaximal levels to enable the specific speeds or actions to be performed, permitting appropriate familiarization and standardization (before and during assessment). (This outlined pattern is usable for *all* types of assessment.)

Isokinetic assessment of most major muscle groups is performed at two or more speeds. The quadriceps and hamstrings are normally evaluated at 60 degrees per second and at a higher velocity such as 180, 240, 300, or more degrees per second. The 60-degree per second peak torque value is frequently cited by the misnomer of strength measure, and the higher-velocity peak torque value is said to relate to function and endurance. In reality, both represent strength (maximal assessment) and are reflective of local and central neural muscular actions.

Isokinetic dynamometry now encompasses multiple systems and units (extremity and trunk). Each isokinetic system is a compromise of maximal speed and torque. The newer "extremity units" have additional accessories to allow multiple-joint and closed kinetic chain exercise and testing (similar to a leg press). Figures 7-6 through 7-10 outline the specific characteristics of the most commonly seen isokinetic systems with additional information available from the manufacturer and references.[5,16]

It is important to utilize the information generated by the computer software in a sensible form (e.g., the numbers should be viewed in relation to clinical data, not in complete isolation). Much information can be generated from these

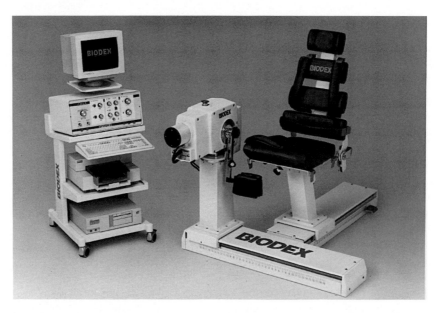

Fig. 7-6. Biodex active system. Modes: passive motion, concentric/eccentric isokinetic, isotonic, isometric (programmable). (Courtesy of Biodex, Shirley, New York; 516/924-9300.)

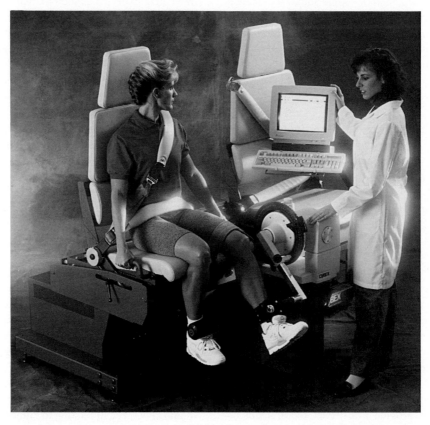

Fig. 7-7. Cybex 6000 active system. Modes: passive motion, concentric/eccentric isokinetic, isotonic and isometric. (Courtesy of Cybex, Ronkonkoma, New York; 800/654-5392.)

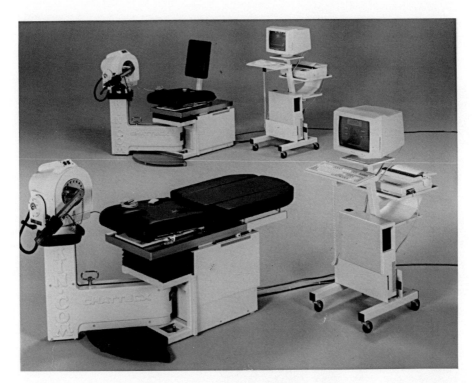

Fig. 7-8. Kin-com series active/interactive. Modes: passive motion, concentric/eccentric isokinetic, isometric, isotonic-sequential protocols. (Courtesy of Chattecx Corp., Hixson, Tennessee; 615/875-5497.)

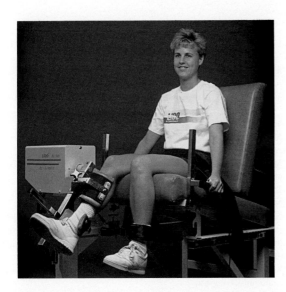

Fig. 7-9. Lido active system robotic. Modes: passive motion, concentric/eccentric isokinetic, isotonic, isometric, isoacceleration. (Courtesy of Loredan Biomedical, West Sacramento, California; 800/729-5436.)

evaluations, and a simple reporting format is recommended rather than too many numbers.

FUNCTIONAL TESTING

In an ideal world, we would always be able to assess the performance of individual patients on specific tasks. This would be the ultimate level of validity, eliminating the problems posed by correlation or representation of a single task to another. The difficulty of this concept is in the multiple complex interactions of the neural, muscular, and skeletal systems. Poor functional performance can be related to inappropriate action in any of the aforementioned systems or a single joint in the kinetic chain, thus making interpretation of this testing much more difficult, particularly when we wish to identify or isolate specific sources of performance variation.

CONCLUSION

Clinicians are becoming more aware of the importance of the integration of dynamic assessment and its place in function through appropriate rehabilitation. Assessment should not be performed in isolation but rather with integration to the performance of actual tasks. It is our recommendation to include functional activities primarily as exercise goals and performance ideals, while using isolated single-joint testing. We thus integrate function (closed-chain activities) with testing (open-chain) procedures. We do not recommend complete reliance on concentric or eccentric or any other specific neural action, but rather recommend asking the neural musculoskeletal system to be faced with a "barrage" of actions that attempt to prepare the individual for the desired activities.

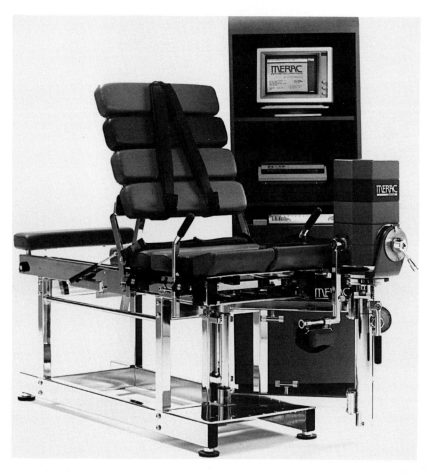

Fig. 7-10. Merac passive system. Modes: Concentric isokinetic, isometric, individualized dynamic variable resistance. (Courtesy of Universal Gym, Cedar Rapids, Iowa.)

REFERENCES

1. Albert M, editor: *Inertial training concepts in eccentric muscle training in sports and orthopedics,* New York, 1991, Churchill-Livingstone.
2. Bohannon RW: Test-retest reliability of handheld dynamometry during a single session of strength assessment, *Phys Ther* 66:206–209, 1986.
3. Bosco C, Komi TV: Potentiation of the mechanical behavior of human skeletal muscle through prestretching, *Acta Physiol Scand* 106:467, 1979.
4. Brown ME, Mayhew JL, Boleach LW: Effect of plyometric training on vertical jump performance in high school basketball players, *J Sports Med Phys Fitness* 26:1–4, 1986.
5. Davies G: *A compendium of isokinetics in clinical usage,* ed 3, La Crosse, Wisc. 1985, S & S Publishers.
6. Feinstein B, et al: Morphologic studies of motor units in normal human muscles, *Acta Anat (Basel)* 23:127–142, 1955.
7. France EP, et al: Preliminary clinical evaluation of the Breg, KAT: effects of training in normals, *Isokinetics Exerc Sci* 2:133–139, 1992.
8. Freeman MAR, Wyke B: Articular reflexes at the ankle joint: an electromyographic study of normal and abnormal influences of the ankle-joint, mechano receptors upon reflex activity in the leg muscles, *Br J Surg* 54:990–1000, 1967.
9. Kegerreis S, Malone T, McCarroll J: Functional progressions: an aid to athletic rehabilitation, *Physician Sports Med* 12:67–71, 1984.
10. Komi TV: *Physiological and biomechanical corelets of muscle function: effects of muscle structure and stretch-shortening cycle on force and speed.* In Terjungrl, editor: *Exercise and sports science reviews,* Lexington, Ky., 1984, Collamore Press.
11. Komi TV, Bosco C: Utilization of stored elastic energy in leg extensor muscles by men and women, *Med Sci Sports Exerc* 10:261, 1978.
12. Komi TV, Buskirk E: Effects of eccentric and concentric muscle conditioning on tension and electrical activity of human muscle, *Ergonomics* 15:417, 1972.
13. Lesmes GR, et al: Muscle strength and power changes during maximal isokinetic training, *Med Sci Sports* 10:266–269, 1978.
14. MacDougall JD, et al: Effects of strength training and immobilization on human muscle fibers, *Eur J Appl Physiol* 43:25–34, 1980.
15. MacDougall JD, et al: Biochemical adaptation of human skeletal muscle to heavy resistance training and immobilization, *J Appl Physiol* 43:700–703, 1977.
16. Malone TR, editor: *Sports injury management, evaluation of isokinetic equipment,* Baltimore, 1988, Williams & Wilkins.
17. Malone TR, Garrett WE: Commentary and historical perspective of anterior cruciate ligament rehabilitation, *J Orthop Sports Phys Ther* 15:265–269, 1992.
18. Moritani T, deVries HA: Neural factors versus hypertrophy in the time course of muscle strength gain, *Am J Phys Med* 58:115–130, 1979.
19. Olson B, Dalpino M, Malone T: Strength changes of the quadriceps in alterations and vertical late measurements after six weeks of training on the Shuttle 2000, *Isokinetics Exerc Sci* 3:57–62, 1993.
20. Rothstein JM: *Measurement in physical therapy,* New York, 1985, Churchill-Livingstone.
21. Shelbourne KD, Nitz P: Accelerated rehabilitation after anterior cruciate ligament reconstruction, *Am J Sports Med* 18:292–299, 1990.
22. Wickiewicztl, et al: Muscle architecture of the human lower limb, *Clin Orthop* 179:275–283, 1983.
23. Wilk KE, Johnson RD, Levine B: A comparison of peak torque values of knee extension and flexor muscle groups using Biodex, Cybex, and Kin-Com isokinetic dynamometers, *Phys Ther* 67:789, 1987 (abstract).
24. Wilk KE, Johnson RD, Levine B: Comparison of knee extensor and flexor muscle groups strength using Biodex, Cybex, and Lido isokinetic dynamometers, *Phys Ther* 68:792, 1988 (abstract).
25. Winters JM, Woo SL, editors: *Multiple muscle systems: biomechanics and movement organization,* New York, 1990, Springer Verlag.

Chapter 8

FORMULATING A
REHABILITATION PROGRAM

W. Ben Kibler
Stanley A. Herring

This book is about *how* to rehabilitate the knee. In subsequent chapters many authors describe techniques for rehabilitation processes for the knee in different injuries and in different sports. This chapter attempts to provide a framework to build these processes on: the phases of rehabilitation, how to establish them, and how to achieve them. In this framework the focus is first on *why* we should rehabilitate and *what* we should rehabilitate. Once these questions have been answered, then *how* to rehabilitate becomes a much easier task. Because the goal of rehabilitation is to restore the knee anatomically, physiologically, and biomechanically to as near a normal situation as possible, the framework must address the entire spectrum of abnormalities that may be found in knee pathologic conditions to give the best results. Anatomic healing is the first prerequisite, but rehabilitation must proceed to physiologic and biomechanical normality before the knee can be considered functionally restored.

Anatomically, the intrinsic pathologic problem in the knee must be treated and rehabilitated. This process includes resolution of knee sprains, treatment of subluxing patellas, repair or resection of torn menisci, and ligament reconstruction. This type of treatment, whether operative or nonoperative, usually addresses most of the clinical symptoms that the athlete presents to the practitioner.

Biomechanically and physiologically, alterations can also occur as a result of intrinsic knee pathology or its treatment. Stiffness of knee ligaments and capsule; inflexibility of the joints causing decreased range of motion; muscle strength, weakness, and/or imbalance; and altered neurologic firing patterns are some physiologic and biomechanical alterations that can be seen as a result of intrinsic knee pathology, ranging from knee sprains to meniscal injuries to ligament injuries. After the intrinsic pathology is anatomically corrected, these alterations must be properly addressed and

corrected to allow the knee to function normally.

However, in addition to the local pathology and local alterations, knee pathology may affect other anatomic areas, because the knee is also a very important link in many kinetic chains of many different athletic activities. Failure to rehabilitate the knee properly so it may work properly in the kinetic chain also may cause abnormal athletic function for the entire kinetic chain. Weakness in the knees following a sprained medial collateral ligament can alter jumping and running patterns, which depend upon proper movement and power in the knee itself. This can hamper performance and possibly put extra stress on other links in the chain. Similarly, shoulder trouble in a throwing athlete can occur as a result of damage to the knee of the plant leg in pitching.

Most of these reasons *why* rehabilitation should be done are fairly evident and are accepted. *What* should be rehabilitated is often a source of confusion. For functional rehabilitation to be most successful, a complete and accurate diagnosis of all problems that exist around the knee following a pathologic problem should be formulated. This includes not only the anatomic problem, such as a torn medial meniscus, but also the functional physiologic and biomechanical alterations that accompany this problem, such as muscle weakness, imbalance, or lack of flexibility. Alterations in other parts of the kinetic chain as well, such as muscle weakness in the hip flexors or gastrocnemius, also must be included in the exercise prescription. Therefore, the search for all of the components that make up the complete and accurate diagnosis may involve looking at other places besides the knee. Very frequently, incomplete knee rehabilitation is the result of limiting the rehabilitation to symptoms only or limiting it to knee abnormalities only. As a result of incomplete rehabilitation, injuries can recur and the rehabilitation process can be frustrating. Incomplete rehabilitation can lead to recurrence of injuries in as many as

77% of individuals who are injured. Also, emphasis on symptom-based rehabilitation leads to misuse of modalities and other types of rehabilitation devices and prolongs the rehabilitation process.

This chapter describes a framework for evaluating "why rehabilitate" and "what should be rehabilitated" and serves as an introduction to the "how of rehabilitation" that is described in the rest of the book.

WHY SHOULD WE REHABILITATE?

The first and most immediate reason for rehabilitation is to resolve the clinical symptoms and the signs that exist at the time of the injury to the knee. The symptoms and signs include swelling, pain, redness, tenderness, decreased motion, lack of muscle strength, and instability. Appropriate modalities such as cold, ultrasound, contrast baths, and immobilization plus the judicious use of nonsteroidal anti-inflammatory medicines are appropriate in achieving the goals of this phase of rehabilitation. If the pathology warrants, surgical intervention may be necessary to resolve the symptoms and signs.

The second reason is to restore function. Functional restoration lies at the heart of the rehabilitation process. Restoration of proper strength and power, flexibility, balance, and performance are the goals of this stage of the rehabilitation process. Restoration of performance of athletic skills requires optimum anatomy but also optimum physiology. Alterations in physiology or incomplete physiologic rehabilitation are more often the source of limitation of performance than are alterations in anatomy.

The third reason to rehabilitate is to decrease the reinjury rate and prevent further injury to the knee. The reinjuries are usually in the same anatomic area, such as repeated medial collateral ligament sprains. Further new injuries may be adjacent, such as medial meniscal tears that can occur in conjunction with old ACL injuries, or may be distant in the kinetic chain, such as plantar fasciitis secondary to prolonged stance phase on the opposite side of an injured knee or shoulder problems in throwers as a result of injury to the plant leg knee. Incompletely rehabilitated injuries are a prime cause of reinjury in the kinetic chain.

The fourth reason to rehabilitate is to maintain other aspects of physical fitness while the knee injury is healing. Upper body strength can be maintained during knee healing, and even opposite leg strength and flexibility training should be continued. At appropriate times of healing, the injured knee can be exercised to maintain aerobic endurance by aqua jogging. In this manner, a higher level of general sports fitness is maintained, decreasing the total rehabilitation time for return to sport.

Finally, a good rehabilitation program shades into a prehabilitation program. The goal of the prehabilitation program, which is preventive and prospective in nature, is to decrease injury risk and increase performance parameters by maximizing the musculoskeletal system's ability to with-

stand the demands inherent in sporting activities. The knowledge and experience gained with the rehabilitation process can be extended to the other knee and to not only normalizing the functional ability of the knee but also improving the ability of the knee above normal. Prehabilitation is usually sport-specific because individual sports have individual demands on the knee.

WHAT ARE WE REHABILITATING?

Rehabilitation of the knee should not be solely concerned with intrinsic pathology in the knee but also concerned with the knee in the context of the entire kinetic chain in which it is participating. Formulating this type of program requires knowledge of the type of injury, its effect on the kinetic chain, and any alterations that exist in the kinetic chain as a result of the injury.

Two major types of intrinsic injuries—macrotrauma injury and microtrauma injury—can occur in the knee. *Macrotrauma injury* is defined by a one-time event and implies a situation in which the anatomic structures were normal before the event and then were distinctly abnormal after the event. The time, place, and mechanism of injury can usually be well documented. Examples of this type of injury would include an ACL tear, a fracture of the femur, or a dislocation of the patella. *Microtrauma injuries* are defined as the result of a process of gradual injury, usually on a basis of overload in which cellular mechanisms are unable to cope with the healing needs. There can be cellular damage, failure of matrix production and repair, and gradual organ functional abnormalities secondary to cellular failure. This is usually a fairly long process that may be accompanied by adaptations in flexibility, strength, biomechanics, and function as the athlete tries to adapt to the abnormal anatomy and physiology. Examples of this type of process are patellar tendonitis, chronic knee sprains, and chondromalacia. The type of injury that occurs in the knee often determines the physiologic and biomechanical alterations as well as the intrinsic pathology. Therefore, emphasis must be placed on understanding the type of injury that occurs so that proper evaluation of the alterations can be obtained prior to starting a rehabilitation program.

Regardless of the type of injury that the athlete sustains, the knee should be rehabilitated in the context of the kinetic chain in which it participates in athletics. The kinetic chain may be defined as a series of links in the body responsible for generation and regulation of the proper amount of force to do athletic activities. The knee is a very important link in the kinetic chain because most running, jumping, and throwing activities involve ground reaction forces transmitted from the ground to the feet and then through the legs (Fig. 8-1). The incompletely rehabilitated knee often "breaks the chain" of normal force generation by decreasing the total force production or making the other links in the chain try to "catch up" by generating extra force to make up for the lack of force generation at the knee (Fig. 8-2).

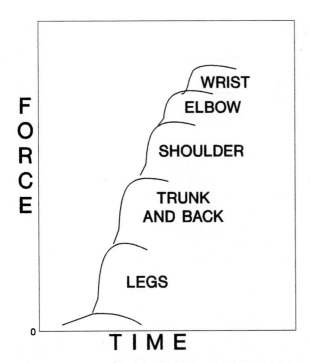

Fig. 8-1. The kinetic chain for force generation in the tennis serve. The knee serves as an important link in transmitting forces from the calf and allowing generation of forces by the quadriceps and hamstring activation.

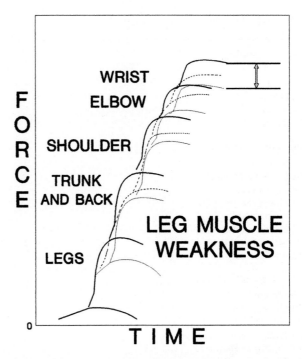

Fig. 8-2. Kinetic chain of the tennis serve showing the decreased force production due to muscle weakness from incomplete rehabilitation around the knee. The functional result would be decreased service velocity or overuse of the smaller muscles of the shoulder, elbow, or wrist in attempts to make up the force decrement.

The force generated through the knee may be used locally, such as in kicking or jumping, or may be used distantly, as in throwing. In either situation, the knee is a very important component of the kinetic chain mechanism.

Another important function of the knee in the kinetic chain is force absorption. In running, the stance leg is responsible for absorbing the force as the runner comes down on the leg by acting as a spring to absorb and store the force to be expended as the leg goes into the push-off phase. Quadriceps muscle activity is at its highest in runners during this early stance phase. Similarly, in baseball throwing, the forward or plant leg is necessary to catch the momentum of the falling body and translate the momentum smoothly so that the body can rotate to deliver the pitch to the plate. Force absorption may be the most important part of the kinetic chain in these activities.

Rehabilitation also needs to be undertaken for alterations that result from the treatment rendered. Meniscal repairs, ACL reconstructions, and sprains all require some type of immobilization for varying periods of time, may involve surgical incisions that require time to heal, and cause pain that alters neurologic firing patterns. These alterations of inflexibility, muscle weakness and imbalance, and impaired neural drive require special attention and work in the rehabilitation program.

To help organize this information and allow a complete understanding of what needs to be rehabilitated, a framework for evaluation can be set up. This framework includes

the clinical symptoms, the anatomic alterations that exist, and the physiologic alterations that occur (Table 8-1). The clinical symptoms include all presenting complaints and apparent signs that relate to the local pathology. The anatomic alterations include all local tissue injury findings of overt nature and all nonovert local and distant tissue overload adaptations that may be present as a result of the microtrauma process. Examples of the local anatomic alterations include patellar tendon damage, torn medial meniscus, or torn anterior cruciate ligament. Examples of the nonovert anatomic alterations include quadriceps muscle tightness, hamstring muscle weakness, or lateral retinacular tightness. The physiologic alterations that exist include biomechanical deficits of inflexibility, strength, and strength balance that may occur as a result of the process leading to the overt injury or as a result of immobilization or repair of the injury. Examples are quadriceps-hamstrings imbalance secondary to immobilization after ligament repair, quadriceps inflexibility secondary to patella baja, and quadriceps strength deficit secondary to inhibition by pain from a torn medial meniscus. Subclinical adaptations occur as the athlete tries to maintain normal performance in the face of injury and/or adaptation. These include alterations in movement patterns and motor firing patterns. Examples of abnormal movement patterns are shortened stance phase in running with patients who have patellar tendonitis, alteration

Table 8-1. Framework for evaluation

Clinical symptoms
Pain
Swelling
Locking
Instability
Decreased motion

Anatomic alterations
Tissue injury
Patellar tendon damage
Torn meniscus
Torn ligament
Tissue overload
Quadriceps (inflexibility)
Hamstring (weakness)
ITB (tightness)

Physiologic alterations
Biomechanical deficits
Muscle weakness
Muscle imbalance
Flexibility imbalance
Subclinical adaptations
Shortened stance phase
No crossover maneuvers
Altered firing patterns

Table 8-2. Acute stage

Clinical symptom and sign resolution
Rest
Modalities
NSAIDs
Surgery
Bracing

Tissue injury damage reduction
Rest
Surgery
Bracing

Criteria for advancement
Pain and swelling reduction
Increased passive range of motion
Tissue damage correction

of weightbearing on landing from a jump in patients who have patellar tendonitis, or avoidance of crossover maneuvers in patients with ACL deficiency. Alterations in motor firing patterns can be seen in abnormal hamstring firing patterns in patients with ACL-deficient knees or in quadriceps inhibition secondary to chondromalacia.

Completion of this evaluation framework for each pathologic problem allows a complete and accurate diagnosis to be made. This diagnosis must be performed before the institution of rehabilitation because it guides the formulation of the exercise prescription, which in turn determines the "how" of rehabilitation. This diagnosis and prescription allow a smoother rehabilitation course with defined stages and goals for rehabilitation and also allow a more functional rehabilitation course because all aspects of knee pathology that contribute to the functional alterations have been included in the diagnosis.

HOW DO WE REHABILITATE?

Many protocols and many rehabilitation tools are illustrated in the various chapters that deal with specific injuries or specific sports. These allow a detailed understanding of the *how* of the rehabilitation process. All of the protocols must go through certain stages that match the normal biologic process of healing and must use appropriate tools in each of the stages. Well-defined criteria must be established to move from one stage to the other, and eventually to return

to play. The framework for evaluation of injuries can be used to establish the components of each stage and give criteria for movement between stages.

Three broad stages can be used to guide progress in rehabilitation. They are the acute stage, recovery stage, and maintenance phase. Reduction or resolution of the symptoms or alterations that are present with a certain injury can be matched to a certain stage. This allows an objective, directed course of rehabilitation, with defined goals.

In the acute stage of rehabilitation (Table 8-2), the major goals should be resolution of the clinical symptoms and signs of pain, swelling, locking or instability, and reduction in the tissue injury damage that has occurred. The clinical symptoms and signs can be dealt with by rest; modalities of cold, heat, ultrasound, or EGS; appropriate anti-inflammatory agents; bracing; and, when indicated, surgery. Tissue injury can be reduced or resolved by the same agents. In acute macrotrauma injuries, such as torn medial menisci, treatment of the clinical symptoms by surgery also completely resolve the tissue injury. However, in chronic microtrauma injuries, such as patellar tendonitis, some tissue injury is still present after the symptoms are eliminated and must be resolved by continuation of therapy into the next stage. Specific criteria for the advancement from this stage are reduction of pain and swelling, improvement of range of motion toward normal, and correction of the tissue injury damage. This stage is usually fairly short, and the goals can usually be seen and achieved. If they are not achieved, however, the subsequent stages become more difficult.

In the recovery stage of rehabilitation (Table 8-3), the tissue injury damage should be completely resolved. The tissues that have been overloaded as a result of the injury or treatment should be normalized, and the physiologic deficits in flexibility, strength, and strength balance should be addressed as part of the continuing effort to rehabilitate beyond the cessation of symptoms. Tissue overloads are

Table 8-3. Recovery stage

Tissue injury damage
Resolved

Tissue overload
Bracing
Flexibility exercises
Specific strengthening exercises

Biomechanical deficits
Quadriceps-hamstrings cocontractions
Eccentric loading
Gastrocnemius strengthening

Criteria for advancement
No pain
Essentially full motion
Good muscle strength and balance

Table 8-4. Maintenance phase

Biomechanical deficits
Normal force couples
Normal flexibility

Subclinical adaptations
Normal stance time
Normal jumping and landing
Normal force transfer

Criteria for return to play
No symptoms
Normal strength
Normal mechanics
Complete functional progressions

usually found in association with chronic microtrauma injuries. Quadriceps inflexibility in patellar tendonitis or quadriceps and hamstring weakness in Osgood-Schlatter disease must be addressed after the acute symptoms are controlled, to prevent reexacerbation of the symptoms. Biomechanical deficits, such as loss of the quadriceps-hamstring force couple as a result of injury or immobilization, or decreased eccentric work capacity in the quadriceps in patellar tendonitis, should be normalized to allow normal force generation and force absorption. Specific criteria for advancement to the next stage of rehabilitation are healing of the tissue injury damage, no pain, normalization of the overloaded tissues that were also involved, and improvement in force couples and biomechanics toward normal.

The final stage of rehabilitation is a maintenance phase (Table 8-4), in which all biomechanical deficits of strength and flexibility are returned to normal and the subclinical adaptations involving movement patterns and motor firing patterns are reduced to normal. The tissues are fairly close to normality, and some athletic activities can be started. After normal flexibility has been achieved and restoration of strength balance has allowed the force couples to generate and absorb force normally, emphasis should be placed on normal movement patterns. Normal local patterns, such as equal stance time on both legs in the running cycle, pushing off and landing on both legs in jumping, and proper force transfer from the push-off leg to the plant leg in throwing, should be achieved. In addition, normal distant patterns in the kinetic chain, such as proper trunk rotation and shoulder motion in the tennis serve, should be reestablished. During this stage, return to play should be considered when specific criteria are met. These are complete resolution of the symptoms and physiologic and anatomic alterations and completion of sport-specific progressions to return to play, whether the activity is running, kicking, jumping, or throwing. These sports-specific progressions involve progressive challenge to the knee and the kinetic chain of the sport. Examples are "long toss–short toss" in throwing, one-legged hop and figure-of-eight drills for basketball, cutting and crossover drills for football, and spider agility drills for tennis. Once these drills are done well in practice, the athlete may return to competition.

CONCLUSION

The process of knee rehabilitation is complex because of the importance of the knee in athletic activities. Knee pathology is important not only in terms of the local effects to the knee but also in its importance as a key part of many kinetic chains of athletic activity. Understanding all of the alterations that occur as a result of knee pathology allows a complete and accurate diagnosis to be made. This diagnosis then becomes the basis for a rational and progressive rehabilitation program to allow return to function as well as cessation of symptoms. As can be seen, cessation of symptoms is only part of the goal of complete rehabilitation of the knee.

REFERENCES
1. Herring SA: Rehabilitation of muscle injury, *Med Sci Sports Exerc* 22:4, 1990.
2. Kibler WB, Chandler TJ, Pace BA: Principles of rehabilitation after chronic tendon injuries, *Clin Sports Med* 11:3.
3. Kibler WB: *Concepts in exercise rehabilitation*. In Leadbetter W, Buckwalter JA, Gordon SL, editors: *Sports induced inflammation*, Chicago, 1990, AAOS.
4. Leadbetter W: *Physiology of tissue repair*. In *Athletic training and sports medicine*, Park Ridge, Ill. 1991, AAOS (Adapted from Ref 3.)
5. Marino M: *Current concepts on rehabilitation in sports medicine and clinical interrelationships*. In Nicholas JA, Hershman EB, editors: *The lower extremity and spine in sports medicine*, St Louis, 1986, Mosby–Year Book.

Chapter 9

THE PSYCHOLOGY OF KNEE INJURIES AND INJURY REHABILITATION

Daniel Gould
Eileen Udry

As a linebacker for a professional football team, T. J. was no stranger to the pain and isolation associated with a season-ending injury. Having undergone reconstructive surgery on his right knee, T. J. had made a successful comeback the following season and thought that the worst was behind him. So when T. J. was hit from the left side and felt that knee buckle beneath him, all he could think was, "This can't be happening to me. I already paid my dues!" In the weeks following his second surgery, T. J. seemed to vacillate over whether he could realistically return to the rigors of professional football. On those days when T. J. felt his chances were reasonable he approached his rehabilitation with fervor. However, there would be days when T. J. would be so despondent over his condition that he would hardly leave his bedroom, much less make it to the training room.

Michelle was a college runner who had undergone surgery for a torn anterior cruciate ligament (ACL) following a car accident. Initially, the sports medicine team was optimistic about Michelle's chances of returning to competitive running relatively quickly. However, in the 4 weeks following her surgery Michelle came into the sports medicine clinic six times with her knee so swollen that she was not able to complete her exercises. It was discovered that Michelle had routinely been doing twice the amount of exercise outlined by the physical therapist, which had resulted in her knee being overstressed. Michelle indicated that she desperately wanted to return to running and was fearful that she would not be able to get back into shape if she did not push herself to her limits. However, because she did not allow her knee adequate rest, Michelle actually recovered more slowly than expected.

Lesley had been under an enormous amount of stress. Recently divorced, she moved to a different city to take a new job. In an effort to reduce her stress levels and lose weight, Lesley joined an athletic club and began doing aerobics after work. However, Lesley's new exercise regimen came to a sudden halt one night in class. A newcomer to the class who was unfamiliar with the routine bumped into Lesley and caused her to land with her foot improperly planted. Lesley immediately felt a sharp pain shoot up

her leg. Despite the obvious fact that her knee was seriously injured, Lesley was still not prepared to hear from her orthopedic physician that her damaged ACL would probably keep her from full aerobics participation for several months.*

These cases clearly illustrate that, despite improvements in training procedures, equipment, and surgical techniques, no one participating in sport or exercise programs is immune to injuries. Noted surgeon and sports medicine physician Richard Steadman has referred to sport injuries as the "greatest equalizer" because, regardless of experience or ability levels, athletes put themselves at risk for injury.[1]

In addition, these cases underscore the importance of considering not only the physiological actors associated with injuries but the psychological aspects as well.[2] Although each of these athletes had similar injuries, they had vastly different psychological responses to them. Furthermore, as we saw in these cases, athletes' psychological responses can have a profound impact on their approach to rehabilitation. Fortunately, there has been a growing awareness among sports medicine providers of the need to consider the psychological factors related to injuries.[3,4] For example, a recent survey of physical therapists indicated that 84% felt limited in their ability to deal with psychological aspects of sport injuries, with 87% of the sample welcoming the opportunity for additional practical information on this subject.[5] Typically, however, sports medicine providers receive minimal training relating to the psychological aspects of injuries. This

*Throughout this chapter the term *athlete* is used. However, it refers to both the "athlete" who participates at the elite or subelite level as well as the individual who might be considered an "exerciser" or recreational athlete.

chapter has been written in an effort to provide the sports medicine provider with an overview of some of the psychological aspects of injuries, particularly knee injuries. More specifically, there are five objectives of this chapter:

1. Providing an overview of the psychological factors identified as psychological antecedents to injury
2. Examining the psychological responses to injury that athletes frequently experience
3. Discussing psychologically based injury rehabilitation strategies
4. Identifying athletes who may face special struggles with injuries
5. Discussing how to integrate psychological strategies into a multimodal injury treatment plan

Before beginning, it seems relevant to clarify the perspective from which this chapter has been written. To this end the interdisciplinary model of knee injury process is presented (Fig. 9-1). Throughout the chapter we will return to this model and provide additional details regarding its specifics. Here we establish the conceptual framework that has guided the remainder of this chapter. The model consists of four interrelated steps. Step 1 focuses on the antecedents of injury; step 2, the physical injury itself; step 3, the athlete's response to the injury; and step 4, injury rehabilitation.

The first aspect of the model to be noted is its interdisciplinary nature. Thus, it is acknowledged that a variety of physical, environmental, and psychological factors influence the individual throughout the injury and rehabilitation process. This chapter focuses on the psychological aspects of injuries, as the physical and environmental aspects are discussed elsewhere in this volume. However, it is our contention that to understand and treat athletic injuries effectively physical, environmental, and psychological factors must be simultaneously considered.

A second characteristic of the model is that it is reciprocal. For instance, an injured athlete may rehabilitate her knee to the point where the medical evidence suggests she is ready to return to competition (step 4 of the model). However, if the athlete does not yet feel psychologically ready to return, she may be prone to "guarding" or "bracing" as she attempts to protect her knee. These subtle protective measures may actually increase the athlete's chances of reinjuring her knee. In the event of reinjury, the athlete returns to step 1 of the model. Thus, the model is reciprocal in the sense that various feedback mechanisms may prevent an athlete from progressing in a linear manner from step 1 to step 4 of the model.

Having looked at a broad overview of this model, we can now turn to a more complete discussion of the individual steps included in it. We begin by discussing step 1 of the model, which relates to precursors of athletic injuries.

PSYCHOLOGICAL ANTECEDENTS OF INJURY

Much of the sports medicine research on antecedents of injuries has focused on two types of factors: (1) *physical factors,* such as training errors, biomechanical deficiencies, and imbalances of strength or flexibility; and (2) *environmental factors,* such as the playing or training surfaces. However, recently a number of *personality and psychosocial factors* have been linked to the incidence of athletic injuries[2,6-8] (see step 1 of Fig. 9-1). This section focuses on these psychological factors, in particular, the psychological antecedents to injury, the mechanisms thought to predispose individuals to injury, and the implications this information has for members of the sports medicine team.

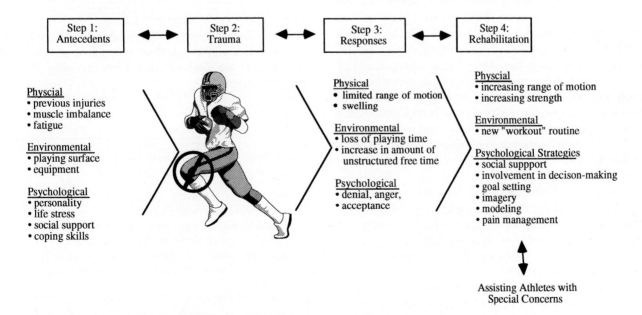

Fig. 9-1. Interdisciplinary model of the knee injury process.

The factors that have most extensively been examined as potential precursors to athletic injuries include personality traits, life stress levels, and a variety of psychosocial factors such as social support and coping skills. The initial wave of research in this area focused on exploring the role of personality traits on the incidence of injuries. It was hypothesized that relatively stable personality dispositions such as individuals' locus of control, self-concept, or degree of introversion or extroversion caused some individuals to be more prone to injury than others.[2] Although there have been few well-designed studies in this area, in general the findings from this line of research have produced equivocal results.[9]

The role of life stress as it relates to the incidence of injuries is an area that has received more attention in the literature and generally produced more consistent results.[8] Because of a number of recent methodologic refinements, researchers can now measure not only major life stress but "daily hassles" and the degree to which individuals interpret these life events as positive or negative. Taken as a whole, the life stress–injury literature has indicated that individuals with higher life stress are more likely to experience injuries.[10] Hence, athletes who have experienced a recent death of a significant other, major move, change in financial status, and/or lead hectic life-styles may increase their risk of injury.

Despite the growing body of literature linking life stress to the occurrence of injuries, it is important to note that recent research hints that the life stress relationship may be more complex that was originally thought.[2] In a comprehensive survey of 452 high school athletes participating in a variety of sports, Smith, Smoll, and Ptacek[7] measured athletes' life event stress, coping skills, and level of social support. These assessments were compared to the number of injuries over the course of a year. These researchers found that when life stress, coping skills, and social support were considered *independently* there were no significant relationships to injury rates. However, one interesting pattern emerged when researchers looked at a subpopulation of athletes who had a particular combination of psychosocial characteristics. More specifically, athletes who experienced high life stress *and* who also were low in coping skills and social support were more likely to become injured.

Taken as a whole, the research suggests it may be possible to develop profiles of "at risk" individuals based on assessments of a number of psychological variables. Although the results of research that encompasses the role of life stress, coping skills, and social support is not yet conclusive, members of the sports medicine team may want to be aware that certain individuals may be psychologically predisposed to injuries. A tentative listing of relevant variables is summarized in the box at right.

Given the growing body of research that has linked psychological factors to the incidence of injury, several follow-up questions have been posed. One has to do with the potential effectiveness of preventive interventions. In other words, researchers have wondered whether it is possible to use psychologically based interventions to reduce the number of injuries that occur in the first place. To date, little research has been conducted in this area. One exception is the work of Davis.[11] Using an archival analysis, injury rates from the previous seasons of two collegiate teams (swimming and football) were determined. Then a progressive relaxation and imagery-based intervention was introduced to these two collegiate teams. A 52% reduction in the number of swimming injuries and a 33% reduction in the number of football injuries were reported. Although caution should be used when interpreting the results of this study because of a number of design flaws, the results suggest that there may be a time when sports medicine professionals would provide educational programs that use psychological strategies as a means of injury prevention.

A second question based on the life stress injury research is, What are the reasons that certain athletes might be more susceptible to injury? Although the underlying mechanisms are not well understood, two explanations have been put forward. One posits that as an athlete's stress levels increase there is a concomitant narrowing of attentional focus.[10] This attentional narrowing of peripheral attention is thought to distract the athlete from task-relevant cues. As an example, a highly stressed soccer player may have a narrower perceptual field that reduces the chances of immediately observing a potential tackler. This reduction of awareness to important peripheral visual stimuli results in an increased risk of injury, which may not occur under less stressful circumstances.

A second explanation that has been posited is that stressed athletes carry unnecessary muscular tension in their bodies.[12] This unnecessary muscle tension is thought to interfere with normal coordination and impede smooth execution. In the case of a basketball player who is going up for a lay-up it would be maintained that, if there is excessive simultaneous contraction of the quadriceps and hamstrings muscles, then a proper landing may not occur. The result may be that the knee or other joints are more likely to become injured.

Potential risk factors associated with an increased risk of injury in athletes

High life event stress (e.g., recent death of significant other, divorce, change in job)

High daily hassles (e.g., chronic interpersonal conflict with coach, financial aid or scholarship hassles)

Low coping skills (e.g., turns to substance abuse, especially alcohol, when stressed; unable to handle constructive criticism)

Low social support (e.g., athlete does not feel other individuals are available to turn to during difficult situations)

Although the attentional narrowing and muscular tension explanations are possible reasons why athletes may become more susceptible to injuries, it should be noted that until further research is conducted these explanations are largely speculative. In addition, it is unlikely that these mechanisms work in isolation from other variables. For instance, although psychological stress brings about increased levels of muscular tension that result in an increased *risk* of injury, an injury may not occur unless other physical and/or environmental variables (e.g., muscle imbalance, previous injuries) are out of alignment as well. Thus, as has been stressed throughout this chapter, there is a need to consider a variety of physical, psychological, and environmental variables as the antecedents of athletic injuries.

Conclusions regarding the psychological antecedents to injuries

In summary, little evidence has supported the conclusion that personality variables are reliable antecedents to injuries. Nonetheless, despite results from life stress–injury research that are far from definitive, the current findings indicate that stress is positively correlated with the incidence of injuries. Understanding this relationship has important implications for the sports medicine team. Certainly the occurrence of an injury may exacerbate the stress response for athletes who are already experiencing high life event stress and lack adequate social support and coping skills. Thus, members of the sports medicine team may need to work especially hard at assisting these at-risk athletes through the rehabilitation process. Sports psychology consultants who are part of a sports medicine team may also want to consider providing routine evaluations of all injured athletes to identify athletes who may be at risk throughout the rehabilitation process. Finally, sports medicine team members involved in coaches' education should stress the importance of the stress-injury relationship and recommend that special attention be given to identifying and reducing stress in at-risk athletes.

Until now the focus of the discussion has been on examining some of the predisposing factors thought to be associated with athletic injuries. Despite the best efforts of coaches, trainers, and athletes to prevent injuries, however, injuries inevitably occur (see step 2 of Fig. 9-1). In the following section we focus on step 3, which deals with athletes' psychological responses to injuries. When members of the sports medicine team understand the psychological consequences of injuries, they are more likely to be able to help the athlete recover optimally, both physically and mentally.

PSYCHOLOGICAL REACTIONS TO ATHLETIC INJURIES

Athletes who experience injuries often find themselves in an emotional maelstrom. Danish[13] has noted that injuries can be particularly stressful for athletes because not only is physical well-being threatened but the athlete's self-concept,

belief system, social network, emotional equilibrium, and in some cases occupational functioning are endangered as well.

As noted in the case studies at the outset of the chapter, the situational details surrounding an injury can vary tremendously. For instance, Michelle's desire to rehabilitate was driven by her perception of competitive pressure, whereas Lesley was primarily interested in returning to exercise for reasons related to stress reduction and weight control. Despite these situation-specific differences, it is generally thought that athletes experience similar psychological reactions following an injury. The most widely recognized framework that has been proposed for understanding this process is the work of Kübler-Ross.[14] Originally developed for work with terminally ill patients, this five-stage grief process model has been applied to work with injured athletes[15-17] (Fig. 9-2).

Denial

During this stage the athlete may say, "This can't be happening to me. It's only a nightmare." It is not uncommon for athletes to downplay the seriousness of the injury and

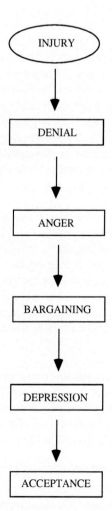

Fig. 9-2. Five-stage grief process model for knee injuries.

its significance at this stage. Despite a tendency to view an athlete who is in the denial stage as not being ready to *begin* rehabilitation, Gordon, Milios, and Grove[5] have observed that some athletes in the denial stage are prone to *overdoing* their rehabilitation. After all, if an injury is not seen by the athlete as being as serious as it really is, then the continuation of high levels of activity would not be perceived by the athlete as detrimental. This overzealous approach to rehabilitation was demonstrated in the case of Michelle, who was doing double the recommended amount of exercise during her rehabilitation.

Anger

Once the reality of the injury becomes apparent, the injured athlete may take a "Why me?" attitude, which focuses on the seeming unfairness of the injury. This can be a difficult time for those close to the athlete, who may vent frustration on anyone in close proximity. When one realizes that this expression of anger is not a personal attack or an indication of lack of character, the anger can be seen for what it more accurately expresses—a sense of loss and frustration.[16]

Bargaining

An athlete who has reached the bargaining phase of the grief process may attempt to rationalize or intellectualize an injury through comments such as "If I can rehab my knee, I'll only play one more year." Pederson[16] has observed that athletes may attempt to draw members of the sports medicine team into the bargaining process (e.g., "I think that my knee would come around faster if I was able to spend more time on the Cybex machine"). Obviously, sports medicine team members must be careful not be persuaded by these requests, which are typically not in athletes' best long-term interests.

Depression

As athletes begin to come to terms with the reality of their injuries and their consequences, it is not unusual for them to withdraw and engage in self-pity. Anderson and Williams[10] have stressed that during this phase those close to the injured athlete should resist the temptation to attempt to get the athlete to "cheer up," as this approach serves only to negate the individual's feelings. A more therapeutic approach includes empathetic listening and emotional support.

Acceptance

At some point most athletes move to the final stage of the grieving process and begin to accept the reality of their injuries. It is thought that rehabilitation efforts will be most effective during this phase because athletes can now take a more action-oriented approach to the rehabilitation.[15,18]

Conclusions regarding the grieving process

Several points bear mention in regard to the grieving process. First, sports medicine team members may be in a prime position to facilitate the grief process as they often have the most frequent contact with the injured athlete. Second, the sports medicine team must show an empathetic, caring attitude toward athletes while recognizing that varied psychological responses are a normal part of the recovery process. Additional assistance may be needed, however, if an athlete becomes stuck at one of the early stages for an extended period of time. Additionally, it is important for those working with athletes to remember that it is not the actual nature or severity of injury that determines individuals' reactions to injury but the individuals' *perception* of the injury and its consequences.[16]

In addition, individuals on the sports medicine team should be aware that athletes may work through the grieving stages at highly variable rates. For example, in the case of T. J. it appeared that he spent a very short period of time in the denial stage but perhaps more than usual in the anger stage. This may have been the result of the fact that he was experiencing a season-ending injury for the second time. Given the diversity of responses to injury, it is sometimes helpful to equate the grief process to a rubber band. Whereas a rubber band holds its same general shape, it can be stretched and bent in different directions. Similarly, whereas athletes experience different emotions at different times following an injury, the same general patterns of grief tend to emerge. Furthermore, although the grief process is presented as a linear model, in reality individuals may move back and forth between stages. For example, while an athlete may appear to be moving from depression to acceptance, a setback in the rehabilitation program may throw the athlete into a temporary emotional tailspin and to withdrawal and depression.

Finally, models other than the Kübler-Ross grief process have been proposed.[16,19] These models generally agree that injured athletes undergo an initial *reactive phase* that is characterized by negative emotions such as denial, anger, and shock. This initial reactive phase is typically followed by an *adaptive phase,* which is marked by more positive emotions such as acceptance, hope, and a sense of confidence.[20]

PSYCHOLOGICALLY BASED INJURY REHABILITATION STRATEGIES

As athletes progress through the injury process, they are involved in some form of rehabilitation (see step 4 of Fig. 9-1). Reports from sports medicine providers have suggested that nonadherence to rehabilitation programs is a significant and complex problem.[16,21] The effects of the most sophisticated medical or surgical techniques can be nullified if individuals do not adhere to their rehabilitation programs. Fortunately, researchers have begun to make some progress toward understanding what types of psychological factors are associated with increased compliance.[21-24] Based on this research, two strategies aimed at creating an atmosphere of compliance are presented: (1) fostering social support and (2) involvement in the decision-making process.

Fostering social support

It has been suggested that one of the most important factors associated with injury rehabilitation is social support.[2,21,22,25] For example, Fisher[21] compared athletes who did and did not adhere to their rehabilitation programs and found that "support from significant others contributed the most to the differentiation between adherers and nonadherers" (p. 49).

Although *social support* has been variously defined, it is often viewed as a type of "social commerce" representing "an exchange of resources between at least two people with a beneficial outcome for the recipient."[26] Social support can be provided in numerous forms, including emotional support, informational support, and tangible support. *Emotional support* encompasses listening from friends, family members, and significant others. *Informational support* includes specific medical information or advice relative to the injury itself and what to expect on the road to rehabilitation. Finally, *tangible support* encompasses financial or material assistance.

Traditionally, sport medicine professionals have tended to provide social support in the form of informational support. While the importance of providing athletes with understandable medical information cannot be overemphasized, members of the sports medicine team often have not realized the degree to which they can assist athletes with other types of social support. For example, athletic trainers or sports psychology consultants can help educate family members on what types of emotional support are likely to be the most helpful throughout the athlete's rehabilitation process. In addition, sports medicine clinics can cultivate social support by forming support groups for injured athletes, that is, forums where injured athletes can meet on a weekly or biweekly basis to discuss their concerns. A strategy with growing popularity, support groups are typically run by a sports psychology specialist and appear to be especially beneficial for athletes who have relatively severe or career-ending injuries.[19]

Whereas the provision of social support is seen as an important element in the rehabilitation environment, it has been suggested that the timing of support may be a relevant consideration.[25] Tacit knowledge suggests that, immediately following an injury, athletes may find emotional support the most helpful. However, as the athlete progresses through the rehabilitation process, the provision of informational or material support may become more appropriate.

The discussion of social support up to now has focused on its positive aspects. However, social support is not an elixir—it can have a negative impact on both the recipient (injured athlete) and the provider (sports medicine team member). With regard to the recipient, some athletes may begin to feel indebted or smothered if they feel they are not able to reciprocate in any meaningful way.[25] There can also be potentially negative aspects of social support as it relates to the sports medicine provider. The most common problem is that providers of social support begin to feel overextended.

If this feeling continues over time, it can lead to feelings of "resource bankruptcy."[25] To reduce the chances that any one person becomes a casualty of emotional exhaustion, it is suggested that several team members be involved in the provision of social support.

Involvement in the decision-making process

Traditionally, sports medicine professionals receive the majority of their training and education with regard to the medical aspects of a injury. Indeed, athletes go to a sports medicine clinic hoping to benefit from this medical expertise and training. However, there has been a growing recognition of the special type of expertise that injured individuals bring with them as they seek medical attention.[23,24] More specifically, individuals' own expertise includes knowledge about their personal resources and successful coping strategies that they have used in the past.[24] Part of the challenge for the sports medicine team lies in eliciting this information from individuals. The goal then is to use this information to engage individuals more actively in their own rehabilitation programs and to increase adherence.

In addition to attempting to involve the injured athlete in the decision-making process, other individuals such as family members or spouses may benefit from being included in the decision-making process. Research has shown that when significant others are involved in and educated about the rehabilitation process, compliance is enhanced.[27] Indeed, the President's Commission of 1982 has suggested that individuals and significant others be viewed as a "unit of care" because of their interdependence.[24] Thus, it is suggested that not only the athlete but also the athlete's significant others should be involved in the medical decision-making process.

Given the importance of involving injured athletes and significant others in the rehabilitation process, what are practical ways of doing so within a sports medicine setting? One suggestion is to conduct a compliance interview with the athlete and significant others prior to the start of the rehabilitation program.[28] This interview can be conducted formally or informally and is an excellent way to obtain information on several issues of importance, for example, how difficult does the athlete feel the rehabilitation program will be to follow? Does the athlete have others to rely on for various forms of emotional, informational, and tangible support? What are the attitudes and perceptions of these significant others toward the rehabilitation process?

In summary, because of this special knowledge that individuals possess, it is important that they be included as much as possible in the decision-making process. It is acknowledged that soliciting input from athletes requires an investment of time on the part of the sports medicine team.[24] However, it is not suggested that the same individual be responsible for providing a diagnosis, developing a rehabilitation program, and developing interventions designed to enhance compliance and recovery rates. Instead, a team approach that includes the athlete is advocated whereby different sources of expertise can be weighed and the most effective *long-term* rehabilitation program designed, based on mutually agreed-upon objectives.

TEACHING PSYCHOLOGICAL SKILLS FOR FACILITATING THE REHABILITATION PROCESS

Research has suggested that the use of psychological strategies, such as goal setting, positive self-talk, and healing mental imagery, are associated with faster recovery times and more positive psychological states in the athlete during rehabilitation.[29,30] Thus, to facilitate the rehabilitation process, members of the sports medicine team should assist athletes in the development and use of certain psychological skills. In the section to follow, five psychological strategies that are thought to be of particular relevance to injured athletes are discussed. These strategies include goal setting, modeling, imagery, self-talk, and pain management.

Goal setting

Although most athletes aspire to return to competition or at least a more active life-style following their injuries, action must be taken for these aspirations to become reality. One strategy that can be used to help athletes turn these dreams into reality is goal setting. Goal setting is thought to facilitate the rehabilitation process by increasing athletes' commitment and persistence to their rehabilitation programs and providing a focus for attention and effort.[31] If utilized correctly, it may also facilitate self-confidence and other important psychological states.[32]

Despite the usefulness of having injured athletes systematically use goal setting, the effectiveness of any goal-setting program is diminished when effective goal-setting principles are not followed. What are cornerstones of an effective goal-setting program? Several elements thought to be essential to effective goal setting are outlined as follows.

Include short-term and long-term goals. As noted previously, the obvious long-term goal of most knee-injured athletes is full recovery and return to competition, but it is important for the athlete to break this goal down into a number of weekly or daily goals. Gould[33] encourages athletes to adopt a stairstep approach whereby a series of sequentially related short-term goals provide a natural progression to one or more long-term goals (see Fig. 9-3). The benefit of using an approach such as the one in Figure 9-3 is that it allows the athlete to see how the incremental progress being made leads to the long-term goals. The ability to see the big picture seems to be especially important during lengthy rehabilitation programs.

Use specific and quantifiable goals. To help athletes make their rehabilitation goals "specific and quantifiable," members of the sports medicine team should encourage athletes to write down their goals, develop a strategy for

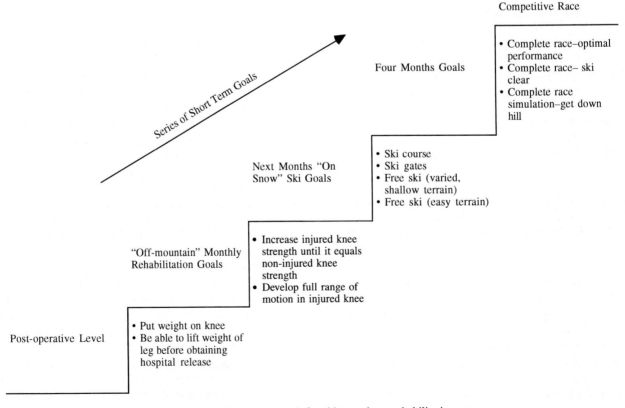

Fig. 9-3. Staircase approach for ski racer knee rehabilitation.

reaching each goal, and have a target date for completion. Thus, a rather vague goal of "wanting to have a knee in good shape for spring football season" would be more effectively restated as "achieve 95% strength in left (injured) knee by doing leg exercises three times daily for 6 weeks until March 1." The injury rehabilitation goal-setting form in the box below has proven useful in this regard.

Help athletes set flexible goals. Sports medicine practitioners are well aware that the rehabilitation process can be plagued by setbacks that can make it impossible for athletes to realize their original goals. For example, an athlete who develops swelling in the knee may not realistically be able to do the preestablished 5 sets of leg lifts on the Cybex machine. If the original goal of completing the leg lifts is seen as carved in stone, the athlete's inability to work toward this goal may serve as an additional source of stress

and frustration. One analogy that has been used to encourage athletes to set flexible goals is to have them think of the recovery process as a rum line in sailing. Just as a sailor tacks back and forth across the wind in order to reach the final destination, so will the injured athlete experience setbacks in the recovery process. The ultimate destination does not change, but the athlete may have to alter the original plan slightly in order to get there.[34]

Assist athletes in setting realistic goals. Athletes can benefit from setting realistic recovery goals. Research in the area of adherence to exercise programs has shown that individuals who did not achieve their goals dropped out of programs at faster rates than those who met their goals. More specifically, after 6 months, 92% of the "non-goal-attainers" had dropped out, and more than 60% of the "goal-attainers" continued with the exercise program.[35] Although

---

Injury rehabilitation goal-setting recovery form

Athlete name: _____   Date: _____

Goal:

_____

_____

_____

_____

Goal achievement strategy (What action must be taken?):

_____

_____

_____

_____

_____

Target date for goal achievement: _____

Goal statement checklist	
_____ Specific	_____ Hard, but realistic
_____ Observable	_____ Performance focused
_____ In my control	_____ Am I committed?

caution is warranted in extrapolating findings from an exercise-adherence setting to a rehabilitation setting, it may be that continued adherence is linked to the degree of progress that individuals feel they are making toward their goals. Obviously, when individuals set realistic goals, they are more likely to be able to meet them.

Modeling

In sports as well as many physical education settings, it is common for athletes to learn motor skills by observing a skilled performer complete the task. Indeed, the work of eminent psychologist Albert Bandura[36] has suggested that this form of learning, called *modeling,* is a powerful means of increasing the observer's self-confidence in completing a task. Furthermore, it has been suggested that the more unfamiliar an individual is with a task, the more advantageous it is to use modeling as a means of increasing the learner's self-confidence.[9]

In the context of a rehabilitation setting, it is not difficult to see how injured athletes, especially those injured for the first time, might benefit from what is known as *peer modeling.* This type of approach typically matches up a newly injured athlete with an athlete who has successfully completed or is nearing the completion of a rehabilitation program for the same or a similar injury.

Many sports medicine clinics already use modeling on an informal basis. However, the efficacy of the systematic use of peer modeling has been studied with positive results. Flint[29] divided athletes who had ACL surgery into two groups: One group periodically viewed videos of other athletes who demonstrated effective coping strategies after undergoing ACL surgery; a second group of athletes simply watched videos that contained neutral information unrelated to their injuries. Athletes who viewed the coping videos were found to have more constructive views toward the rehabilitation, to be more knowledgeable about the rehabilitation process, and to have greater insight into the demands of rehabilitation. These results suggest that sports medicine clinics may want to incorporate modeling on a systematic basis. Moreover, video technology may be an efficient and cost-effective method of utilizing peer models.

Whereas modeling is often viewed within the context of its potential benefits to observers, it has been noted that there may also be benefits to athletes who act as models.[36] More specifically, athletes who serve as role models are able to develop a sense of the progress that they have made through the rehabilitation process.

Imagery

Imagery or visualization is a psychological strategy in which individuals call upon *all* their senses (visual, auditory, kinesthetic, etc.) to create an image in the mind of an experience.[8] It is frequently used in conjunction with relaxation exercises, as it is thought that the mind is more receptive to new information when it is in a relaxed state. There are

a number of ways imagery can be used in conjunction with the injury rehabilitation process. One approach is to have athletes use imagery to prevent the deterioration of performance skills that occurs during the time the athlete is not physically able to practice. In cases where videotapes of preinjury performance are available, this medium can be used to facilitate athletes' recall of their performances.[37] Some sports medicine practices actually set up videocassette recorders in their rehabilitation areas so that athletes can watch tapes of their preinjury performances while they do rehabilitation and conditioning exercises (e.g., riding a stationary bike). Used in this way, videotapes provide powerful visual and auditory images for athletes to focus on during the rehabilitation process. Therefore, having video playback units installed in rehabilitation areas may be a useful strategy.

Another way that imagery has been used is an attempt to assist in the healing process. For instance, an athlete who has surgery on a knee may imagine that the surgical repair is slowly being filled with cement, which is adding to the strength of the knee.[38] This type of healing mental imagery has been used in a variety of other types of medical settings, including work with cancer patients.[39] Although research in this area has been plagued by a lack of well-controlled studies, the initial results have been encouraging. Ievleva and Orlick[30] found that among a group of athletes who had knee and ankle injuries those who used healing mental imagery had faster healing rates.

Changing self-talk and negative beliefs

All of us engage in what is referred to as *self-talk* or *internal dialogue.* The self-talk that we use is closely tied to our belief systems, which in turn influence our behavior. In and of itself, self-talk is neither good nor bad. Self-talk becomes destructive only when it is based on an irrational belief system.[40] For example, if an athlete believes that the injury is the most devastating thing ever to happen and that there is no possibility of returning to competitive sport, the chances of this athlete making a successful recovery are diminished. As an example of a such a pattern, an athlete might be saying, "Just my luck. I get the injury that ends it all for me."

Changing negative self-talk patterns to more rational and productive ones involves three steps. First, athletes must become aware of their self-defeating thought patterns. Individuals are often not conscious of the frequency with which they engage in negative thought processes during the course of a day. Therefore, eliciting an awareness of the frequency of the negative thoughts is a necessary and useful first step. Having the athlete log or keep a record of negative thoughts that accompany rehabilitation is a good way to bring about this awareness.

In the second step of the process, athletes develop a cue word or image that signals them to short-circuit their negative thought cycle and replace their irrational, negative thoughts with more positive ones. The replacement with more positive thoughts is thought to help in the development of more productive coping skills and problem-solving behaviors.[8] Thus, an athlete who makes an overgeneralization such as "I always get injured in the critical part of the season" might develop a cue such as seeing an oversized pair of scissors cut up the negative statement or something as simple as a stop sign. The athlete is taught, any time the negative thoughts begin, to call up the stop cue to short-circuit the negative thought cycle before it becomes self-fulfilling.

Having short-circuited the negative thought processes, the athlete initiates the third step. The athlete replaces the former statement with a more rational statement, such as "I have come back from some tough injuries before and I can do it again." These replacement thoughts are of the utmost importance because they refocus the athlete's attention on something more constructive.

Pain management

Pain is an integral part of the sport experience. Athletes often hold deeply ingrained beliefs concerning the importance of pushing themselves to their physical limits, as evidenced by axioms such as "No pain, no gain."[2] In addition, athletes often receive conflicting messages regarding the appropriateness of playing with pain. As a case in point, during the preliminary rounds of the 1993 Wimbledon, Pete Sampras was suffering from an injured rotator cuff. Although the American Tennis Professionals (ATP) tournament training staff acknowledged that continuing to play without rest could result in further damage to the shoulder, one training staff member was quoted as saying, "It [the shoulder] is very tender . . . under ideal circumstances you wouldn't play, but this is Wimbledon."[41] Statements such as this send conflicting messages to athletes regarding the value of their long-term health as compared to the potential short-term gains of competition.

It has been shown that athletes tend to have higher pain thresholds than nonathletic populations[42] and that experienced athletes are less likely to overestimate the seriousness of their injuries.[43] Thus, it may be that athletes learn to block out certain types of pain. However, given the complex and multidimensional nature of pain, it is too simplistic to assume that all athletes in sports medicine settings are adequately equipped to deal with the pain of rehabilitation. Thus, several pain management strategies are introduced here; more detailed coverage can be found in the excellent work of Heil and Fine[44] and Heil.[19]

One of the most important things that members of the sports medicine team can do is to help athletes learn to distinguish between the "normal" pain of rehabilitation and pain that is counterproductive to the rehabilitative process. Fisher, Domm, and Wuest[21] found that athletes who adhered more to their rehabilitation programs were less bothered by pain. These researchers speculated that those who adhered less to their rehabilitation programs had not learned what type of pain to expect from their treatment program. Certainly, if athletes misinterpret their pain as a sign of reinjury, they are not likely to continue to rehabilitate and may erroneously be labeled as unmotivated.[44] For this reason discussing "normal" versus "abnormal" pain with injured athletes and having peer models discuss this topic can be very useful strategies.

A variety of self-regulation strategies can be used to help in the pain management process; the two techniques presented here deal with attentional focusing. When an attentional focusing strategy is used, the athlete adopts what is referred to as either a *dissociative* or *associative* attentional focus.[19] When a dissociative focus is used, the athlete intentionally directs his or her attention away from the pain and toward a more pleasant external image. Thus, an athlete may imagine being at a beach enjoying the water and sun and not the knee pain. This type of attentional focus has been demonstrated to be relatively easy to learn as well as effective for the majority of individuals.[19] This approach may be very helpful after surgery, when an athlete is trying to deal with the pain resulting from a surgical procedure.

In contrast to the use of dissociative strategies, pain can also be managed through the use of an associative strategy. This approach entails having the athlete intentionally focus on the sensations of pain. The individual then attempts to modify various aspects of pain, which, if successful, allows the pain to be reinterpreted in a more positive way. The efficacy of this approach seems to be linked to the feelings of control the individual achieves when some measure of control is achieved over the pain.[19] Associative strategies may work better for certain individuals under specific conditions. For example, although dissociative strategies are thought to have wider clinical applicability, some individuals seem to prefer and respond more favorably to associative strategies. In addition, at certain points during the rehabilitation process, the treatment provider may want the injured athlete to monitor the amount of pain experienced and adjust workloads accordingly. Under these circumstances, the use of a dissociative strategy that encourages the athlete to focus away from the pain would be inappropriate.

Conclusions regarding the use of psychological skills for the rehabilitation process

To summarize, there are a wide variety of psychological skills that athletes can use throughout the rehabilitation process. One might be tempted to conclude that many athletes would already be familiar with techniques such as imagery and goal setting, as they are frequently used in athletic settings for performances-enhancement purposes. However, some athletes are so physically gifted they may not have ever developed these psychological strategies for performance-enhancement purposes.[45] In other instances, athletes may have a difficult time transferring psychological skills they use on the athletic field to a rehabilitation setting. For these reasons many injured athletes would benefit from the systematic use of one or more of these strategies during the rehabilitation process.

ASSISTING INJURED ATHLETES WITH SPECIAL CONCERNS

Whereas the psychological strategies in the previous sections are thought to be applicable for the majority of injured athletes, some athletes may have concerns that warrant special consideration from members of the sports medicine team. In this section two areas of concern are addressed: (1) athletes who show signs of poor adjustment and (2) the malingering athlete. Because of the complex nature of these areas, this discussion focuses only on the identification of these situations. For a more comprehensive discussion, the reader is referred to work of Petitpas and Danish[46] on maladjustment in athletes and the work of Rotella, Olgivie, and Perrin[47] on malingering athletes.

Poor adjustment

In a previous section several models of the grief process (e.g., Kübler-Ross) were discussed. A common characteristic of these models is that they are thought to describe a "normal" grief response in athletes following injury. However, some individuals encounter more profound psychological difficulties following injuries. The reasons for these difficulties are varied but often result when athletes have an inordinate amount of their personal identity tied to athletic participation or they experience a career-ending injury.[2] How can members of the sports medicine team determine when athletes are displaying signs of poor injury adjustment? The box on this page contains a checklist of symptoms that can be used to assist sports medicine team members in this process. This checklist has been adapted from the work of Petitpas and Danish,[46] who have extensive counseling experience with injured athletes.

There are several important points regarding the information in the box at upper right. First, sports medicine providers are more likely to be able to detect these symptoms if they have developed good rapport with athletes. Certainly, an athlete whose self-esteem is threatened by a physician or athletic trainer is unlikely to reveal feelings of psychological distress.

In addition, it is important to note that the presence of any *one* of the symptoms would not necessarily indicate an athlete in need of further psychological assistance. Rather, members of the sports medicine team would be looking for the presence of multiple symptoms that persist over a period of time. Once it is thought that an athlete is not adjusting normally, it is important to make a referral to the appropriate sport psychology specialist or counselor.

Petitpas and Danish[46] have cautioned that sports medicine team members should not conclude that athletes are coping effectively with their injuries based solely on whether athletes are keeping medical appointments or adhering to their rehabilitation program. In some cases an athlete may be able

---

Signs of potential adjustment problems in athletes
Rapid mood swings
Fatalistic view toward recovery
Withdrawal from significant others
Repeatedly returning too soon to activity and experiencing reinjury
Obsession over when will be able to return to play
Exaggerated bragging about accomplishments
Dwelling over minor physical complaints
Guilt over letting other team members down
Feelings of denial/anger/confusion over an extended time period

Adapted from Petitpas A, Danish S: *Psychological considerations in the care of athletic injuries.* In Murphy S, editor: *Clinical sport psychology,* Champaign, Ill, Human Kinetics, in press.

to handle the practical considerations of the rehabilitation process, yet still experience trouble dealing with the sense of loss, anger, and isolation of the injury. In these instances it may be more appropriate to make an assessment based on whether the individual's interpersonal relationships have suffered.

Malingering

The case studies introduced at the outset of this chapter all depicted instances in which the athletes were very anxious to return to their previous level of activity as quickly as possible. This motivation is thought to be typical of the vast majority of athletes. However, in some cases athletes may feel there is more to be gained from continuing to remain "injured." For instance, the athlete may view the injury as an escape from the rigors of training, a way to obtain more attention, or a face-saving mechanism if poor performance was apparent prior to the injury.[19,23,47] In such cases malingering may be a problem that the sports medicine team has to contend with.

Strictly speaking, *malingering* is defined as the intentional production or gross exaggeration of symptoms, which is motivated by external incentives or personal gain.[48] Malingering tends to be suspected in those cases in which the medical reports differ from those of the athlete, the athlete is resistant or uncooperative, or the rehabilitation process is plagued by problems and setbacks.[30] Despite these relatively clearcut definitions, it is widely maintained that the ambiguity associated with malingering creates one of the most challenging situations for the sports medicine team.[19,47]

In terms of attempting to come to some decision about whether an athlete is malingering, it has been suggested that the "total picture" be considered.[19] More specifically, it is considered appropriate to look not just at the individual's personality but also at previous performance level, playing time, and likelihood of any secondary gains to be made from continuing to be injured. Rarely does a single factor

---

An approach for dealing with a malingering athlete

In approaching the athlete the sports medicine team members should:
- Acknowledge his/her confusion in attempting to understand the athlete's situation
- Present the concerns honestly and openly (e.g., "I know this is a difficult time for you, but I have some concerns that I was hoping we could talk about.")
- Avoid attacking the athlete or making accusations
- Attempt to find a mutually agreeable situation (e.g., "I have some thoughts on some things we might try to change, but first I would like to hear what you think would be the best solution in the long run.")
- Spell out the boundaries of acceptable behavior (e.g., "OK, so we have agreed that talking to your coach is something that you will do tomorrow.")
- Define consequences if unacceptable behavior surfaces (e.g., "If you do not talk to your coach tomorrow, I will need to speak to him/her directly myself.")
- Focus on reinforcing positive change!

Adapted from Rotella R, Heil J: *Psychological aspects of sports medicine.* In Reider B, editor: *Sports medicine: the school-aged athlete,* Philadelphia, 1991, WB Saunders.

provide enough information to make a sound decision.

In the event that all competing hypotheses for the athlete's behavior have been logically dismissed, it may be appropriate to approach the athlete on the issue of malingering. Rotella and Heil[17] suggest approaching the situation as one might when faced with other types of interpersonal conflict, that is, as a time when trust building is needed. Specific suggestions for the sports medicine team members are found in the box above.

Although malingering is certainly not to be encouraged, under extremely limited circumstances it is actually considered an adaptive form of behavior.[48] For instance, a child who is not motivated to participate in sports may be under inordinate parental pressure to do so.[19] Because of the power differential between parent and child, there may be no other viable options for the young athlete but to play. However, the child may view having to leave the sport or decrease involvement in it because of an injury as a golden opportunity. Under these circumstances the focus of the sports medicine team members must shift from treatment of the malingerer to changing the behavior of the parent.

INTEGRATING SPORTS PSYCHOLOGY SPECIALISTS INTO A MULTIMODAL TREATMENT PLAN

Throughout this chapter, the role that psychological factors play in the injury process have been highlighted. However, it is somewhat ironic that the majority of sports medicine clinics do not employ someone who has received training in this area. Fortunately, the inclusion of sports

psychology specialists as members of the sports medicine team is an approach that has gained increasing support.[46] It is suggested that sports psychology consultants would be able to provide the following services if integrated into the sports medicine team.[8,46]

1. Assess athletes' responses to injury and their coping resources, and identify those athletes who show evidence of needing more comprehensive psychological services and make referrals as appropriate.
2. Educate injured athletes on the use of psychological strategies (e.g., pain management) that may enable them to reduce some of the psychological distress that often accompanies injuries.
3. Educate family members, significant others, and coaches about what type of responses are most likely to facilitate athletes' recovery.
4. Interface with other members of the sports medicine team to help ensure that clients receive clear and understandable information and feedback about their injuries and their rehabilitation progress.

CONCLUSION

The past several decades have witnessed a tremendous advance in medical knowledge, surgical procedures, and rehabilitation equipment—all of which have been extremely useful in decreasing the amount of time that athletes are sidelined by knee injuries. Not only have significant advances regarding our understanding of the physical aspects of knee injuries occurred but also our understanding of the psychological aspects has vastly improved. This chapter was written to provide members of the sports medicine team with an appreciation of these psychological factors as well as practical suggestions for how they can more effectively work with injured athletes. It is our contention that optimal rehabilitation only occurs when the physical and psychological aspects of knee-injured athletes are treated in an interdisciplinary, multifaceted fashion. Hence, the information in this chapter must be integrated with the other information in this text if the most effective rehabilitation program is to be formulated and implemented. By doing so, the probability of optimal recovery will be maximized in the knee-injured athlete.

REFERENCES

1. Steadman R: *A physician's approach to the psychology of injury.* In Heil J, editor: *Psychology of sport injury,* Champaign, Ill, 1993, Human Kinetics.
2. Gould D, Weinberg R: *Foundations of sport and exercise,* Champaign, Ill, Human Kinetics, in press.
3. Weiss M, Troxel R: Psychology of the injured athlete, *Athletic Training* 21:104–109, 1986.
4. Wiese D, Weiss M: Psychological rehabilitation and physical injury: implications for the sports medicine team, *Sport Psychol* 1:318–330, 1987.
5. Gordon S, Milios D, Grove R: Psychological aspects of the recovery process from sport injury: the perspective of sport physiotherapists, *Aust J Sci Med Sport* 23:53–60, 1991.
6. Kerr G, Minden H: Psychological factors related to the occurrence of athletic injuries, *J Sport Exerc Psychol* 10:167–173, 1988.

7. Smith R, Smoll F, Ptacek J: Conjunctive moderator variables in vulnerability and resiliency research: life stress, social support, coping skills, and adolescent sport injuries, *J Pers Soc Psychol* 58:360–370, 1990.
8. Williams J, Roepke N: *Psychology of injury and injury rehabilitation.* In Singer R, Murphy M, Tennant L, editors: *Handbook of research in sport psychology,* New York, 1993, Macmillan.
9. Feltz D: *Self-confidence in sport performance.* In Pandolf K, editor: *Exercise and sport science reviews,* New York, 1988, Macmillan.
10. Anderson M, Williams J: A model of stress and athletic injury: prediction and prevention, *J Sport Exerc Psychol* 10:29–306, 1988.
11. Davis J: Sport injuries and stress management: an opportunity for research, *Sport Psychologist* 5:175–182, 1991.
12. Nideffer R: The injured athlete: psychological factors in treatment, *Orthop Clin North Am* 14:373–385, 1983.
13. Danish S: *Psychological aspects in the case and treatment of athletic injuries.* In Vinger P, Hoerner E, editors: *Sport injuries: the Unthwarted epidemic,* Boston, 1986, PSG.
14. Kübler-Ross E: *On death and dying,* London, 1969, Macmillan.
15. Lynch G: Athletic injuries and the practicing sport psychologist: practical guidelines for assisting athletes, *Sport Psychol* 2:161–167, 1988.
16. Pederson P: The grief response and injury: a special challenge for athletes and athletic trainers, *Athletic Training* 21:312–314, 1986.
17. Rotella R, Heil J: *Psychological aspects of sports medicine.* In Reider B, editor: *Sports medicine: the school-aged athlete,* Philadelphia, 1991, WB Saunders.
18. McDonald S, Hardy C: Affective response patterns of the injured athlete: an exploratory analysis, *Sport Psychol* 4:261–274, 1990.
19. Heil J: *Psychology of sport injuries,* Champaign, Ill, 1993, Human Kinetics.
20. Hardy C, Crace K: Dealing with injury, *Sport Psychol Training Bull* May/June:1–8, 1990.
21. Fisher A, Domm M, Wuest D: Adherence to sports-related rehabilitation programs, *Physician and Sportsmedicine* 16:47–52, 1988.
22. Duda J, Smart A, Tappe M: Predictors of adherence in the rehabilitation of athletic injuries: an application of personal investment theory, *J Sport Exerc Psychol* 11:367–381, 1989.
23. Dunbar-Jacob J: Contributions to patient adherence: is it time to share the blame? *Health Psychol* 12:91–92, 1993.
24. Rothert M, Talarczyk G: Patient compliance and the decision-making process of clinicians and patients, *J Compliance Health Care* 2:55–71, 1987.
25. Hardy C, Crace K: *The dimensions of social support when dealing with sport injuries.* In Pargman D, editor: *Psychological basis of sport injuries,* Morgantown, W Va, 1993, Fitness Information Technology.
26. Hardy C, Richman J, Rosenfeld L: The role of social support in the life-stress/injury relationship, *Sport Psychol* 5:128–139, 1991.
27. Erling J, Oldridge N: Effect of spousal support program on compliance with cardiac rehabilitation, *Med Sci Sports Exerc* 18:531–540, 1985.
28. Geronilla L: Handling patient non-compliance using reality therapy, *J Reality Therapy* 5:2–13, 1985.
29. Flint F: *Seeing helps believing: modeling in injury rehabilitation.* In Pargman D, editor: *Psychological basis of sport injuries,* Morgantown, W Va, 1993, Fitness Information Technology.
30. Ievleva L, Orlick T: Mental links to enhanced healing, *Sport Psychol* 5:25–40, 1991.
31. Locke E, Shaw K, Latham G: Goal setting and task performance, *Psychol Bull* 90:125–152, 1981.
32. Burton D: *The Jekyll/Hyde nature of goals.* In Horn T, editor: *Advances in sport psychology,* Champaign, Ill, 1992, Human Kinetics.
33. Gould D: *Goal setting for peak performance.* In Williams J, editor: *Applied sport psychology: personal growth for peak performance,* Palo Alto, Calif, 1992, Mayfield.
34. Wiese-Bjornstal D, Smith A: *Counseling strategies for enhanced recovery of injured athletes within a team approach.* In Pargman D, editor: *Psychological basis of sport injuries,* Morgantown, W Va, 1993, Fitness Information Technology.
35. Danielson R, Wanzel R: *Exercise objectives of fitness program dropouts.* In Landers D, Christina R, editors: *Psychology of motor behavior and sports,* Champaign, Ill, 1977, Human Kinetics.
36. Bandura A: *Social foundations of thought and action: a social cognitive theory,* Englewood Cliffs, NJ, 1986, Prentice-Hall.
37. Rotella R, Heyman S: *Stress, injury, and psychological rehabilitation of athletes.* In Williams J, editor: *Applied sport psychology: personal growth to peak performance,* Palo Alto, Calif, 1993, Mayfield.
38. Green L: *The use of imagery in the rehabilitation of injured athletes.* In Pargman D, editor: *Psychological basis of sport injuries,* Morgantown, W Va, 1993, Fitness Information Technology.
39. Simonton C, Simonton S, Creighton J: *Getting well again,* New York, Bantam.
40. Ellis A: *Self-direction in sport and life.* In Orlick R, Partington J, Salmela J, editors: *Mental training for coaches and athletes,* Ottawa, 1988, Coaching Association of Canada.
41. Smith D: Sore shoulder might slow top seed against Aggassi, *USA Today,* June 30, 1993, 1C.
42. Jaremko M, Silbert L, Mann T: The differential ability of athletes and nonathletes to cope with two types of pain: a radical behavioral model, *Psychologist* 31:265–275, 1981.
43. Crossman J, Jamieson J: Differences in perceptions of seriousness of disrupting effects of athletic injury as viewed by athletes and their trainer, *Percept Mot Skills* 61:1131–1134, 1985.
44. Heil J, Fine P: *The biopsychology of injury-related pain.* In Pargman D, editor: *Psychological basis of sport injuries,* Morgantown, W Va, 1993, Fitness Information Technology.
45. Petrie G: *Injury from an athlete's point of view.* In Heil J, editor: *Psychology of sport injury,* Champaign, Ill, 1993, Human Kinetics.
46. Petitpas A, Danish S: *Psychological considerations in the care of athletic injuries.* In S Murphy, editor: *Clinical sport psychology,* Champaign, Ill, Human Kinetics, in press.
47. Rotella R, Olgivie B, Perrin D: *The malingering athlete: psychological considerations.* In Pargman D, editor: *Psychological basis of sport injuries,* Morgantown, W Va, 1993, Fitness Information Technology.
48. American Psychiatric Association: *Diagnostic and statistical manual of mental disorders,* 3rd ed., rev., 1987.

Chapter 10

USE OF PROTECTIVE DEVICES

Mark G. Kowall
Lonnie E. Paulos

In the fall of 1984, the Sports Medicine Committee of the American Academy of Orthopaedic Surgeons conducted a symposium on knee bracing to classify the types of knee braces available and to review the existing research.[1] This sports medicine committee developed three categories to describe the various types of knee braces available: prophylactic, rehabilitative, and functional. Prophylactic knee braces were described as those designed to prevent or reduce the severity of knee injuries. Rehabilitative knee braces were described as those designed to allow protective motion of injured knees treated operatively or nonoperatively. Functional knee braces were described as those designed to provide stability for unstable knees. The conclusions of this symposium were that, despite a large number of braces available from a variety of manufacturers, there was a disappointing lack of research validating the manufacturers' claims. Unfortunately, there continues to be confusion regarding the data collected on knee braces, as well as the indications for their use. In this chapter, we attempt to summarize the data as well as give our preferred use of braces. We concentrate on the prophylactic, the rehabilitative, and the functional, as well as braces for patellofemoral instability.

PROPHYLACTIC LATERAL KNEE BRACING

Prophylactic knee bracing was introduced to reduce the number and severity of knee injuries. Since their introduction in the late 1970s, these braces have gone through a period of widespread popularity and use, followed by an increase in skepticism as to their effectiveness.

Prophylactic knee braces are of two design types. The first consists of a lateral bar design with a single axis, dual axis, or polycentric hinges fitted with a hyperextension stop. Examples include the McDavid Knee Guard (McDavid Knee Guard, Clarendon Hills, Illinois), Anderson Knee Stabilizer (Omni Scientific, Martinez, California), and the Protective Knee Guard (Don Joy Orthopedic, Carlsbad, California) (Fig. 10-1). The second type consists of plastic cups

with polycentric hinges; this type is often custom-fitted. Examples include the Losee Knee Defender (Don Joy Orthopedics), Am-Pro Knee Guard (American Prosthetics, Davenport, Iowa), and the Iowa Knee Orthosis (Am-Pro Knee Guard) (Fig. 10-2).

Early Clinical Data

George Anderson, head trainer of the then Los Angeles Raiders, was the first to introduce a brace designed to augment taping for an athlete with a medial collateral injury. This original brace, later termed the Anderson Knee Stabilizer brace, was not intended for prophylactic use on uninjured knees, but rather as a device to protect a previous knee collateral injury.[2] After its introduction sparked interest in the potential benefits of preventing knee injuries, within a relatively short period of time, more and more manufacturers developed braces designed for protecting against knee injuries, and prophylactic knee braces were commonplace.

Initial studies on the efficacy of prophylactic knee braces encountered several difficulties. Among these were methods of data collection in the rapidly changing rules of football and the changing methods of treating MCL injuries of the knee.

Schriner[3] reported in 1985 on 1246 high school football players at 25 different schools. This early study reported no MCL or ACL injuries in braced players and concluded that prophylactic bracing substantially reduced injury risk. However, because of the large number of schools involved as well as the method of data gathering, the accuracy of reporting injuries is questioned.

Three longitudinal studies analyzing the rate of football injuries presented in 1986 had the advantage of limitation to a single school.[4-6] The first study carried out at the University of Arizona in Tucson by Hewson et al.[4] spanned 8 years. The authors concluded that the use of prophylactic knee bracing had no effect on the rate of injuries. A similar study was conducted by Rovere et al.[5] at Wake Forest University during the years 1981 to 1985 using the Anderson

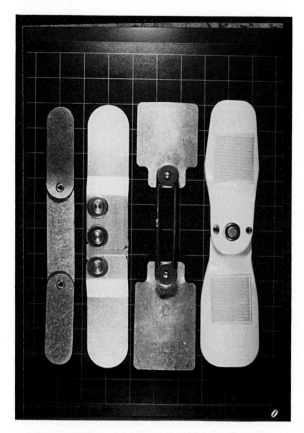

Fig. 10-1. Examples of the lateral bar design prophylactic knee brace.

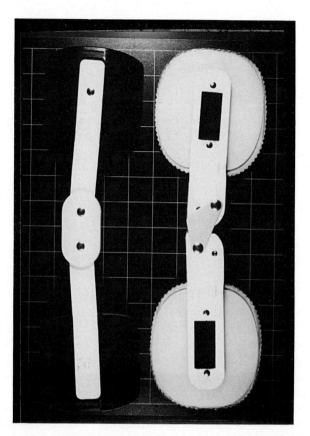

Fig. 10-2. Examples of the plastic cups with polycentric hinge design prophylactic knee brace.

Knee Stabilizer. These authors concluded that the Anderson Knee Stabilizer was ineffective as a prophylactic knee brace. At the University of North Carolina, Chapel Hill, Taft et al.[6] found no change in the numbers of ACL or MCL injuries. They did, however, observe a decrease in surgically treated MCL injuries. These authors concluded that lateral bracing may reduce the number of severe MCL injuries. However, during this period there was a decrease in the surgical treatment of MCL injuries, which may have affected the results in this study.

Teitz et al.[7] collected data from 71 NCAA 1 football teams (6307 players) in 1984 and 61 similar schools (5445 players) in 1985 regarding prophylactic knee brace use. This study found no significant difference in the incidence of all injuries between braced and unbraced players. It did, however, find significantly more MCL injuries among braced players. There was no significant difference in the grades of these MCL injuries. The authors concluded that prophylactic braces were not useful in preventing injuries and may even be harmful. This study involved four different prophylactic knee braces and found no significant difference among them.

In 1987, Garrick and Requa[8] presented a review of six clinical prophylactic brace studies published or presented up to that time. They pointed out several inconsistencies from study to study. These include the fact that some studies

report all injuries, whereas others report only MCL injuries; this is important in that prophylactic braces are designed to limit MCL injuries. Other problems included injury rate reporting. Some studies report rates per number of players, whereas others report incidence per "exposure." The authors also pointed out that the North Carolina study showed 74,400 exposures in 5 years and the Wake Forest study showed less than half that in 4 years. This fact definitely raises the specter of inaccurate reporting methods.

Laboratory data

To better understand the role of preventive knee bracing in injury prevention, Paulos and France in 1987 published a two-part biomechanical investigation using fresh, frozen cadaver knees.[9-11] In the first part of the investigation, two braces, the McDavid Knee Guard and the Omni Anderson Knee Stabilizer, were evaluated.[11] The effects of lateral bracing were analyzed according to valgus force, joint line opening, and ligament tensions. In this study, valgus applied forces to the cadavers, with or without braces, consistently produced medial collateral ligament (MCL) disruptions at ligament tensions higher than the anterior cruciate ligament (ACL) and higher than or equal to the posterior cruciate ligament (PCL). More importantly, no significant protection could be documented with the two preventive braces used (Fig. 10-3). The authors also identified four potentially ad-

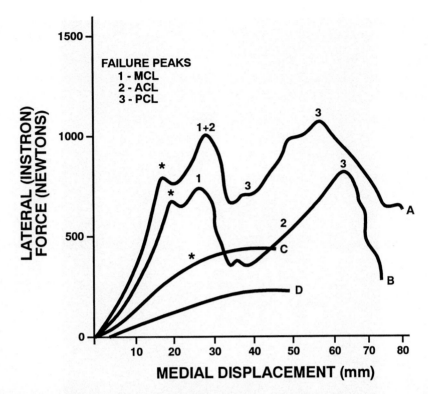

Fig. 10-3. Typical failure pattern for matched knee cadaver testing. *A,* Braced knee; *B,* unbraced knee; *C,* Omni brace alone; *D,* McDavid brace alone. * = Point of first ligamentous failure or permanent deformation. (From Paulos LE, et al: The biomechanics of lateral knee bracing, part I: response of the valgus restraints to loading, *Am J Sports Med* 15:425, 1987.)

verse effects of lateral bracing. The first, *ligament preload,* was characterized as an increased static MCL strain associated with brace application. The second potentially adverse effect, *joint line contact,* represents premature contact of the center member of the brace with the lateral bony structures of the knee. This contact significantly decreases brace efficiency by reducing the effect of the lever arm. Also, depending upon brace design, joint line contact may concentrate forces normally distributed along the lateral surface of an unbraced leg directly into the knee joint. Concentration of force at the joint line may inflict more damage to knee ligaments than incurred in the unbraced knee condition. The third potentially harmful consequence of lateral bracing, *center axis shift,* refers to a shift of the axis of valgus rotation from approximately the center of the knee laterally toward the brace. During valgus loading, this shift places the ACL under tension sooner than the unbraced knee. The final problem observed was *brace slippage,* which concerns the fit and fixation of the brace on the knee. It is influenced by knee varus or valgus angulation, paddle contour, hinge design, and brace fixation technique.

In the second part of this study, the authors examined specifically preload and lateral joint line contact.[10] Six commercially available brace types (manufactured by Don Joy, Omni Scientific, Stromgren-Scott, Mueller, Tru-Fit, and McDavid) were tested on an anatomically correct surrogate

knee model instrumented to measure ligament-tendon tension and medial joint opening (Fig. 10-4). Results of this study were (1) brace-induced MCL preload in vivo was negated by joint compressive forces, (2) the "ideal" brace should increase the lateral force at MCL injury by 80%, (3) at 1000% strain per second rate, MCL failure force was increased by 28%, and (4) on the average only one brace exceeded the minimum impact safety factor (ISF), which represented an MCL load reduction of 30% (Fig. 10-5). Conclusions of this two-part study were that prophylactic braces were probably not harmful but of questionable value in preventing injury during sports.

Further biomechanical studies of prophylactic braces have been performed by Baker et al.[12,13] In these two studies, the authors concluded that functional braces were able to limit abduction stresses and angles, but that prophylactic braces were of little or no protective effect. They also concluded that the prophylactic braces studied had a limited capacity to protect the MCL from direct lateral stress with the knee in full extension. In flexion or with the change in direction of the load, the protective effect is further reduced.

Carlson and French[14] conducted studies on 11 commercially available knee orthoses in terms of their ability to protect the knee from externally applied valgus moments. The authors related two aspects of design, orthosis length and orthosis rigidity, to the effectiveness of protecting

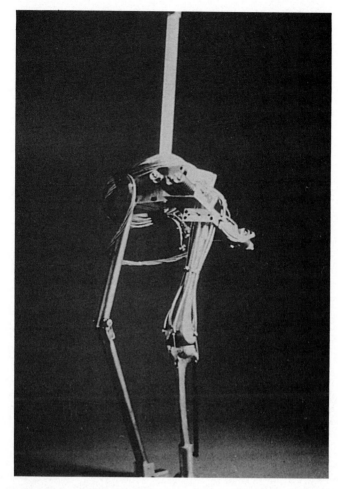

Fig. 10-4. Surrogate knee used in brace investigation. (From Paulos LE, et al: Impact biomechanics in lateral knee bracing: the anterior cruciate ligament, *Am J Sports Med* 19:338, 1991.)

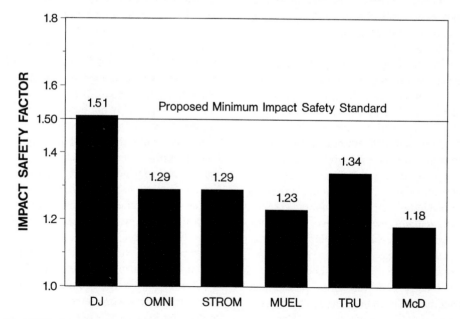

Fig. 10-5. Impact safety factor for braces tested averaged over all test conditions. (From France EP, et al: The biomechanics of lateral knee bracing, part II: impact response of the braced knee, *Am J Sports Med* 15:436, 1987.)

against knee valgus overload injuries. They concluded that a completely rigid, perfectly fitted knee brace must be at least 50 cm long to prevent MCL injuries. Because no brace is completely rigid or fits perfectly, it is unlikely that a knee brace shorter than 50 cm can approach significant protection for the MCL.

As a follow-up to the two-part biomechanical study conducted by Paulos and France, these authors conducted an experiment specifically designed to study the effect of prophylactic knee bracing on the ACL and the suspected center axis shift phenomenon.[15] Using the previously designed mechanical surrogate model, they concluded that no significant center axis shift occurred with any of the four prophylactic braces studied. Braces that were stiff enough to delay joint line contact protected the ACL better than the MCL. The lack of significant center axis shift was ascribed to soft tissue compliance, allowing axial shift to the tibia and femur as medial joint line opening occurred.

Recent clinical studies

In an attempt to mitigate the shortcomings of early clinical studies, later clinical evaluations of prophylactic braces have concentrated on prospective controlled matched subjects in well-controlled populations. Grace et al[16] studied 330 athletes wearing either single-hinge or double-hinge prophylactic knee braces. Each of these players was a high school varsity or junior varsity player from the Albuquerque or Santa Fe, New Mexico, school systems. Each was matched for size, weight, and position with a player who did not wear a knee brace. Players at different levels (i.e., varsity or junior varsity) were matched with players at similar levels. Players were also matched within 1 inch of height and 7 pounds in weight. There was no statistically significant difference in the severity of the injuries. In addition, the authors found an alarming increase in other major injuries of the same limb as that which incurred a knee injury. The conclusion was drawn that a single, upright, double-hinged brace did not decrease the incidence of knee injuries and that the use of a single, upright, single-hinged prophylactic brace was associated with increased rate of injury to the knee. Both types of prophylactic braces were associated with an increased injury rate to the ipsilateral ankle and foot.

Two recent studies seemed to support the use of a prophylactic knee brace in college football. Rudner,[17] with the use of survival analysis methods, showed a decreased rate of injury per exposure for braced players. Additionally, an excellent study from the United States Military Academy at West Point[18] attempted to control variables through the use of a tightly controlled uniform patient population. The study subjects were 1396 cadets taking part in an eight-man intramural tackle football program; 691 players wore prophylactic knee braces, and 705 did not. All braced players used the Protective Knee Guard from Don Joy Orthopedics. All injured players were evaluated for severity of MCL and ACL injuries. A greater number of knee injuries was found in the control group than in the prophylactic brace group. This was statistically significant only among defensive players. Fifty-two percent of the injuries were to the MCL and 22.5% to the ACL. A statistically greater number of MCL injuries occurred in controls, but there was no statistical significance in the ACL injuries. The authors stated that the size of the players in their study was comparable to high school football players. They concluded that their findings may be applicable to high school play, but not to intercollegiate or professional football. They also identified a trend that the efficacy of prophylactic braces may be dependent upon the height and weight of players and the level of play experienced.

Conclusions

Despite more than a decade of use of prophylactic knee braces, a clear scientific and clinical consensus has not been reached regarding the efficacy of these braces. Trends in the use of these braces have been from widespread use based on anecdotal reports with little scientific data to decreased use based on epidemiologic and biomechanical studies showing no protective effect and possibly harmful results. As braces and investigative studies become better, newer evidence seems to point to a role for prophylactic braces in specific populations based on level of play, the size of players, and possibly the position played, rather than universal use in all contact sports.

Our opinion, based on current research, is that prophylactic knee bracing is a viable concept and that, at the present time, the use of presently available prophylactic knee brace designs should not be discouraged for contact sports in selected positions within these sports. The use of these braces should be voluntary, and a system must be in place to assure that they are properly applied and maintained in good condition at all times.

REHABILITATIVE BRACES

Rehabilitative braces are designed for protected and controlled motion of injured knees. In particular, protection of the postoperative knee is necessary to prevent excessive tension or disruption of the ligaments and to allow them to heal in their corrected position. Rehabilitative braces play a vital role in the long-term goals of rehabilitation, which include (1) returning the patient to activity in the shortest period of time, (2) minimizing the harmful effects of joint immobilization, and (3) preventing overload of tissues.

Prior to the advent of rehabilitative braces, early methods of postoperative stabilization included splints, hinged cast bracing, and above-knee or cylinder casts.[19-21] However, the deleterious effects of long-term joint immobilization led to an aggressive attempt at early range of motion following surgery.[22-25] Additionally, studies by Krackow and Vetter[26] showed that long leg casts applied over minimal or no padding allowed significant varus/valgus, anterior, posterior, and rotatory motion at the knee when manipulated manually.

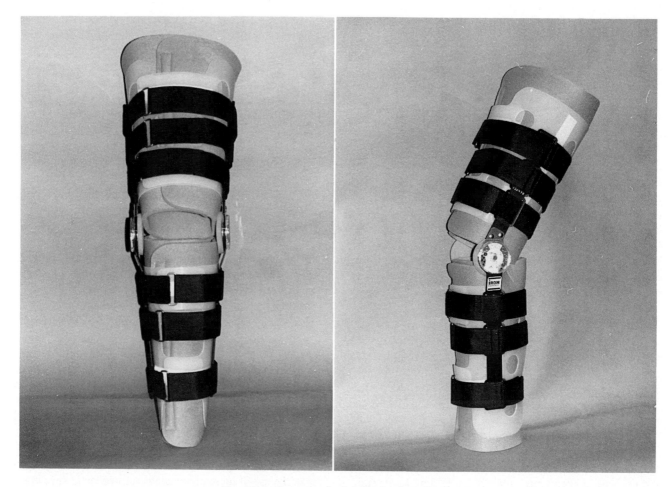

Fig. 10-6. Example of rehabilitative knee brace.

Medial opening to valgus stress ranged from 64% to 100% more after casting than the amount of instability present prior to casting. Legs with normally contoured thighs were not protected against anterior instability after casting, and an average of 48% of precasting rotational instability remained after casting. Orthotic knee braces were introduced to provide early and controlled range of motion of injured knees while also allowing control of range of motion (Fig. 10-6).

Despite the importance of rehabilitative braces, little research has been done comparing the various braces. Two studies recently performed, however, have investigated the differences in the various types of rehabilitative braces.[27,28] Hofman et al.[28] compared the ability of six commercially available orthotic knee braces to stabilize ligamentous injuries using fresh cadaver specimens. Anterior, valgus, and rotational forces were applied to the intact knee after the anterior cruciate ligament and medial collateral ligaments were cut and again after application of the knee braces. Although all braces provided increased stability compared to unbraced knees, the majority of braces did not duplicate natural ligamentous stability. Of the six braces tested, they found a significant difference between them and their ability to stabilize the knee. They concluded that the difference in

performance was most likely due to differences in brace design. Lateral and medial molded supports seemed to provide better stability than single, posterior, or posteroanterior supports. Increased sidebar rigidity also generally seemed to result in greater stability, but these observations were not quantitative. The authors did point out the problem that cadavers were used with their study. Tissue tone in the cadaver is significantly altered from the physiologic norm, and the viscoelastic response of the tissue mass does not approximate what is found in the clinical situation. Cawley et al.,[27] in an effort to overcome the shortcomings of using a cadaver model, used a specially constructed mechanical surrogate of the lower limb to test and compare eight different rehabilitative braces. The braces tested were felt to be representative of a variety of different designs available at the time. The braces tested were Zimmer Flex Tex (Zim), Don Joy ROM Splint (ROM), Medical Technology Bledsoe Brace (MED TECH), Medical Designs Universal Leg Bracing System (MED DES), Don Joy ROM Splint with shells (ROM-S), Orthopaedic Systems Inc. Limited Motion Functional Knee Brace (OSI), 3-D Orthopaedic Two-Way Brace (3-D), and Orthopaedic Technology Inc. Universal Brace (OTI). They found that most of the braces significantly reduced both translation and rotation relative to unbraced

Table 10-1. Mean data for passive extension

Condition	Mean start angle	SD	Mean end angle	SD
ROM	71	± 1.73	64.6	± 0.54
MED DES	60	± 0	46.6	± 0.54
Zim	63	± 5.24	45.8	± 2.16
3-D	68	± 4.63	49.4	± 2.07
ROM-S	62	± 1.73	53.8	± 0.44
OTI	68	± 0	60.0	± 0

From Cawley PW, France EP, Paulos LE: Comparison of rehabilitative knee braces: a biomechanical investigation, *Am J Sports Med* 17:144, 1989.

Table 10-2. Valgus rotation mean displacements 30 degrees of knee flexion

Condition	14 N/m	SD	20 N/m	SD
Unbraced	8.8 (9.24)	± 1.24	21.75 (22.83)	± 0.89
3-D	9.05 (9.5)	± 2.23	13.8 (14.49)	± 1.65
MED DES	6.1 (6.4)	± 0.73	10.55 (11.0)	± 1.69
ROM	4.75 (4.98)	± 0.90	8.05 (8.45)	± 1.62
OTI	6.0 (6.3)	± 0	10.2 (10.71)	± 0.27
MED TECH	8.4 (8.82)	± 1.35	13.25 (13.19)	± 1.06
ROM-S	4.1 (4.3)	± 0.65	6.9 (7.24)	± 0.65
Zim	9.1 (9.55)	± 1.47	16.0 (16.8)	± 1.41
OSI	6.43 (6.75)	± 2.23	9.93 (10.4)	± 3.33

From Cawley PW, France EP, Paulos LE: Comparison of rehabilitative knee braces: a biomechanical investigation, *Am J Sports Med* 17:144, 1989.

Table 10-3. Mean total AP translation 30 degrees of knee flexion

Condition	93 N	SD	155 N	SD
Unbraced	12.3	± 0.97	18.55	± 0.83
OTI	7.45	± 1.29	12.9	± 1.43
ROM	3.8	± 0.83	12.8	± 1.43
ROM-S	6.125	± 1.31	12.55	± 1.31
OSI	9.2	± 0.30	14.7	± 0.74
3-D	7.3	± 0.83	13.9	± 0.41
MED TECH	8.9	± 0.51	15.15	± 0.90
Zim	11.72	± 1.01	17.45	± 1.89
MED DES	9.52	± 0.30	15.4	± 0.39

From Cawley PW, France EP, Paulos LE: Comparison of rehabilitative knee braces: a biomechanical investigation, *Am J Sports Med* 17:145, 1989.

ularly those in a more active stage of rehabilitation.

In summary, the most important design feature for the rehabilitative brace is a controlled range of motion including flexion, extension, varus/valgus, and rotation. Also important are the design features to protect the knee from accidental loading from falls in the early postoperative period. Comfort, size adjustability, and cost-effectiveness are also important considerations in the choice of the rehabilitative brace.

FUNCTIONAL KNEE BRACING
History of the functional knee brace

Functional bracing of the knee is a relatively recent phenomenon. Prior to the late 1960s, functionally unstable knees were stabilized with cumbersome orthoses primarily designed for patients with neuromuscular diseases.

In the early 1970s, Nicholas of Lenox-Hill Hospital developed the first functional or "derotation" brace, which was used for the chronically unstable knee.[30] The original Lenox-Hill brace was specifically engineered for anteromedial rotatory instability.[31]

Prior to the advent of functional knee bracing, taping was used by most trainers for stabilizing unstable knees. Since the introduction of the Lenox-Hill brace, at least 25 functional braces have been marketed.

In 1984, Paulos introduced the descriptive classification system for functional braces. Two basic constructions were identified: the hinge-post, strap type of brace and the hinge-post, shell type. Examples of the hinge-post, strap variety include the Lenox-Hill (Lenox-Hill Brace Shop), Feanny (Medical Design, Westerville, Ohio), and Don Joy 4-Point (Don Joy Orthopedic, Carlsbad, California) (Fig. 10-7); the hinge-post shell type includes the Generation II polyaxial (Generation II Orthotics, Vancouver), C.Ti. (Innovation Sports), and Don Joy RKS (Fig. 10-8). In addition to the two construction types, there are now three different styles of ACL braces: the "off-the-shelf," the adjustable or postoperative, and the custom-molded ACL brace. The MVK and Don Joy 4-Point are examples of "off-the-shelf" braces; the Dual Stage brace is an example of the adjustable ACL

limbs under static conditions, although differences between braces did exist. Tables 10-1 through 10-3 show the mean data collected on the eight braces tested. They pointed out, however, that the loads applied in their test conditions were well below physiologic loading conditions and may be clinically relevant only in those patients who are nonweightbearing or partially weightbearing. In this study, Cawley et al. pointed out the principal factors affecting the choice of rehabilitation braces. They found that the brace straps fared better that interlock with the sidebars, creating a strong single functional unit. Brace hinges having a positive stop mechanism using a shear pin were able to resist higher loads. They also found that how the individual components of the brace were attached together (glued, Velcro, riveted, welded, or sewn) and how each of the components resists the forces of fall were relevant. As the brace is used, many of the attachments become less effective in completing their function through normal use and wear. They also found that both the location of the hinge and the hinge design played a very important role in limiting flexion and extension motions. They, as well as Stevenson et al.,[29] found that subjects were able to achieve 15 to 20 degrees more extension than the hinge allowed. Because of this, the authors recommend that an extension stop of at least 10 to 20 degrees greater than the desired limit be employed for all patients, partic-

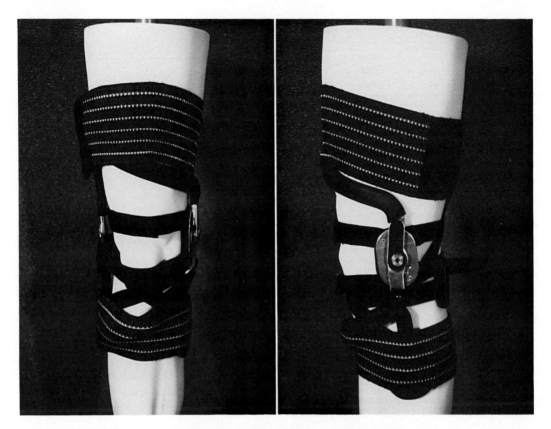

Fig. 10-7. Example of hinge-post strap type of functional knee brace.

brace; and the Lenox-Hill is an example of the custom-molded ACL brace.

Several general review articles on functional bracing are particularly helpful in the clinical situation that requires an overview of concepts or types of braces available.[32-36] The recent review articles by Cawley et al.[34] and Branch and Hunter[32] are particularly useful in analyzing the different aspects of research performed on functional braces.

Subjective assessment

Numerous studies have analyzed the effect of functional braces on controlling instability or "giving way" episodes during athletic performance.[37-45] Bassett and Fleming[37] in their study of the Lenox-Hill brace found that 70% of patients with anterolateral rotatory instability still complained of episodic giving way episodes in spite of using the brace. The majority of these patients participated in sports requiring jumping, twisting, or cutting. Colville et al.,[39] in a similar study of 45 patients using the Lenox-Hill brace, found that 62% still complained of knee instability in the brace. However, nearly 70% of their patients felt that it improved their athletic performance and 91% felt that the brace was beneficial to them. In a study by Mishra et al.[42] comparing four designs of functional knee braces in 42 patients with arthrometer-documented increased anterior laxity, 31 of whom had arthroscopically proven ACL injuries, only 60% of those questioned had experienced giving way after their injury.

However, when wearing the brace, 15% stated that they still had episodes of giving way. It appeared that 25% of those patients experiencing giving way without a brace also experienced it with a brace. They also found that, during functional testing with a one-legged hop and a 40-yard shuttle run, subjective assessment was not significantly changed by brace usage. They found that the most common complaints for brace users in this study were related to brace slippage, bulk, and heat retention.

Overall, these studies report that functional braces are effective in reducing the number of giving way episodes but not in eliminating such episodes. The effectiveness of the braces in controlling instability is related to the degree of instability and the athletic demands placed on it. Events that require stop-start, cutting, pivoting, or jumping maneuvers have an increased likelihood of giving way episodes experienced by the patient.

Mechanical stability

Multiple papers have addressed the ability of the functional knee brace in terms of controlling tibial translation relative to the femur.[37-39,44-50] Two papers investigated this effect via standard manual clinical examination techniques, specifically the drawer test, Lachman test, and pivot shift test.[37,51] The concerns about using standard examination techniques to evaluate the effects of functional knee bracing are that (1) it is difficult to quantify manual tests, particularly

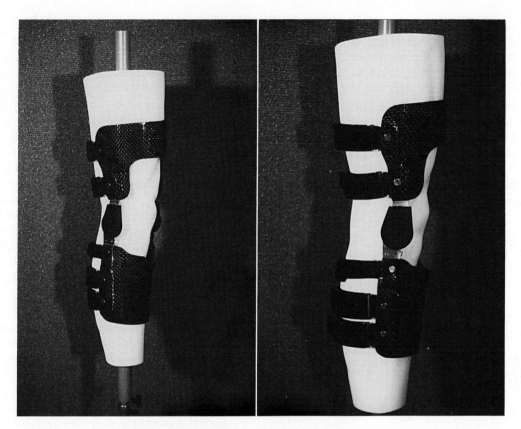

Fig. 10-8. Example of hinge-post shell type of functional knee brace.

when a brace is interposed on the knee; (2) the loads applied must necessarily remain below what must be considered the physiologic norm because of concerns over liability; and (3) there are some significant doubts regarding the performance of the pivot shift maneuver with the brace in place. In that this test requires an induced valgus maneuver, some braces by the nature of their design might actually exaggerate this maneuver.[34]

The introduction of the knee arthrometer prompted numerous studies evaluating the effect of functional braces in terms of reducing anterior translation.* Beck et al.[46] studied the ability of seven functional braces to control anterior tibial translation in three severely lax ACL-deficient knees with the use of two instrumented testing devices. The braces tested were the Don Joy 4-Point, Generation II, RKS, Lenox-Hill, Feanny, C.Ti., and Lerman. Of the seven braces tested, some were more effective in controlling anterior tibial translation than others; the hinge-post, shell design outperformed the hinge-post, strap design, with the exception of the Don Joy 4-Point, which ranked first in the KT-1000 testing (Table 10-4). They also found variations in the measured translations between the two instruments used, a point that must be considered when interpreting the repeatability of the knee arthrometer.

Mishra et al.[42] also used the arthrometer to evaluate four designs of knee braces in 42 patients with unilateral knee injuries. They performed the test with an 89-N passive anterior displacement, high-load passive anterior displacement, and a quadriceps contraction active displacement. They also found that, although the use of a brace decreased the measured pathologic anterior displacement on all tests, there were differences between brands of braces and their ability to reduce laxity (Table 10-5).

Aside from the difficulties related to operator error, questions of the validity of the applied load and the technique of measurements arise. Loads possible with the arthrometers are at the extreme lower limit of what would occur in dynamic physiologic activity. In addition, testing with these instruments for the most part is static in a nonaxial loaded limb. Again, this does not reflect the physiologic condition.

A kinematic analysis involving the study of the six degrees of freedom of the knee joint in the ACL-deficient knee joint has been studied. Knutsen and co-workers[53,54] completed a two-part study comparing seven ACL-deficient subjects with several normal controls during physiologic loading conditions by using an electrogoniometer and force platform. In both studies the authors found that tibial rotation was reduced with the application of a functional brace. The authors conclude, however, that a reduction in total knee flexion with a consequent reduction in automatic axial rotation probably accounts for this finding. In their second

*References 38, 39, 42, 45, 46, 49, and 52.

study, the authors found that the functional braces evaluated also reduced total varus/valgus motion of the surgical knee. Branch et al.[47] measured the compensatory kinematic changes during a side-step cutting maneuver performed in an ACL-deficient subject both with and without bracing. Without bracing, the ACL-deficient subject had a cumulative external rotation of the hip, knee, and ankle that translated to a compensatory early turning of the body toward the side of the step cut. For ACL-deficient subjects wearing a functional knee brace, the authors found no statistically significant difference in rotation, flexion-extension, or varus-valgus rotation in any major joint in the body. However, they found that the knee total rotation of the planted limb in the strap type of brace was closer to the normal subjects' pattern, whereas that in the shell type of brace was closer to the pattern of ACL-deficient subjects.

The results from the kinematic data, specifically, that the functional brace may modify the total degree of freedom that the knee normally experiences, lead to the authors' opinion that the effectiveness of functional braces lies in the control of "coupled motion." *Coupled motion* refers to a combination of the normal six degrees of motion present in the knee. As stated earlier, these involve three rotations (flexion-extension, varus-valgus, and internal-external rotation) and three translations (anterior-posterior shear, medial-lateral shear, and joint compression distraction). Although the functional brace has been proven to be ineffective in the laboratory in terms of controlling straight anterior displacement with higher loads, we feel that a functional brace worn by an ACL-deficient patient is successful in controlling hyperextension as well as varus-valgus motion. By controlling knee motions, the total "envelope" of motion about the knee is reduced. The control of coupled motion is our primary rationale for using functional braces in the ACL-reconstructed knee.

Biomechanical studies

Several biomechanical studies have been attempted to quantify directly the strain on both the ACL and MCL in vitro and in vivo.[12,13,55,56]

Table 10-4. KT-1000 values (mm) for braces tested

Brace	20-lb Anterior	20 Total	Maximum anterior	Active anterior drawer
Don Joy 4-Point	0.33	−1.13	2.00	1.07
Generation II	1.07	−0.20	5.13	2.17
RKS	1.93	0.70	5.93	1.83
Lenox-Hill	1.90	3.30	7.57	2.00
Feanny	2.80	2.30	5.73	2.10
C.Ti.	2.23	1.90	6.47	3.03
Lerman	2.47	1.70	6.33	3.57

From Beck C, et al: Instrumented testing of functional knee braces, *Am J Sports Med* 14:254, 1986.

Table 10-5. Anterior displacement: comparison of mean side-to-side differences (mm) of normal knees versus braces tested

Group	n	Side to side difference	Displacement force 89 N	Displacement force Manual maximum	Displacement force Quadriceps active
Normal knees	120	Greater minus lesser	0.80 ± 0.80	0.80 ± 1.00	0.80 ± 0.60
All braces	42	I − N	5.00 ± 2.04	6.45 ± 2.36	4.06 ± 1.71
		B − N	1.41 ± 2.25	2.75 ± 2.32	1.70 ± 1.65
		*p**	<.001	<.001	<.001
Don-Joy 4-Point	20	I − N	5.16 ± 1.46	6.29 ± 2.32	4.05 ± 1.94
		B − N	0.47 ± 1.98	1.97 ± 1.70	1.37 ± 1.58
		*p**	<.001	<.001	<.001
C.Ti.	9	I − N	4.75 ± 4.31	7.42 ± 1.50	5.08 ± 2.06
		B − N	1.17 ± 2.04	2.58 ± 2.29	1.25 ± 1.97
		*p**	<.05	<.006	<.003
Lenox-Hill	6	I − N	5.07 ± 1.43	6.79 ± 2.93	4.29 ± 0.95
		B − N	3.00 ± 2.06	4.07 ± 2.32	3.07 ± 1.30
		*p**	<.006	<.001	<.043
RKS	7	I − N	4.75 ± 1.56	5.51 ± 2.58	3.13 ± 0.88
		B − N	2.44 ± 2.29	3.56 ± 3.17	1.63 ± 1.53
		*p**	<.001	<.009	<.003

*Matched *t*-tests (injured no brace minus normal) versus (injured with brace minus normal).
(From Mishra DK, Daniel DM, Stone ML: The use of functional knee braces in the control of pathologic anterior knee laxity, *Clin Ortho Rel Res* 241:218, 1989.)

Arms et al.[55] quantified the strain on the ACL with the use of the Hall strain transducer in braced and unbraced cadaver knees. Their results suggested that bracing did not protect the anterior cruciate ligament when anterior shear loads were applied across the tibial-femoral joint. Instead, they found that the strain on the anterior cruciate ligament was increased when the knee was braced in all positions from 0 to 90 degrees of flexion. They suggested that the functional brace may actually cause an anterior displacement of the tibia that may increase the strain on the anterior cruciate ligament.

Baker et al., in a two-stage project,[12,13] also attempted to measure the strain on the anterior cruciate and medial collateral ligaments with and without prophylactic and functional braces. In the first stage of their project, a static abduction, external rotation force was applied to a cadaver knee, simulating a fixed foot with upper body contact. Force transducers were placed on the MCL and ACL, and four functional braces and two prophylactic braces were tested. The results were that (1) functional braces had some capacity to control abduction angle, whereas prophylactic did not; (2) in certain loading situations, prophylactic bracing had no effect on reducing the MCL transducer loads; and (3) there was an increased ACL load above the no-brace measurement when one prophylactic brace was applied, suggesting a prestressing effect. In the second stage of the experiment, similar measurements were obtained in cadavers in which a direct lateral impact load was applied, simulating a clipping injury. Results revealed that in the unbraced knee, the largest MCL and ACL forces occurred at full extension when the impact was a direct lateral or anterior oblique blow. They found that the functional and prophylactic braces had some capacity to reduce knee abduction angle to a limited extent, but that the functional braces were always more effective than the prophylactic braces, regardless of the direction of impact or the flexion angle. With lateral impact loading, external tibial rotation was decreased by the functional braces with the MCL intact, but the protective effect of the functional braces was reduced to near zero with the MCL cut. Prophylactic braces provided little or no protection against external rotation stresses.

The results of these cadaver studies are limited because of the changes in soft tissue compliance of the thigh and calf and the lack of active muscle contraction that have been shown to affect the strain on the anterior cruciate ligament in previous studies.

In a recent study quantifying the strain on the ACL in a functionally braced knee in vivo, Beynnon et al.[56] tested seven functional braces in 13 patients undergoing arthroscopy for partial meniscectomy. They found that, at low anterior shear loads, some functional braces were able to provide a strain-shielding effect compared with the no-brace knee. This strain-shield effect did not occur at higher loads. More important, they found that in this group of patients who had intact anterior cruciate ligaments and were sub-

jected to static loads, there was no increased strain on the anterior cruciate ligament as a result of wearing a functional brace.

In summary, these biomechanical studies suggest that functional braces have some capacity to protect the medial collateral ligament and may have some effect on controlling external rotation. Although most functional braces have some stress-shielding effect on the anterior cruciate ligaments at low static loads, their effect is less pronounced at physiologic loads.

Energy expenditure

The effect of wearing a brace on energy expenditure and associated physiologic measures has been the subject of many reports. Houston and Goemans[57] reported that wearing knee braces increased the blood lactate concentration during a 15-minute endurance ride on a cycle ergometer at a heart rate of 170 beats per minute by 41%. Soule and Goldman[58] reported that adding weights to the feet produced a higher energy expenditure response than adding weights to other parts of the body. They demonstrated that wearing a 6-kg weight on each foot while walking at 93 m per minute (3.43 miles per hour) caused a 420% increase in energy expenditure. Using a rough extrapolation of energy expenditure from this study, Zetterlund et al.[59] suggested that a 2-lb weight on one foot would produce a 30% increase in energy consumption. Moving it to the knee and increasing the gait speed to 161 m per minute (6 miles per hour) resulted in a predicted increase of 5%.

Zetterlund et al.[59] looked at the differences in energy expenditure and associated physiologic measures in ten patients with ACL deficiencies who were wearing a Lenox-Hill functional brace. They concluded that (1) young adult males with ruptured ACL exhibit a small but significant (4.58%) increase in oxygen consumption while wearing the Lenox-Hill brace and running at 161 m per minute when compared with running without the brace, and (2) heart rate was also increased significantly (5.1%) while wearing the brace under these conditions. Although the differences in physiologic parameters at relatively low levels of exercise appeared to be low, one has to consider the effect on energy expenditure during high levels of exercise for prolonged periods of time.

Proprioception

Proprioception, or the ability of the central nervous system to interpret the position of the knee, has been a focus of interest in the ACL-deficient knee. In studies by Schultz et al.[60] and Schutte et al.,[61] mechanoreceptors were found to be within the substance of the cruciate ligaments. Barrack et al.[62] first quantified proprioception in a group of ACL-deficient patients. In these patients compared with an age-matched control group, they found a significantly higher mean threshold value for detecting a change in the position of the knee joint. They speculated that ACL-deficient patients may experience a decline in proprioceptive function that may contribute to the progressive instability and disability that occur over time. A study utilizing dynamic EMG during walking in ACL-deficient patients revealed increased activity of the hamstrings and decreased activity of the quadriceps and gastrocnemius muscles during joint loading in the transition from the swing phase to the stance phase of gait.[63] This increased hamstring activity was interpreted to be a protective mechanism for the ACL-deficient knee and presumed to be the result of stimulation of capsular or tendinous mechanoreceptors. These mechanoreceptors may be stimulated by the abnormal strain experienced in an ACL-deficient knee.

Proprioceptive feedback is one of the two most popular theories as to what produces the subjective improvement seen in ACL-deficient patients who wear functional braces. The other popular theory is that of mechanical stability controlling the giving way episodes. The proponents of the proprioceptive feedback theory feel that the brace can provide information to the central nervous system about the position of the knee during activity that can thus alter motor control of the surrounding knee musculature and provide joint stability.

Cook et al.[40] used both a force platform and high-speed photography to perform a dynamic, in vivo, functional analysis of the C.Ti. brace in 14 athletes who had arthroscopically proven absent ACLs. The authors concluded that the C.Ti. brace allows for significantly better running and cutting performances from those who had deficient ACLs. They also found that athletes who had not achieved 80% of the quadriceps strength as measured by Cybex testing showed even more improvement while wearing the functional brace than those patients who had achieved normal strength.

Branch and co-workers[64] designed a study to determine if bracing altered muscle-firing amplitude, duration, or timing or created improved dynamic stability. In their study they looked at 10 ACL-deficient patients and 5 normal controls. Two braces, the Lenox-Hill and the C.Ti., were evaluated. Using foot switches and dynamic EMGs, they evaluated each subject during the performance of a sidestep, cutting maneuver. In the unbraced situation, subjects as compared with normal controls, demonstrated a significant increase in lateral hamstring activity during the swing phase. During the stance phase, subjects showed a significant decrease in quadriceps and gastrocnemius activity and an increase in medial hamstring activity (Fig. 10-9). The combined decreased quadriceps-gastrocnemius activity with increased hamstring activity, also demonstrated by Limbird et al.,[63] could have a protective effect on the ACL-deficient knee. The increased stance-phase activity of the medial hamstrings, also reported by Tibone et al.,[65] suggests that the medial hamstrings may be more important than the lateral hamstrings in preventing a pathologic anterior drawer produced by an active quadriceps contraction. In comparing braced versus unbraced ACL-deficient subjects, the braced subjects showed significant decreases in medial hamstring activity during the stance and swing phases and decreased quadriceps activity during the stance phase (Fig. 10-10). The authors suggest that the braced knee may require less stabilization created by the agonist-antagonist cocontraction. Additionally noted in the braced versus nonbraced situation was no significant difference in the timing of muscle firing in the braced knee. This suggests that a brace does not appear to provide proprioceptive feedback to improve dynamic knee stability.[32,64] The theory of bracing providing proprioceptive feedback has yet to be proven conclusively.

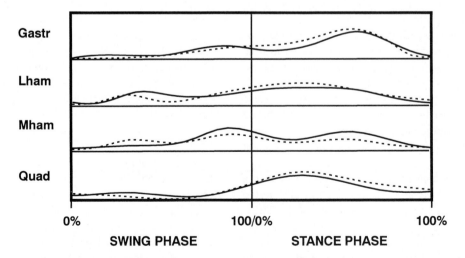

Fig. 10-9. Mean swing and stance phase curves for controls and subjects without bracing: Straight line = normal; dash line = ACL deficient. (From Branch TP, Hunter RE, Donath M: Dynamic EMG analysis of anterior cruciate deficient legs with and without bracing during cutting, *Am J Sports Med* 17:38, 1989.)

Authors' preference for postoperative ACL bracing

At our institution, patients are placed into a type of rehabilitative brace for the first 3 weeks. Based on our laboratory investigation, we found that the postoperative rehabilitation brace that interlocks with the sidebars and has hinges with a positive stop mechanism using a shear pin was the most effective and efficient in terms of providing flexion-extension, anterior-posterior, and varus-valgus support. Its disadvantages are that it tends to slip down the leg and is more difficult to apply than some of the others.

The key features one should look for in the postoperative brace are the presence of femoral and tibial circumferential shells, association with hinges that control motion every 10 degrees, and straps that run circumferentially around the leg and should interconnect or interweave with the brace struts so that no slippage occurs.

At 3 weeks, the rehabilitative brace is designed to break down into the interim or "transitional" brace (Fig. 10-11). This interim brace provides continued control of motion, specifically hyperextension and varus-valgus for the healing ligament, but allows progression of the rehabilitative process, including muscle strengthening and increasing girth.

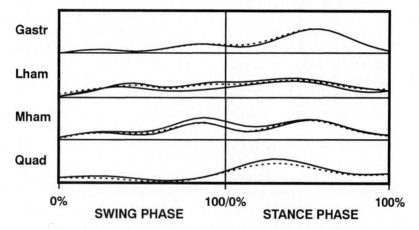

Fig. 10-10. Mean swing and stance phase curves for subjects with and without each brace. Thick line = no brace; thin line = C.Ti. brace; dash line = Lenox-Hill brace. (From Branch TP, Hunter RE, Donath M: Dynamic EMG analysis of anterior cruciate deficient legs with and without bracing during cutting, *Am J Sports Med* 17:39, 1989.)

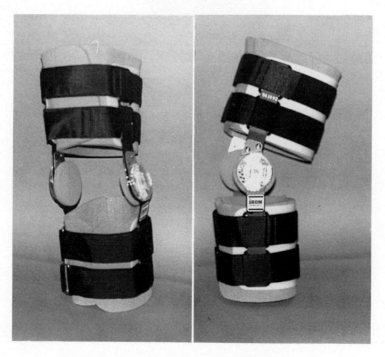

Fig. 10-11. Example of transitional rehabilitative brace.

At approximately 9 to 12 months postoperatively and continuing for the first year upon return to sports, patients are fitted for the functional brace. At this period their limb girth and muscle strength are usually at an acceptable level.

Functional braces can be divided into three levels. Level one braces are designed to control hyperextension only. These braces have collapsible hinge supports without thigh or tibial shells. These braces are not designed to provide medial or lateral support and are also the least effective in controlling flexion-extension motion. We prefer to use this type of brace in patients who have only a grade I or II isolated ACL ligament injury. Examples of this type of brace include the Cincinnati Brace and the TS7 Brace (Fig. 10-12).

Level two braces have tibial and thigh shells that connect rigidly to hinge supports. These braces are represented by the OTI, Lenox-Hill, Don Joy 4-Point, and C.Ti. braces. We use these braces when a grade III ACL, grade III ACL-MCL, or another combination injury is present. These braces provide more varus-valgus support but tend to be bulkier and less comfortable.

Level three braces are designed to control AP excursion, as well as varus-valgus for combined and global laxities. These injuries usually include both anterior and posterior cruciate ligament rupture. No level three braces are now on the market that control both anterior and posterior drawer; therefore, custom-made orthoses are the only ones available. These orthoses usually extend from ankle to hip and include knee cages and extension and flexion stops (Fig. 10-13).

Bracing for PCL instability

The majority of functional braces are designed for the ACL-deficient knee. Many of these braces have been described by the manufacturer as treating all forms of knee instability, including that attributed to a PCL deficiency. It is important to evaluate each brace in terms of its orthotic design and material properties for posterior instability. Posterior instability problems require special design characteristics to treat the instability effectively. The primary purpose is to treat the posterior dropback or sag in the nonsurgical cases and to preload anteriorly or protect the graft from these forces postoperatively in surgical cases. However, because the PCL brace must direct its force through the soft tissue mass of the calf musculature, it is less effective than the ACL brace, which directs its force on the anterior tibia.

Quadriceps rehabilitation is of utmost importance for these patients and is started as soon as possible after diagnosis. During quadriceps exercises, the patellofemoral joint reactive forces are increased; with the effect of the posterior dropback from a PCL deficiency, these forces are increased even more. Patients often complain of patellofemoral pain during functional training sessions. The ability of

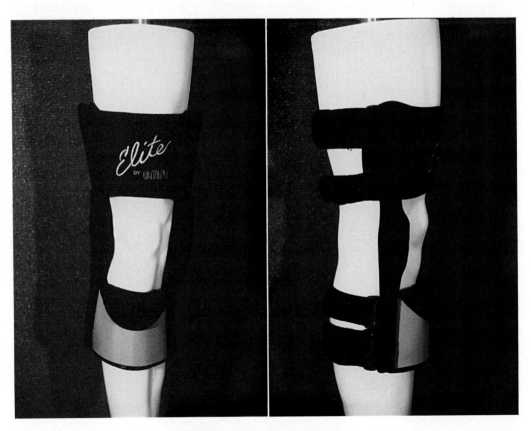

Fig. 10-12. Example of level I brace.

the functional brace to help reestablish the relationship of the knee joint in the PCL-deficient knee has been helpful during the rehabilitative process.

PATELLOFEMORAL BRACES

Patellofemoral pain is a common complaint in both the athletic and nonathletic populations. There are many etiologies of patellofemoral pain, but the most frequent cause has been associated with patellofemoral malalignment.[66]

Malalignment is seen clinically as patellar hypermobility leading to patellar subluxation or dislocation. Additionally, malalignment can be seen as patellar tilt leading to lateral patellar compression syndrome (LPCS). Oftentimes both problems are seen together, leading to an especially difficult treatment dilemma.

The initial treatment of patellar malalignment is conservative, consisting of activity modification, nonsteroidal anti-inflammatories, and physical therapy to strengthen the quadriceps and hence improve patellar tracking.[66-69] In an attempt to improve patellar tracking, several devices have been used, including straps, sleeves, braces, and taping (Fig. 10-14).

The use of braces in the treatment of patients with pa-

tellofemoral subluxation and dislocation has been controversial. Braces for the prevention of dislocating or "slipping" patella were first described by MacAusland and Sargent,[70] who used a split kneecap pad held in place with a Jones knee brace for treatment. They combined the brace treatment with baking and massage to give tone to relaxed ligaments and exercises to shrink muscles for postural strength. Pearson[71] developed a poroplastic, felt "kneecap pad" in the treatment of patellofemoral dislocation.

Levine in 1978[72] described the results of an infrapatellar strap used for patients with anterior knee pain. In this study, 24 knees in 17 patients with "straightforward symptoms of chondromalacia" were reviewed. The brace was found to be successful in all but one patient with pronounced "squinting patella." The following year, Levine and Splain[73] again reported on the use of this infrapatellar strap. In this study, which consisted of 57 patients with 79 symptomatic knees, they found that 77% of patients experienced enough pain relief to resume normal activity. However, the authors do not comment on the preoperative diagnosis of the patient, specifically patellar hypermobility or lateral patellar compression syndrome, nor is a follow-up stated. In 1981,

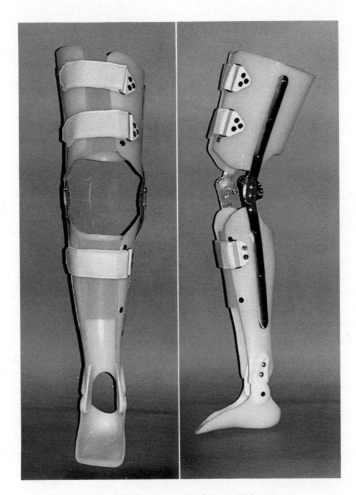

Fig. 10-13. Example of level III brace.

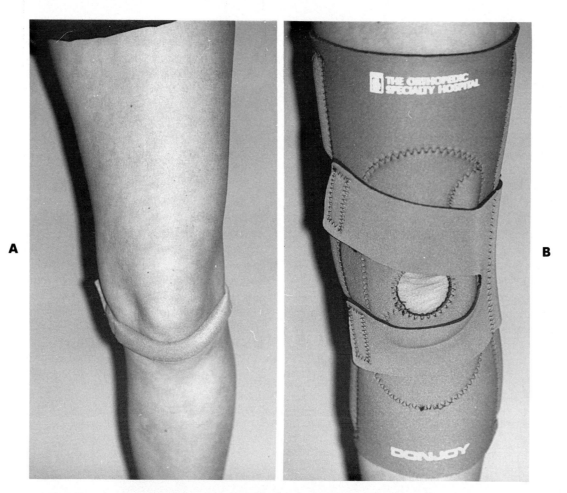

Fig. 10-14. Different types of patellar bracing, including straps **(A)**, sleeves **(B)**, devices with pressure pads **(C)**, and taping **(D)**.

a preliminary report on the Palumbo dynamic patellar brace stated that symptoms were reduced in 93% of 62 patients who had patellofemoral dysfunction.[74] This device is designed to provide a medially displacing force to the lateral border of the patella and to maintain constant pressure during flexion, extension, and rotation of the knee. It was reported to be useful in the diagnosis of suspected subluxation in the treatment of patellar subluxation and patellofemoral arthritis, and in the prevention and treatment of chondromalacia and patellar tendonitis. However, no documentation of these benefits were given. Moller and Krebs found similar symptomatic improvement of patellofemoral pain using patellar braces.[75]

Lysholm et al.[76] performed one of the few studies to objectively evaluate the use of an elastic patellar brace in patients with patellofemoral arthralgia. In this study they attempted to analyze the quadriceps muscle strength with the Cybex II Isokinetic Dynamometer in patients with patellofemoral arthralgia with and without a patellar brace. In the 24 patients studied, 88% improved their performance with the use of a brace. Based on the results of this study, the authors endorsed the use of a brace as a supplement to

quadriceps rehabilitation, specifically, isotonic and isokinetic exercise.

In 1985, Villar[77] was unable to reproduce Levine's success rate for decreasing patellofemoral pain by using the infrapatellar brace. In this study, which involved 37 active-duty military recruits with patellofemoral pain, only 24% demonstrated some improvement in symptoms at 1 week, and 22% at 1 year following brace application.

McConnell, a physical therapist from Australia, in an effort to improve patellar maltracking, suggested a program utilizing a taping technique to improve patellofemoral malalignment.[68] In addition to addressing the medial-lateral glide component of maltracking, this taping technique is designed to address patellar tilt and rotational abnormalities. In her original article, she states a 92% success rate in 35 patients with a mean duration of symptoms of approximately 5 years. Eighty-three percent of these patients reportedly experienced no pain in eight or fewer treatment sessions. However, these initial results do not contain a control group and lack objective evidence to support the use of taping. Recently, Kowall et al.,[78] in an attempt to objectively evaluate the use of a patellar taping program, found no change

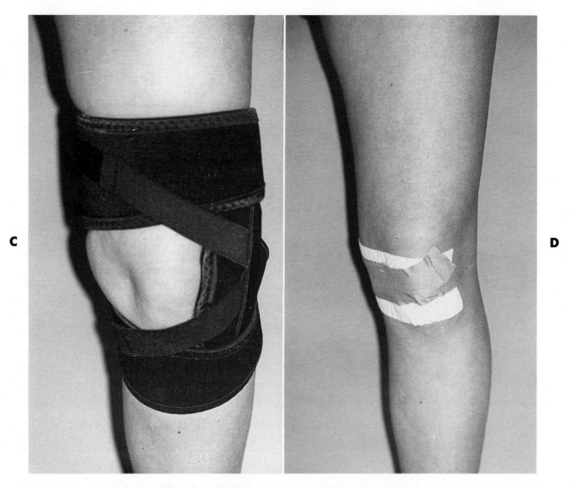

Fig. 10-14, cont'd. For legend see opposite page.

in subjective improvement, quadriceps isokinetic strength, or EMG activation in patients who had a patellar taping program added to a formal physical therapy program. Although statistical significance was achieved, the numbers in this study were low.

Patients with patellofemoral pain occasionally demonstrate a significant gait abnormality while walking or running. As James et al.[79] and McKenzie et al.[80] have pointed out, sometimes this abnormality is linked to the feet. They have stated that appropriate footwear and orthotics may be helpful to certain patients with patellofemoral pain.

A review of these articles on patellar braces offers an incomplete evaluation of their efficacy and few concrete guidelines as to their use. The orthopedic literature lacks well-controlled prospective studies on specific clinical uses of these orthoses. The exact function of many of the different patellar orthotics is unclear. These braces may help alleviate knee pain for a variety of reasons. The warmth the device provides to the knee may be therapeutic. Sensory feedback may be altered, which might reduce the patient's awareness of discomfort. Possible alteration in circulation is another potential effect of these devices. These are very nonspecific

mechanisms of patellar brace function that may help explain their potential effectiveness.

The mechanical function of these devices seems limited to applying a medial force to the lateral aspect of the patella in patients with tracking problems. This is one function of patellar bracing that is based on sound biomechanical principles. To assume that this principle might be applicable in treating other types of knee pain is speculative.

At our institution, we use patellar orthotics in conjunction with a well-supervised patellar protection and strengthening program emphasizing quadriceps strengthening and hamstring stretching. We use off-the-shelf knee sleeves and braces with medially directed forces in those patients who demonstrate patellar hypermobility with subluxation. In those patients who demonstrate severe hypermobility, patellar subluxation, and genu recurvatum, we have been using a recently developed patellofemoral brace (Lenox-Hill, New York City) that controls extension and provides a medially directed force (Fig. 10-15). The purpose of this patellofemoral brace is to block abnormal lateral subluxation of the patella when the knee approaches extension. The major component of this brace includes a single-hinge system to

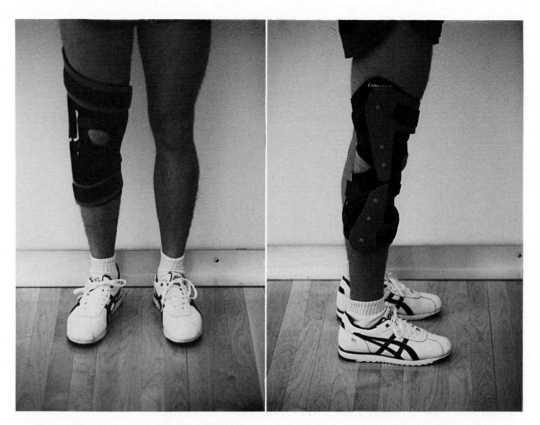

Fig. 10-15. Example of patellofemoral brace to control patellar subluxation and genu recurvatum.

facilitate bilateral application of the brace that also controls varus-valgus rotation. Also, a tibial and femoral shell system is integrated with a three-dimensional-strength undersleeve. The undersleeve contains a patellar buttressing system that is integrated through straps with the lateral hinge bar. The rigid portion of this brace is applied to the knee, utilizing a special strapping system that helps maintain the position of the lateral hinge. The biomechanical forces are applied to the patella when the knee moves toward full extension to produce a medial force on the patella, moving the patella medially. The rigid brace system blocks the knee in extension at about 15 to 20 degrees, thus improving patellofemoral congruity. Initial clinical reports with this brace at our institution are encouraging.

In conclusion, anterior knee pain secondary to patellofemoral maltracking is common. The initial treatment of these problems is conservative, consisting of quadriceps strengthening and activity modification. Patellar orthotics are used in selected cases with specific physical findings and well-defined clinical goals.

REFERENCES

1. American Academy of Orthopaedic Surgeons: *Knee braces seminar report,* Chicago, Ill, 1984, American Academy of Orthopaedic Surgeons.
2. Anderson G, Zeman SC, Rosenfeld RT: The Anderson Knee Stabler, *Physician Sportsmed* 7:125–127, 1979.
3. Schriner J: The effectiveness of knee bracing in preventing knee injuries in high school athletes, *Med Sci Sports Exerc* 17:254, 1985 (abstract).
4. Hewson GF, Mendini RA, Wang JB: Prophylactic knee bracing in college football, *Am J Sports Med* 14:262–266, 1986.
5. Rovere GD, Haupt HA, Yates CS: Prophylactic knee bracing in college football, *Am J Sports Med* 15:111–116, 1987.
6. Taft TN, Hunter S, Fundurbeck CH: Presented at the American Orthopaedic Society for Sports Medicine, July 1, 1985, Nashville.
7. Teitz CC, et al: Evaluation of the use of braces to prevent injury to the knee in college football players, *J Bone Joint Surg [Am]* 69:2–9, 1987.
8. Garrick JG, Requa RK: Prophylactic knee bracing, *Am J Sports Med* 15:471–476, 1987.
9. France EP, Paulos LE: In vitro assessment of prophylactic knee brace function, *Clin Sports Med* 9:823–841, 1990.
10. France EP, et al: The biomechanics of lateral knee bracing, part II: impact response of the braced knee, *Am J Sports Med* 15:430–438, 1987.
11. Paulos LE, et al: The biomechanics of lateral knee bracing, part I: response of the valgus restraints to loading, *Am J Sports Med* 15:419–429, 1987.
12. Baker BE, et al: A biomechanical study of the static stabilizing effect of knee braces on medial stability, *Am J Sports Med* 17:182–186, 1989.
13. Baker BE, et al: The effect of knee braces on lateral impact loading of the knee, *Am J Sports Med* 17:182–186, 1989.
14. Carlson JM, French J: Knee orthoses for valgus protection, *Clin Orthop* 247:175–192, 1989.

15. Paulos LE, France EP, Cawley PW: Impact biomechanics in lateral knee bracing: the anterior cruciate ligament, *Am J Sports Med* 19:337–342, 1991.

16. Grace TG, et al: Prophylactic knee braces and injury to the lower extremity, *J Bone Joint Surg [Am]* 70:422–427, 1988.

17. Rudner M: Football players who wear knee braces show fewer incidents of serious injury, *Big 10 Conference News Service Bureau* 2:6, 1988.

18. Sitler J, et al: The efficacy of a prophylactic knee brace to reduce knee injuries in football: a prospective randomized study at West Point, *Am J Sports Med* 18:310–315, 1990.

19. Bassett FH, Beck JL, Weiker G: A modified cast brace: its use in nonoperative and postoperative management of serious knee ligament injuires, *Am J Sports Med* 8:63–67, 1980.

20. Haggmark T, Eriksson E: Cylinder or mobile cast brace after knee ligament surgery, *Am J Sports Med* 7:48–56, 1979.

21. Sandberg R, Nilsson B, Westlin N: Hinged cast after knee ligament surgery, *Am J Sports Med* 15:270–274, 1987.

22. Enneking WF, Horowitz M: The intra-articular effects of immobilization of the human knee, *J Bone Joint Surg [Am]* 54:973–985, 1972.

23. Noyes FR: Functional properties of knee ligaments and alterations induced by immobilization, *Clin Orthop* 123:210–242, 1977.

24. Salter RB, Field P: The effects of continuous compression on living articular cartilage, *J Bone Joint Surg [Am]* 42:31–49, 1960.

25. Salter RB, et al: The biological effect of continuous passive motion on the healing of full-thickness defects in articular cartilage: an experimental investigation in the rabbit, *J Bone Joint Surg [Am]* 62:1232–1251, 1980.

26. Krackow KA, Vetter WL: Knee motion in a long leg cast, *Am J Sports Med* 9:233–239, 1981.

27. Cawley PW, France EP, Paulos LE: Comparison of rehabilitative knee braces: a biomechanical investigation, *Am J Sports Med* 17:141–146, 1989.

28. Hofman AA, et al: Knee stability in orthotic knee braces, *Am J Sports Med* 12:371–374, 1984.

29. Stevenson DV, et al: *Rehabilitative knee braces control of terminal knee extension in the ambulatory patient,* presented at the 34th ORS Meeting, Atlanta, February 1–4, 1988.

30. Nicholas JA: Bracing the anterior cruciate ligament deficient knee using the Lenox-Hill derotational brace, *Clin Orthop* 172:137–142, 1983.

31. Nicholas JA: The five-one reconstruction for anteromedial instability of the knee, *J Bone Joint Surg [Am]* 55:899–922, 1973.

32. Branch TP, Hunter RE: Functional analysis of anterior cruciate ligament braces, *Clin Sports Med* 9:771–797, 1990.

33. Butler PB, et al: A review of selected knee orthosis, *Br J Rheumatol* 22:109–120, 1983.

34. Cawley PW, France EP, Paulos LE: The current state of functional knee bracing research: a review of literature, *Am J Sports Med* 19:226–233, 1991.

35. Nelson KA: The use of braces during rehabilitation, *Clin Sports Med* 9:799–811, 1990.

36. Podesto L, Sherman MF: Knee bracing, *Orthop Clin North Am* 19:737–745, 1988.

37. Bassett GS, Fleming BW: The Lenox-Hill brace in anterolateral rotatory instability, *Am J Sports Med* 11:345–348, 1983.

38. Branch T, Hunter R, Reynolds P: Controlling anterior tibial displacement under static load: a comparison of two braces, *Orthopedics* 2:1249–1252, 1988.

39. Colville MR, Lee CL, Civillo JV: The Lenox-Hill brace: an evolution of effectiveness in treating knee instability, *Am J Sports Med* 14:257–261, 1986.

40. Cook FF, Tibone JE, Redfern FL: A dynamic analysis of a functional brace for anterior cruciate ligament insufficiency, *Am J Sports Med* 17:519–524, 1989.

41. Marans HJ, et al: Functional testing of braces for anterior cruciate ligament deficient knees, *CJS* 34:167–172, 1991.

42. Mishra DK, Daniel DM, Stone ML: The use of functional knee braces in the control of pathologic anterior knee laxity, *Clin Orthop* 241:213–220, 1989.

43. Tegner Y, Lysholm J: Derotational brace and knee function in patients with anterior cruciate ligament tears, *J Arth Rel Surg* 1:264–267, 1985.

44. Wojtys EM, et al: A biomechanical evaluation of the Lenox-Hill brace, *Clin Orthop* 220:179–184, 1987.

45. Zogby RG, et al: A biomechanical evaluation of the effect of functional braces on anterior cruciate ligament instability using the Genucom knee analysis system, *Trans Orthop Res Soc* 14:212, 1989.

46. Beck C, et al: Instrumented testing of functional knee braces, *Am J Sports Med* 14:253–256, 1986.

47. Branch TP, et al: Kinematic analysis of anterior cruciate ligament–deficient subjects during side-step cutting with and without a functional knee brace, *Clin J Sports Med* 3:86–94, 1993.

48. Markoif K, Kochan A, Amstutz H: Measurement of brace stiffness and laxity in patients with documented absence of the anterior cruciate ligament, *J Bone Joint Surg [Am]* 66:242–253, 1984.

49. Mortenson WW, et al: An in-vivo study of functional knee orthoses in the ACL disrupted knee, *Orthop Res* 13:520, 1988.

50. Wojtys EM, et al: Use of a knee-brace for control of tibial translation and rotation, *J Bone Joint Surg [Am]* 72:1323–1329, 1990.

51. Coughlin L, Oliver J, Berretta G: Knee bracing and anterolateral rotatory instability, *Am J Sports Med* 11:161–163, 1983.

52. Rink PC, et al: A comparative study of functional bracing in the anterior cruciate deficient knee, *Orthop Rev* 18:719–726, 1989.

53. Knutsen KM, Bates BT, Hammil J: A biomechanical analysis of two functional knee braces, *Med Sci Sports Exerc* 19:303–309, 1987.

54. Knutsen KM, Bates BT, Hamill J: Electrogoniometry of post-surgical knee bracing in running, *Am J Phys Med* 62:172–181, 1983.

55. Arms S, et al: The effect of knee braces on anterior cruciate ligament strain, *Trans Orthop Res Soc* 12:245, 1987.

56. Beynnon BD, et al: The effect of functional knee braces on strain on the anterior cruciate ligament in vivo, *J Bone Joint Surg [Am]* 74:1298–1312, 1992.

57. Houston ME, Goemans PH: Leg muscle performance of athletes with and without knee support braces, *Arch Phys Med Rehabil* 63:431–432, 1982.

58. Soule RG, Goldman BF: Energy cost of loads carried on the head, hands and feet, *J Appl Physiol* 27:687–690, 1969.

59. Zetterlund AE, Serfuss C, Hunter RE: The effect of wearing the complete Lenox-Hill derotation brace on energy expenditure during horizontal treadmill running at 161 meters per minute, *Am J Sports Med* 14:73–76, 1986.

60. Schultz RA, et al: Mechanoreceptors in human cruciate ligaments, *J Bone Joint Surg [Am]* 66:1072–1076, 1984.

61. Schutte MJ, et al: Neural anatomy of the human anterior cruciate ligament, *J Bone Joint Surg [Am]* 69:243–247, 1987.

62. Barrack RL, Skinner HB, Buckley SL: Proprioception in the anterior cruciate deficient knee, *Am J Sports Med* 17:1–6, 1989.

63. Limbird TJ, et al: EMG profiles of knee joint musculature during walking: changes induced by anterior cruciate ligament deficiency, *J Orthop Res* 6:630–638, 1988.

64. Branch TP, Hunter R, Donath M: Dynamic EMG analysis of anterior cruciate deficient legs with and without bracing during cutting, *Am J Sports Med* 17:35–41, 1989.

65. Tibone JE, et al: Functional analysis of anterior cruciate ligament instability, *Am J Sports Med* 14:276–284, 1986.

66. Fulkerson JP, Shea KP: Current concepts review: disorders of patellofemoral alignment, *J Bone Joint Surgery [Am]* 72:1424–1429, 1990.

67. DeHaven K, Dolan W, Mayer P: Chondromalacia patella in athletes: clinical presentation and conservative management, *Am J Sports Med* 7:5–11, 1979.

68. McConnell JS: The management of chondromalacia patella: a long term solution, *Aust J Physiotherapy* 32:215–223, 1986.
69. Paulos LE, et al: Patellar malalignment: a treatment rationale, *Phys Ther* 60:1624–1632, 1980.
70. McAusland W, Sargent A: Recurrent dislocation of patella, *Surg Gynecol Obstet* 35:35–41, 1922.
71. Pearson C: After treatment of lateral dislocation of the patella by a new form of kneecap, *Lancet* 1:1984.
72. Levine J: A new brace for chondromalacia patella and kindred conditions, *Am J Sports Med* 3:137–140, 1978.
73. Levine J, Splain SH: Use of the infrapatella strap in the treatment of patellofemoral pain, *Clin Orthop* 139:179–181, 1979.
74. Palumbo PM: Dynamic patellar brace: a new orthosis in management of patellofemoral disorders, *Am J Sports Med* 9:45–49, 1981.
75. Moller BN, Krebs B: Dynamic knee brace in the treatment of patellofemoral disorders, *Arch Orthop Trauma Surg* 104:377–379, 1986.

76. Lysholm J, et al: The effect of a patella brace on performance in a knee extension strength test in patients with patellar pain, *Am J Sports Med* 12:110–112, 1984.
77. Villar R: Patellofemoral pain and the infrapatellar brace, *Am J Sports Med* 5:313–315, 1980.
78. Kowall MG, et al: *Patellar taping in the treatment of patellofemoral pain: a prospective randomized study,* presented at the American Orthopaedic Society for Sports Medicine, San Francisco, February 21, 1993.
79. James S, Bates G, Osternig L: Injuries to runners, *Am J Sports Med* 6:40, 1978.
80. McKenzie D, Clement DB, Taunton JE: Running shoes, orthotics and injuries, *Sports Med* 2:334–347, 1985.

Part III

PRACTICAL APPLICATIONS: INJURY-SPECIFIC REHABILITATION PROGRAMS

Chapter 11

PATELLOFEMORAL JOINT INJURIES

Kevin P. Shea
John P. Fulkerson

Injuries to the patellofemoral joint and supporting soft tissue structures are quite common in the athlete. The patella protrudes in front of the knee and is often the first structure contacted in a collision with the ground. Athletes who engage in sport without proper conditioning (inadequate strength in the quadriceps and lack of flexibility in the iliotibial band and hamstrings) are prone to overuse injuries. Finally, as many as 20% of adolescents have some degree of asymptomatic patellofemoral malalignment that may become painful with rigorous athletic activity. Simple avoidance of athletic competition is not sufficient to relieve pain. Specific rehabilitation is required to alleviate symptoms and restore function in the athlete's knee.

To properly rehabilitate the injured patellofemoral joint, it is critical that the treating physician (1) understand the anatomy and biomechanics of the patellofemoral joint mechanism; (2) correctly diagnose the cause of the anterior knee pain; (3) recognize pre-existing patellofemoral malalignment and its contributions, if any, to the pain in the anterior knee; and (4) understand the rationale behind the modalities and therapeutic exercises used to rehabilitate patients with injuries to the patellofemoral joint.

ANATOMY AND BIOMECHANICS OF THE PATELLOFEMORAL JOINT

The patellofemoral joint is composed of the bony patella, which articulates with the femur via the V-shaped femoral trochlea, and the supporting soft tissues. The patella not only functions to increase the lever arm of the quadriceps mechanism but also serves to protect the deeper structures.[1] During normal knee motion, the patella is usually centered congruently in the femoral trochlea by 20 degrees of knee flexion and remains centered throughout further knee flexion.[2] In the nonpathologic knee, no excessive translation (medial or lateral) or tilting of the patella occurs after 20 degrees of knee flexion.[2] As knee flexion progresses, the area of contact of the patellar articular cartilage that contacts the femoral trochlea moves proximally on the patella; that is, different areas of the patellar articular cartilage contact the femoral trochlea in different degrees of knee flexion[3] (Fig. 11-1).

The patellofemoral joint is stabilized by the quadriceps, the medial and lateral retinacula, and the patellar tendon. The magnitude and direction of the combined forces in these tissues, in conjunction with the resistance offered by the lateral femoral trochlea, determine patellar motion during active knee flexion and extension (Fig. 11-2). The quadriceps muscles exert a vector pull on the patella that is directed superiorly and slightly laterally to the midline of the thigh. The lateral retinaculum prevents excessive medial translation of the patella. However, when the lateral retinaculum becomes pathologically shortened, it also exerts a lateral vector pull on the patella. The patellar tendon stabilizes the patella in a downward direction. However, when the tibial tubercle is laterally displaced (a tubercle sulcus angle not equal to zero), this patellar tendon may also exert a laterally directed force on the patella during active motion.[4] Femoral anteversion, pronated feet, and quadriceps contraction while actively changing direction (cutting) may all dynamically increase knee valgus and increase the lateral displacement vector on the patella. The sum of these forces tends to result in one large superiorly and laterally directed force. The superiorly directed force motors knee extension. In the nonpathologic knee, laterally directed force on the patella is counteracted predominantly by the vastus medialis obliquus (VMO) and the lateral wall of the femoral trochlea. Thus, injuries to the VMO unbalance the forces that prevent the patella from moving laterally and potentially precipitate a painful malalignment syndrome, particularly in patients with preexisting but asymptomatic malalignment.

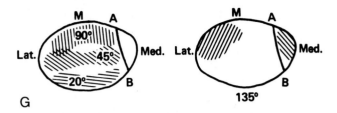

Fig. 11-1. The area of the patella in contact with the femur changes with the degree of knee flexion. (From Hungerford DS, Barry M: Biomechanics of the patellofemoral joint, *Clin Orthop* 144:11, 1979.)

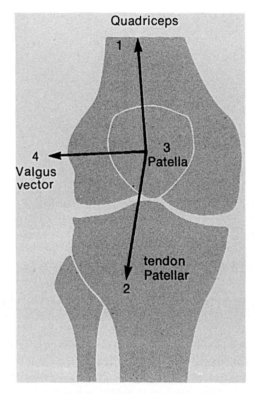

Fig. 11-2. Summation of forces that influence patellar motion. (From Fulkerson JP, Hungerford DS: *Disorders of the patellofemoral joint,* ed 2, Baltimore, 1990, Williams & Wilkins.)

Chronic lateralization of the patella tends to shorten the lateral retinaculum and may lead to excessive lateral patellar tilt.[5,6] Repetitive, forced knee flexion, which is common in many athletic activities, may stretch this already shortened lateral retinaculum, leading to pain. Small nerve injury (presumably from repetitive stretching and scarring) may form the basis of pain in the lateral retinaculum.[7]

The patellar articular cartilage is subject to compressive forces greater than body weight during active knee extension. Patellofemoral joint reaction force is primarily the sum of the vector forces acting to compress the joint contributed by the pull in the quadriceps mechanism and the patellar tendon[8] (Fig. 11-3). Active quadriceps extension with the knee in 40 to 70 degrees of knee flexion results in the highest joint reaction forces for a given level of quadriceps effort.[8] The patellar articular cartilage is the thickest in the body

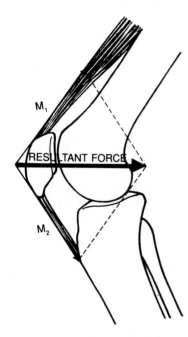

Fig. 11-3. Summation of forces that contribute to pressure across the patellofemoral joint. (From Fulkerson JP, Hungerford DS: *Disorders of the patellofemoral joint,* ed 2, Baltimore, 1990, Williams & Wilkins.)

and very resistant to damage. If the articular cartilage becomes damaged through either prolonged malalignment or direct contusion, contraction of the quadriceps increases the patellar joint reaction force and may cause pain. Grood et al.[9] have shown that terminal extension (i.e., the last 15 degrees of knee extension) requires large quadriceps forces to achieve full extension. Exercises done in this range tend to aggravate preexisting areas of inflammation in the quadriceps tendon and the patellar tendon and may also aggravate lesions on the distal patellar joint surface.

Thorough understanding of these mechanical factors, which affect patellar motion and contribute to concentrated stress to various areas of the patellofemoral joint mechanism, is important not only to understanding the basis of anterior knee pain but also to provide a framework from which to design a rehabilitation program for the patellofemoral joint.

PATELLOFEMORAL SYNDROMES

Hopefully, the era in which all anterior knee pain was attributed to chondromalacia patella has passed. Anterior knee pain arises from many sources, some of which are better understood than others.[10] Anterior knee pain in the athlete can be divided into two broad categories: (1) that which is primarily related to overuse (even though minor trauma may have occurred), including patellar tendonitis and patellofemoral malalignment syndromes; and (2) that associated primarily with trauma, including patellar fracture, patellar dislocation, and traumatic contusion to the patella (traumatic chondromalacia patellae). Exact determination of the cause of the anterior knee pain aids the physician in designing a successful rehabilitation program.

Overuse syndromes

The most common cause of anterior knee pain in the athlete is *overuse*. The athlete complains of a dull ache in the anterior aspect of the knee that may be accentuated by climbing stairs or prolonged sitting with the knee bent (movie sign). Although these symptoms may occur during sport, pain and stiffness usually start 12 to 24 hours after activity. Pain in the back of the knee, particularly the hamstring origin or in the midbelly of the posterior thigh, is also common. The complaints may be gradual at first, but become accentuated if the early symptoms are ignored. Crepitus, knee effusion, and "giving way" are uncommon findings in pure overuse syndromes. If any of these findings is present, one should seek another diagnosis. Prolonged avoidance of treatment may result in diminished performance and pain with everyday activities. The more advanced the symptoms, the greater the length of treatment that is required.

Commonly, the athlete who presents with these symptoms is improperly trained and enters an athletic contest with leg muscles that lack the proper strength, flexibility, and endurance. The quadriceps is particularly sensitive to overuse and can become quite painful. Tightness in the hamstring and quadriceps can concentrate stress on the patellofemoral joint and surrounding tissues during vigorous activity. Muscles become tighter as they fatigue, accentuating the stress on the peripatellar area. This effect becomes amplified when the athlete's quadriceps and hamstrings lack the endurance necessary to safely engage in athletics. Prolonged stress may lead to soft tissue breakdown, particularly in the patellar tendon. Small nerve injury may also occur.

On examination, the athlete will usually have poor resting tone in the quadriceps muscle. When the quadriceps is contracted, the VMO may be atrophic. The thigh circumference may be diminished compared to the contralateral side. Flexibility tests often reveal tightness in the quadriceps, hamstrings, and iliotibial band, and attempts to passively stretch each muscle may reproduce pain. Sometimes the anterior knee tenderness is difficult to localize. In the adolescent, tenderness may be present in the tibial tubercle (Osgood-Schlatter disease) or at the apophyses of the distal pole of the patella (Sinding Larsen Johannson syndrome). Factors that predisposed the patellofemoral malalignment should be sought. Isokinetic testing to document weakness often aggravates the symptoms and should not be performed.

Foundations of rehabilitation in these overuse syndromes are (1) avoidance or modification of activities that precipitate pain until the muscle-tendon units are properly rehabilitated, (2) nonsteroidal anti-inflammatories to reduce inflammation, (3) appropriate strengthening (described later) to rehabilitate the quadriceps mechanism and VMO with gradual return to

sport, (4) taping and modalities to support therapeutic exercises, and (5) correction of soft tissue contractures, most notably hamstrings, quadriceps, iliotibial band, and lateral retinaculum. Iontophoresis with 10% hydrocortisone cream may reduce pain and inflammation in recalcitrant cases of patellar tendonitis and in patellar tendonitis where a discrete area of localized tenderness is found.[11] The most common areas are the proximal patellar tendon, inferior pole of the patella, lateral retinaculum, and VMO insertion onto the patella.

Every effort should be made to aid the athlete in maintaining cardiovascular fitness while rehabilitation is ongoing. Swimming, emphasizing the upper body, may produce little pain in the anterior knee and is to be encouraged. Walking or running in the pool may have the added effect of strengthening the leg muscles without placing undue stress on the patellofemoral joint. Isotonic, open-chain knee extension exercises and short-arc quadriceps exercises are to be avoided, as they place undue stress on the extensor mechanism. Of primary importance is to individualize strengthening techniques and to work all muscles through a pain-free range of motion.

Before the athlete returns to competition, effort should be made to restore proper alignment and strength to the trunk and hip musculature. Failure to address weakness in the ipsilateral hip may lead to further overuse of the quadriceps mechanism and further injury.

Surgery is almost never indicated as treatment for these overuse syndromes except in cases where there is recalcitrant patellar tendonitis[12] or overuse associated with patellofemoral malalignment that does not respond to extensive conservative management.[13]

Lateral patellar tilt

Excessive lateral patellar tilt may cause progressive pain and disability in the athlete. The athlete may complain of pain in the anterior aspect of the knee, which, when further investigated, is really located either in the lateral retinaculum, the VMO, or both. He often states that he has only a dull ache in the knee at rest but a dramatic increase in his pain after exertion. Early in the course of this syndrome, the pain often persists for only a few hours after activity. Later, the symptoms may persist for 2 or more days after athletic exertion and may be constant. Daily activities such as stairclimbing and even walking on level ground may be affected. Swelling and effusion are usually not present unless the articular cartilage of the patella is degenerated. Giving way may occur primarily because of quadriceps inhibition secondary to pain.

On physical exam the patella often appears laterally tilted. The lateral retinaculum is tight and may be tender. Attempts to correct the patellar tilt, with downward pressure on the medial aspect of the patella, may precipitate pain.[6] Pain may be further aggravated by forced flexion of the knee (Fig. 11-4). The VMO insertion on the patella may be tender

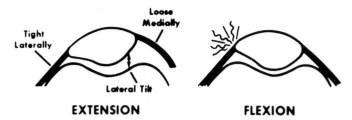

Fig. 11-4. Pain in pathologic patellar tilt emanates from the lateral retinaculum, which is stretched during knee flexion. (From Fulkerson JP: The etiology of patellofemoral pain in young, active patients, *Clin Orthop* 79:132, 1983.)

from overuse. The VMO is usually atrophic and there may or may not be signs of co-existing patellar subluxation. The knee should be checked for signs of meniscal damage or ligamentous injury as well, and those injuries treated accordingly.

The initial treatment for patellar tilt is similar to that for overuse injuries. Modalities and soft tissue mobilization should concentrate on the pathologically tight lateral retinaculum. McConnell[14] taping (see next section) has been extremely helpful in attempting to control patellar alignment. In many cases, the athlete experiences immediate relief of symptoms with taping alone. The tape may be worn 24 hours a day and changed every day. Taping should be used in conjunction with mobilization techniques to gradually correct tightness in the lateral retinaculum. Muscular rehabilitation should emphasize closed kinetic chain activities to strengthen the quadriceps (VMO) and hamstring muscle groups through a pain-free range. In recalcitrant cases, it may be necessary to use electrical stimulation or biofeedback techniques in order to train the athlete's VMO to contract at appropriate times. Open-chain knee extension exercises should be avoided.

Rehabilitation of excessive patellar tilt syndrome may require up to 6 months to restore the athlete to a pain-free state. However, return to sports should be individualized. The athlete may return with some pain as long as the extensor mechanism is satisfactorily strengthened and normal flexibility is achieved. The use of a patellar stabilizing brace may be of some benefit during the early return to sport.

If rehabilitation is not successful and the athlete continues to exhibit pain with exertion, a computed tomography (CT) scan should be obtained to look for evidence of patellofemoral malalignment, specifically patellar tilt.[2] Lateral release has been shown to be effective in more than 90% of cases in which tilt is documented preoperatively by CT scan and the articular cartilage is not yet degenerated under the lateral facet.[15] Lesser results are obtained with lateral release if advanced articular cartilage changes are encountered, and alternate methods such as tibial tubercle anteromedialization may be necessary.[15]

Patellar subluxation

Occasionally an athlete may complain of feelings of giving way of the patella, the feeling that the patella has skipped out of joint, or obvious recurrent patellar dislocations. There may be a history of a traumatic onset, but usually symptoms develop insidiously. The athlete may frequently state that the knee feels stable except during high-speed cutting or twisting maneuvers with the foot planted. These maneuvers tend to accentuate the normal valgus in the knee and increase the laterally directed vector on the patella. Subluxation episodes may be transient or have sequelae of pain and stiffness that last for 1 or more days after each occurrence. Effusion may be present, particularly if synovial or articular cartilage damage co-exist.

On examination, the medial or lateral retinaculum or both may be very tender, particularly if a major subluxation has just occurred. The patella is usually very mobile both medially and laterally. Apprehension with laterally directed pressure on the medial portion of the patella is usually present. The examining physician should look for signs of excessive femoral anteversion and a laterally rotated tibial tubercle. The tubercle sulcus angle is usually abnormal (Fig. 11-5).[4] These findings tend to increase the lateral vector on the patella and may precipitate subluxation with large quadriceps forces. In addition, the VMO frequently has a high insertion on the patella or exhibits signs of atrophy and disuse.

Treatment of recurrent patellar subluxation should consist of avoidance of activities that precipitate symptoms and restoration of flexibility and muscle strength, as previously described. McConnell taping[14] may stabilize the patellofemoral joint and reduce the frequency of subluxation episodes. A patellar stabilizing brace may also produce the same effect. Emphasis on hip flexibility, primarily the elimination of internal rotation contractures, may lessen the dynamic Q-angle and further aid in reducing exertional symptoms. Biofeedback techniques to teach the athlete to control the VMO may be extremely useful. These biofeedback techniques can be utilized as isolated exercises or in conjunction with closed-chain exercises such as bicycling, stairclimbing, or cross-country skiing (see section later).

The athlete may return to sport once appropriate strength has been achieved in the quadriceps mechanism, appropriate flexibility has been restored to all muscles in and around the knee, and the athlete's symptoms are minimized. The athlete should be instructed that he or she may have a predisposition to recurrent subluxations because of structural abnormalities either in the hip or in the knee and to continue knee conditioning to remain active in athletics.

If symptoms of subluxation are not relieved by conservative means, a CT scan should be performed through the mid-patella transverse plane to document subluxation.[5] If symptoms have persisted longer than 1 year and the athlete remains symptomatic, surgery may be undertaken to restore

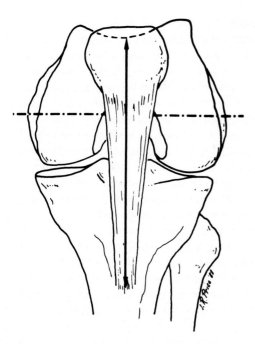

Fig. 11-5. Measurement of the tubercle-sulcus angle. (From Ko-lowich PA, et al: Lateral release of the patella: indications and contraindications, *Am J Sports Med* 18:361, 1990.)

alignment of the patellofemoral joint to normal. Surgery should include a lateral release and a distal realignment if necessary.[16] At this time it is unclear what role excessive femoral anteversion plays in the development of patellar subluxation, and surgery to correct this abnormality is not indicated.

Immediately after surgery, rehabilitation should begin, emphasizing active flexion and passive extension exercises. Quad sets maintain tone in the quadriceps and pliability of the peripatellar tissues in the early postoperative period. Full range of motion should be sought as soon as possible. Exercises should be done daily to maintain the range of motion. Active quadriceps rehabilitation can begin once the tubercle osteotomy has healed at approximately 6 weeks postoperatively. Closed kinetic chain exercises should be performed until adequate restoration of quadriceps strength has been achieved. The athlete is typically returned to sport at 12 to 16 weeks after surgery. A patellar stabilizing brace may be worn if the athlete prefers.

Acute lateral patellar dislocation

Acute lateral traumatic patellar dislocation occurs often in an athletic setting. The athlete is frequently planted and moves into an opponent who contacts the medial portion of the patella and causes a traumatic patellar dislocation. The diagnosis is usually obvious, and the immediate treatment is to extend the knee gently and manually manipulate the patella back into its trochlear sulcus. Patients typically have hemarthrosis, and they may have traumatic extensor lag.

Radiographs should be taken to ensure that no loose body formation has occurred.

The majority of the orthopedic literature suggests that acute patellar dislocation should be treated conservatively with immobilization for a period of 3 to 6 weeks and then gradual rehabilitation with range-of-motion and progressive resistance exercises.[8] If loose bodies are noted in the joint, usually from either the medial facet fracture, lateral femoral trochlea, arthroscopy should be performed to remove the loose bodies and repair the fractured facet, and a lateral release performed if indicated. Rehabilitative exercises should begin immediately.

There is some emerging thought that all first-time traumatic patellar dislocations should be examined arthroscopically. Thompson[17] has suggested that up to 60% of patients suffering a first-time traumatic lateral patellar dislocation have loose body formation or articular cartilage lesions that can be treated arthroscopically. Others have suggested that acute repair of the VMO allows early mobilization of the injured knee, leading to more optimal results. At this time these reports must be considered preliminary and not the gold standard.

Traumatic chondromalacia patella

Contusion to the anterior portion of the knee, such as from a fall directly on the patella or direct collision with another player, can produce a variety of pain patterns from transient bruising pain to prolonged severe pain with knee motion. Very little is known about the physiologic effects of direct contusion on the patella. Dye and Boll[18] have shown that bone remodeling can take place after patellar contusion for up to 2 years, as evidenced by a technetium-99 bone scan. Others have shown that direct contusion to the patella can produce a variety of articular cartilage changes that range from transient articular cartilage swelling to permanent fissuring in the articular surface, which ultimately results in patellofemoral arthritis. At the time of injury to the patella, it is difficult if not impossible to predict which course these traumatic injuries will take.

The athlete should be placed on nonsteroidal anti-inflammatories and a rehabilitation program that minimizes stress on the patellofemoral joint. Therapeutic modalities (which are discussed later) have little if any effect on symptoms in this disorder. Attempts should be made to optimize patellofemoral mechanics by encouraging adequate muscle strength and flexibility while avoiding those exercises that tend to place undue stress across the patellofemoral joint. Closed kinetic chain exercises should be emphasized. Patellar taping may be effective in relieving the stress on an injured area of the patellar cartilage. Findings associated with patellofemoral malalignment (i.e., excessive patellar tilt, laterally displaced tibial tubercle and VMO atrophy) should be identified and treated as outlined later to minimize the stress on the injured patellofemoral joint. If a specific point of tenderness appears in the retinaculum, an injection of local anesthetic and corticosteroid, if performed early, may be of some benefit.

The long-term results of conservative treatment of traumatic chondromalacia patella are inconsistent. Some athletes may recover quite quickly, while others may go on to painful degeneration of the patellofemoral joint, characterized by severe pain with knee extension, effusion, retropatellar crepitus, and inability to actively use the leg. Reflex sympathetic dystrophy may develop in susceptible patients.

Surgery is not usually helpful in treatment for traumatic chondromalacia patella. Surgery should be undertaken if symptoms persist for more than 1 year. If patellar malalignment is noted by CT scan, realignment may be appropriate. Tibial tubercle anteriorization may relieve stress on the injured articular cartilage, particularly if the inferior portion of the patella is primarily involved. Patellectomy may be indicated if symptoms persist for more than 2 years, the patient is incapacitated with pain, and a bone scan indicates that there is increased bone turnover in the patella compared to the surrounding structures. The results of patellectomy, however, are disappointing in many patients, particularly in athletes, and patellectomy, therefore, should be considered only as a salvage procedure.

Patellar fractures

Patellar fractures in the athlete should be treated as patellar fractures in any other patient would be treated, and the reader is referred to standard orthopedic fracture texts. Of importance is that rigid internal fixation should be achieved, if possible, so that immediate range-of-motion exercises can be started. The quadriceps mechanism, particularly the VMO, can rapidly lose strength and flexibility, making rehabilitation difficult after patellar fracture.

Other conditions

Medial shelf syndrome,[19] lateral patellar plicae,[20] and retinacular neuromas[6] may also cause anterior knee pain in the athletic population. Treatment of these conditions relies on appropriate diagnosis. Direct injection of corticosteroids into the soft tissue, in conjunction with range of motion, flexibility, and strengthening exercises, may relieve pain or allow the pathologically tightened intra-articular soft tissue to stretch out. Should the athlete fail to respond, particularly if the symptoms are temporarily relieved by a small injection of local anesthetic, surgery may be undertaken to remove the medial shelf, cut the plicae, or excise the painful retinacular tissue (scar, neuroma). Postoperative rehabilitation should follow the guidelines developed later in this chapter.

SPECIFIC REHABILITATIVE TECHNIQUES

The goal of successful patellofemoral joint rehabilitation is restoration of flexibility and strength in the muscles surrounding the patellofemoral joint.[22] Although it has long been recognized that restoration of strength in the quadriceps

mechanism, specifically the VMO, is of critical importance to restoring patellofemoral joint function, many commonly used strengthening techniques only aggravate pain symptoms in the anterior knee and lead to unsuccessful results. Failure to recognize flexibility deficits, particularly in the hamstring groups can also hamper progress. Adjuncts to strengthening and flexibility training include patellar taping, biofeedback techniques, modalities to temporarily relieve pain, patellar stabilization braces and straps to control symptoms during activities, nonsteroidal anti-inflammatories, and cardiovascular training to maintain the athlete's physical fitness while rehabilitating from the injury. A slow, supervised return to sport is usually advisable.

Once it is determined that the athlete's injury is to the patellofemoral joint, a decision should first be made as to whether the athlete can continue with sport at all or continue with sport on a reduced level. This must be an individualized decision. Factors that enter into this decision should be the amount of pain that the athletics cause, whether any effusion is present (athletes with significant effusion should not be allowed to participate in any vigorous athletic activity[23]), and, most important, how the athlete feels about continuing to participate in athletics. Quite often peer pressure is placed on the athlete to continue with the sport, and the treating physician should be prepared to support the athlete's decision to go on the disabled list for a period of time. At times the physician can "take the blame" for this decision, taking all the pressure off the athlete and allowing him or her to safely rehabilitate the knee injury. If a decision is made to take the athlete out of sport, a cardiovascular program should be designed that does not aggravate the knee symptoms but provides cardiovascular conditioning so the athlete will be as fit as possible once a decision to return him to the athletic field has been made.

Flexibility and strength

Flexibility. The knee should be assessed as described in the previous section and a determination made as to the exact nature of the athlete's injury, such as patellar tilt or overuse. The flexibility of the soft tissues, primarily the hamstrings, quadriceps, and iliotibial band, should be assessed in the following fashion: With the athlete supine, the athlete is asked to take both hands and hold the hip in 90-degree flexion. He is then asked to actively extend the knee as fully as possible. The angle formed between the calf and the thigh is then measured as the popliteal angle. The tighter the hamstring muscle groups, the lower the popliteal angle and the greater the resultant stress on the patellofemoral joint and patellar tendon from hamstring contracture. Optimally, the athlete should be able to straighten the knee completely in this position (Fig. 11-6, A).

The quadriceps tightness is then measured with the patient in the prone position. The examiner straightens the contralateral knee and flexes the ipsilateral knee with the hip remaining fully extended. The distance between the buttock and the patient's heel is measured. Optimally this would be less than 5 inches (Fig. 11-6, *B*).

Finally, the iliotibial band (ITB) flexibility is measured. The patient is placed in the lateral position. The leg to be examined is superior. The lower hip is slightly flexed, and the knee is flexed 90 degrees. The upper knee is extended, and the entire leg is lined up with the trunk at body height. The upper leg is externally rotated so that the patella rotates upward. The leg is then lowered to the ground. If the leg does not touch the ground, the ITB is tight (Fig. 11-6, *C*).

If the patella is tilted on visual inspection, the lateral retinaculum may be tight. The examiner should compress the medial aspect of the patella in an attempt to reduce the tilt to neutral. The amount of resistance offered by the lateral retinaculum, in conjunction with the amount of pain produced in the lateral retinaculum with this maneuver, is subjectively recorded as lateral retinacular tightness.

Any soft tissue tightness should be gradually corrected as part of the rehabilitation program. The stretching exercises described later in this chapter should be held for a count of at least 4 before tension is released. The patient should be encouraged to stretch the muscle to the point where stretching is felt, but *not to the point of pain*. Stretching to the point of discomfort or forceful bouncing is to be discouraged as it can lead to further muscle injury. Flexibility is much more easily achieved with slow, sustained stretches than with forceful bouncing as well.

Many older athletes may tell the examiner that they have always had difficulty with their flexibility, particularly in the hamstrings. Others often state that they are aware that they are "tight individuals" and that this tightness has not been a problem in the past. It has been our experience that once patellofemoral symptoms develop, adequate flexibility needs to be achieved through therapeutic stretching, or very little pain relief and improved athletic performance will occur.

Hamstring stretching should be performed in the seated position with the affected leg straight out in front of the athlete (Fig. 11-6, *D*). If the athlete's hamstrings are excessively tight, both legs should be placed straight out in front of the athlete. Otherwise, the contralateral hip should be externally rotated, and the contralateral foot should be placed flush with the affected knee. The athlete then gently stretches his hands toward the foot in attempts to bring his nose to the kneecap. Although this exercise does stretch the hamstrings, the lumbar spine is also flexed. Athletes with co-existing back pain may have difficulty with this exercise. If back pain develops, stretching should be performed in the seated position with the lumbar spine in neutral or slightly extended posture. More aggressive hamstring stretching can be performed in the standing position with the ipsilateral leg positioned on a bench or a bar at waist level. Stretching again proceeds with the athlete trying to touch his hands to his feet and his nose to the patella. Traditional "hurdlers'" stretches (i.e., seated with the contralateral hip internally rotated and the knee flexed behind the patient) are to be avoided because these exercises may excessively strain the knee and hip ligaments. Stretching exercises can be done in sets of 10 or 15. Stretching should be done only until a sensation of stretching is felt in the muscle. Stretching should never be excessively painful. Pain may indicate tearing of muscle tissue at the musculotendinous junction that may cause further injury.

The quadriceps may be stretched either in the standing position or in the prone position. The ipsilateral hip is extended and then the ipsilateral ankle is brought to the buttock (Fig. 11-6, *E*). If the stretching is done in the standing position, care must be taken to avoid hip flexion, which decreases the stretching on the quadriceps muscle.

To stretch a tight ITB, the previously detailed position for ITB testing is needed. The leg to be stretched is lowered to the ground or table and left unsupported, stretching the ITB.

Stretching of the lateral retinaculum is quite difficult to achieve by oneself. Attempts at gentle stretching of the lateral retinaculum are usually met with involuntary resistance from quadriceps contraction. Patellar taping for tilt may be helpful in slowly stretching out the lateral retinaculum. Otherwise, the patella should be mobilized with the assistance of an athletic trainer or therapist. In this technique, the athlete is sidelying, and the therapist or trainer with the thumbs gently glides the patella medially, while gentle massage of the lateral retinaculum may increase its pliability. Patellar mobilizations must be done gently, particularly if the lateral retinaculum is very painful. Excessive mobilizations may cause longlasting soft tissue pain and prevent rehabilitation from going any further.

Strength. The mainstay of rehabilitation of patellofemoral joint injuries is restoration of strength in the quadriceps mechanism. The quadriceps mechanism is the main dynamic stabilizer of the patellofemoral joint and the VMO and the major dynamic force that counteracts the tendency toward lateral displacement of the patella during knee motion. In most, if not all, patellofemoral joint syndromes, the VMO is atrophied and unable to participate in active patellar motion; in many instances the VMO may be tender because of overuse.

The strategy for knee rehabilitation is to restore strength in the VMO gradually but painlessly, first in a seated posture and then in a standing posture. Once proficiency at muscle contraction is achieved in standing, stairclimbing and then sport-specific rehabilitation can continue. A major theme of this chapter is that isokinetic knee extension exercises should not be used in rehabilitation of patellofemoral joint injuries because of the stress that they place across the patellofemoral joint and the strain that these exercises produce in the patellar tendon and periretinacular tissues. Isokinetic exercises may be used, however, in elite strengthening of the quadriceps mechanism and hamstring muscles once painless range of motion and painless function have been achieved.

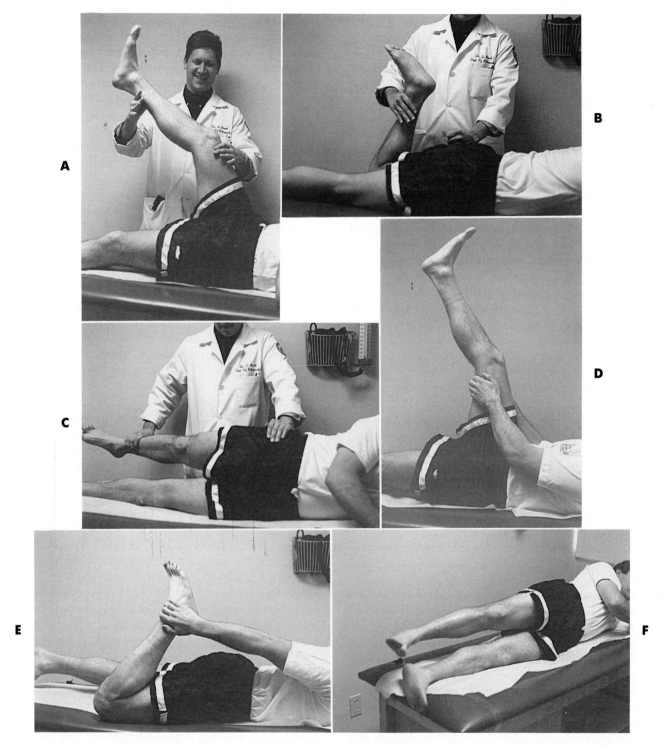

Fig. 11-6. Authors' preferred methods for measuring flexibility in the **(A)** hamstrings, **(B)** quadriceps, and **(C)** iliotibial band and for correcting tightness in the **(D)** hamstrings, **(E)** quadriceps, and **(F)** iliotibial band.

In the beginning of the therapeutic program, the quadriceps mass should be objectively measured. Measurements of thigh girth 4 to 5 cm above the superior pole of the patella usually suffice. In the supine position, the patient is asked to contract the quadriceps mechanism. The bulk of the quadriceps and specifically the VMO is assessed as compared to the contralateral side. Comparisons to the contralateral side may not be helpful if the patellofemoral pain is bilateral.

Initially, strengthening is done with quadriceps contraction and straight leg raising. The ability to contract the VMO is the foundation of treatment. If the VMO contraction does not occur with quadriceps contraction, the athlete must be taught to contract the VMO. The athlete is instructed to compress the medial thigh tissue to the femur with his hand and actively flex and extend the knee (Fig. 11-7). The VMO is activated in various degrees of knee flexion and extension. This maneuver usually causes the VMO to contract. Lateral movement of the patella that is observed on unassisted knee flexion and extension will disappear. A biofeedback electrode can be placed over the VMO, and the athlete can be taught to contract the VMO voluntarily. The strengthening programs described here may produce more pain in the knee unless VMO contraction occurs during quadriceps contraction. Electrical stimulation may be necessary for muscle reeducation.

Once the athlete is able to straight leg raise and hold the knee extended with minimal pain, the process is repeated in the sitting position. The knee is fully flexed, and the athlete is asked to extend the knee fully against gravity. The therapist or trainer should pay specific attention to the timing of VMO contraction and the tracking of the patella. If the VMO is not contracting during knee extension, the therapist needs to use specific suggestive techniques to help the patient selectively contract the VMO. We employ a biofeedback device that informs the patient that the VMO is contracting during knee extension. If this device is not available, the manual pressure technique described previously may be employed.

This process should not be painful. If pain develops during the course of strengthening, the patella should be assessed for evidence of malalignment. Selective patellar taping may be necessary to temporarily realign the patella (see next section). Modalities may be used to decrease the pain temporarily while the strengthening continues.

Once adequate quadriceps contraction and VMO contraction are achieved in the supine and sitting positions, standing and weight shifting are attempted. Again, attention should be directed to contraction of the VMO during standing and weight shifting from the ipsilateral to contralateral leg to ensure that the quadriceps is functioning properly. Gait training emphasizing proper alignment of the spine and hips in conjunction with ambulation then proceeds.

In minor patellofemoral joint injuries in the athletic population, these steps may all be accomplished quickly on an initial evaluation. If the injury is serious and painful, the

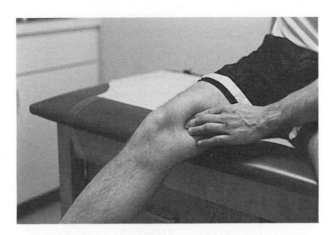

Fig. 11-7. McConnell's method for educating the VMO to contract with knee extension.

process may take several weeks to achieve. By no means should strengthening in a squatting position, stairclimbing, or other methods be initiated unless the athlete can demonstrate proper VMO contraction during normal gait and weight shift. Strengthening exercises can then proceed in a variety of positions. Step-down, rather than step-up, exercises on the painful knee can be performed in sets of 10 or 15. The ipsilateral foot is placed on a step with a height of approximately 9 inches and the athlete then steps up onto the apparatus. The level of the step may be varied to achieve more strengthening if necessary. During the initial phases the therapist or trainer needs to assess the mechanics of stepping. Improper weight shifting either toward or away from the injured leg alters stresses on the patellofemoral joint and may lead to pain. The biofeedback apparatus may be used to ensure proper VMO contraction as occurring during the strengthening exercises (Fig. 11-8). Other exercises can include squatting without weights until the thigh is parallel to the ground or bouncing on a trampoline. The objective of all these exercises is to begin using the quadriceps and hamstring muscles in a closed kinetic chain by working the muscles against gravity alone.

Once the athlete is able to do these simple strengthening exercises, more challenging exercises on either a stationary bicycle, simulated cross-country ski machine, or motorized stairclimbing machine can be performed. Isotonic exercises with a leg press machine, which requires the use of both the quadriceps and the hamstring muscles to move the weight, may also be performed in a painless arc of motion. It should be continually emphasized that the exercises may be performed until the muscle if fatigued, but pain should not occur during any of these exercises. Again, no open-chain knee extension exercises should be performed as part of the rehabilitation.

Finally, once the strengthening exercises are performed adequately, the thigh girth is reassessed. The athlete is ques-

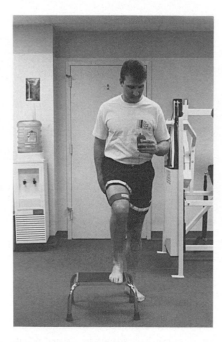

Fig. 11-8. Patient using a biofeedback apparatus to ensure that the VMO is contracting with knee strengthening.

tioned about symptoms of patellofemoral pain, and adjustments in taping and modalities may be made. Before a decision is made on return to sport, activities frequent in the athlete's specific sport are recreated in the gymnasium or physical therapy center. The athlete is encouraged to go through specific maneuvers such as cutting lateral movements, climbing, or backpeddling as required of his specific sport. A slide board may be very useful in simulating side-to-side sports. Again, it is useful to wear the biofeedback apparatus in order to be reassured that the VMO is contracting appropriately. However, by this point the quadriceps mechanism and VMO are usually contracting in concert on a subconscious level, and there is little cause for concern of dysfunction. Only once the athlete is felt to be fully rehabilitated should isokinetic testing be considered. If isokinetic testing is done, it should be at higher speeds only. The goals of strengthening exercises should be to restore the quadriceps to between 80% and 100% of the peak body weight ratio, and the hamstrings should be at least 65% of the quadriceps strength. As long as this strength is achieved, flexibility in the quadriceps, hamstrings, and iliotibial band is restored, and there are minimal to no symptoms, the athlete can return to the sport.

Patellar taping

McConnell[14] has introduced the concept of skin taping to correct symptomatic malalignment in the patellofemoral joint. Early results have been encouraging; some athletes gain relief from their pain immediately after application of the tape. Others find that therapeutic strengthening is much less painful and much more easily performed. At this time,

it is unclear whether patellar taping is curative (i.e., whether prolonged taping can stretch out a pathologically tight lateral retinaculum) or merely palliative. Furthermore, it is unclear whether the beneficial effects of taping diminish with time.

McConnell has identified four components of patellar orientation that may be abnormal and that can be corrected by skin taping. These components may be present statically or dynamically. In all cases the patient is supine and the femur parallel to the table.

1. *Patellar glide* measures the centering of the patella in the femoral sulcus. To measure *static glide,* place each index finger at the femoral condyles so that the thumbs meet at the center of the patella. The patella should lie in the midline between the two condyles. To measure *dynamic glide,* the patient performs an isometric quadriceps contraction. The patellar pull should be in line with the femur. Carefully note the timing of the contraction of the VMO as compared to the vastus lateralis.
2. *Tilt* measures the orientation of the patella in the transverse plane. To measure *static tilt,* compare the height of the medial and lateral patellar borders. Both borders should be parallel with the frontal plane. *Dynamic tilt* observes whether an increase in tilt occurs with quadriceps contraction.
3. *Rotation* measures the rotation of the patella in the frontal plane. A line is constructed connecting the superior and inferior poles of the patella. This line should be parallel to the long axis of the femur. Abnormal rotation is named according to the direction in which the inferior pole is displaced, that is, internal or external rotation.
4. *Anterior-posterior component* measures the orientation of the patella in the coronal plane. To measure *statically,* place one finger along the superior border of the patella and another along the inferior border. A line connecting the two usually demonstrates that the inferior pole is tilted posteriorly. *Dynamically,* palpate the inferior pole of the patella and have the athlete contract the quadriceps. If the inferior pole disappears into the fat pad, *inferior tilt* is present. This finding is commonly associated with pain on knee extension or hyperextension.

Once the abnormal patellar orientation is identified, specific taping techniques are used to restore normal patellar orientation. White Hypafix tape (Homedco, West Hartford, Connecticut) is placed over the patella and over the skin of the medial retinaculum. Brown Leuko Sports tape (Foster Medical, Hartford, Connecticut) is then used to control the malalignment. The white tape can also be used to reinforce the brown tape. The tape is worn every day for 2 weeks. It should be removed and the skin cleaned every night. It is normal for the skin to be reddened underneath the tape. If skin breakdown occurs, the taping should be stopped and a patellar stabilizing brace used instead.

After 2 weeks of use, the result from the taping technique

should be assessed. Muscle strengthening exercises should be performed during this 2-week period, and progressive gains should be seen. If this is the case, the athlete should begin to be weaned off the tape by taping every other day, for sports activities only, and the like. This progressive weaning should be individualized, depending on how well stretching and strengthening are progressing. The goal is to keep the athlete pain-free and to keep the rehabilitation process advancing.

Taping techniques

1. To control *glide,* secure one end of the tape to the lateral patellar border. Glide the patella medially with your thumb while maintaining tension in the tape. Lift the medial soft tissue (skin) toward the patella (several skin folds appear), and secure the tape medially and across the knee (Fig. 11-9).
2. To control *lateral patellar tilt,* secure the tape at the upper middle portion of the patella and pull the tape medially to lift the lateral patellar border, correcting the tilt. Lift the medial soft tissues as indicated previously and secure tape.
3. To control *external patellar rotation,* secure one end of the tape at the middle of the inferior border of the patella. Rotate the patella internally (inferior pole rotates medially), keeping tension of the tape. Lift the medial soft tissue and secure tape to it. If the patient also has *inferior tilt,* apply the same principles, but tape from the superior patellar pole, so as not to irritate the fat pad.
4. *Inferior tilt (anterior-posterior component)* is usually combined with one of the other orientation abnormalities noted previously. It is usually controlled by improving the glide or tilt component. With modification of the *rotation correction* technique (paragraph 3), tape placed in the superior half of the patella tends to lift the inferior pole of the patella out of the fat pad.

Modalities

Modalities play an important role in the treatment of patellofemoral joint injuries. Few modalities, if any, have been scientifically proven to be curative alone. However, modalities can enhance a well-designed program of therapeutic flexibility and strengthening exercises.

Heat applied to the knee (hydrocollator packs, towels soaked in warm water, electric heating pads, or even a warm shower) increases local blood flow, which is thought to accelerate edema resorption. Heat application also increases soft tissue pliability, facilitating stretching of the quadriceps, hamstrings, and patellar retinaculum. Warm-up exercises (e.g., calisthenics, stationary bicycle) also increase the soft tissue temperature and should be encouraged at the start of a rehabilitative session, as long as knee pain is not provoked.

Cryotherapy (ice) has the opposite effect as heat application. Local vasoconstriction slows edema formation.

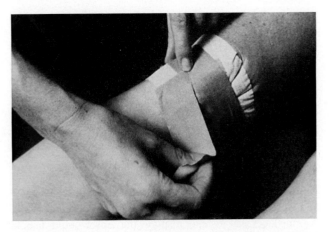

Fig. 11-9. McConnell method of patellar taping. (From Fulkerson JP, Hungerford DJ: *Disorders of the patellofemoral joint,* ed 2, Baltimore, 1990, Williams & Wilkins.)

However, soft tissue pliability is lessened, temporarily reducing overall knee flexibility. In our opinion, cold modalities should be used almost exclusively at the end of a workout, athletic practice, or game. Continued athletic activity may lead to further soft tissue injury because of decreased knee flexibility, possible alteration in joint mechanics brought on by this flexibility loss, and the anesthetic effect of icing masking pain. Very few exceptions to this rule exist.

Phonophoresis, the use of ultrasound waves, and *iontophoresis,*[11] the use of low-voltage electrical current, have both been shown to have significant short-term benefits in directly reducing soft tissue pain and muscle spasm and in mobilizing soft tissue edema. Both modalities can enhance the gains from a therapy session, decreasing pain associated with stretching exercises in particular. Another advantage is that pharmaceuticals can be delivered through the skin to the injured soft tissues by either phonophoresis or iontophoresis. The authors currently favor an iontophoresis regimen with a 10% cortisone cream for a total of 10 treatments over a 3-week period to augment the treatment of patellar tendonitis and quadriceps tendonitis. Treatments should be discontinued if no benefit is achieved after five or six treatments. Iontophoresis can cause skin burns underneath the electrodes. It should be used with caution in dark-complected athletes, as cortisone can alter local melanocyte function, leading to local skin color changes that can be permanent. It has been suggested that ultrasound waves can disrupt bone healing. Thus, phonophoresis is to be avoided if a patella, femur, or tibial tubercle fracture is suspected.

Electrical stimulation to reeducate muscle contraction may be vital as a first step in restoring quadriceps strength. Often, the patellofemoral joint is so painful that the quadriceps is involuntarily inhibited. All attempts to strengthen the quadriceps are thwarted. Electrical stimulation in conjunction with biofeedback techniques usually bring voluntary control again. At this time, it is unclear whether electrical stimulation alone can build muscle strength.

Biofeedback techniques to selectively train the VMO to contract have greatly assisted patellofemoral joint rehabilitation. The VMO is the only structure that dynamically counteracts the structural laterally directed vector on the patella during normal knee motion. In many subacute and chronic patellofemoral joint injuries, the VMO is weakened and atrophic. Thus, the foundation of rehabilitation of the patellofemoral joint is restrengthening the VMO. More traditional methods to strengthen the VMO (see previous section on strengthening) may fail.

In the biofeedback technique, an electrode that measures the intensity of muscle contraction is placed over the VMO and a grounding electrode is placed elsewhere on the body. A transducer that visually displays the sensor output is held in the patient's hand. The therapist or trainer then encourages quadricep contraction until the VMO is activated. Slowly, the athlete learns how to selectively contract the VMO and is "rewarded" with a handheld visual display indicating success. Once this technique is mastered in a seated position, closed kinetic chain exercises can be started using the biofeedback loop. Stepping, climbing, bicycling, and selective weightlifting can be performed, using the biofeedback sensor to assure that the VMO is contracting during these activities.

Transverse friction massage (TFM) is used by many physical therapists and athletic trainers to assist soft tissue healing. In theory, vigorous massage transverse to the orientation of collagen fibers enhances soft tissue healing and encourages fibroblasts to orient new collagen directly in line with the existing collagen, instead of in the random array that can characterize scar tissue. The theoretical advantage of TFM is that the resultant collagen architecture is oriented in a mechanically advantageous direction, making the collagen less likely to be reinjured. Although this phenomenon has been observed in a laboratory setting, clinical efficacy is not yet proven. In addition, the manual pressure provided by the therapists' fingers is quite high and can be extremely painful to the patient.

Patellar stabilizing braces

Patellar stabilizing braces can be beneficial in alleviating patellar pain associated with exercise.[23,24] Although biomechanical studies have not shown actual correction of patellar malalignment by the brace, athletes have reported decreased pain and increased athletic performance with brace use. We encourage the use of a patellar stabilizing brace with rehabilitation and sports in patients with anterior knee pain who cannot tolerate patellar taping (because of skin breakdown or other reasons).

Straps have been developed to treat painful syndromes in the distal patellar tendon and tibial tubercle (Osgood-Schlatter disease).[25] Theoretically, these straps should decrease stress on these areas that occurs with quadriceps contraction. In our experience, the beneficial effects are inconsistent.

Nonsteroidal anti-inflammatory agents

Nonsteroidal anti-inflammatory agents may be used in therapeutic doses for all athletes with musculoskeletal injuries who do not have any predisposition to gastrointestinal disorders. A short course of anti-inflammatory agents (1 to 2 weeks) may diminish pain and decrease the associated inflammation. In addition, having therapeutic doses of anti-inflammatory agents on board during rehabilitative exercises may decrease the amount of inflammation and swelling caused by the therapeutic exercises. Some animal studies have suggested that use of anti-inflammatory agents may accelerate the repair and healing in musculoskeletal tissues, although this has not been proven in humans.

AUTHORS' PREFERRED REHABILITATION SCHEME

Most patellofemoral joint injuries can be rehabilitated according to our algorithm as outlined here. Specific alterations are discussed in the preceding text.

1. Identification of specific patellofemoral joint injury
2. Determination of whether the athlete can continue the sport
3. Evaluation of patellar orientation
   a. Specific taping as required
4. Stretching of hamstrings, quadriceps, and iliotibial band
5. Modalities as indicated
   a. Iontophoresis with 10% cortisone cream for patellar tendonitis
6. Nonsteroidal anti-inflammatory agents
7. Quadriceps strengthening, specifically VMO
   a. Seated
   b. Standing
   c. Stepping
   d. Bicycling
   e. Leg press
   f. Sports-specific
8. Return to sport
   a. Taping or patellar bracing as required
   b. Continued strengthening
   c. Slow weaning from tape and other treatment, according to individual needs

ACKNOWLEDGMENTS
The authors wish to thank Charlotte Stavnitzky, Kim Cubeta, and Sue Philo for their assistance in the preparation of this manuscript.

REFERENCES
1. Kaufer H: Mechanical function of the patella, *J Bone Joint Surg [Am]* 53:1551, 1971.
2. Schutzer SF, Ramsby GR, Fulkerson JP: Computerized tomographic classification of patellofemoral pain patients, *Orthop Clin North Am* 17:235–248, 1986.
3. Hungerford DS, Barry M: Biomechanics of the patellofemoral joint, *Clin Orthop* 144:9–15, 1979.
4. Kolowich PA, et al: Lateral release of the patella: indications and contraindications, *Am J Sports Med* 18:359–365, 1990.

5. Fulkerson JP, Shea KP: Current concepts review: disorders of patellofemoral alignment, *J Bone Joint Surg [Am]* 72:1424–1429, 1990.

6. Fulkerson JP: Awareness of the retinaculum in evaluating patellofemoral pain, *Am J Sports Med* 10:147–149, 1982.

7. Fulkerson JP, et al: Histologic evidence of retinacular nerve injury associated wth patellofemoral malalignment, *Clin Orthop* 197:196–205, 1985.

8. Fulkerson JP, Hungerford DS: *Disorders of the patellofemoral joint*, ed 2, Baltimore, 1990, Williams & Wilkins.

9. Grood ES, et al: Biomechanics of knee extension, *J Bone Joint Surg [Am]* 66:725–734, 1984.

10. Radin EL: A rational approach to the treatment of patellofemoral pain, *Clin Orthop* 144:107–109, 1979.

11. Glass J, Stephen R, Jacobsen S: The quantity and distribution of radiolabeled dexamethasone delivered to tissues by iontophoresis, *Int J Dermatol* 19:519–525, 1980.

12. Martens M, et al: Patellar tendonitis: pathology and results of treatment, *Acta Orthop Scand* 53:445–450, 1982.

13. Fulkerson JP, Schutzer SF: After failure of conservative treatment for painful patellofemoral malalignment: lateral release or realignment? *Orthop Clin North Am* 17:283–288, 1986.

14. McConnell J: The management of chondromalacia patella: a long-term solution, *Aust J Physiother* 32:215–223, 1986.

15. Shea KP, Fulkerson JP: Pre-operative computed tomography scanning and arthroscopy in predicting outcome after lateral retinacular release, *Arthroscopy* 8:327–334, 1992.

16. Post WR, Fulkerson JP: Distal realignment of the patellofemoral joint, *Orthop Clin North Am* 23:631–643, 1992.

17. Thompson N: Personal communication, 1988.

18. Dye S, Boll D: Radionuclide imaging of the patellofemoral joint in young adults with anterior knee pain, *Orthop Clin North Am* 17:249–262, 1986.

19. Dandy DJ: Anatomy of the medial suprapatellar plica and medial synovial shelf, *Arthroscopy* 6:79–85, 1990.

20. Patel D: Plica as a cause of anterior knee pain, *Orthop Clin North Am* 17:273–277, 1986.

21. Fisher RL: Conservative treatment of patellofemoral pain, *Orthop Clin North Am* 17:269–272, 1986.

22. Kennedy JC, Alexander IJ, Hayes KC: Nerve supply of the human knee and its functional importance, *Am J Sports Med* 10:329–335, 1982.

23. Moller RN, Krebs B: Dynamic knee brace in the treatment of patellofemoral disorders, *Arch Orthop Trauma Surg* 104:377–379, 1984.

24. Lysholm J, et al: The effect of a patellar brace on performance in a knee extension strength test in patients with patellar pain, *Am J Sports Med* 12:110–112, 1984.

25. Levine J, Kashap S: A new conservative treatment of Osgood-Schlatter disease, *Clin Orthop* 158:126–128, 1981.

Chapter 12

MENISCAL INJURIES

Gregory E. Lutz
Russell F. Warren

Traditionally, rehabilitation of patients after meniscal injuries was limited. The menisci, not thought to be a key functional component to the human knee, were surgically removed when injured.[1] After the wound had healed, patients gradually returned to their functional activities with minimal short-term disability.[2] However, as time passed, many of these patients developed advanced degenerative arthritis, and clinicians began to report the disappointing long-term consequences of this treatment approach.[3–9] This realization, coupled with an increased understanding and appreciation for the vital structure-function role of the menisci in load transmission,[10–14] joint stability,[8,15,16] lubrication, and articular cartilage nutrition,[7] has led to more conservative surgical approaches to patients with meniscal injuries. Arthroscopy and arthroscopic surgical techniques have contributed significantly to this trend, allowing for preservation of as much meniscal tissue as possible and thus resulting in less short- and long-term morbidity.

The role of rehabilitation in restoring function to the meniscal-injured knee has become better recognized. Yet, the application of sound biomechanical principles in rehabilitation protocol has been lacking. Typically, rehabilitation programs were divided into phases[18] that were based more on the temporal relationship to a surgical procedure than to actual rehabilitation principles (see box on p. 135). In the past, many patients were immobilized for prolonged periods in the hopes of protecting the repaired meniscus or graft.[19–22] This practice led to joint contractures and poor articular cartilage nutrition. When rehabilitation was implemented, much of the program focused on reversing the deleterious effects of prolonged immobilization rather than on restoring function to the injured knee. When strengthening exercises were prescribed, they tended to consist primarily of straight leg raises and leg extensions. Exercises that do not follow the specificity-of-training principle and produce nonphysiologic loading of the knee joint result in potentially harmful effects on the healing structures and precipitate patellofemoral symptoms in many patients. Frequently, rehabilitation programs did not include proprio-

ceptive and agility exercises, which are important for a safe and successful return to functional activities. The need for a long-term commitment to exercise was not emphasized to patients, and short-term gains were lost when the program was discontinued prematurely. Last, traditional rehabilitation programs consisted mainly of "cookbook protocols" that were not designed to meet the specific needs of the patient and often resulted in inefficient use of both the patient's and the therapist's time and effort.

As our awareness of the importance of rehabilitation to the nonoperative and postoperative care of patients with knee injuries continues to increase, so does our knowledge of the efficacy of various rehabilitative techniques. As rehabilitation practitioners, we need to continue to analyze and validate which rehabilitative techniques are safe and efficient in limiting disability while restoring function to patients with musculoskeletal injuries. In this chapter, we discuss our current rehabilitative techniques for patients with meniscal injuries that are managed either nonoperatively or operatively. These techniques are based on established principles of rehabilitation, clinical experience, and new information about the potential forces generated on the healing menisci during various therapeutic exercises.

MANAGEMENT OF MENISCAL INJURIES
Clinical findings

Most meniscal injuries are noncontact and usually involve a compression force coupled with a rotational force to an already flexed knee. The injury can be a result of an acute traumatic event associated with a high-level activity such as cutting, or it can be the result of a chronic degenerative process manifested during a nonspecific low-level activity such as squatting and rotating. A knee effusion usually develops gradually over 48 to 72 hours. Acute knee effusions that develop within a few hours of the event are more commonly associated with anterior cruciate ligament tears, osteochondral fractures, patellar dislocations, or epiphyseal or physeal fractures. Other symptoms associated with meniscal tears are joint-line pain, morning stiffness, intermittent locking and catching, and giving way episodes.

The physical examination begins with evaluation of the patient's gait and alignment. Patients with meniscal injuries frequently have an antalgic gait and increased pain with deep squatting and duckwalking. Depending upon the duration, effusion or quadriceps atrophy may or may not be present. Testing of active knee range of motion may reveal a deficit due to pain inhibition, preexisting soft tissue contracture, or an intra-articular blockage from a displaced meniscal fragment. The patient can be placed in a prone position with the legs off the end of the examining table to test for subtle losses of extension. A springy end feel on a bounce test is suggestive of a displaced meniscal fragment. Palpation of the medial joint line is best performed with the knee flexed. Palpation of the lateral joint line is best performed with the knee in a figure-of-four position. Joint-line tenderness with a positive McMurray's, Steinmann's, or Apley's test is highly suggestive of a meniscal injury. A complete examination of the ligamentous structures and patellofemoral area is necessary to rule out associated injuries.

Diagnostic tests

Radiographic examination of the knee is routinely performed and includes anteroposterior, lateral, notch, and Merchant's views. In older patients, standing (anteroposterior views at 0 degrees and posteroanterior views at 45 degrees) is helpful in evaluating for associated degenerative changes. Double-contrast arthrography has been largely replaced by magnetic resonance imaging, which offers a non-invasive means of confirming a suspected meniscal injury; however, the most objective test remains arthroscopy. Continued advances in smaller-diameter arthroscopes are enabling these procedures to be performed cost-effectively under local anesthesia in the office setting.[23] Direct visualization and probing of the meniscus offers a definitive diagnosis, allows for accurate classification, and directs treatment.

Classification of meniscal tears

There are four basic patterns of meniscal tears: longitudinal, oblique, radial, and horizontal. Tears may be full thickness, partial thickness, or a combination. It is also very helpful to accurately define the actual location of the meniscal tear by using a zone classification system (Fig. 12-1). The radial zones are lettered *A, B,* and *C* for the medial meniscus and *D, E,* and *F* for the lateral meniscus. The circumferential zones are as follows: 0, meniscal-synovial junction; 1, outer third; 2, middle third; and 3, inner third.

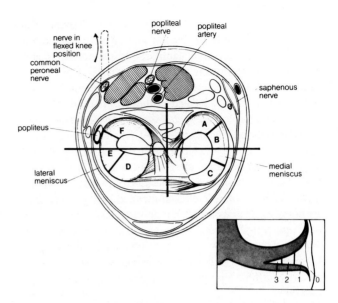

Fig. 12-1. The zone classification system for defining tears of the menisci. Radial zones A through C are in the medial meniscus and D through F are in the lateral meniscus. The circumferential zones 0 through 3 indicate the depth of the tear. (From Warren RF, Hanley S, Bach BR: In Parisien JS, editor: *Arthroscopic surgery,* New York, 1988, McGraw-Hill.)

Treatment options

The goal of treatment is to eliminate the symptoms associated with a meniscal injury while preserving as much meniscal tissue as possible. This is accomplished by first accurately defining the pathology and then deciding on whether operative intervention is warranted. Not all meniscal injuries require operative treatment. Tears that can be initially managed nonoperatively are[24] (1) asymptomatic tears, (2) tears smaller than 1 cm located in the peripheral third (zones 0 and 1) that are stable to probing and have a good chance of healing on their own, (3) partial-thickness tears stable to probing, (4) short radial tears, and (5) young patients with meniscal tears who are not experiencing mechanical symptoms. This last group of patients can be approached nonoperatively at first in an attempt to preserve as much meniscal tissue as possible. Because the vascular penetration of the skeletally immature meniscus is greater than that in the adult, meniscal tears in young people have a greater potential for spontaneous healing if managed properly. It is important to emphasize that nonoperative treatment does not mean no treatment. These patients need the same rehabilitation attention that is given to patients who have had surgery in order to maximize their function and potentially prevent reinjury.

If a meniscal tear is not suitable for a nonoperative approach, the next step is to determine whether the tear can be repaired. The vascular supply of the human menisci, which has been studied extensively, exists primarily at the peripheral 10% to 25% of the lateral meniscus and 10% to

30% of the peripheral medial meniscus.[25,26] Branches from the superior and inferior medial and lateral geniculate arteries form a perimeniscal capillary plexus that supplies the peripheral borders of the menisci. In general, tears that are suitable for meniscal repair are acute longitudinal tears larger than 1 cm and located in the peripheral third (zones 0 and 1) in a stable knee.[27,28] If there is an associated injury to the anterior cruciate ligament (ACL) and a reconstruction is not performed, the chance of a successful repair is diminished.[29] Under these circumstances an ACL reconstruction, if clinically indicated, would help protect the repaired meniscus and is therefore recommended. Although attempts are being made to repair other types of meniscal tears (radial, flap, and complex tears) using vascular enhancement techniques, the long-term success of this subgroup has yet to be scientifically validated.[30] If the meniscal tear cannot be repaired, arthroscopic partial meniscectomy is usually performed.

Although the goal of treatment is to preserve as much meniscal tissue as possible, some meniscal injuries require subtotal or total meniscectomy. Because of the potential deleterious effects of total meniscectomy on the knee joint, alternative treatment methods are being sought, including replacement of the removed meniscus with an allograft or possibly a synthetic prosthesis.[31–33]

REHABILITATION AFTER MENISCAL INJURY

Many of the current rehabilitative techniques used for patients with meniscal injuries have been adopted from advances made in the rehabilitation of athletes after ACL reconstruction.[16] Our rehabilitation program is divided into five functional stages based on rehabilitation and biomechanical principles (see box, upper right). The length of the rehabilitation program varies from weeks to months, depending on the initial extent of injury, surgical procedure performed, and motivation of the patient. These stages are intended to provide a foundation from which the specific rehabilitative interventions can then be modified to meet the individual's pathology and functional goals. As in other areas of rehabilitation, a team approach offers comprehensive patient care, and communication among the physician, therapist, and patient is needed to ensure a successful outcome.

Stage I: early protected mobilization

The potential advantages of early mobilization include decreasing the effects of disuse, retarding capsular contracture, maintaining nutrition in the articular cartilage, and allowing early controlled forces on healing collagen tissues. Rehabilitation can be effective only when postoperative pain and swelling are decreased to a level that allows comfortable, coordinated motion with the avoidance of substitution patterning—an incorrect and inefficient muscular pattern that hinders recovery and may lead to reinjury.[34] An important point to remember throughout the rehabilitation pro-

Current stages of meniscal rehabilitation	
Stage I.	Early protected mobilization
Stage II.	Kinetic chain strength training
Stage III.	Neuromuscular proprioceptive training
Stage IV.	Functional activity training
Stage V.	Return to activity and maintenance program

gram is that pain and effusion inhibit muscle activation and decrease strength. The distention of the knee joint by fluid can reflexly inhibit quadriceps contraction. Neuroreceptors in the joint respond to changes in the capsular tension and constitute the afferent limb of a reflex arc that, in turn, inhibits the lower motor neurons supplying the quadriceps muscle. A "no pain, no gain" attitude should be avoided by the patient and therapist.

Therapeutic modalities are particularly useful early in the rehabilitation program.[34,35] Cryotherapy (ice packs, massage, and compression devices) causes a decrease in postoperative and postexercise pain and swelling. Many forms of electrotherapy (interferential current, microcurrent, TENS) may play a role in pain modulation. Electrical muscle stimulation produces isometric contraction, which, by itself, may not be transferable to functional activities but aids in early neuromuscular reeducation of the quadriceps and hamstring muscles. Biofeedback, which provides the patient with both visual and auditory signals in response to muscle activation, is also a useful modality in reeducating the quadriceps and hamstring muscles.

If there are no contraindications, nonsteroidal anti-inflammatory drugs (NSAIDs) are routinely prescribed to aid in further controlling the inflammatory response and facilitate the rehabilitation program. Double-blinded studies of NSAIDs versus placebo in patients following meniscectomy have demonstrated significantly less effusion and discomfort, as well as earlier return to work or athletic activities, in patients who received NSAIDs.[36,37] The median time for return to sports was 22.5 days for the NSAID group and 56 days for the placebo group.

The main therapeutic exercises used during this stage are range-of-motion exercises. These exercises can be performed passively, with active assistance, or actively. Passive range-of-motion (PROM) exercises are implemented immediately and can be performed by continuous passive motion (CPM) machines or by the use of the unaffected leg to provide support for the affected leg. Early passive full range of motion is encouraged. CPM machines are not used routinely for patients following meniscal surgery. These machines are usually reserved for the following circumstances: (1) after meniscal repair or allograft transplantation, (2) after associated chondral injuries and chondroplasty, (3) after associated anterior cruciate ligament injury and reconstruction, and (4) in patients with preexisting degenerative joint disease who may have difficulty in initiating early motion on their own. Active-assisted range-of-motion exercises and active range-of-motion (AROM) exercises are initiated early. Gentle, prolonged, pain-free stretching exercises at end ranges may be necessary to achieve full range of motion, particularly in patients with preexisting flexion contractures. Isotonic strengthening exercises for the upper body (particularly the crutch-walking muscles), contralateral leg, and hip and ankle musculature of the affected leg are all encouraged.

A rehabilitation brace is used for patients who require a greater degree of protection during the rehabilitation program. Patients who have had a meniscal repair, a meniscal allograft, or an associated reconstruction of the anterior cruciate ligament are placed in a rehabilitation brace set at 0 degrees during ambulation with gait aids and opened to 0 to 90 degrees during *active* rehabilitation exercises. Early *passive* full extension is encouraged. The brace is worn during all weightbearing activities and discontinued at 6 weeks after meniscus repair and 8 weeks after meniscal allograft. Most patients with symptomatic meniscal injuries require some form of gait aid (cane, crutches, or walker) and training in its use. Table 12-1 summarizes the recommended guidelines for early protected mobilization based on the treatment option chosen. The progression from touch weightbearing to full weightbearing depends on the surgical procedure performed and the degree of protection required. The least restricted patients are those who are managed nonoperatively or have had simple partial meniscectomies in which the gait is initiated with partial weightbearing and advanced to full weightbearing as tolerated over a relatively short period of time. Patients who have had a meniscal repair with an ACL reconstruction are started at partial weightbearing and advanced to full weightbearing gradually over a 6-week period; those with isolated meniscal repairs are advanced to full weightbearing more rapidly (1 to 2 weeks). We and others have not noticed any adverse effects from this approach.[27,38] The most restricted patients have undergone meniscal allograft transplantation. During the healing period, weightbearing is restricted to touch only. After approximately 4 weeks, gait is then advanced to partial weightbearing; only after 6 weeks is full weightbearing allowed. It takes time for the peripheral borders of the menisci to become securely anchored to the surrounding structures. We have found that overaggressive weightbearing early on in the rehabilitation program leads to development of recurrent knee effusions that may ultimately retard the recovery process. Independent of the time the patients are in a protected weightbearing status, a symmetric gait pattern with normal swingthrough is encouraged while using crutches. In addition, the patients need to be instructed in safe techniques of ascending and descending stairs.

Cardiovascular endurance can be maintained by the use of one-legged cycling, rowing, pool walking, swimming, or an upper body ergometer early on in the rehabilitation program. Bicycling is a valuable rehabilitative exercise that

Table 12-1. Early protected mobilization

Treatment option	Recommended guidelines
Nonoperative	No brace, crutches partial to full weightbearing as tolerated 0-1 weeks
Partial meniscectomy	No brace, crutches partial to full weightbearing as tolerated 0-2 weeks
Meniscal repair	Rehabilitation brace AROM exercises 0-90 degrees first 6 weeks PROM exercises full range after 6 weeks Crutches partial weightbearing 0-2 weeks Crutches advanced to full weightbearing 2-6 weeks
Meniscal allograft	Rehabilitation brace 0-6 weeks AROM exercises 0-90 degrees PROM exercises full range Crutches touch weightbearing 0-6 weeks Crutches partial weightbearing 4-6 weeks Full weightbearing after 6 weeks

improves knee range of motion, muscular endurance, and lower extremity coordination. Two-legged cycling can be started before full weightbearing, once the patient has achieved at least 100 degrees of knee motion.

Stage II: kinetic chain strength training

Therapeutic exercises can potentially create extremely high repetitive loads on the menisci, which may jeopardize the healing process after injury or repair. The mechanical response of menisci to applied loads is dependent upon their material properties and shape, the shape and alignment of the tibiofemoral joint, associated soft tissue attachments and muscular forces, and the magnitude and direction of the applied force. These are important elements to consider in designing a rehabilitation program that protects healing structures while restoring function through therapeutic exercises.

The menisci are composed primarily of type I collagen bundles, which are arranged in a characteristic orientation.[39] The deep bundles are oriented circumferentially, and the more superficial radially oriented bundles function as tierods to improve the structural integrity of the menisci. Although the menisci resist large compression forces in the knee, the circumferential hoop tensile stress that develops under a load probably dominates their function and their failure. The menisci, when viewed from an axial orientation, are C-shaped structures. The medial meniscus is larger in diameter than the lateral meniscus. The peripheral border of each meniscus is thick and convex; the central portion is thin and concave. This wedge shape (as viewed from the sagittal plane) is felt to play an important role in resisting shear forces at the tibiofemoral joint, particularly in the ACL-deficient knee.

Levy and co-workers[15,40] analyzed the effects of the medial meniscectomy on the anterior-posterior motion of the cadaveric knee. They demonstrated that isolated medial meniscectomy had little effect on anterior-posterior motion of the knee. However, when the ACL was resected, there was a significant increase in the degree of displacement, particularly at 60 degrees of knee flexion. They postulated that the thick wedge shape and firmly attached posterior horn of the medial meniscus assume a greater role in resisting forces when the ACL is injured than does the less firmly attached posterior horn of the lateral meniscus. It is conceivable that during in vivo conditions, when forces at the tibiofemoral joint include both shear and compression, the role of the menisci in resisting shear forces becomes even more important. Shoemaker and Markolf[41] demonstrated that the amount of anterior tibial displacement in the ACL-deficient cadaveric knees with intact menisci was significantly reduced if concomitant compression forces were applied. They felt that the higher compression forces improved joint congruency and thereby limited the amount of anterior translation of the tibia.

The exact amount of force that the menisci can assume before failure is unknown.[42] However, the amount of force potentially generated on these structures during rehabilitative exercises is becoming better understood.[38,43-46] Knowledge of tibiofemoral shear and compression forces generated during different types of rehabilitative exercises is important in designing rehabilitation programs that do not place excessive loads on the injured meniscus.

In the rehabilitation program, a distinction is made between open and closed kinetic chain exercises. The kinetic chain terminology was originally derived for mechanical engineering purposes and has since been adopted to describe human body kinematics.[47] Steindler observed that when the foot or hand was fixed ("closed kinematic chain") joint motion and muscular recruitment patterns differed from when the foot or hand was mobile ("open kinematic chain"). This terminology has more recently been used to describe biomechanical differences in commonly employed knee rehabilitation exercises.[16,38] More specifically, in a closed kinetic chain (CKC) exercise, the foot is fixed and knee motion is accompanied by motion in the other joints along the kinetic chain (hip and ankle). Examples of such exercises are the squat and leg press, which strengthen the quadriceps and hamstring muscles simultaneously. In contrast, with an open kinetic chain (OKC) exercise, the foot is mobile, and motion of the knee joint occurs in isolation and independently from the other joints located along the kinetic chain. Examples of such exercises are the leg extension and leg curl, which strengthen the quadriceps and hamstrings in isolation, respectively.

Clinical,[48] cadaveric,[43] and biomechanical[38,44,46] studies have all demonstrated significant shear and compression forces generated by OKC exercises that may potentially create deforming forces not only on reconstructed cruciate ligaments but also on healing meniscal injuries, repairs, or transplanted allografts. The forces generated during CKC exercises have not been as extensively studied. However, Lutz et al.[38] used a two-dimensional biomechanical model to calculate differences in tibiofemoral shear and compression force between open and closed kinetic chain exercises. They demonstrated that the CKC exercise produced significantly less tibiofemoral shear force when compared to the OKC exercises. Analysis of tibiofemoral compression forces revealed that the closed kinetic chain exercises produced significantly higher compression forces at the very angles where the OKC exercises produced maximum shear forces. Electromyographic analysis of quadriceps and hamstring cocontraction revealed significantly higher degrees of cocontraction during the CKC exercise. They proposed that the reduction in shear force seen during the CKC exercise was a result of the more axial orientation of the applied force and the cocontraction of the hamstrings.

This information is useful in designing rehabilitation programs not only for patients with ACL injury or reconstruction[16,38] but also for patients with meniscal injuries. The goal of rehabilitation is to restore function through therapeutic exercise while protecting healing structures from excessive shear forces. For this reason CKC exercises are emphasized and OKC extension exercises are discouraged for quadriceps strengthening. It has been stated that the menisci resist 30% to 70% of the compression force transmitted at the tibiofemoral joint during weightbearing activities.[10-14] Ahmed and Burke[10] demonstrated that, as knee flexion increased, the menisci assumed a greater proportion of the compression force. Based on this information, we do not allow our patients to perform CKC exercises past 90 degrees of flexion. Of additional interest is that during an OKC flexion exercise, which strengthens the hamstrings, the compression forces are very low. However, the amount of posterior shear force generated can be very high (2000 N).[38] We are cautious in prescribing these exercises to patients with meniscal repairs or allograft transplantations that need to be protected from excessive shear forces.

CKC exercises not only make sense biomechanically but also follow important rehabilitation principles. The specificity of training principle is well accepted in the rehabilitation community.[34] This principle states that the most efficient means of restoring function is to use those exercises that most closely resemble the activities the patients are expected to perform. CKC exercises more closely resemble these activities than do OKC exercises. CKC exercises provide more functional training of much of the musculature along the so-called kinetic chain. In addition, these exercises offer the enhanced neuromuscular training benefits of speed, balance, and coordination—key components of most functional activities.

Guidelines for the progression of CKC strengthening exercises are presented in the box at right. Manual resistance exercise is a form of strengthening in which the resistance is applied by the therapist to either a dynamic or static muscular contraction. This allows the therapist to establish a qualitative baseline level of strength and pain-free arcs from which progress can be measured. These exercises are initially performed in the anatomic planes of motion and progressed to diagonal patterns known as proprioceptive neuromuscular facilitation (PNF) techniques.[34] Although this form of training is time-consuming for the therapist, we have found it to be helpful early on in the rehabilitation program when a controlled type of closely monitored strengthening is required. CKC types of manual resistance strengthening can be performed and are emphasized. CKC multiangled isometrics can be initiated early in the rehabilitation program (Fig. 12-2). Patients are instructed to perform submaximal isometric cocontractions of the quadriceps and hamstrings against steps of varying heights that place the knee at approximately 30, 60, and 90 degrees.

Once the patient has achieved better muscular control of the knee, and pain and effusion are minimal, isotonic CKC exercises are begun. These exercises can be performed parallel to the floor so that the actual compression loads placed on the knee are probably less than if performed in a weight-bearing position (Fig. 12-3). These exercises are initially performed with double limb and then single limb support, isolating the affected limb. High repetitions and light weights allow the patient to perform the movement safely and efficiently. Once the weightbearing restriction has been lifted, the patient can progress to higher-level types of full weightbearing CKC exercises. The use of a sport-cord initially during these CKC activities provides the patient with some assistance. The patient can perform sport-cord assisted squats (Fig. 12-4) and advance to sport-cord assisted lunges (Fig. 12-5). The patient can perform bodyweight squats initially without and then with added resistance. Machine-based squats (Fig. 12-6) usually precede free-weight squats because patients learn these exercises more easily and can use their upper extremities for balance support. Progression to the higher-level CKC free-weight strengthening exercises, such as power squats (Fig. 12-7), front squats (Fig. 12-8), and lunges (Fig. 12-9), depends upon a patient's goals and abilities. These exercises are technically demanding and require proper instruction by the therapist or trainer. Lighter weights and higher repetitions are again emphasized while the patient is learning the exercise. Only after the patient has demonstrated proper execution of the exercise is the amount of weight increased.

During this stage the patient needs gait reevaluation and reeducation regarding normal symmetric ambulation with the avoidance of excessive heel strike. Gait aids and rehabilitation braces are discontinued once this has been established and the period of protection is over. In addition to the CKC strengthening exercises, a variety of CKC aerobic exercises may be added (Fig. 12-10). If there has been

---

> **Progression of closed kinetic chain strengthening exercises**
>
> Manual resistance and multiangled isometrics
> Isotonic double limb support leg presses
> Isotonic single limb support leg presses
> Sport-cord assisted squats
> Sport-cord assisted lunges
> Machine power squats
> Free-weight power squats
> Free-weight front squats
> Free-weight lunges

---

an associated ACL reconstruction, the patient is usually fitted with a functional derotational brace at this time.

Stage III: neuromuscular proprioceptive training

In the past, rehabilitation programs focused primarily on strengthening and paid little attention to the neuromuscular-proprioceptive training of the knee joint.[19-22] In fact, many current rehabilitation programs still neglect this stage of rehabilitation.[18] Simple muscle strengthening does not necessarily improve the speed, the degree, and the quality of muscle contraction necessary for maintaining dynamic knee stability.

Studies of human meniscal specimens have demonstrated the presence of three morphologically distinct mechanoreceptors:[49,50] Ruffini endings, Golgi tendon organs, and Pacinian corpuscles. Axons have been identified and shown to penetrate from the perimeniscal tissue into the outer and middle thirds of the menisci, but not the inner third. The presence of these receptors suggests that the menisci may play an important role in providing afferent sensory information to the central nervous system in order to delicately regulate the biomechanical function of the knee. The meniscal horns that become taut at the extremes of flexion and extension were found to have higher concentrations of neural elements. This arrangement may allow for protective postural muscular reflexes that modulate joint compression and alignment in order to ensure safe and efficient functional activities. Studies have demonstrated significant impairments in knee proprioception in patients with injuries to the ACL or osteoarthritis of the knee.[51,52] Whether patients with isolated meniscal injuries also have proprioceptive deficits is unknown; however, many of these patients do have associated ACL injuries[53-55] or preexisting osteoarthritis and can benefit from proprioceptive training. It is conceivable that injury to the meniscus, particularly if it involves the richly innervated peripheral third, would result in deficits in proprioception. However, this possibility needs further scientific investigation.

The role of the menisci in providing "dynamic knee stability" is further supported by their soft tissue relationships with the quadriceps, semimembranosus, and popliteus mus-

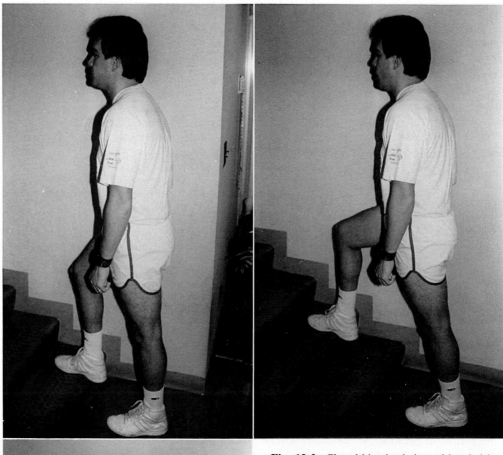

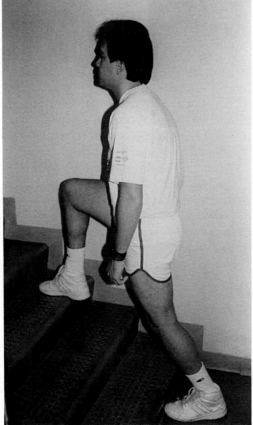

Fig. 12-2. Closed kinetic chain multiangled isometric step-up exercises at varying step heights.

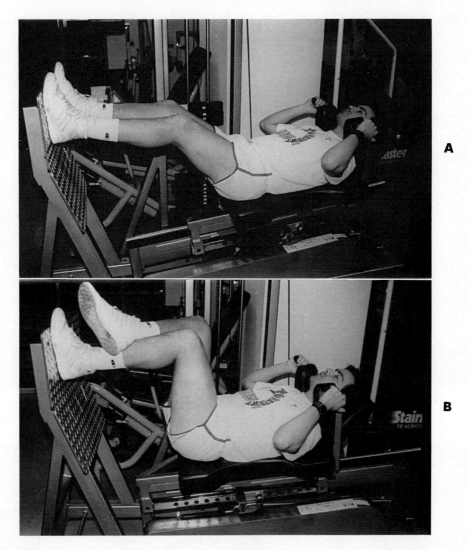

Fig. 12-3. Closed kinetic chain leg press in **A,** double limb support, and **B,** in single limb support positions.

cles. Kapandji[56] proposed that during knee extension the menisci are pulled anteriorly by meniscopatellar fibers, and during knee flexion they are pulled posteriorly by the semi-membranosus and popliteus expansions. Certainly the menisci do not function in isolation within the knee joint, and although their contribution to dynamic knee stability is not well understood, it should not be underestimated. This information has strong implications regarding rehabilitating patients with meniscal injuries. It is important to restore soft tissue flexibility as well as neuromuscular proprioception and coordination in order to regain function and prevent reinjury.

The neuromuscular-proprioceptive training of patients after meniscal injuries is accomplished with a variety of balance board, profitter, sliding board, and minitrampoline exercises. Guidelines for the progression of these exercises are provided in the box on p. 146. These exercises are

initiated once the patient has achieved full range of knee motion and demonstrated pain-free cocontraction of the quadriceps and hamstrings during the CKC strengthening exercises. These exercises create changes in joint position and pressure that stimulate joint neuroreceptors to provide afferent stimulation to the central nervous system, which, in turn, exhibits descending control on muscular contraction. Under the supervision of a therapist or trainer knowledgeable in these techniques, the patient is instructed to maintain a degree of quadriceps and hamstrings cocontraction during various limb positions. Initially, these exercises can be performed in a seated position and then standing with partial and then full weightbearing single limb stance on the balance board. The addition of biofeedback to the hamstrings facilitates cocontraction of the hamstrings (Fig. 12-11). Ihara and Nakayama demonstrated significant improvements in reaction time of the hamstrings after a 3-

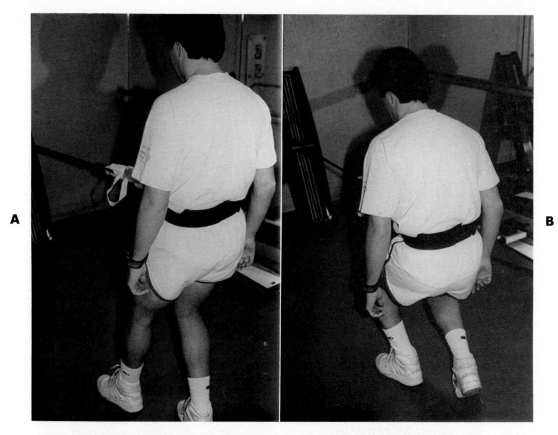

Fig. 12-4. Sport-cord assisted squatting exercise emphasizes controlled eccentric and concentric muscle training. **A,** Starting position. **B,** Descending position.

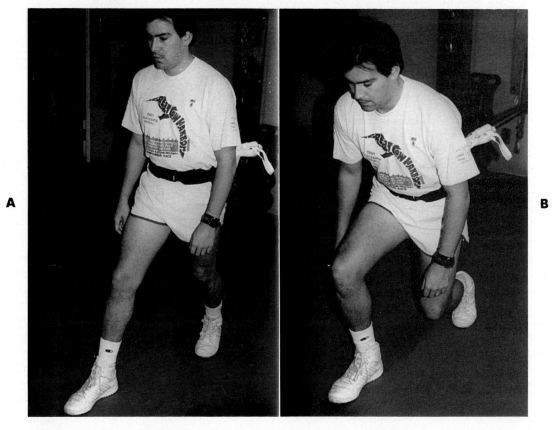

Fig. 12-5. Sport-cord assisted lunges allow for improved isolation of affected limb. **A,** Starting position. **B,** Descending position.

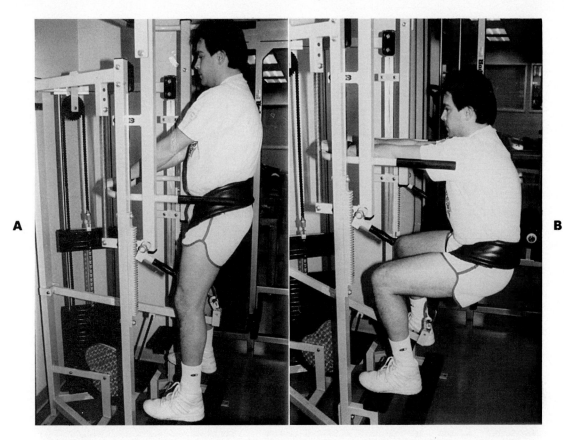

Fig. 12-6. Power squats on a machine. **A,** Starting position. **B,** Descending position, with patient holding on for balance support.

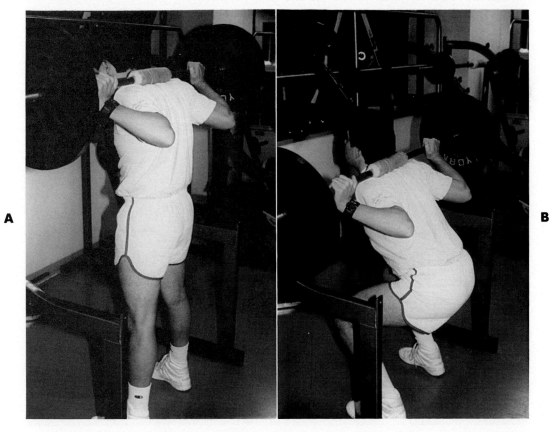

Fig. 12-7. Power squats using free weights require greater degrees of concentration and coordination. **A,** Starting position. **B,** Descending position.

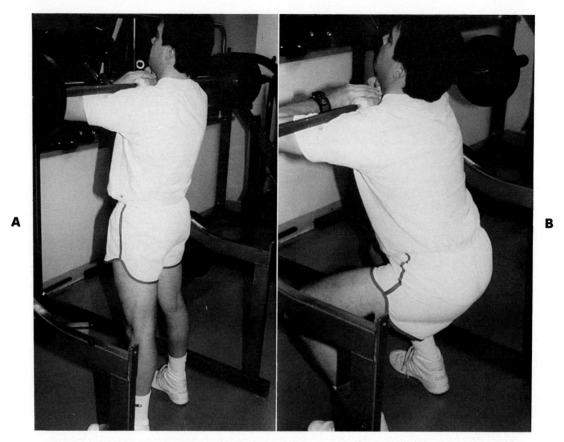

Fig. 12-8. Front squats using free weights are more difficult than the power squats and are performed with less weight. **A,** Starting position. **B,** Descending position.

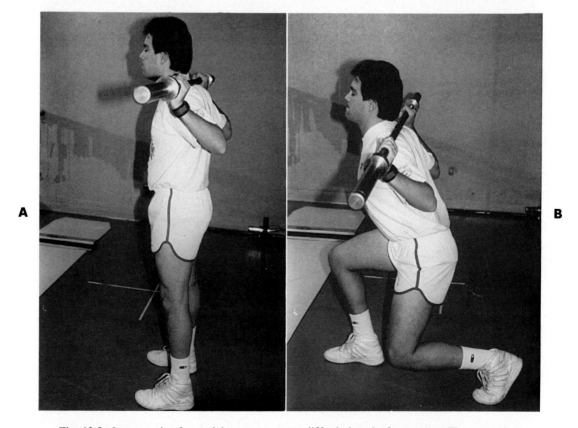

Fig. 12-9. Lunges using free weights are even more difficult than the front squats. These exercises isolate the affected limb and require greater degrees of coordination and strength. **A,** Starting position. **B,** Descending position.

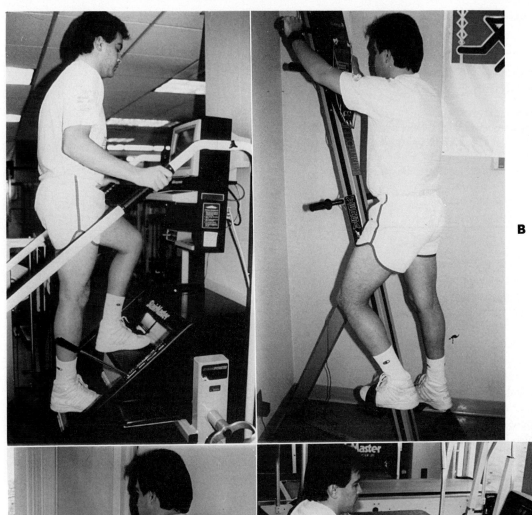

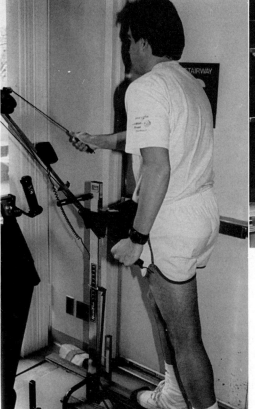

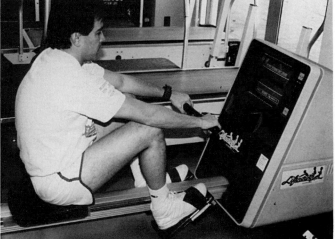

Fig. 12-10. Examples of closed kinetic chain aerobic exercise machines. **A,** Stairmaster. **B,** Versaclimber. **C,** Nordic Track. **D,** Rowing.

Guidelines for progression of neuromuscular proprioceptive exercises

Seated balance board exercises
Standing partial weight balance board exercises
Standing full weight balance board exercises (double limb support)
Standing full weight balance board exercises (single limb support)
Sliding board and profitter exercises
Minitrampoline exercises

---

month program utilizing these types of exercises.[57]

The premise of our dynamic knee stabilization program is that the repetitive microtrauma or macrotrauma experienced by the intra-articular structures during functional activities is eliminated or minimized through the concept of muscle fusion or cocontraction.[58-60] Anatomically the key muscles that control shear and rotational forces on the knee are the quadriceps and hamstrings. Once patients have achieved dynamic stability during the balance board activities, they can apply this to more functional activities. In our experience, these exercises not only improve dynamic knee control but also instill in the patient a greater level of confidence, which is necessary for the subsequent stage of rehabilitation.

Stage IV: functional activity training

For many patients with meniscal injuries, the rehabilitation program ends here, and they are instructed in a maintenance program. They have developed the necessary strength, endurance, and proprioception for the standard activities of daily living. In patients who have had a total meniscectomy and/or meniscal transplantation, a certain degree of activity modification is needed to further protect the already damaged articular surfaces and subchondral bone. These patients need to be educated in the avoidance of repetitive high-loading activities. The maintenance program under these circumstances emphasizes low-impact activities such as pool walking or swimming, bicycling, Stairmaster, Versaclimber, or Nordic Track. A walking program is encouraged, but proper shoes with an impact-absorbing orthosis are recommended.

For the athlete who places higher functional demands on the knee, sport-specific agility training is necessary in order to ensure a safe return to athletic competition. The athlete with a significant knee injury must relearn the skill patterns required for the sport. These skill patterns consist of "coordination engrams." An engram is hypothesized to represent the neurologic organization that accounts for the memory of preprogrammed automated multimuscular movements.[34] Engrams are not inherent and can be formed only by thousands of repetitions of the precise multimuscular movement. The most efficient way to develop these coor-

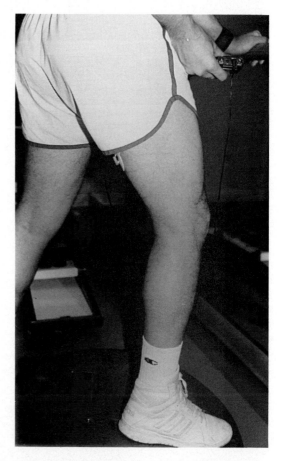

Fig. 12-11. Neuromuscular proprioceptive training using a balance board and EMG biofeedback to emphasize hamstrings cocontraction.

dination engrams is to begin with slow, methodical repetitions of the specific task or tasks to be performed.

Before these agility exercises are begun, the athlete must have met the following criteria: (1) Pain-free full range of knee motion is possible, (2) affected limb strength on 20-repetition maximum single leg CKC leg press is within 10% of the unaffected limb, (3) good dynamic joint control is demonstrated with full weight single leg balance board activities, and (4) if there has been an associated ACL reconstruction, serial KT-1000 arthrometer measurements have not shown an interval increase greater than 3 mm. Because of the high shear forces generated and the minimal amount of functional information obtained, OKC isokinetic strength testing is not routinely performed.[44]

In general, the athlete is started on level-surface straight-ahead running activities before cutting or jumping types of activities are introduced. When the athlete has demonstrated greater degrees of precision with these movements, speed and force can be increased. Plyometric training can be added, with special attention to avoid overtraining. Good communication between all the members of the rehabilitation team (physician, therapists and trainers, patient, and coach) needs to be continued. If knee pain or swelling develops, the athlete needs to be reevaluated by the physician.

Stage V: return to activity and maintenance program

Once the patient has achieved a preinjury level of performance, return to work or athletic competition is permitted. Prevention of reinjury is an important issue for patients with meniscal injuries. The menisci have come to be regarded as valuable structures of the knee that need to be protected. Muscular strength, endurance, and dynamic knee stability need to be maintained to minimize the risk of future injuries. Patients are instructed in knee-safe postures. Proper posture may play a role in preventing further injury to the knee joint during higher-level running, jumping, and cutting types of activities by avoiding a "heel-locked" position and pivoting on the ball of the foot. The maintenance program continues to emphasize CKC exercises for strengthening and endurance training at least twice weekly. By this time in the rehabilitation program, patients should have an excellent understanding of their exercise program and are encouraged to continue in a more independent fashion with routine follow-ups. In addition to a stretching program to maintain soft tissue flexibility, patients are instructed in proper warm-up and cool-down principles.

SUMMARY

Many variables affect the rehabilitation of patients after meniscal injury. Our treatment program is based first on obtaining an accurate diagnosis and then on defining the extent of pathology. The rehabilitation program presented is comprehensive and meant to provide guidelines for the rehabilitation practitioner. Each patient needs to have a rehabilitation program designed specifically to address his or her pathology and functional goals. Patients should not be given unrealistic promises about premature return to functional activities. Rather, they should be educated about the goals of each of the five stages. Progression from one stage to the next depends on the patient's compliance and objective knee findings, not an arbitrarily set time frame. Rehabilitation can be a very powerful therapeutic tool that contributes greatly to the nonoperative and postoperative care of patients with meniscal injuries. However, it needs to be based on scientific principles and implemented by knowledgeable practitioners.

REFERENCES

1. Smillie J: *Injuries of the knee joint,* vol 4, Edinburgh, 1971, Churchill Livingstone.
2. Perey O: Follow-up results of meniscectomy with regard to working capacity, *Acta Orthop Scand* 32:457–469, 1962.
3. Allen P, Denham R, Swan A: Late degenerative changes after meniscectomy: factors affecting the knee after operation, *J Bone Joint Surg [Br]* 66:666–671, 1984.
4. Baratz M, Fu F, Mengato R: Meniscal tears: the effect of meniscectomy and of repair on intra-articular contact areas and stresses in the human knee, *Am J Sports Med* 14:270, 1986.
5. Cox J, et al: The degenerative effects of partial and total resection of the medial meniscus in dogs' knee, *Clin Orthop* 109:179–183, 1975.
6. Dandy D, Jackson R: The diagnosis of problems after meniscectomy, *J Bone Joint Surg [Br]* 57:349, 1975.
7. Fairbanks T: Knee joint changes after meniscectomy, *J Bone Joint Surg [Br]* 30:664–670, 1948.
8. Krause W, et al: Mechanical changes in the knee after meniscectomy, *J Bone Joint Surg [Am]* 58:599–604, 1976.
9. Zaman M, Leonard M: Meniscectomy in children: a study of fifty-nine knees, *J Bone Joint Surg [Br]* 60:436–437, 1978.
10. Ahmed A, Burke D: In vitro measurement of static pressure distribution in synovial joints, part I: tibial surface of the knee, *J Biomech Eng* 105:216–225, 1983.
11. Kettlekemp D, Jacobs A: Tibiofemoral contact area determination and implications, *J Bone Joint Surg [Am]* 54:349–356, 1972.
12. Radin E, Delamotte F, Maquet P: Role of the menisci in the distribution of stress in the knee, *Clin Orthop* 185:290, 1984.
13. Voloshin A, Wosk J: Shock absorption of meniscectomized and painful knees: a comparative in vivo study, *J Biomed Eng* 5:157, 1983.
14. Walker P, Erkman M: The role of the menisci in force transmission across the knee, *Clin Orthop* 109:184–192, 1972.
15. Levy I, Torzilli P, Warren R: The effect of medial meniscectomy on anterior-posterior motion of the knee, *J Bone Joint Surg [Am]* 64:883–888, 1982.
16. Lutz G, Stuart M, Sim F: Rehabilitative techniques for athletes after reconstruction of the anterior cruciate ligament, *Mayo Clin Proc* 65:1322–1329, 1990.
17. Johnson R, Pope M: *Functional anatomy of the meniscus: AAOS symposium on reconstruction of the knee,* St Louis, 1978, Mosby–Year Book.
18. Vander-Schilden J: Improvements in rehabilitation of the postmeniscectomized or meniscal-repaired patient, *Clin Orthop* 252:73–79, 1990.
19. Dehaven K, Black D, Griffiths H: Open meniscus repair: technique and 2 to 9 year results, *Am J Sports Med* 17:788–791, 1989.
20. Morgan C, Cascells S: Arthroscopic meniscal repair, *Arthroscopy* 2:1, 1986.
21. Rosenberg T, Scott S: Arthroscopic meniscal repair evaluated with repeat arthroscopy, *Arthroscopy* 2:1, 1986.
22. Scott G, Jolly B, Henning C: Combined posterior incision and arthroscopic intra-articular repair, *J Bone Joint Surg [Am]* 68:847, 1986.
23. Halbrecht J, Jackson D: Office arthroscopy: a diagnostic alternative, *Arthroscopy* 8:320–326, 1992.
24. Weiss C, et al: Non-operative treatment of meniscal tears, *J Bone Joint Surg [Am]* 71:811–822, 1989.
25. Arnoczky S, Warren R: Microvasculature of the human meniscus, *Am J Sports Med* 10:90–95, 1982.
26. Arnoczky S, et al: *Meniscus.* In Woo S, Buckwalter J, editors: *Injury and repair of the musculoskeletal soft tissues,* Chicago, 1987, AAOS.
27. Cooper D, Arnoczky S, Warren R: *Arthroscopic meniscal repair,* vol 9, 1990.
28. Warren R: Arthroscopic meniscal repair, *Arthroscopy* 1:170, 1985.
29. Warren R: Meniscectomy and repair in the anterior cruciate ligament–deficient patient, *Clin Orthop* 252:55–63, 1990.
30. Arnoczky S, Warren R, Spivak J: Meniscal repair using an exogenous fibrin clot, *J Bone Joint Surg [Am]* 70:1209, 1988.
31. Arnozcky S, Warren R, McDevitt C: Meniscal replacement using a cryopreserved allograft: an experimental study in the dog, *Clin Orthop* 252:121–128, 1990.
32. Garrett J, Stevenson R: Meniscal transplantation in the human knee: a preliminary report, *Arthroscopy* 7:57–60, 1991.
33. Henning C: Current status of meniscus salvage, *Clin Sports Med* 9:567–576, 1990.
34. Kottke F, Lehman J: *Krusen's handbook of physical medicine and rehabilitation,* ed 4, Philadelphia, 1990, WB Saunders.
35. Scott S: Current concepts in the rehabilitation of the injured athlete, *Mayo Clin Proc* 17:154–160, 1984.
36. Arvidsson I, Eriksson E: A double blind trial of NSAID versus placebo during rehabilitation, *Orthopedics* 10:1007, 1987.

37. Ogilvie-Harries D, Baver M, Correy P: Prostaglandin inhibition and the rate of recovery after arthroscopic meniscectomy, *J Bone Joint Surg [Br]* 67:567, 1985.

38. Lutz G, et al: Comparison of tibiofemoral joint forces during open and closed kinetic chain exercises, *J Bone J Surg* 1992.

39. Bullough P, et al: The strength of the menisci of the knee as it relates to their fine structure, *J Bone Joint Surg [Br]* 52:564–570, 1970.

40. Levy I, Torzilli P, Warren R: The effect of lateral meniscectomy on motion of the knee, *J Bone Joint Surg [Am]* 71:401–406, 1989.

41. Shoemaker D, Markolf K: Effects of joint load on the stiffness and laxity of ligament-deficient knees, *J Bone Joint Surg [Am]* 67:136–146, 1985.

42. Frankel V, Burstein A, Brooks D: Biomechanics of internal derangement of the knee: pathomechanics as determined by analysis of instant centers of motion, *J Bone Joint Surg [Am]* 53:945–962, 1971.

43. Grood E, Noyes F, Butler D: Biomechanics of the knee extension exercise, *J Bone Joint Surg [Am]* 66:725–734, 1984.

44. Kaufman K, et al: Dynamic joint forces during knee isokinetic exercise, *Am J Sports Med* 19:305–316, 1991.

45. Smidt G: Biomechanical analysis of knee flexion and extension, *J Biomech* 79–92, 1973.

46. Yasuda K, Tetsuto S: Exercise after anterior cruciate ligament reconstruction, *Clin Orthop* 220:275–283, 1987.

47. Steindler A: *Kinesiology of the human body under normal and pathological conditions,* Springfield, Ill, 1955, Charles C Thomas.

48. Henning C, Lynch M, Glick K: An in vivo strain gauge study of elongation of the anterior cruciate ligament, *Am J Sports Med* 13:22–26, 1985.

49. Day B, et al: The vascular and nerve supply to the human meniscus, *Arthroscopy* 1:58–62, 1985.

50. Zinny M, Albright D, Dabeziew E: Mechanoreceptors in the human medial meniscus, *Acta Anat (Basel)* 133:35–40, 1988.

51. Barrack R, Skinner H, Buckley S: Proprioception in the anteric cruciate deficient knee, *Am J Sports Med* 17:1–6, 1989.

52. Barrett D, Cobb A, Bentley G: Joint proprioception in normal, osteoarthritic, and replace knees, *J Bone Joint Surg [Br]* 73:53–56, 1991.

53. Cerabona F, et al: Patterns of meniscal injury with acute anterior cruciate ligament tears, *Am J Sports Med* 16:603–609, 1988.

54. Indelicato P, Bittar E: A perspective of lesions associated with ACL insufficiency of the knee: a review of 100 cases, *Clin Orthop* 198:77–80, 1985.

55. Noyes F, et al: Arthroscopy in acute traumatic hemarthrosis of the knee: incidence of anterior cruciate tears and other injuries, *J Bone Joint Surg [Am]* 62:687–695, 1980.

56. Kapandji I: *The physiology of the joints, lower limb,* Edinburgh, 1970, Churchill Livingstone.

57. Ihara H, Nakayama A: Dynamic joint control training for knee ligament injuries, *Am J Sports Med* 14:309–315, 1986.

58. Baratta E, Solomonow M, Zhou B: Muscular coactivation: the role of the antagonist musculature in maintaining stability, *Am J Sports Med* 16:113–122, 1988.

59. Solomonow M, Baratta R, D'Ambrosia R: The role of the hamstrings in the rehabilitation of the anterior cruciate ligament-deficient knee, *Sports Med* 7:42–48, 1989.

60. Walla D, et al: Hamstring control and the unstable anterior cruciate ligament–deficient knee, *Am J Sports Med* 13:34–39, 1985.

Chapter 13

LIGAMENTOUS INJURIES

K. Donald Shelbourne
Thomas E. Klootwyk
Mark S. De Carlo

Injuries to the ligamentous structures of the knee make up a large part of a sports medicine practice. The ability to accurately assess, examine, diagnose, and treat the injured knee is important in ensuring a successful return to athletic competition. Once the diagnosis has been made, the cornerstone of treatment of a ligamentous knee injury is rehabilitation. In the last decade, we have seen great advancements in nonoperative and postoperative knee ligament rehabilitation programs. Our purpose with this chapter is to review our present rehabilitation of the commonly injured ligaments of the knee.

REHABILITATION OF MEDIAL COLLATERAL LIGAMENT INJURIES

The medial collateral ligament (MCL) is a commonly injured structure of the knee. The treatment of this injury has advanced tremendously over the last 10 to 15 years. No longer is operative treatment indicated for an MCL tear. The advancement of nonoperative treatment of MCL injuries has been led by Indelicato.[1,2] It is now known that, with appropriately guided rehabilitation, the athlete who sustains an MCL injury can rapidly return to the field of play in a safe manner and without long-term consequences of clinical instability.

Anatomy review

The anatomy of the medial side of the knee has been well described by Muller[3] and by Warren and Marshall.[4] Anatomically there are three layers of the medial capsuloligamentous complex. Layer I is the superficial layer and encompasses the deep fascia from the patellar tendon anteriorly to the popliteal fossa posteriorly. Anteriorly this layer joins the periosteum of the tibia. Posteriorly it joins the posteromedial capsule and the posterior oblique ligament of the knee. The tibial collateral ligament, layer II, has fibers in the more posterior aspect that are oriented more obliquely and, as the fibers approach the posteromedial corner of the

knee, they blend with the deep capsular ligament (layer III). This forms the "posterior oblique ligament" of the knee as noted by Hughston and Eilers. The semimembranosus tendon also helps reinforce the posteromedial corner of the knee. Layer III is the true capsule of the knee and a distinct entity in its anterior two thirds, but it helps form the posterior oblique ligament in its posterior third. The medial meniscus is firmly attached to this deep layer (layer III) of the medial side of the knee.

Mechanism of injury

Injuries to the MCL can be from contact with a direct blow to the lateral side of the thigh or leg or from noncontact with a valgus force transmitted through to the knee. Studies show that the majority of major MCL injuries arise from contact. Two separate reviews have demonstrated that the majority of the higher-grade MCL injuries occur through direct contact. Hughston and Barrett[5] reported that 86% of knees treated for anteromedial instability sustained the injury as a result of contact.

We have found that the majority of third-degree MCL injuries occur through direct contact, but that second-degree MCL injuries frequently occur through indirect rotational forces associated with a valgus movement to the knee. Both of these injuries are seen in association with third-degree anterior cruciate ligament (ACL) tears, but in this section we discuss only isolated MCL injuries.

Clinical evaluation

History. As in all areas of medicine, the evaluation of a patient with a knee injury begins with the history of the injury. The presence of a valgus contact injury should raise suspicion of damage to the medial collateral ligament complex. To determine the severity of the injury and also to aid in the determination of additional ligamentous injuries, pertinent questions need to be asked. Did you hear or feel a pop in your knee? Was there significant swelling within 1 to 2 hours? Did you feel as if your knee came apart? Did you feel that you had significantly injured your knee? Were you able to continue to play? The patient's ability to localize pain to the medial side of the knee can also aid in the history-taking aspect of the evaluation.

Physical exam. The physical exam begins with observation of the patient's gait pattern. The patient who has sustained a tear of the ACL ambulates with a bent-knee gait because of the large hemarthrosis that accompanies this injury and the pain of extending the knee against traumatized tissue in the notch. Although not always the case, the patient with an injury to the MCL usually ambulates with a vaulting gait pattern during which the quadriceps actively splints the knee in extension as a means of preventing further injury to the medial collateral ligament and of attempting to control pain.

The normal uninjured knee should always be examined first for baseline measurements and to allow the patient to experience the knee exam without discomfort.

The evaluation of the knee for an effusion is the next step in the examination sequence. Our experience has been that when an effusion is associated with an isolated injury to the MCL it is minimal to moderate. In a few cases it can be large. In the case of a larger effusion, it is important to rule out associated injuries that more typically produce larger effusions such as an associated ACL or posterior cruciate ligament (PCL) tear or an osteochondral fracture.

The patella is the next area of the knee examined. It is important to rule out a patellar subluxation or a reduced patellar dislocation. With either of these injuries, the medial patellofemoral ligament can be injured and can produce medial knee pain. Simple palpation of the medial peripatellar capsule and medial patellar facet and performing a patellar lateral apprehension test can assist in ruling out a patellar subluxation or dislocation. In addition, patellar dislocations are frequently associated with tearing of the vastus medialis obliquus insertion on the femoral epicondyle. Tenderness at this location above the MCL attachment is seen in most acute patellar dislocations.

Palpation of the medial collateral ligament along its entire course is the next step in the knee evaluation. With injury to the MCL, there is tenderness isolated to the ligament itself. It is important to determine the exact location of maximal tenderness. We have found that the patient is most comfortable and therefore can more easily relax if the knee is supported in approximately 20 to 25 degrees of flexion and the hip of the ipsilateral extremity is allowed to relax into external rotation. The ability to minimize any discomfort during the exam can gain patient confidence and thereby assist in the patient's ability to relax the injured extremity in allowing an accurate assessment of the injured knee. The point of maximal tenderness can indicate the site of the injury to the MCL, which may have implications in the patient's ability to regain range of motion (ROM) during

the rehabilitation process. Those patients who have sustained an MCL injury near the femoral insertion site have a greater tendency to have stiffness and a slower return of their ROM during the rehabilitation process.[6]

Because testing the integrity of the MCL in this acutely injured knee may be painful, additional testing to rule out other ligamentous injuries must be performed prior to valgus stress testing. Palpation of the lateral aspect of the knee is performed. Knee range of motion is measured and documented. We use three numbers to measure ROM and record these as a, b, and c. The a represents the degree of hyperextension the knee is able to obtain. The b represents any degree short of extension, and c represents the degree of knee flexion. After measuring the ROM, a Lachman exam to evaluate the ACL is performed. If enough flexion exists in the injured knee, a posterior drawer test is performed to evaluate the PCL; if not, a posterior Lachman test is used to help evaluate PCL integrity.

The most important test to evaluate the MCL is valgus stress testing in full extension and 30 degrees of flexion. Grood has demonstrated that at 25 to 30 degrees of flexion the MCL is the primary stabilizing structure.[7] As the knee is moved into extension, the secondary restraints including the ACL and the PCL assume greater responsibility in preventing excessive medial opening. It is important to correlate the degree of valgus opening with the amount of flexion that the knee is in when being tested.

The amount of medial knee opening of the injured knee compared to the contralateral knee is a direct measure of damage to the medial capsuloligamentous complex.[1] We have found it easier to evaluate the medial instability with the leg positioned off the side of the table and the knee secured by one of the examiner's hands and thigh (Fig. 13-1). This allows the patient to better relax the injured extremity and allows the examiner to evaluate the medial ligaments by applying a gentle rocking valgus force to the knee without needing to stabilize the ipsilateral thigh in midair.

It has been noted that the rotation during valgus stress testing can play a role in the detected instability. Muller states that the tibial collateral ligament is tight in extension and external rotation.[3] A normal amount of internal rotation of the tibia occurs as the knee flexes from full extension to approximately 30 degrees of flexion. This results in a slight amount of laxity in the tibial collateral ligament. This normal amount of medial laxity with valgus stress with the tibia in internal rotation can be incorrectly interpreted as an indication of medial instability. Therefore, the tibia should be maintained in external rotation to evaluate the medial capsuloligamentous complex.

A ligament evaluation should document the "quality" of the "end point." A firm or good-quality end point is an indication that an injury to the medial ligamentous complex is of grade I (mild) or II (moderate) severity. The lack of a

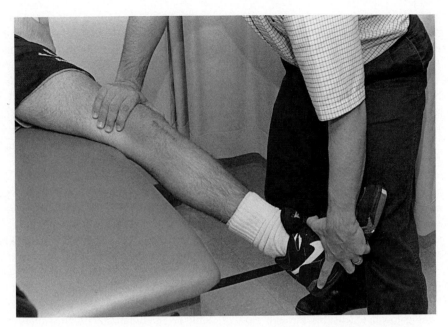

Fig. 13-1. Valgus stress testing to evaluate the medial capsuloligamentous complex.

good-quality end point with valgus stress prior to the ACL being loaded is indicative of a grade III (severe) injury to the medial capsuloligamentous complex.

Valgus stress applied to the knee in full extension with resultant medial opening is indicative of damage to at least the deep capsular ligament, the tibial collateral ligament, and the posterior oblique ligament. If the finding of gross medial instability is noted, then damage to one or both of the cruciate ligaments should also be suspected.[1] Valgus stress applied to the knee in 30 degrees of flexion with resultant medial opening is indicative of damage to the tibial collateral ligament, the underlying mid-third portion of the deep medial collateral ligament, and also possibly damaged are the anterior fibers of the posterior oblique ligament.[1]

The rating scale of MCL injuries represents a continuum of injury to the medial capsuloligamentous complex from mild to severe. We use a grade I (mild) description of an MCL injury for those patients who have a history of a contact or noncontact valgus knee injury, physical exam findings of tenderness along the course of the MCL, and valgus stress testing revealing minimal medial joint opening with a good-quality end point. Grade II (moderate) MCL injuries have a history and physical exam findings similar to grade I injuries with the exception that with valgus stress testing there is a noted increase in medial joint opening with a detectable end point still present. Grade III (severe) MCL injuries are often associated with more swelling and pain than grade I and II injuries. The distinguishing finding of grade III MCL injuries is the lack of a quality end point with valgus stress testing of the knee in 30 degrees of flexion.

Treatment

Nonoperative treatment of isolated MCL injuries was originally investigated by Indelicato.[1,2] Conservative management of all grades (I, II, III) of isolated MCL injuries is now considered standard treatment. Once an associated injury to the ACL and PCL has been ruled out and an isolated MCL injury has been diagnosed, the rehabilitation process begins. The rehabilitation program for MCL injuries can be divided into three phases. The treatment for grade I and II injuries is identical, and the treatment for grade III injuries is very similar. The rehabilitation time depends on the degree of injury and the aggressiveness of the athlete. Phases of the rehabilitation program can be overlapped depending on the demands and rehabilitation progress of the individual athlete.

Grade I and II injuries

Phase I. The initial phase of rehabilitation focuses on control of pain, swelling, and inflammation. We use the knee Cryo/Cuff (AirCast, Summit, New Jersey) throughout the rehabilitation process. The Cryo/Cuff is able to provide cold and compression to the injured knee. The cold helps alleviate the patient's pain, and the compression helps to control knee swelling and give the patient a feeling of stability. By controlling pain and swelling, other clinical variables including gait, range of motion, and strength can be emphasized.

With lower-grade injuries, the need for knee support with a knee immobilizer is unlikely, but occasionally, when an athlete has significant pain associated with this injury, a few days of immobilization are of benefit. Along similar lines, most patients with lower-grade injuries are able to ambulate without a significant limp. When patients do demonstrate a significant antalgic gait, crutch use with weightbearing as tolerated is recommended until the patient can resume a normal gait pattern. Physical therapy is focused on the gait until the patient can consistently ambulate without a limp. It is important for the patient to realize that limping can become a habit and must be consciously avoided. With the control of pain, swelling, and a normal gait, ROM is emphasized.

The restoration of full ROM is of critical importance. Nearly all normal knees possess some degree of hyperextension. Our goal is to restore the full hyperextension to the injured knee. This is accomplished through towel extensions and prone hangs. Towel extensions are performed with the patient in a supine position on a table and the heel of the affected extremity propped on a rolled towel high enough to evaluate the thigh and calf off the table. This exercise is performed passively initially; as quadriceps strength and leg control improve, patients are encouraged to actively extend the knee while performing towel extensions through isometric quadriceps setting (see Fig. 13-4). Prone hangs are performed on a table. A small ankle weight can be added to the affected extremity to assist the effectiveness of the prone hang (see Fig. 13-5).

Improvement in flexion is accomplished through three separate exercises. Wall slides (see Fig. 13-6), heel slides (see Fig. 13-7), and active assisted flexion in a seated position (see Fig. 13-8) all assist the patient in the return of flexion. Wall slides are performed while lying in a supine position with both legs extended up the side of a wall. The injured knee is allowed to slide slowly down the wall into flexion with assistance from the uninjured leg. Active assisted knee flexion is performed in a seated position with the noninvolved leg placed across the front of the injured leg. This exercise is typically performed while sitting off the end of a table so that the patient's knee can flex beyond 90 degrees. Heel slides are started once the patient has at least 90 degrees of active knee flexion. This exercise involves passively flexing the knee while in a long sitting position on the table or floor. The patient grasps the ankle of the involved leg and passively pulls the knee into flexion.

With an injury to the MCL, isometric quadriceps strengthening is started soon after the injury. Once the patient is relatively comfortable, initial exercises of quadriceps setting and straight leg raises are instituted. As the patient improves, limited-range isotonic exercise with light resistance is started.

By the end of phase I, the patient should have minimal swelling, full ROM, and a baseline of quadriceps strength restored to allow good leg control and a normal gait.

Phase II. The primary emphasis of phase II of the rehabilitation program is advanced strengthening with the use of closed-chain exercises. Weightroom workouts emphasize functional activities in addition to closed-chain strengthening. High repetitions with light weights are employed early, and the patient is progressed to low repetitions with higher weight. Specific exercise instruction includes knee bends, step-ups, leg press, hip sled use, and squats. It is important to use a well-balanced strengthening program for all lower-extremity musculature. A fast-speed strengthening program is also introduced in phase II of the rehabilitation program. This includes bicycling, StairMaster (Tri-tech, Tulsa, Oklahoma), and swimming, as well as exercise modalities such as the Fitter (Fitter International, Calgary, Alberta), shuttle, and the slide board.

Phase III. The focus of phase III is on a functional return to the previous activity level. At this point in the rehabilitation process the athlete should have full ROM without pain. Minimal swelling should be present. Muscular strength can be evaluated with isokinetic testing. With strength in the 80% to 90% range of the uninjured extremity, a functional progression is instituted, along with a progressive running program. The functional progression is based on the sport, position, and athletic demand of the injured athlete. The functional progression is an organized sequence of activities of increasing difficulty that enables the athlete to reacquire the skill necessary for safe and effective return to sporting activities. It is important that each successive activity in the functional progression be performed without pain, significant increase in swelling, or antalgic running pattern. With an injury to the MCL, an athlete is started with fast speed walking and advanced to jogging, jumping, and finally sprinting activities. As the initial drills are performed without symptoms, the subsequent drills are made progressively harder. Final additions of the functional progression include figure-of-eight drills, along with sport-specific drills using half- and full-speed cutting off the injured extremity. Once all the steps of the functional progression have been completed, the athlete is ready to resume full athletic activity.

In the area of supportive brace use with MCL injuries, we will comment only briefly, as a separate chapter has been devoted to the use of various braces and their applications in rehabilitation of athletic injuries. We have found that the demands of the athlete, coupled with the grade of the MCL injury, determine the need for postinjury bracing. We have noted success using double upright medial and lateral support braces. Two examples are the DonJoy Playmaker (Smith and Nephew Donjoy, Carlsbad, California) (Fig. 13-2) and the Pro Hinged Brace (Pro Orthopedic Devices, Tucson). The braces are issued during phase II of the rehabilitation process and are used through the remainder of the rehabilitation program and as the athlete returns to the field of play.

Summary

The medial capsuloligamentous complex is a commonly injured structure of the knee. The usual mechanism of injury is by direct contact. There no longer exists a need for operative treatment of the isolated MCL injury. Our rehabil-

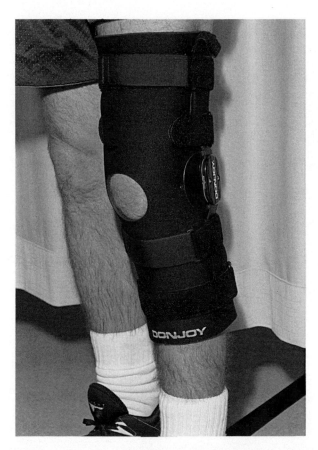

Fig. 13-2. The Don Joy Playmaker Brace, an example of a double upright brace used in the rehabilitation of MCL and ACL injuries.

itation is divided into three phases. The first phase is devoted to control of pain, swelling, and restoration of range of motion. The second phase concentrates on strengthening the injured knee. The third and final phase is centered around the return of the athlete to competitive sport.

ACL RECONSTRUCTION REHABILITATION

During the last decade we have noted extensive advancement in the area of postoperative ACL rehabilitation. Today the physician and the physical therapist work closely together to ensure that the reconstructed knee is properly rehabilitated from the time of the injury until the athlete returns without limitation to the field of play. Our preoperative rehabilitation process begins as soon as the patient tears the ACL, and our postoperative rehabilitation is begun on the same day as the reconstructive procedure.

We divide our ACL rehabilitation program into four phases. Each phase has particular criteria that must be met before the athlete is allowed to progress to the next phase. The first part of the rehabilitation process is the preoperative phase. The second phase starts at the time of the reconstructive procedure and covers the first 2 weeks after the reconstruction. The third phase includes the third, fourth, and fifth weeks following the reconstruction. The final phase

encompasses the time from the end of the third phase until the athlete returns to the field of play for full competition.

Preoperative phase

Perhaps the greatest advancement in the last 10 years in ACL rehabilitation has been in the area of preoperative rehabilitation. The importance of resolution of postinjury swelling and the restoration of full ROM prior to proceeding with ACL reconstruction is now realized. No longer is immediate surgery recommended for the isolated ACL-injured knee. Shelbourne has demonstrated an unacceptable increased incidence of postoperative arthrofibrosis when reconstructing acutely injured knees.[8,9] In place of proceeding with an immediate reconstruction, patients are started immediately in preoperative rehabilitation. The preoperative rehabilitation is separated into two areas. The first area is the rehabilitation of the injured knee. The second area is the mental preparation of the patient for the reconstructive procedure, including a detailed explanation of the operative reconstruction and the postoperative rehabilitation program.

Knee rehabilitation. The initial attention in the rehabilitation of the acutely injured ACL knee is focused on controlling the postinjury swelling. We have found the knee Cryo/Cuff to be extremely valuable in this phase of the rehabilitation. The "cold" of the Cryo/Cuff aids in the control of postinjury pain, and the compression assists in the control of the hemarthrosis. With appropriate control of pain and reduction in swelling, the rehabilitation program can be advanced to work on ROM, gait, and strength.

Most knees possess some degree of hyperextension (Fig. 13-3). Obtaining full ROM, including full hyperextension, is important prior to surgical reconstruction of the injured knee. The prerequisite of full preoperative ROM is achieved through a few simple exercises. Towel extensions and prone hangs are ways to regain normal full hyperextension following ACL injuries just as they were used following MCL injuries. Towel extensions are performed with the towel rolled high enough to elevate the calf and thigh off the table (Fig. 13-4). In addition, the patient is in the supine position to relax the hamstring tendons that passively tighten while sitting. A 2½-lb weight may be added to the anterior tibia or femur to assist in regaining full hyperextension. Isometric quadriceps contractions are performed while the patient is working on towel extensions. We feel that this quadriceps setting into terminal extension assists in gaining leg control and therefore improves the normalization of the gait pattern. An additional way to achieve full extension is prone hangs. Prone hangs can also be performed with the use of a light ankle weight (Fig. 13-5).

Just as after MCL injuries, wall slides, heel slides, and active assisted knee flexion in the seated position are all exercises that are utilized in the preoperative phase of the rehabilitation to restore knee flexion. Wall slides are accomplished with the patient lying supine on a table with both legs extended up the wall. With assistance from the

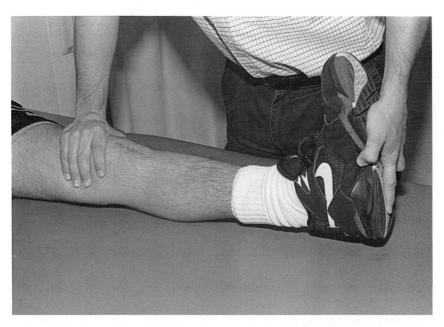

Fig. 13-3. Normal knee hyperextension that most knees possess.

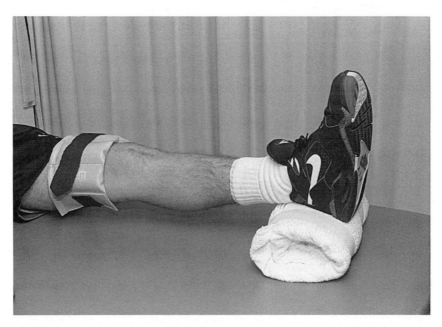

Fig. 13-4. Towel extensions are used to achieve passive hyperextension of the knee. The towel must be high enough to elevate the thigh and calf off the table.

uninjured leg, the injured knee is allowed to slide down the wall into a flexed position (Fig. 13-6). When the patient has 90 degrees of flexion, heel slides are added. Heel slides are accomplished by having the patient grasp the ankle of the involved extremity and passively pull the injured knee into a flexed position (Fig. 13-7). The final exercise used to improve flexion is active assisted knee flexion. With the patient in a seated position at the end of a table, the uninjured leg is placed in front of the injured leg to facilitate knee

flexion. It is important to be seated at a table that allows the knee to flex beyond 90 degrees (Fig. 13-8).

The final phase of the preoperative knee rehabilitation program is the restoration of a normal gait and strength work. After the acute injury to the ACL, our patients usually use crutches in a partial weightbearing pattern. Patients are encouraged to progress their weightbearing status as tolerated. We allow our patients to discard crutches as soon as they are able to ambulate without a limp. Strength work is

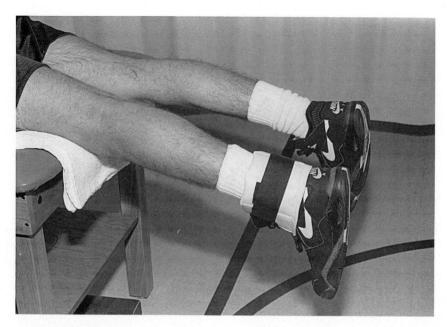

Fig. 13-5. Prone hangs with ankle weight added to the affected extremity. This exercise assists in regaining full hyperextension.

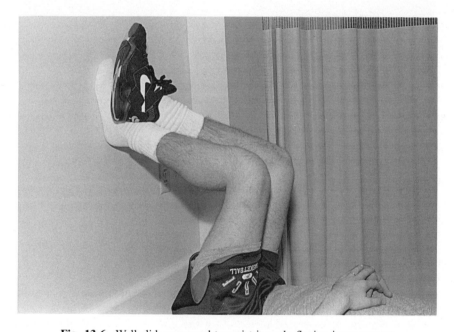

Fig. 13-6. Wall slides are used to assist in early flexion improvement.

initiated once patients have decreased their swelling, regained full ROM of the injured knee, and resumed a normal gait. We recommend starting with closed-chain exercises such as knee bends, step-ups, and calf raises. Next the athlete progresses to the weightroom activities of leg press, the hip sled, and squats.

Our preoperative goals of the knee rehabilitation are to have the patient with an ACL-deficient knee present to the operating room for reconstructive surgery with no swelling, full knee ROM, and a normal gait.

Preoperative mental preparation. In addition to the rehabilitation of the knee prior to operative reconstruction, the mental preparation of the patient is also critically important in properly preparing the patient for surgery. The patient should have a complete understanding of the operative procedure and the postoperative rehabilitation. We

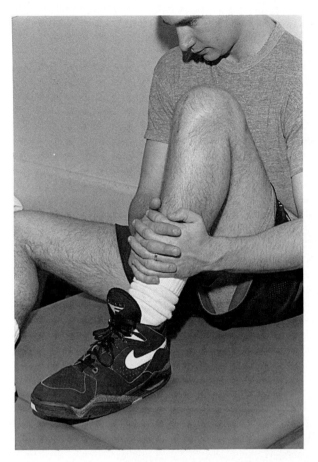

Fig. 13-7. Heel slides are used to gain the terminal degrees of flexion.

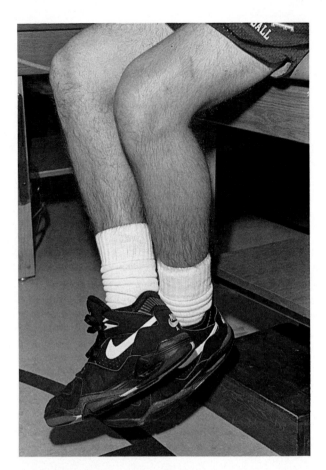

Fig. 13-8. Active assisted knee flexion is an additional activity to improve flexion in the injured knee.

utilize knee models to demonstrate the autogenous central third patellar tendon ACL reconstruction that we perform. A picturebook of the postoperative rehabilitation is reviewed with the patient, and all questions concerning the rehabilitation process are answered. All patients are given detailed written information outlining the postoperative ACL rehabilitation.

The procedure should be performed at a time that is convenient for the patient and family. School, work, and family schedules need to be arranged so that during the initial days after the reconstruction the patient can concentrate completely on rehabilitation of the reconstructed knee. In regard to school schedules, we often schedule surgery for a vacation break or delay the surgery until the completion of a semester. It has also been well documented that an appropriate delay in surgery with the patient fully rehabilitating the injured knee decreases the incidence of postoperative arthrofibrosis.[8-10] Waiting until the patient is mentally prepared for surgery only adds to the likelihood of achieving a successful rehabilitation postoperatively.

Data collection. The preoperative collection of data is extremely helpful in accurately and objectively evaluating our patients postoperatively. Documentation of ROM, KT-

1000 (Medmetric, San Diego) stability testing, isokinetic strength evaluation, and single leg press strength should be done prior to reconstructive surgery.

Postoperative rehabilitation

The following discussion pertains to those patients who undergo ACL reconstruction using securely fixed autogenous patella tendon grafts.

Phase I (0–2 weeks)

Hospital rehabilitation. The initial 2 weeks after ACL reconstructive surgery comprise the most important phase of the postoperative rehabilitation program. The term *accelerated* has been associated with our rehabilitation program, but in reality the first 2 weeks after reconstruction provide a time of relative rest with attention directed at only five important parameters: (1) maintain full hyperextension, (2) control postoperative swelling with rest and leg elevation, (3) allow the operative wounds to heal, (4) maintain good quadriceps leg control, and (5) obtain 90 degrees of flexion. Although patients can be up and about on an unlimited basis after surgery, we have noted that this may lead to excessive swelling with resultant stiffness and pain and delay the overall rehabilitation process. The goal of the entire rehabilitation program is to avoid problems rather than treat them once they have been allowed to occur.

The postoperative phase of rehabilitation actually begins in the operating room. Once the new ligament is in place, the knee is taken through a full ROM including full hyperextension and full flexion. With full ROM confirmed in the operating room, the surgeon can be assured that the new ligament has not captured the joint, and full ROM of the reconstructed knee is possible postoperatively. Part of our postoperative dressing applied in the operating room is the knee Cryo/Cuff. We have found that the Cryo/Cuff applied in this timely manner greatly reduces the amount of postoperative swelling and assists in postoperative pain control.

Once the patient arrives in the hospital room, the reconstructed knee is placed into a CPM machine. The CPM fulfills two goals in our postoperative rehabilitation: predictable extremity elevation and gentle ROM of the knee. The knee elevation is important to assist in the control of swelling, whereas gentle ROM may assist the patient in regaining knee ROM after the reconstruction. The CPM machine is set at 0 to 30 degrees. The 0-degree setting reflects the importance of obtaining full hyperextension after surgery. We limit flexion to 30 degrees because flexion beyond 30 degrees with the Cryo/Cuff in place can cause excessive tightness of the thigh sleeve. Also, repeated early flexion to 90 degrees leads to excessive swelling in the acute postoperative time frame and delay in the overall rehabilitation program.

Full hyperextension. Emphasis on full postoperative knee hyperextension begins on the same day as the reconstructive procedure. This early extension work allows the newly reconstructed ligament to mold itself perfectly into the notch. The potential space of the notch in front of the ligament can fill with fibrous scar tissue and may become a permanent block to full hyperextension if the knee is allowed to remain in a flexed position after surgery. Therefore, by obtaining full hyperextension immediately and routinely after surgery, this potential space does not fill with scar tissue and become a block to future full hyperextension. The routine of obtaining full hyperextension is initiated a few hours after the patient arrives in the hospital room. The patient lifts his or her own leg out of the CPM and props the heel on the end of the padded bed frame. The reconstructed knee is then allowed to relax into full hyperextension. This process can be assisted by the addition of a small ankle weight to the front of the proximal tibia. This exercise of achieving full hyperextension is performed for 10 minutes each waking hour. The process of hourly passive hyperextension that is started in the hospital is continued on an identical schedule once the patient arrives home after discharge.

Control of swelling. Although the rehabilitation program is often referred to as *accelerated,* the initial 2 weeks after the reconstruction is a time of knee elevation and rest. Patients are permitted to bear weight as tolerated, but they are cautioned to be up and about for bathroom use and meals only. Patients who do not follow this rest and elevation guideline and walk for extended periods develop excessive knee swelling, increased pain, and knee stiffness and overall delay the rehabilitation process. By limiting the amount of postoperative swelling, the surgical wounds are allowed to heal, and the rehabilitation program can be advanced.

Quadriceps leg control. The maintenance of good quadriceps leg control is an additional area of early emphasis in our postoperative rehabilitation protocol. This early emphasis is reflected in the functional strengthening exercises started on the same day as the reconstructive procedure. Independent straight leg raises are coordinated with the work on full hyperextension. The mobilization of the patella and the restoration of the patellar tendon to its full length are direct results of this early quadriceps contraction activity. Our opinion is that the early quadriceps activity assists in preventing the postoperative complication of patellar contraction syndrome. In addition to performing a straight leg raise each hour in conjunction with the passive extension exercises, isometric quadriceps contractions are also performed. This early quadriceps activity aids in the restoration of the extensor mechanism of the knee and leads to an easier obtainment of a normal gait pattern.

On the second postoperative day, patients are instructed on gait training with crutch assistance. Patients are allowed to bear weight as tolerated. Initially patients are encouraged to ambulate with the Cryo/Cuff and a Tecnol (Tecnol, Fort Worth, Texas) immobilizer in place (Fig. 13-9). As noted previously, patients are encouraged to limit their ambulation in the early postoperative period. With gait training completed, the patient is discharged from the hospital.

Flexion. Flexion is the final area of emphasis during this initial postoperative rehabilitation program. Work on flexion begins on the first postoperative day. With continued emphasis on full hyperextension, flexion is worked on only three times per day during this early postoperative time frame. The patient allows the knee to bend gently over the side of the bed. With the goal of the entire first 2 weeks after the reconstruction to achieve 90 degrees of flexion, the patient is easily able to obtain this with a three times per day schedule. Attempting additional flexion work leads only to increased swelling and therefore an overall delay in the rehabilitation program. In conjunction with the work on flexion, patients perform short arc quadriceps activity in the range of 90 to 30 degrees.

Upon arrival home from the hospital, the patient continues the routine of hourly passive extension with straight leg raises and isometric quadriceps exercises, along with three times per day flexion with short arc quadriceps activity.

Discharge from the hospital. Criteria for discharge from the hospital are (1) full passive hyperextension, (2) good quadriceps leg control, (3) minimal swelling, and (4) adequate flexion in the range of 90 degrees. A 2-day hospital stay is important to prevent postoperative complications.

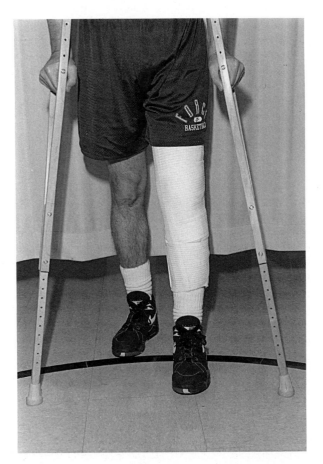

Fig. 13-9. Postoperative weightbearing is allowed. Crutches are used until the patient is able to ambulate without a limp.

We would rather prevent complications with our rehabilitation than treat complications that are allowed to occur.

Patients are directed to rest, keep the reconstructed knee elevated, and use the CPM and Cryo/Cuff. Ambulation should be limited to assist in the control of swelling. This early approach facilitates the acceleration of the rehabilitation program at 2 weeks after surgery.

Early office and therapy visits. We insist on seeing our patients 1 week after the reconstruction. These early visits are important in detecting any potential complications such as lack of full hyperextension, excessive swelling, or poor leg control. If problems are detected, they can be adequately addressed and corrected in the first few days after surgery.

Week 1. At this first office visit, the same criteria used to evaluate patients for discharge from the hospital are used: (1) full hyperextension, (2) good quadriceps leg control, (3) flexion of approximately 90 degrees, and (4) minimal knee swelling with surgical incision healing.

Full hyperextension must be obtained in the first 2 weeks after the reconstruction. If full hyperextension is not achieved in this time frame, this space fills with scar tissue and, along with resultant posterior capsular tightness, becomes a permanent block to hyperextension.

The patient's gait pattern is also assessed. Patients are allowed to stop crutch-assisted ambulation as soon as they are able to assume a normal gait pattern. At this time the majority of patients are able to ambulate with only one crutch, although a few have already resumed a normal gait pattern.

The initial session with physical therapy reinforces the previously reviewed areas of importance, along with the introduction of a few additional rehabilitation exercises. As always, full hyperextension remains the focus of the rehabilitation. The patient now starts utilizing prone hangs with the use of a small ankle weight. Wall slides and some work with active assisted flexion are used to achieve 90 degrees of flexion. Normalization of the gait pattern is an important part of the first postoperative therapy visit. Leg control is emphasized. Additional leg control rehabilitation includes bilateral knee bends and calf raises, all closed-chain exercises (Fig. 13-10). Control of swelling guides the patient's activity between the first and second week. As long as swelling is controlled and knee ROM is improving, the patient is allowed to increase his or her daily activities.

Week 2. The next postoperative visit is at 2 weeks after surgery. Full hyperextension remains the most critical parameter to be evaluated. With proper wound healing, the sutures are removed. Other expectations at this stage in the rehabilitation process include a normal gait pattern without crutch assistance, flexion easily to 90 degrees, and minimal knee swelling. It is important for the patient to understand the importance of swelling control. A knee effusion does not prohibit full knee hyperextension, but it makes flexion improvement difficult. The patient must understand that activity increases need to be undertaken on a gradual basis so as not to significantly increase swelling of the knee and impede improvement in knee flexion.

Throughout the next few weeks, while maintaining full knee hyperextension, knee flexion is approached with greater vigor. Improvements in flexion are accomplished through the use of wall slides, heel slides, and active assisted knee flexion as previously described. Heel slides can be started when the patient has at least 90 degrees of comfortable knee flexion.

Additional strengthening exercises are introduced at the 2-week office visit. The therapist adds unilateral knee bends (Fig. 13-11), the stationary bike, and the StairMaster or a similar closed-chain kinetic vertical climbing machine (Fig. 13-12) to the rehabilitation program. Lateral step-ups are introduced when the patient is able to perform unilateral knee bends without difficulty. The lateral step-up involves standing in a full weightbearing position with the reconstructed extremity on a 2- to 4-inch step. The operative knee is slowly flexed until the nonoperative leg touches the floor. Then the patient slowly extends the operative knee to full hyperextension (Fig. 13-13). The emphases on full hyperextension, early leg control, and the normalization of ambulation with early appropriate functional activities set the

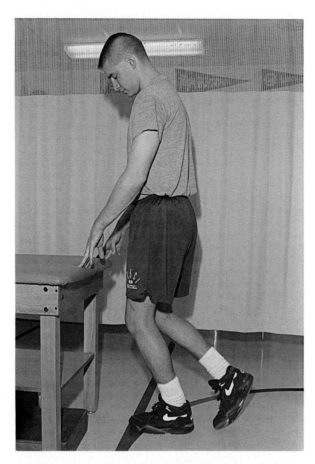

Fig. 13-10. Early strength work using knee bends is started after the second week of postoperative rehabilitation.

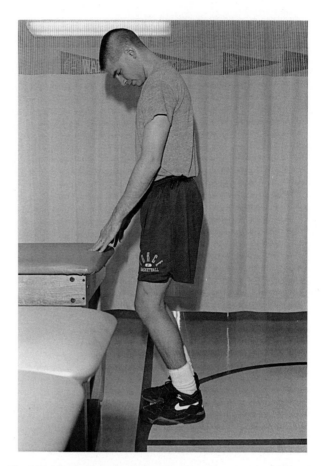

Fig. 13-11. Unilateral knee bends are added as an additional means of improving leg strength.

tone for the remainder of the rehabilitation program, and they are of foremost importance in ensuring a successful outcome.

Lack of full hyperextension. The importance of early and frequent postoperative follow-up is realized if a patient at 2 weeks after the reconstruction does not have full hyperextension. Although this problem is rare, we treat it very aggressively. All efforts are directed at obtaining full hyperextension, and shifting the rehabilitation focus to flexion is postponed. The consequences of a long-term flexion contracture with a resultant bent knee gait and a painful knee with athletic activity are reviewed with the patient. The purpose of full hyperextension with the molding of the newly reconstructed ligament into the notch is also reviewed. We then proceed with aggressive treatment of the flexion contracture. The same day that the problem is identified, the therapist works with the patient to achieve as much extension as possible through prone hangs and manual hyperextension. As soon as the patient's knee is as straight as possible, the operative extremity is placed into a cylinder full-leg hyperextension cast that is molded with forceful hyperextension. The patient leaves this cast in place for 24 hours and is allowed to bear weight as tolerated in the confines of the

cast. The patient returns to the office the next day for cast removal, additional extension stretching, and replacement in a new hyperextension cast. This entire process is repeated until the reconstructed knee has obtained full hyperextension, which usually takes 2 or 3 days. With full hyperextension obtained, the patient no longer is required to wear the cast during the day but continues to wear a univalved hyperextension cast at night for 1 to 2 weeks. The hyperextension prevents the reconstructed knee from assuming a flexed position while the patient sleeps. This greatly assists the patient's ability to maintain full hyperextension and allows a gradual refocus of the rehabilitation to flexion and an eventual normal progression of the overall rehabilitation program.

Phase II (3–5 weeks). The second phase of the postoperative ACL rehabilitation program has the following goals: (1) maintain full hyperextension, (2) increase flexion, (3) begin progressive strengthening, (4) maintain a minimal amount of swelling, and (5) resume normal activities of daily living. During this phase patients increase the activities of daily living as long as they maintain full hyperextension and minimal swelling. Again, the goal of the rehabilitation program is preventing complications rather than treating

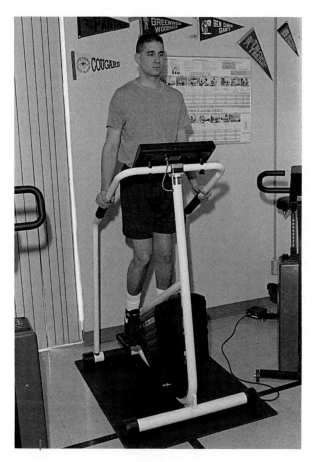

Fig. 13-12. The StairMaster functions as an excellent closed-chain functional rehabilitation activity.

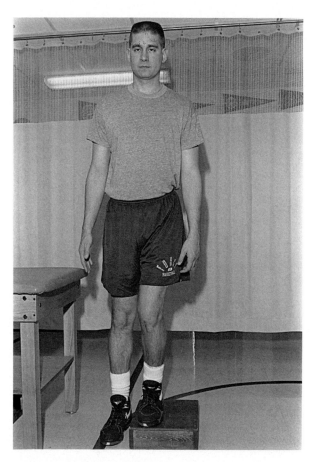

Fig. 13-13. Additional strength work utilizing the lateral step-up is employed in the second week of the rehabilitation process.

them once they occur. The importance of swelling control is that it allows faster and steadier increases in flexion. Strength work is added as long as a compromise in knee ROM is not noted. It is difficult for patients to focus on different areas of rehabilitation at the same time. Our philosophy is to add progressive activities to the rehabilitation process without compromising previously accomplished goals. Our opinion is that the resumption of a normal gait pattern is the first and most important activity to improve strength in the early phase of rehabilitation. As noted, we also utilize the StairMaster, bike, step-ups, and leg press to assist the patient in early strength gains with the initial goal of a normal ambulation pattern.

Our therapists assist the patient in ways to avoid an antalgic gait pattern such as minimizing shoulder sway, instructing in proper heel-to-toe gait, and emphasizing quadriceps contracture at heel strike.

Original concerns expressed over possible fixation failure or early graft weakness being limiting factors to a rapidly progressive rehabilitation program have not been realized. With more than 3000 ACL reconstructions performed at our clinic, we have not observed graft failure or fixation failure because of this early postoperative time period. The goals and demands of the patient are the determinants for our

recommendations of activity level during this period of the rehabilitation. Those patients who are adamant about a quick return to athletic activity need to be guided to obtain full knee ROM before they begin an intense program to regain strength. It has been our finding that it is difficult, if not impossible, for patients to obtain full knee ROM if they are concentrating on a vigorous strength program. Because ROM is more easily obtained in the early phases of rehabilitation, we stress full ROM prior to earnest strength work. We have noted that if patients maintain full hyperextension, achieve full flexion, ambulate without a limp, and maintain minimal swelling, strength gains can be accomplished quickly.

As far as the final flexion gains are concerned, heel slides achieve the majority of the terminal range of flexion. Lowering the seat on a stationary bicycle is also a way to assist in the improvement of flexion. Simple strengthening activities including single leg kneebends, lateral step-ups, and calf raises are continued. More traditional weightroom training can also be added: quarter-squats, calf raises, and the leg press with the flexion angle no greater than 90 to 100 degrees (Fig. 13-14). We also recommend the hip sled during this phase.

The next addition to the rehabilitation in this phase is

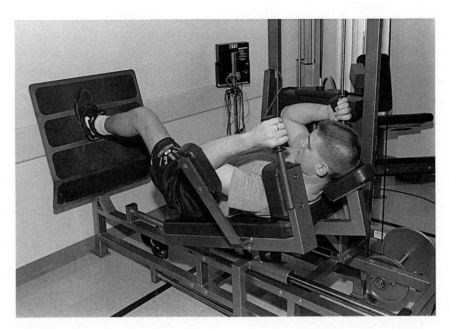

Fig. 13-14. Strength exercises using the leg press are added in the second phase of the rehabilitation program. Flexion beyond 100 degrees is discouraged.

fast-speed strengthening. When the patient has at least 100 to 110 degrees of flexion, the bicycle can be utilized for faster-speed strength workouts. Swimming using the free-style and flutter kick is instituted at this time. A fast-speed pace using the water vest in the deep end of the pool can be started. The StairMaster work is of longer duration and higher intensity. We also utilize the Fitter and Shuttle machines as means of introducing fast-speed weightbearing activities.

Limited solo athletic activities are started when the patient has near normal ROM, good leg control, and improving confidence in his or her newly reconstructed knee. The time when patients are allowed to return to full activities is determined by the individual's drive, goals, and the resultant morbidity of utilizing an autogenous patellar tendon graft. We tailor our rehabilitation program to emphasize to patients what they are able to do and not so much what they are not allowed to do. We do not follow a traditional time format for reintroduction of certain progressive activities. Instead, we recommend that they achieve certain rehabilitation goals, maintain those accomplishments, and progressively advance themselves through the rehabilitation program as rapidly as their reconstructed knee allows and as quickly as they are motivated to do so.

At the completion of phase III of the rehabilitation program, the patients have easily returned to all activities of daily living without compromise. They demonstrate full hyperextension, nearly full flexion, adequate quadriceps strength to allow the knee to actively extend into the terminal range of extension, and ability to ambulate without an antalgic gait. The last phase of the rehabilitation program is the return of the athlete to competition.

Phase III (5 weeks–return to sport). As has been stated previously, the accelerated rehabilitation program was developed to prevent complications rather than to treat complications once they occur. In the past we noted that our noncompliant patients advanced activities beyond recommendation and yet they were performing better and earlier in their postoperative rehabilitation program than those patients on whom we were placing unfounded restrictions. During the mid-1980s we recommended traditional advancement of activities based on the published data of animal studies regarding ligament healing and decline in ligament strength in the early postoperative time period.[11] Although we never encouraged our patients to return to athletic activities early in their rehabilitation, we found that most patients advanced their activities as they were able by closely following their course and probing for answers. Of great interest to us was that these noncompliant patients suffered no ill effects from their nonprescribed aggressive behavior. They performed better than those patients who had strictly followed their postoperative activity restrictions. These noncompliant patients had returned to vigorous sporting activity on their own without failure or detriment to the graft. We therefore have noted that the initial fears of a graft being too weak to withstand early aggressive activity have been unsupported.

The recommendations for phase III of the rehabilitation are not based on laboratory data but on more than 3000 ACL reconstruction patients having demonstrated what can be safely accomplished in an appropriate aggressive manner without jeopardizing graft integrity or long-term stability. We do not actively encourage our patients to accelerate their rehabilitation program, but we do not prevent those patients who desire to push themselves from doing so as long as they maintain the criteria of full hyperextension, full flexion, good leg control, a normal gait, and minimal swelling.

The initial postoperative testing occurs at either the 1- or 2-month postreconstruction visit. At this time, KT-1000 and isokinetic strength testing are performed. Whether this testing is done at 1 or 2 months is determined by the obtainment of full knee ROM and the aggressiveness of the patient. With full ROM and an athlete's desire to accelerate a return to competitive sport, these tests are usually performed at 1 month after the reconstruction. The importance of possessing full ROM, especially full hyperextension prior to stability testing, derives from our belief that an attempt at assessing ligamentous stability prior to the time when full hyperextension has been returned leads to falsely low KT-1000 measurements. When testing is performed, the difference between preoperative and postoperative stability scores is recorded for each patient.

The evaluation of postoperative strength is also performed at this time. We use isokinetic strength measurements to determine the advancement of the patient's running program. Through clinical experience gained with follow-up of our patients, we have noted those athletes who initiate a running program with isokinetic strength of the quadriceps of less than 70% are prone to develop patellar tendonitis, knee effusions, and a resultant decrease in knee flexion. Therefore, if strength evaluation reveals quadriceps strength less than 70% of the nonoperative leg, we recommend avoidance of running until leg strength can be improved. At this time we are also evaluating additional methods of determining postoperative strength. Leg press and single leg hop are two of the alternate strength tests.

With our postoperative isokinetic strength evaluation, we use an antishear device to control anterior shear in the knee. To block terminal extension, a 20-degree block is utilized. Also, at the first postoperative evaluation, isokinetic evaluations are done at 180 and 240 degrees per second only.

When testing with the leg press, the patient is instructed to perform as many repetitions as possible with the operative and then the nonoperative leg. The weight used is the patient's body weight, and the patient is encouraged to work to maximum fatigue in each leg tested. The strength index is calculated by dividing the number of repetitions of the operative leg by the number of repetitions of the nonoperative leg. The single leg hop test involves the patient performing a single leg hop off each leg with the distance jumped measured. Patients are instructed to jump off and land on a single leg only. The distance jumped with the reconstructed leg is divided by the distance jumped by the normal leg and a hop index is reported.

We use a 60% isokinetic strength level in both the quadriceps and hamstring muscle groups as a value the patient must be above before the postoperative light functional progression program is started. These agility drills include lateral shuffles, cariocas, and jumping rope. Simple sporting activities performed by the patient alone are also progressed

at this time. These include hitting a tennis ball or racquetball off a wall or shooting a basketball. These early agility drills improve the patient's strength and speed, as well as aiding in restoring quickness and proprioception in the early phase after reconstruction. These activities are also of benefit in restoring the patient's confidence in the recently reconstructed extremity. We have noted that in performing these early agility drills instead of running, with its associated reactive ground forces, the reconstructed knee develops less swelling and soreness.

A postoperative brace is utilized on those patients who take a more aggressive approach to return to athletic competition. The brace assists their confidence in the reconstructed knee. We fit our athletes with a polycentric molded brace. The patient is fitted for the brace at the first office visit and picks the brace up for use at the second-week postoperative visit. After a few weeks of wearing the brace for outside or school activities, the brace is utilized for athletic activity only.

The leg press, hip sled, safety squat, and squat rack are the weightroom exercises performed during this phase of the rehabilitation. Increased resistive work is done on the StairMaster and bicycle and with swimming in an effort to increase fast-speed strengthening.

At this point in the rehabilitation, the office and physical therapy visits are scheduled depending on how the patient is performing. If a problem exists in the patient's rehabilitation, then more frequent visits are arranged. Otherwise, follow-up is routinely scheduled at 5 weeks, 3 months, 6 months, and 1 year, with long-term follow-up at 2 and 5 years. KT-1000 stability, isokinetic strength, and functional testing are done at each of these routine visits. In regard to the isokinetic testing, the 20-degree extension block is removed starting at the 3-month follow-up.

More aggressive workouts are conducted as the patient's strength and confidence improve. Additional activities include figure of eights, running backward, and jogging, with progression to half-speed sprinting. The patient is allowed to work back to full activity on his or her own pace as long as it is done in a stepwise progressive manner without developing unacceptable knee swelling or stiffness. The criteria we utilize for return to unrestricted sporting activity is completion of all functional activities that are specific to the sport in which they are involved and quadriceps strength of 80% compared to the nonoperative leg, at all speeds tested. We counsel our patients that, with the return to athletic competition, they will require at least 3 to 4 months of sport-specific play before they gain full confidence in their reconstructed knee.

Summary

The accelerated rehabilitation program has been developed over the last 10 years in treating more than 3000 ACL reconstructions using an autogenous patellar tendon graft. The protocol has been advanced through close and careful follow-up and by evaluating our patients and advancing the rehabilitation when more aggressive noncompliant patients were noted to have a lower incidence of postoperative complications than less active, more compliant patients. We are aware of the laboratory and animal studies that traditional ACL rehabilitation protocols are based on, but we have adjusted our program based on our clinical findings and patient results. Fixation failure or graft weakness have not been problems with our reconstructive surgery or our postoperative rehabilitation.

The focus of the development of the rehabilitation program has been to prevent complications from occurring rather than treat them once they are allowed to occur. Certain previous postoperative restrictions that we placed on our patients have been noted to be unnecessary. Our present approach is to avoid inappropriate timing of surgery by not operating in the acute phase of the injury and performing early and detailed postoperative follow-up to detect any problems as they arise.

Our ACL rehabilitation program has been developed to decrease the occurrence of postoperative complications. Our goals are to ensure long-term stability in a knee that possesses full ROM and to provide a timely and safe return to sporting activity. The rehabilitation program is divided into four phases: preoperative and phases I, II, and III postoperatively. The preoperative control of swelling, restoration of full ROM, and mental preparation of the patient for surgery, along with phase I postoperative emphasis on full hyperextension, good quadriceps leg control, and control of swelling are the cornerstones of the rehabilitation program. As always, we continue to critically evaluate the rehabilitation protocol, closely and objectively evaluate our results, and allow our patients to continue to guide us through additional advancements in our rehabilitation program.

POSTERIOR CRUCIATE LIGAMENT INJURY REHABILITATION

The rehabilitation of posterior cruciate ligament (PCL) injuries is covered here briefly. Our experience in dealing with PCL injuries is significantly less than that with the more common MCL and ACL injuries. The rehabilitation goals of full range of motion and normalization of gait remain the same. The manner of achieving these goals is also similar.

The rehabilitation of PCL injuries is divided into three phases: phase I is the control of pain and swelling, phase II is the restoration of full ROM and normalization of ambulation, and phase III is the return of the athlete to normal activities of daily life and eventually athletic competition. For those competitive athletes involved in collision sports, we utilize a postinjury PCL brace when they return to athletic competition.

Our PCL postoperative rehabilitation program is slower than the ACL reconstruction rehabilitation program. In the PCL program, emphasis is placed on posterior tibial support and a resting splint with the leg in full extension. Aggressive

flexion is postponed for up to 6 weeks after the PCL reconstructive procedure. Other postoperative activities are also introduced at a slower rate.

LATERAL LIGAMENTOUS COMPLEX REHABILITATION

An isolated injury to the lateral ligamentous complex of the knee is extremely uncommon. When the diagnosis is made, it is important to rule out other ligamentous injuries in addition to evaluating the knee for damage to the posterolateral complex. A rehabilitation of isolated lateral ligamentous injuries follows the same previously outlined principles of pain and swelling control, restoration of motion, normalization of gait pattern, functional strengthening activities, and return to activities.

SUMMARY

It is evident with the completion of this chapter that our basic rehabilitation principles are the same, regardless of which ligament of the knee has been injured. The initiation of the rehabilitation involves control of postinjury pain and swelling. The second part of the rehabilitation is restoration of full ROM and normalization of ambulation. The final phase involves strengthening with emphasis on closed-chain functional activities and a safe return of the athlete to the field of play. We continue to make advancements in all areas of rehabilitation by closely evaluating our patients and their results.

REFERENCES

1. Indelicato PA: Injury to the medial capsuloligamentous complex. In Feagin Jr JA, editor: *The crucial ligaments,* Churchill Livingstone, 1988, New York.
2. Indelicato PA: Non-operative treatment of complete tears of the medial collateral ligament of the knee, *J Bone Joint Surg [Am]* 65:323-329, 1983.
3. Muller W: *The knee: form, function, and ligament reconstruction,* New York, 1983, Springer-Verlag.
4. Warren LF, Marshall JL: The supporting structures and layers on the medial side of the knee: an anatomical analysis, *J Bone Joint Surg [Am]* 61:56-62, 1979.
5. Hughston JC, Barrett GR: Acute anteromedial rotary instability: long-term results of surgical repair, *J Bone Joint Surg [Am]* 65:145-153, 1983.
6. Rubinstein RA, Shelbourne KD: Management of combined instabilities: anterior cruciate ligament/medial collateral ligament and anterior cruciate ligament/lateral side, *Operative Tech Sports Med* 1:66-71, 1993.
7. Grood ES, et al: Ligamentous and capsular restraints preventing straight medial and lateral laxity in intact human cadaver knees, *J Bone Joint Surg [Am]* 63:1257-1269, 1981.
8. Shelbourne KD, et al: Arthrofibrosis in acute anterior cruciate ligament reconstruction: the effect of timing of reconstruction and rehabilitation, *Am J Sports Med* 19:332-336, 1991.
9. Shelbourne KD, et al: Postoperative cryotherapy for the knee, *Orthopedics* (in press).
10. Arnoczky SP, Tarvin GB, Marshall JL: Anterior cruciate ligament replacement using patellar tendon, *J Bone Joint Surg [Am]* 64:217-224, 1982.
11. Clancy WG, et al: Anterior and posterior cruciate ligament reconstruction in rhesus monkeys: a histological, microangiographic, and biomechanical analysis, *J Bone Joint Surg [Am]* 63:1270-1284, 1981.

SUGGESTED READINGS

Cabaud HE, Rodkey WG, Feagin JA: Experimental studies of acute anterior cruciate ligament injury and repair, *Am J Sports Med* 7:18–22, 1979.

Feagin JA: The syndrome of the torn anterior cruciate ligament, *Orthop Clin North Am* 10:81–90, 1979.

Feagin JA, Lambert KL: Mechanism of injury and pathology of anterior cruciate ligament injuries, *Orthop Clin North Am* 16:41–46, 1985.

Fetto JW, Marshall JL: The natural history and diagnosis of the anterior cruciate ligament insufficiency, *Clin Orthop* 147:29–38, 1980.

Hughston JC, et al: Classification of knee ligament instabilities, part I: The medial compartment, *J Bone Joint Surg [Am]* 58:159–172, 1976.

Hughston JC, et al: Classification of knee ligament instabilities, part II. The lateral compartment, *J Bone Joint Surg [Am]* 58:173–179, 1976.

Hunter LY, Funk FJ, editors: *Rehabilitation of the injured knee,* St Louis, 1984, Mosby–Year Book.

Jones KG: Reconstruction of the anterior cruciate ligament: a technique using the central one-third of the patellar ligament, *J Bone Joint Surg [Am]* 45:925–932, 1963.

Noyes FR, et al: Biomechanical analysis of human ligament grafts used in knee ligament repairs and reconstructions, *J Bone Joint Surg [Am]* 66:344–352, 1984.

Noyes FR, et al: Intraarticular cruciate reconstruction; part I. perspectives on graft strength, vascularization, and immediate motion after replacement, *Clin Orthop* 172:71–77, 1983.

Noyes FR, et al: The symptomatic anterior cruciate deficient knee: part I, The long-term functional disability in athletically active individuals, *J Bone Joint Surg [Am]* 65:154–162, 1983.

Paulos LE, et al: Intraarticular cruciate reconstruction: II. replacement with vascularized patellar tendon, *Clin Orthop* 172:78–84, 1983.

Paulos LE, et al: Knee rehabilitation after anterior cruciate ligament reconstruction and repair, *Am J Sports Med* 9:140–149, 1981.

Shelbourne KD, Klootwyk TE, DeCarlo MS: Update on accelerated rehabilitation after anterior cruciate ligament reconstruction, *J Orthop Sport Phys Ther* 15:303–308, 1992.

Shelbourne KD, Nitz P: Accelerated rehabilitation after anterior cruciate ligament reconstruction, *Am J Sports Med* 18:292–299, 1990.

Shelbourne KD, Wilckens JH: Current concepts in anterior cruciate ligament reconstruction, *Orthop Rev* 19:957–964, 1990.

Chapter 14

OTHER SOFT TISSUE INJURIES
OF THE KNEE

Champ L. Baker, Jr.

BURSITIS

A *bursa* is defined as "a sac-like cavity filled with a viscid fluid and situated at places in the tissues at which friction would otherwise develop."[1] The function of the bursa is to reduce the amount of friction between surrounding surfaces as they rub over each other during a joint's range of motion. Inflammation of this fluid-filled sac is described as *bursitis*. Bursitis can be classified as either acute or chronic and can result from either a traumatic episode or repeated minor traumas.

Prepatellar bursitis

The prepatellar bursa is located between the subcutaneous layer and the anterior surface of the patella. The location of the bursa makes it susceptible to trauma from a fall or a direct blow to the anterior aspect of the knee. A secondary cause of irritation is repeated minor trauma that can develop from repeated kneeling or crawling on the knee. Chronic prepatellar bursitis is sometimes referred to as *housemaid's knee* because of the increased incidence of bursal inflammation in people who are engaged in activities that require repeated kneeling. It is a common problem in wrestlers.

Acute prepatellar bursitis. Acute prepatellar bursitis, or hemorrhagic bursitis, is usually the result of a single episode of trauma to the knee. A common cause is a fall on the flexed knee. The patient presents with localized swelling above the knee that is ballottable. Erythema may be present. Close inspection of the knee reveals that the effusion is not usually intra-articular and does not restrict motion of the joint. The sudden onset of symptoms after a direct blow to the knee is caused by blood in the bursa from the rupture of an artery or vein. The examiner should look for lacerations or skin abrasions that could lead to a secondary infection.

Initial radiographs should include anteroposterior and lateral views of the knee as well as a skyline view of the patella to rule out a fracture.

The differential diagnosis includes cellulitis, or a secondary infection. If an infection is suspected, fluid from the bursa should be aspirated using a sterile technique, examined, and sent for cultures and sensitivity. It is important to prevent contamination of the knee joint during aspiration or drainage of the bursa. *Staphylococcus* is the most common organism in suppurative prepatellar bursitis,[2] but anaerobic organisms have also been cultured from the bursa. Broad-spectrum antibiotics should be given until specific culture results are available. If the bursa is infected, surgical drainage should be performed through a longitudinal incision adjacent to the patella.[3]

The initial treatment for acute bursitis involves ice, compression, and nonsteroidal anti-inflammatory medications. The compression bandage should be applied above the patella to place constant pressure over the bursa. Depending on the patient's symptoms, immobilization with the knee in extension may be indicated initially, and crutches can be used for protected weightbearing.

Swelling of the bursa is a localized phenomenon; however, rehabilitation of the entire lower extremity and the quadriceps muscles in particular must begin immediately to maintain tone and prevent reaccumulation of fluid in the bursa. The patient must continue to wear a compression wrap to decrease the potential space and minimize return of swelling. The patient is instructed in the proper technique of quadriceps setting and straight leg raising exercises to maintain quadriceps tone and to work in conjunction with the compression dressing to force fluid from the bursa. After 48 hours, the knee should be reexamined. If there is marked diminution of the size of the bursal sac or minimal reaccumulation of fluid after aspiration, the compression wrap can be kept on and the patient started on gentle, passive range-of-motion exercises to regain flexion. Patients should also continue to use crutches until full quadriceps control has been regained and they can walk with no limp.

Chronic prepatellar bursitis. Chronic prepatellar bursitis is more commonly seen than acute prepatellar bursitis. It is the result of repeated episodes of minimal trauma. The diagnosis is based on the patient's history and the clinical examination of the knee. Often, the skin shows evidence of chronic irritation, such as callosities or thickening. The bursa is usually palpable and is seldom tender (Fig. 14-1).

Aspiration, compression, and protective wraps to prevent additional trauma have been used to treat this condition, usually without complete success. Maintaining good quadriceps tone and strength helps to keep the bursa from becoming too distended. However, if the bursal sac is chronically thickened and fluid tends to reaccumulate easily, aspiration alone is unsuccessful. If an infection has been ruled out, a corticosteroid can be injected into the bursal sac to decrease inflammation. A compression wrap should be applied and worn continuously to decrease the joint space and lessen the likelihood of fluid reaccumulation.

Often, chronic prepatellar bursitis requires surgical excision to resolve the problem completely. The bursa should be sharply resected from its adherence to the subcuticular tissue and removed in toto. It is important to remove the entire sac; otherwise, fluid will continue to accumulate and a secondary sac will form. A postoperative drain should be inserted to keep fluid from reaccumulating, and a compression wrap should remain in place for 48 to 72 hours after surgery. Occasionally, drainage continues after excision of a chronic prepatellar bursa, and care must be taken to prevent secondary infection.

Chronic bursitis, whether it is treated conservatively or surgically, can recur; therefore, it is important for the patient to wear a compression bandage and protective pad when returning to sports. Maintaining quadriceps strength and lower extremity mobility is equally important. Chronic prepatellar bursitis often causes abnormal function of the extensor mechanism and changes in patellofemoral joint mechanics. This can lead to decreased quadriceps tone and circumference, problems that should be treated with appropriate strengthening exercises to minimize symptoms before the patient returns to sports. To be able to return to normal activities, a patient should have achieved full range of motion and full flexion without discomfort, and have good quadriceps tone and strength. The athlete should keep a protective pad and compression bandage over the superior aspect of the knee to prevent further trauma and effusion.

Deep and superficial infrapatellar bursitis

The patellar tendon attaches to the distal portion of the patella and inserts onto the anterior tibial tuberosity. A deep bursal sac lies behind the patellar tendon and in front of the

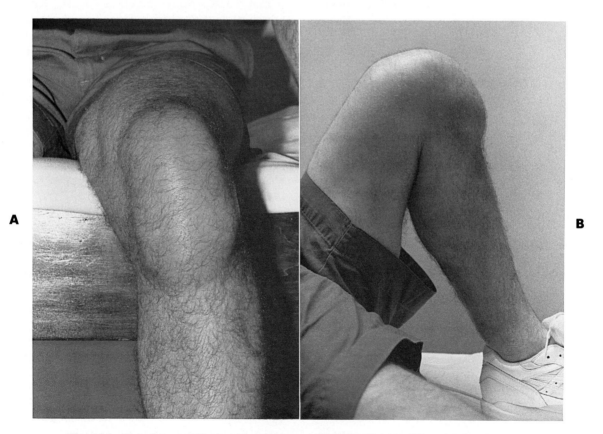

Fig. 14-1. Chronic prepatellar bursitis is characterized by localized swelling. **A,** Anterior view. **B,** Lateral view.

infrapatellar fat pad that lines the anterior surface of the tibia (Fig. 14-2). The superficial infrapatellar bursa lies between the skin and the anterior surface of the patellar tendon. These bursae can become irritated by either direct trauma (the superficial) or overuse from friction between the tendon and anterior aspect of the tibia (the deep). The physical findings are indistinguishable from those related to Osgood-Schlatter disease. The age of the patient and the presence of tibial tubercle apophysitis helps to distinguish this irritation of the tubercle from the deep-seated inflammation of the infrapatellar bursa.

Examination reveals localized pain and tenderness to palpation. The diagnosis is usually made by direct palpation of the area of maximal involvement, either superficial or deep to the tendon (Fig. 14-3). Often, a patient with superficial infrapatellar bursitis has swelling anterior to the tendon.

Treatment is the same as for prepatellar bursitis and includes application of a compression wrap, nonsteroidal anti-inflammatory medications, and ice. The use of localized heat decreases inflammation. Again, a compression wrap is used to help decrease the size of the bursa and to prevent further injury. An injection of corticosteroid into this area is not advisable because of the bursa's close proximity to the patellar tendon and the possible deleterious effects on the tendon. Surgical correction is rarely, if ever, indicated.

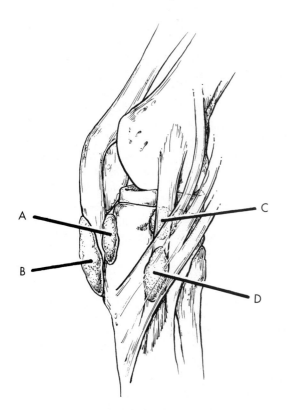

Fig. 14-2. Lateral view of the knee showing bursae. *A,* Deep infrapatellar bursa; *B,* superficial infrapatellar bursa; *C,* tibial collateral ligament bursa; *D,* pes anserine bursa.

A good range of knee motion and sufficient quadriceps power to help maintain full extension are the hallmarks of rehabilitating the knee to competition level. Protective support and compression wraps should be used to prevent recurrence of localized irritation to the bursa (Fig. 14-4).

Pes anserine bursitis

Another superficial bursa on the medial aspect of the knee lies superficial to the tibial collateral ligament and between the tendons of the sartorius, gracilis, and semitendinosus muscles (see Fig. 14-2). These three tendons insert on the anteromedial aspect of the proximal tibia and their tendinous insertion resembles a goose's webbed foot, thus, the *pes anserine*. The pes anserine bursa lies approximately 2 cm distal to the medial joint line; when inflamed, tenderness is noted on palpation of the bursa below the level of the joint line (Fig. 14-5). Thus, it can be distinguished from tibial collateral ligament bursitis, a meniscal tear (medial joint line pain), or irritation of the semimembranosus tendon.

Irritation of the bursa develops from friction or direct injury. An injury to the knee that causes quadriceps atrophy may place unusual stress on the hamstring muscles, and resultant weakness translates to increased friction at the level of the attachment. Marked hamstring tightness is another cause for increased friction over the anteromedial aspect of the tibia at the attachment. In selected instances, the anteromedial portion of the tibia is a site for osteochondromal formation, which presents as a mass over which the pes anserine tendons must pass during flexion and extension of the knee.

Localized pain and tenderness are the hallmark of the diagnosis, as well as discomfort during external rotation of the flexed knee. Crepitus can often be elicited with palpation. Valgus stress to the knee usually does not cause or increase discomfort over the pes anserine bursa, thus allowing the examiner to distinguish this problem from a medial collateral ligament injury.

Symptomatic pes anserine irritation often results from weakness in the hamstring muscles and causes an abnormal strain on the tendons. Treatment is symptomatic and usually consists of ice, nonsteroidal anti-inflammatory medications, and strengthening exercises for the quadriceps. The hamstring muscles are often tight, and stretching and strengthening are important aspects of treatment (Fig. 14-6). Bursitis under the pes anserine tendons often resolves if etiologic factors, such as quadriceps atrophy and weakness, hamstring tightness, or intra-articular disorders of the knee, are eliminated. If a meniscal tear is present causing abnormalities in the extensor mechanism and secondary pes anserine bursitis, the tear may need to be treated arthroscopically. Rehabilitation helps to resolve the secondary bursitis. Local corticosteroid injections are rarely indicated, but may be helpful in recalcitrant cases and in treating symptoms localized in the bursa.

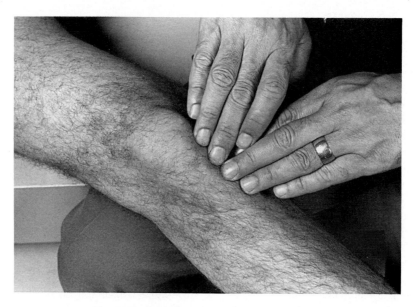

Fig. 14-3. Palpation of deep infrapatellar bursa.

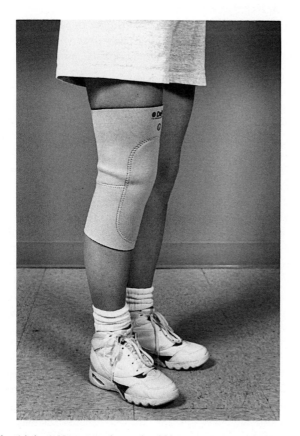

Fig. 14-4. A Neoprene sleeve should be worn to prevent recurrent irritation of the bursa.

Tibial collateral ligament bursitis

In 1988, Kerlan and Glousman[4] reintroduced the concept of irritation of the tibial collateral ligament bursa as a cause of medial knee pain. Brantigan and Voshell[5] initially described this bursa 45 years ago, but the relationship of medial knee pain to irritation of the bursa was not reported in the literature until recently. The diagnosis is made based on the history of isolated medial knee pain at the level of the tibial collateral ligament with no history of injury. Examination of the patient's knee elicits tenderness at the level of the medial joint line that is exacerbated with valgus stress. The site of the tenderness is the distal insertion of the tibial collateral ligament (Fig. 14-7) and should be differentiated from tenderness at the joint line due to meniscal injury or tenderness of the tibial arm of the semimembranosus due to tendinous irritation.

Similarly, as with the treatment process for other types of bursitis in the knee, it is extremely important to develop good quadriceps strength to help maintain normal gait and correct this laxity of the medial ligaments that may be contributing to the irritation of the tibial collateral ligament attachment. One cubic centimeter of short-acting steroid and lidocaine is injected into the bursa with the patient sitting with the affected leg hanging over the edge of the table. After the injection, the patient can be reexamined. If the tenderness is eliminated, the diagnosis is confirmed. More than 60% of patients in Kerlan and Glousman's[4] study improved with nonsurgical treatment.

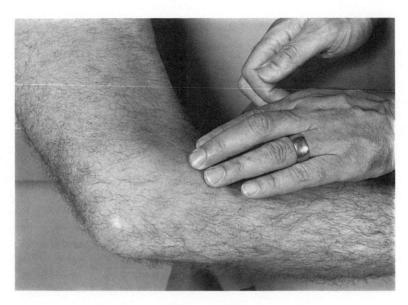

Fig. 14-5. Palpation of the pes anserine bursa.

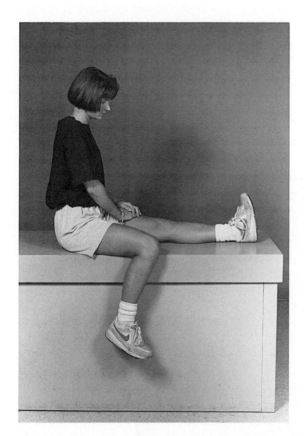

Fig. 14-6. Hamstring stretching corrects the weakness and tightness of the muscles that strain the tendons and irritate the pes anserine bursa.

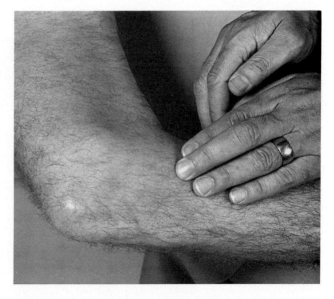

Fig. 14-7. Palpation of the tibial collateral ligament bursa.

Iliotibial band friction syndrome

The iliotibial tract, or band, receives tendinous reinforcements from the tensor fascia lata muscle and the gluteus maximus muscle. With flexion and extension of the knee, the thickest portion of the band, which is located adjacent to the lateral femoral condyle, moves from a position posterior to one anterior to the axis of motion in the last 30 degrees of extension. There is a bursa deep to the band overlying the prominence of the lateral femoral condyle, and its irritation is the cause of iliotibial band friction syndrome.

The iliotibial band friction syndrome is commonly seen in runners, particularly during downhill running, or in anyone who participates in an activity that requires repetitive flexion and extension of the knee. Symptoms are exacerbated by climbing hills or stairs and may be precipitated by contusion or injury. Training errors, such as a rapid increase in mileage or running too far in a single run, can aggravate the condition. In runners, there is often an aching sensation in the lateral aspect of the knee that increases as the athlete increases his or her mileage. Pain is initially present when the athlete is running and often occurs in the same spot during the workout. The pain may be present while the athlete is walking and training. Centered over the lateral femoral condyle, it occasionally radiates distally to the tibial attachment or proximally to the lateral thigh. There is localized tenderness to palpation 2 to 4 cm proximal to the lateral joint line over the lateral femoral condyle (Fig. 14-8). The pain is often aggravated at 30 degrees of knee flexion but is more intense when the leg comes in contact with the ground at foot strike.[6]

Diagnosis of iliotibial band friction syndrome can be made from the patient's history and a clinical examination that reveals localized tenderness over the lateral femoral condyle, particularly while moving the knee through the last 30 degrees of flexion to full extension. Noble[7] described a compression test to elicit the pain of this syndrome. The patient is in the supine position with the affected knee flexed to 90 degrees. Digital pressure is applied over the proximal prominence of the lateral femoral condyle as the knee is extended. At 30 to 40 degrees of flexion, the patient experiences pain similar to that experienced while running. Renne[8] described a maneuver in which the athlete stands on the affected leg with the knee flexed 30 to 40 degrees (Fig. 14-9). This position can also reproduce the pain because it brings the iliotibial band into tight contact with the lateral femoral condyle. Pain may be further accentuated by having the patient hop in this knee-flexed position.

Other factors that can cause this irritation include training errors in running; biomechanical malalignments, such as genu varum that cause extensive tightness of the band at the knee or leg-length inequalities; and excessive running on hills or a cambered road. The examiner often finds associated tightness in the iliotibial band. The Ober test demonstrates this tightness and is diagnostic.

The differential diagnosis includes lateral meniscal tears or cysts. Strains of the fibular collateral ligament or mid-third lateral collateral ligament can also be confused with this syndrome. The most common misdiagnosis is popliteal tenosynovitis, which is irritation of the popliteal tendon insertion on the lateral femoral condyle. The diagnoses can be made by differentiating tenderness or pain localized at the popliteus insertion that does not increase with flexion and extension from tenderness over the lateral condyle that varies with flexion and extension of the knee.

Treatment of iliotibial band friction syndrome consists

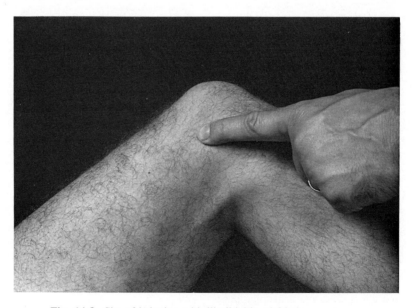

Fig. 14-8. Site of irritation with iliotibial band friction syndrome.

of first eliminating the factors that cause the irritation. Running and training should be reduced to the point of minimal or no pain with adequate rest between training cycles. Hill running should be avoided until the patient is asymptomatic. When running on a cambered road or indoor track, the athlete should alternate running cycles. Leg-length inequality should be corrected with orthotics such as lateral sole wedges. An injection of steroids into the area of maximum tenderness may be used if other modalities are not successful. In rare instances, surgical release of the posterior fibers of the tract may be necessary.

Successful treatment of this syndrome always includes stretching of the iliotibial tract. Passive gravity stretches are done initially (Fig. 14-10). Active stretching can then be performed (Fig. 14-11). These stretches should be a permanent addition to the athlete's warm-up regimen.

Bicipital bursitis

Analogous to the tibial collateral ligament bursa on the medial aspect, the lateral bicipital, or bicipitofibular, bursa lies between the fibular collateral ligament and the fibular attachment of the biceps femoris. As with most bursitis, direct trauma or overactivity can cause irritation of this small bursa.

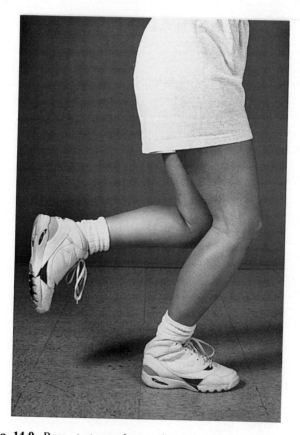

Fig. 14-9. Renne test reproduces pain of running in patients with iliotibial band friction syndrome.

Diagnosis rests with the examiner's eliciting point tenderness at the site of the bursa and ruling out ligamentous or meniscal injuries (Fig. 14-12). Localized swelling is often seen. Steroid injections are seldom indicated for a localized bursal irritation. Treatment is primarily conservative with emphasis on stretching and strengthening of the long and short heads of the biceps femoris. Ice or moist heat and anti-inflammatory medications can also be helpful; however, successful treatment usually consists of stretching the tightness of the iliotibial band and tract and stretching the lateral hamstrings to eliminate direct pull on the biceps attachment.

Popliteal bursitis

A popliteal cyst, commonly called a Baker's cyst, is a localized collection of fluid in the posterior fossa of the knee. The cyst may be caused by extension of the semimembranosus bursa in the interval between the medial head of the gastrocnemius and the semimembranosus muscle belly. Fluid accumulates in the bursa as a result of chronic effusion that has increased the articular pressure over a period of time. The most common cause of this effusion in a nonrheumatoid knee of an adult is a torn meniscus or degenerative arthritis. The cyst is usually noticed by the patient as a palpable mass on the posterior aspect of the knee that is often tense in flexion (Fig. 14-13). Usually, no tenderness is present, but rather an ache in the posterior aspect of the knee. Because of the bursa's location, the patient may experience discomfort during knee flexion or extension.

Differential diagnoses include arteriovenous malformations, hemangiomas, or soft tissue tumors. Occasionally, calcification and loose bodies are present in the popliteal area. Radiographs are not usually helpful, but the diagnosis can be made definitively with ultrasound, arthrography, or magnetic resonance imaging (MRI). These studies can detect the abnormality that has caused the formation of the symptomatic bursa.

Treatment focuses on correcting the primary knee disorder. In some patients, aspiration of the cyst is also needed. It usually reveals a jellylike substance or clear synovial fluid. Exercises are inadequate to fully treat the cyst, which usually abates when the primary disorder is treated. Arthroscopy is often indicated to treat intra-articular injuries, and the cyst is allowed to resolve. However, if the cyst does not resolve, excision may be required.[9]

Once the cause of the popliteal cyst has been treated, it usually disappears. Meniscal tears and degenerative changes can often be successfully treated with an aggressive rehabilitation program that negates the need for surgical intervention. In this situation, continued emphasis on exercises for the hip flexors and quadriceps musculature is important with regard to both maintaining quadriceps tone and strength and eliminating any extensor lag that may be causing symptoms (Fig. 14-14). It is important for the patient to stretch

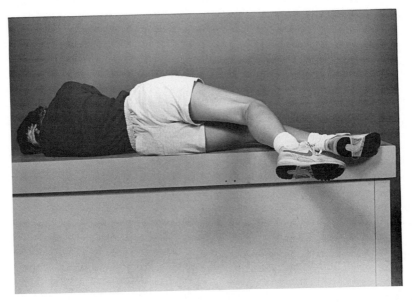

Fig. 14-10. Passive gravity stretch for iliotibial band tightness. The athlete lies on the unaffected side with the leg flexed to stabilize the pelvis and maintain perpendicular orientation of ASIS to the surface he or she is lying on. The affected leg is in extension at the hip, and the knee is allowed to hang over the edge of the table and passively adducted under the influence of gravity. The position is held for 15 minutes with a rest period, if needed, to reduce discomfort.

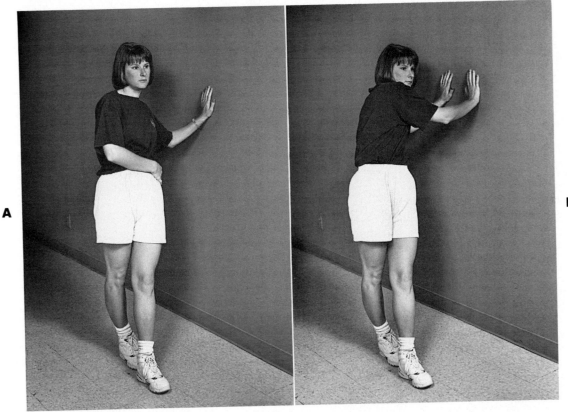

Fig. 14-11. Iliotibial band stretch. **A,** The athlete stands with both knees fully extended, and the affected leg is extended at the hip and adducted as far as possible. **B,** The athlete then either side-flexes the trunk maximally to the unaffected side or rotates the waist away from the affected side while attempting to touch the heel of the unaffected leg.

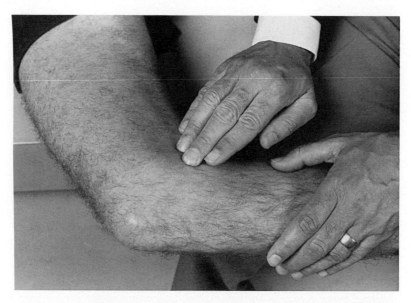

Fig. 14-12. Site of bicipital bursitis tenderness.

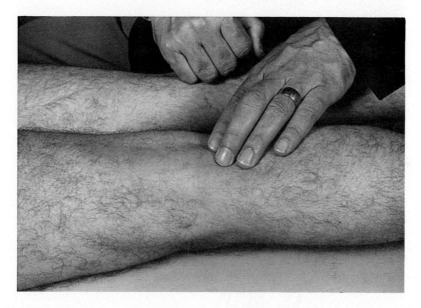

Fig. 14-13. Location of the semimembranosus bursa. Aching in this area associated with a palpable mass suggests a Baker's, or popliteal, cyst.

out the hamstring muscles, although care must be taken not to aggravate the palpable posterior mass. Aspiration of the cyst is not indicated in all but a few selected cases. Compression wraps or bulky bandages are rarely needed because the cyst is protected by its posterior position in the knee. Compression wraps generally do not help to decompress this cyst.

TENDONITIS

Tendonitis, an injury to the substance of the tendon, is usually secondary to degenerative changes or cumulative microtrauma. It is often the result of repetitive loading or overloading or as a compensation for other problems about the knee. The four most common tendinous irritations about the knee are semimembranosus tendonitis, medially; popliteal tenosynovitis, laterally; biceps femoris tendonitis, laterally; and patellar tendonitis, anteriorly.

Patellar tendonitis

The most common tendonitis about the knee is irritation of the extensor mechanism, specifically the patellar tendon. The term *jumper's knee* refers to inflammation of the patellar

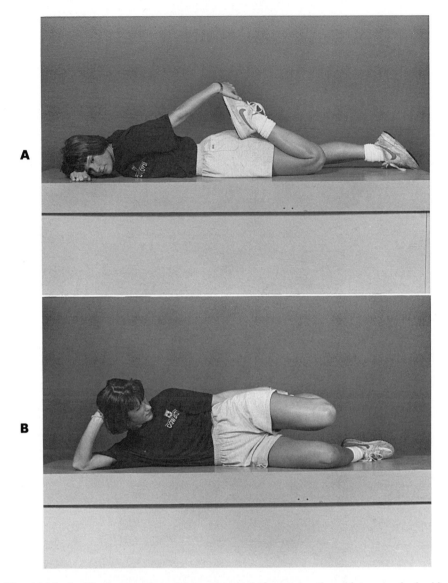

Fig. 14-14. A, Hip flexor and quadriceps stretch. Lying prone, the athlete extends the hip and simultaneously flexes the knee. **B,** Modified hip flexor and quadriceps stretch. Lying on the unaffected side allows the athlete to be in a position of less hip extension and knee flexion if muscle tissue is tender and less flexible immediately after an injury.

or quadriceps tendon, and it is a functional overload syndrome usually seen in athletes who are subjected to intense repeated loading. It is particularly prevalent in volleyball, basketball, high jumping, weightlifting, soccer, and cycling. The most common precipitating extrinsic factors are the duration and intensity of training sessions and the playing surface. Less commonly involved are intrinsic factors such as the athlete's body weight, height, presence of patella alta, and flexibility of the knee.

The presenting symptom is pain that often becomes activity related. Blazina et al.[10] classified patellar tendon disorders in stages secondary to activity-related symptoms. Stage I is pain after activity only with no functional impairment. Stage II is pain at the beginning of activity that disappears after warm-up and reappears with fatigue. Stage III is pain during and after activity that impairs function, and patients are unable to participate in sports at their previous levels. Stage IV is complete rupture of the tendon. This staging and classification are based on a patient's symptoms, including a gradual increase in pain until activity must be ceased. The hallmark of the examination is pain to palpation, usually at the tibial tubercle insertion or in the skeletally immature patient at the level of the apophysis. Rarely is there associated swelling and erythema over the tendon itself. With Osgood-Schlatter disease, there may be an enlargement of the tubercle.

Radiographs are usually negative, but pertinent positive findings may include bipartite patella, ossification of the inferior pole of the patella, or osteochondritis of the tibial tubercle insertion.

Treatment is based on the classification as described by Blazina et al.[10] Treatment for stages I, II, and III is non-operative. Patients with stage I, which is pain with activity only, are advised to increase their warm-up before training, use ice after the activity, and take oral anti-inflammatory medications. Therapy includes exercise to increase hamstring flexibility and to strengthen the quadriceps. Elastic knee supports may be beneficial. Injections are contraindicated.

With stage II tendonitis, a hot pack or heating pad may be used to assist in the warm-up phase before activity. Again, cooling down, stretching, and an ice massage are indicated after activity. Rest and limitation of activities may be indicated in stage II.

In patients who have stage III tendonitis, prolonged rest is the most important part of treatment. Cessation of sports in conjunction with the treatment protocol outlined for stages I and II helps to diminish symptoms.

Physical therapy is an extremely important part of the treatment of patellar tendonitis. Because most problems are related to excessive extrinsic loading with repetitive abnormal stress on the patellar tendon, extrinsic exercises should be included as part of the quadriceps strengthening program. As with rehabilitation of other types of tendonitis around the knee, flexibility should be emphasized to reduce the stress on the extensor mechanism. Eccentric loading can be achieved by having the patient perform minisquats (Fig. 14-15) or, more dynamically, by bouncing on a trampoline.

Patellar taping as described by McConnell[11] is thought by some practitioners to be advantageous in the treatment of patellar tendonitis. This is recommended particularly in cases of hypermobility of the patella or as a means to reeducate the muscles by a tactile biofeedback mechanism. Braces and wraps can be helpful, and a patellar tendon strap (Fig. 14-16) often helps to diminish symptoms.

Some patients with stage III tendonitis require surgical intervention, particularly if bone scans or MRIs show focal tendon degeneration. Patients who have symptoms that are unresponsive to nonoperative treatment and who have discontinued participation in sports for an extended period of time may require surgical treatment. Surgery involves making a longitudinal split in the peritenon and identifying and removing the abnormal area in the patellar tendon. The patellar tendon defect is then closed with absorbable sutures, and the leg is immobilized for 4 weeks with weightbearing as tolerated. Both isometric and isotonic exercises can be performed during this time. At 6 weeks, once 90 degrees of knee flexion has been achieved, the patient can begin more aggressive exercises. It may be 3 to 4 months before the patient can return to sports after surgery.

Stage IV, or complete tendon rupture, requires surgical

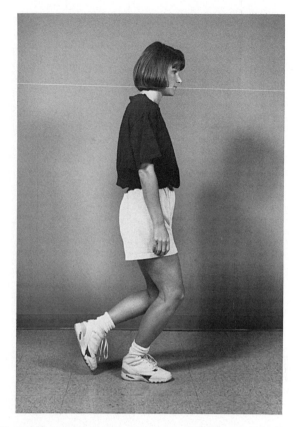

Fig. 14-15. Initially, minisquats are done holding onto a table or chair for support. The athlete bends at the knees to about a 45-degree angle, pauses, and then returns to the standing position. Rehabilitation progresses to no support and using only the involved leg.

treatment and extensive rehabilitation to regain motion and strength.

Osgood-Schlatter disease. Osgood-Schlatter disease, or inflammation of the patellar tendon apophysis, occurs in girls between the ages of 8 and 13 years and in boys between the ages of 10 and 15 years. The proximal epiphysis of the tibia projects downward over the metaphysis, and one or two ossification centers appear in young adolescents. These tendons eventually form the tuberosity with closure occurring at age 18 or 19 years.

Continued pain and inflammation can result in an excessively large tibial tubercle, or there can even be separation of loose bodies into the tendon itself (Fig. 14-17). The disease is benign with treatment related to symptoms of pain.

Treatment of Osgood-Schlatter disease consists of modifying one's activities. As with patellar tendonitis in the adult, adolescents must temporarily eliminate or decrease participation in jumping, kicking, and running activities. Acetaminophen, aspirin, or ibuprofen is used to treat this condition over a short period of time. A rapid acceleration in growth can precipitate or accentuate symptoms related to the apophysitis. As this occurs, increasing flexibility of hamstring muscles and the gastrocnemius muscle group is im-

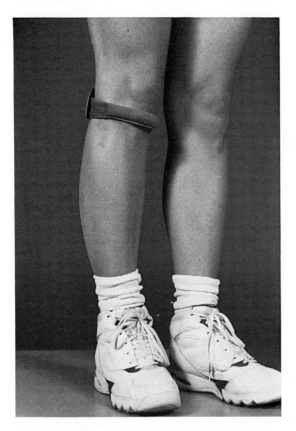

Fig. 14-16. A patellar tendon strap can be worn to relieve symptoms of patellar tendonitis.

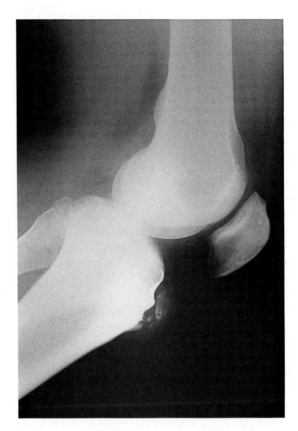

Fig. 14-17. Osgood-Schlatter disease. Ossicles can be seen in the patellar tendon.

portant. Often, the symptoms abate following a simple static stretching program for the hamstring muscles coupled with a mild decrease in activity. Occasionally, a knee sleeve is helpful; even less frequently, immobilization for several weeks is used to decrease symptoms.

Although a loose ossicle may occasionally require surgical excision, no surgery is appropriate until the apophyses are closed—at which time symptoms have usually resolved. Surgery should be considered only if a loose ossicle continues to produce pain with bending or kneeling and if irritation of the bursa develops. This is a self-limiting disease, and patient education and modification of activities are the hallmark of treatment.

Semimembranosus tendonitis

The semimembranosus muscle-tendon unit is an important dynamic stabilizer of the medial aspect of the knee. It acts as a powerful flexor and medial rotator of the knee with its five arms that insert in the posteromedial corner of the knee. These five attachments connect to the posterior aspect of the capsule and to the medial meniscus and medial flare of the tibia. The capsular and bony attachments enable this musculotendinous unit to play a key role in dynamic knee stability.

The tibial arm of the semimembranosus lies in a groove of the anteromedial aspect of the tibia inferior to the medial

joint line. Semimembranosus tendonitis causes persistent aching pain at the posteromedial aspect of the knee that is most often noticeable after strenuous activity. It is common among runners and among athletes who overexert themselves.

The examination reveals maximum tenderness to palpation at the posteromedial aspect of the knee just below the joint line (Fig. 14-18). Here the tibial arm of the semimembranosus tendon can be readily palpated. Tenderness in this tendon can be easily differentiated from medial joint line pain or pain from the tibial collateral ligament bursa or the pes anserine bursa. Quadriceps atonia and marked tightness of the hamstring tendons may be present as well. Initially, radiographs may be negative, but a bone scan can show an inflammatory response at the tibial insertion.

Tendonitis usually occurs as an isolated entity, although it may be associated with degenerative joint disease or tears of the medial meniscus. It is often overlooked as the cause of pain and should be considered in patients with no history of trauma who have tenderness over the medial joint line after running or overuse. Ray and co-workers[12] emphasized the importance of considering semimembranosus tendonitis as a cause of medial joint pain in their study of 115 patients. Patients were categorized as acute (less than 2 weeks), subacute, or chronic (more than 6 weeks) based on the duration of symptoms. All patients were initially

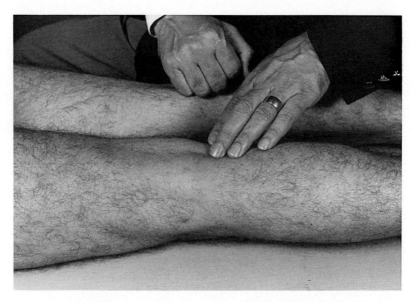

Fig. 14-18. Site of pain with semimembranosus tendonitis.

treated with rest, hamstring stretching exercises, and oral nonsteroidal anti-inflammatory medications. When symptoms persist, they recommended a bone scan to aid in making the diagnosis. They believe a positive bone scan with increased uptake of the posteromedial corner correlates with a diagnosis of semimembranosus tendonitis, which was defined as either primary or secondary. With primary tendonitis, there was no other associated knee abnormality. Secondary tendonitis indicated the presence of a significant knee abnormality with the development of tendonitis as a compensatory mechanism. The authors believe that semimembranosus tendonitis is not uncommon and is often overlooked as a cause of posteromedial knee pain. It often occurs as an isolated overuse syndrome, and most patients respond well to nonoperative treatment.

Rehabilitation focuses on static stretching of the hamstring muscles; stretching is the most important component in removing stress from the tendinous attachment. Localized modalities such as phonophoresis, iontophoresis, or ice and friction massage (Fig. 14-19) may be helpful in eliminating the source of pain. Occasionally, transcutaneous electrical nerve stimulation or a localized injection of soluble steroid may be beneficial.

Ray and co-workers[12] performed surgery on 10 of 115 patients who had semimembranosus tendonitis over a 5-year period. In these 10 patients, surgical exploration yielded histologic findings of tendon degeneration in all specimens. At surgery, the area of necrosis is excised with several longitudinal excisions into the tendon to stimulate a healing response. The insertional site is usually drilled with a small K-wire to promote bleeding. The direct head and proximal portion of the tendon are pulled up, parallel to the posterior edge of the medial collateral ligament, and sutured to it,

redirecting the semimembranosus tendon. At 1 year after surgery, nine patients had no complaints; one patient had persistent patellofemoral problems but no medial joint line pain. All of these patients returned to their usual occupations.

Biceps femoris tendonitis

A source of tenderness at the lateral aspect of the knee is irritation of the insertion of the long head of the biceps femoris tendon. The diagnosis is made by detecting tenderness to palpation at the insertion of the tendon on the fibular head. Tenderness may be more proximal if there is crepitation of the tendon sheath. It may be difficult to differentiate between tendonitis and irritation of the bursa of the fibular collateral ligament.

Treatment of biceps femoris tendonitis is similar to the treatment of irritation of bicipital bursitis. However, the attachment of the long or short head of the biceps femoris may be treated aggressively with local modalities centered on the point of irritation. Stretching and strengthening of the lateral supporting ligaments of the knee must be emphasized as well (Fig. 14-20). Ice and nonsteroidal anti-inflammatory medications are helpful, but primarily this problem can be corrected with aggressive physical therapy.

Popliteal tenosynovitis

The popliteal tendon arises from the lateral femoral condylar groove just inferior to the epicondyle and anterior to the fibular collateral ligament. The tendon passes through the hiatus and capsule adjacent to the lateral meniscus and passes deep to the fibular collateral ligament to attach to the posterosuperior aspect of the tibial condyle. The function of the popliteal tendon is the internal rotation of the tibia

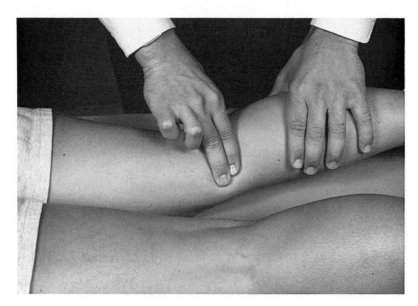

Fig. 14-19. Deep friction massage. The therapist uses two fingers to apply increasing pressure to the skin over the semimembranosus tendon.

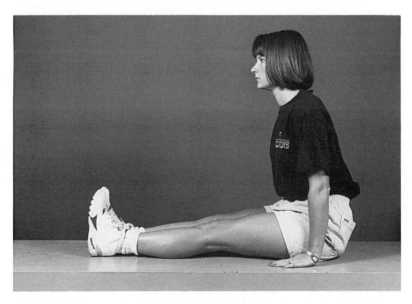

Fig. 14-20. Double hamstring stretch. With knees flat and back straight, hold the stretch for 6 to 10 seconds.

that assists in the locking mechanism of the knee.[13] It also helps to retract the posterolateral portion of the meniscus during flexion and extension, and it works with the posterior cruciate ligament to prevent forward displacement of the femur during deceleration and downhill running.[14] The popliteal tendon is often involved in traumatic ligamentous injuries of the knee that include the posterolateral corner and result in posterolateral rotatory instability. The most common cause of popliteal tenosynovitis is chronic overuse in runners, particularly those who engage in downhill running.[15] The most characteristic symptom is pain localized

in the lateral aspect of the knee on weightbearing with the knee flexed 15 to 20 degrees. Popliteal tenosynovitis is often difficult to distinguish from iliotibial band friction syndrome. In most patients, symptoms begin within a few minutes to 24 hours after excessive walking or running. Symptoms usually cease when the activity is limited or by walking stiff-legged.

Examination reveals tenderness over the popliteal tendon insertion immediately anterior to the fibular collateral ligament (Fig. 14-21). Radiographs are usually negative, although there may be radiodensity in the area of the popliteal

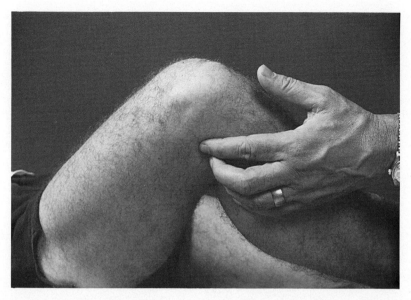

Fig. 14-21. Patient positioning to detect popliteal tenosynovitis. With the knee flexed to 90 degrees, the patient's hip is flexed, abducted, and externally rotated by placing the foot of the involved leg on the opposite knee. This position opens the lateral joint and allows the examiner to palpate nearly 2 cm of the tendon from its femoral origin distal to the fibular collateral ligament.

tendon. The differential diagnosis includes iliotibial band friction syndrome and lateral meniscal tears. Patients with meniscal disorders usually relate a definite episode of trauma, whereas patients with iliotibial band friction syndrome have localized tenderness over the lateral femoral condyle, particularly with the knee in 30 degrees of flexion.

Treatment for popliteal tenosynovitis involves cessation of running—particularly downhill running—and decreasing the pace and distance of the run. Symptoms are usually transient; if these symptoms persist, however, local injections of steroids can be beneficial. Although stretching exercises are not as helpful as they are in other types of tendonitis because of the position of the insertion of the popliteus, stretching can help to alleviate other symptoms related to the posterolateral corner of the knee. Stretching the gastrocnemius-soleus muscle complex helps to eliminate the pull on the posterolateral corner (Fig. 14-22). The irritation at the areas of insertion of the popliteus can be treated with local measures, such as friction massage, steroid injections, ice massage, and iontophoresis.

Quadriceps tendonitis

A variation of jumper's knee involves irritation of the interface of the patella and quadriceps tendon. Quadriceps tendonitis arises from the same precipitating factors as true jumper's knee, or patellar tendonitis. Quadriceps tendonitis is an overuse syndrome associated with running and jumping sports. It is often precipitated by a blow to the quadriceps muscle mass with the knee flexed. This injury can cause weakness of the extensor mechanism and continuation of flexion types of activities can cause symptoms referable to the quadriceps insertion rather than to the patellar tendon.

Treatment is the same as for patellar tendonitis with the same grading system of symptoms, ranging from stage I, symptoms with forced activity only, to stage IV, a ruptured quadriceps tendon. Treatment is nonoperative and consists of reduction of activity and emphasis on eccentric and concentric exercises.

Quadriceps contusion

Quadriceps strains can range from a simple bruise of the thigh to a rupture of the muscle with localized bleeding. A contusion of the quadriceps femoris muscle group is caused by a blow to the anterior, medial, or lateral thigh. Most often, it occurs in contact sports, such as football, rugby, or soccer, when one player's helmet or knee hits another player's unprotected anterior thigh. Often, the severity of the contusion is underestimated. The injury can cause disability and preclude a return to sports for a prolonged period. At the time of injury, the patient may experience pain in the thigh area and an inability to bear weight without discomfort. Localized swelling may become apparent because of hematoma formation (Fig. 14-23). In the immediate postinjury period, examination reveals localized pain, restricted range of motion, and, in particular, an inability to flex the knee past 90 degrees. There may be a palpable mass caused by the hematoma, and the patient may be unable to perform a straight leg raise or a quadriceps contraction. Discoloration may occur; at times, sympathetic effusion develops in the knee.

The severity of the injury is classified by the patient's range of motion of the knee at 24 to 48 hours after the injury

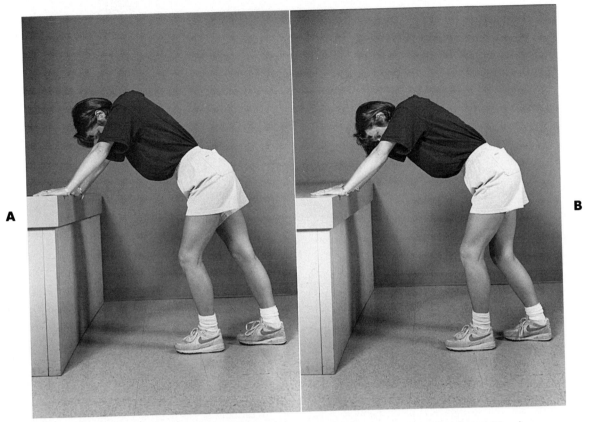

Fig. 14-22. A, The gastrocnemius is stretched by placing one foot in front of the other and leaning forward. The heel of the back foot is kept flush with the floor. **B,** The soleus is stretched in the same way the gastrocnemius is stretched, except the knee of the affected leg is bent.

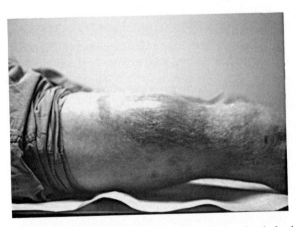

Fig. 14-23. Quadriceps contusion can vary from a simple bruise to a large, deep hematoma.

(Table 14-1). Treatment protocol is based on this classification, which is usually a good predictor of the length of recovery. The object of therapy for a quadriceps contusion is to limit swelling and hemorrhaging, thereby minimizing the formation of scar tissue. Initial treatment focuses on the prevention of further injury. The player is usually taken from the field, ice packs and pressure are used to minimize swelling, and crutches are used for protective weightbearing.

Table 14-1. Classification of quadriceps contusion

Severity	Range of motion
Mild	>90° of flexion
Moderate	45° to 90°
Severe	<45°

From Reid DC: *Sports injury assessment and rehabilitation,* New York, 1992, Churchill Livingstone.

Anti-inflammatory medications can be started after 24 hours. After the severity of the injury is classified, treatment can be started.

Recently, Ryan and others[16] reviewed the treatment protocol instituted at West Point in 1973 following a study of quadriceps contusions by Jackson and Feagin,[17] and the treatment was updated.

In the initial West Point study, Jackson and Feagin[17] reported that patients' legs were immobilized in extension. Ryan et al.[16] recommended altering this treatment because of their results, which showed that the most difficult motion to regain after a severe contusion was flexion. Therefore, in the initial phase of the injury, they recommended that the hip and knee be flexed as far as pain permits. An ice pack

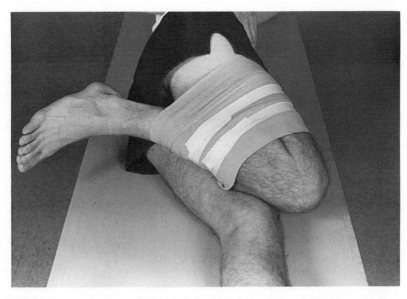

Fig. 14-24. In the initial phase of a quadriceps contusion injury, a compression dressing is used to keep the knee flexed. Maximum flexion stretches quadriceps muscle fibers to prevent excessive bleeding into the muscle, which produces adhesions.

is then applied to the thigh and a compression dressing applied (Fig. 14-24). Keeping the limb in a flexed position is conducive to restoring and maintaining a normal range of motion. A continuous passive motion machine can be used for severe injury, but most patients can keep their hips and knees flexed with the use of pillows or cushions.

Treatment is now divided into three phases. The purpose of the first phase is to limit hemorrhage; therefore, rest, ice, and a compression wrap are used, along with elevation and flexion of the knee. Within 24 to 48 hours after injury, the patient should be pain-free at rest and the thigh girth stabilized.

In phase two, the object is to restore motion to the involved lower extremity. The use of ice and the whirlpool are continued, but active flexion and extension exercises should be begun, with weight-bearing as tolerated. Gravity-assisted and active-assisted exercises help to achieve a functional range of motion as muscle discomfort abates (Fig. 14-25). Usually, crutches can be discarded when the patient achieves 90 degrees of motion with no limp and good quadriceps control.

Phase three is the functional rehabilitation phase. Strength, motion, and endurance are emphasized. Cycling, swimming, walking, and aquatics are used in a pain-free rehabilitation program. Rehabilitation advances to the next phase when full active motion and squat can be achieved with no pain. A thigh girdle with an anterior pad for protection from reinjury is used by the patient when partici-

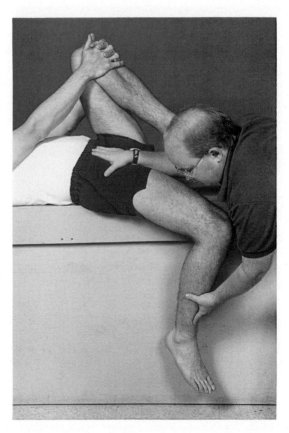

Fig. 14-25. Manual rectus femoris stretch for early treatment of a quadriceps contusion.

pating in contact sports for the next 3 to 6 months.

It is important for the patient to regain full motion as well as flexibility in the quadriceps musculature. Following contusion to the quadriceps, there will be shortening of the muscle. Concentric and eccentric exercises are helpful in restoring flexibility and strength to the muscles. The Ely test is used to detect rectus femoris tightness (Fig. 14-26). If the patient's pain has subsided, the modified Ely test can be used to measure range of motion (Fig. 14-27). A therapist can help the patient perform active-assistive and passive stretching exercises. Mobilization and hold-relaxed techniques, as well as static stretching, can be helpful to improve contractures that may have developed in the quadriceps musculature.

There are several procedures that should not be part of the treatment of quadriceps contusions: heat massage, steroidal injections, or forceful stretching of the muscle should be avoided. A premature return to sport and reinjury to the same area may predispose the patient to heterotopic bone formation and myositis ossificans. In the study by Ryan et al.,[16] no cadet who had knee motion greater than 120 degrees developed myositis ossificans. Overall, in 11 of 117 patients who developed myositis ossificans in their study, five risk factors were identified: initial range of motion of less than

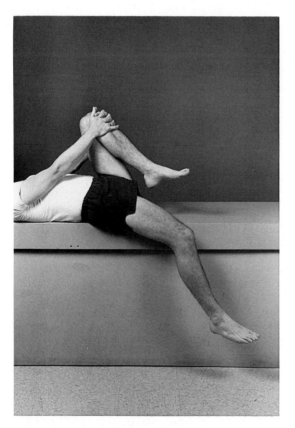

Fig. 14-26. The Ely test with the patient supine. When the unaffected knee is grasped and flexed, tightness in the rectus femoris causes extension of the affected knee.

120 degrees, injury occurred in football, history of quadriceps injury, delay in treatment greater than 72 hours, and an ipsilateral knee effusion. Heterotopic bone formation should be suspected in patients who have a decrease in range of motion during the early treatment period and an increase in pain. The hematoma may also become harder and firmer.

Radiographs may show ossification as early as 20 days after the injury, although bone scans can detect the development even earlier. If myositis ossificans develops, range-of-motion exercises and resistive exercises should be discontinued, the patient should be given ibuprofen, and activity should be decreased. Progress is usually slow, but as the thigh mass starts to soften and motion returns, rehabilitation and stretching can begin. The patient's thigh should be protected when he or she returns to sports. In some selected instances, the mass may need surgical excision. This can be done after the bone mass has matured, usually at 6 months. If the excision is done too early, the mass may recur. A bone scan should be negative prior to excision of the mass.

Included in the differential diagnosis of a quadriceps contusion are muscle rupture, arterial bleeding, and, occasionally, thigh compartment syndrome. Once myositis ossificans has developed and can be seen radiographically, the differential diagnosis includes osteosarcoma and periosteal osteosarcoma. A history of trauma before bone maturation is detected on radiographs suggests a diagnosis of myositis ossificans.

The criteria for return to sport after a quadriceps contusion are restoration of normal quadriceps strength, flexibility, and muscle power and pain-free full range of motion. A protective pad should be worn over the area of injury upon return to sports.

Hamstring strain

The posterior muscles of the thigh—the semimembranosus and semitendinosus medially and the biceps femoris laterally—are collectively called the *hamstring muscle.* Hamstring strains or injuries are usually caused by a rapid contraction of the muscle secondary to violent stretching. This leads to some degree of tearing within the musculotendinous unit, causing pain and resultant disability (Fig. 14-28). These injuries are commonly seen in runners, sprinters, and soccer players. The hamstrings are thought to be the most frequently strained muscle group in the body, and strains have a tendency to recur.

Each of the hamstring muscles has either a medial or lateral attachment on the proximal tibia, and symptoms can be referable to the distal insertion either through bursitis or tendonitis. The musculature of the hamstring has a high proportion of type II fibers that are involved with high-intensity exercises. This increased force production and forced extrinsic stretching secondary to high-velocity movement is thought to be the cause of tears in the hamstring musculature.

The function of the hamstring muscle is to extend the hip and flex the knee. The biceps femoris rotates the flexed knee laterally, whereas the semimembranosus and semitendinosus help to rotate the flexed knee medially. They also cocontract with the quadriceps to stabilize the knee and work to accelerate the leg during running. Strains occur most often during running and specifically during the late forward-swing phase and the take-off phase. Two mechanisms of injury are proposed: (1) an excessive antagonistic force on a relaxed muscle that causes overstretching and (2) a stretching of the muscle with elongation of the hamstring and a rapid protective contraction that tears the muscle fibers.

Therefore, both overstretching or rapid contraction can play a role in the injury. Other causes are muscle imbalance, tightness or weakness, poor conditioning, improper warm-up, and inadequate healing of preexisting injuries.

The most common site of injury is the junction of the muscle and tendon, although tears may occur proximally with an avulsion off the ischium. Tears rarely occur in the distal half of the thigh. As a general rule, if the injury is more proximal, the healing time is longer. However, all tears are subject to healing with scarring in the muscle belly and, therefore, have a tendency to recur.

Hamstring avulsions or tears in the musculature can heal;

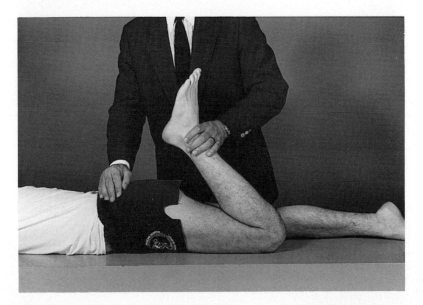

Fig. 14-27. Modified Ely test is done with patient prone, the hip extended, and the knee flexed. Tightness in the rectus femoris causes the buttock to rise when the affected knee is flexed.

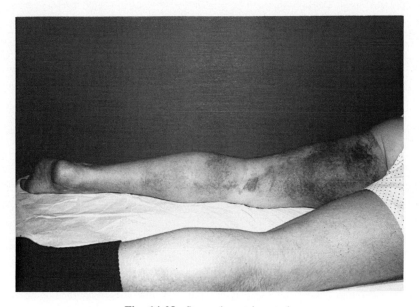

Fig. 14-28. Severe hamstring strain.

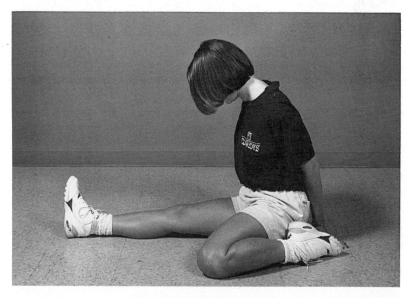

Fig. 14-29. The hurdler's stretch maintains flexibility. One leg is extended and the opposite leg is abducted at the hip and flexed at the knee. The athlete leans forward and holds the stretch for 10 seconds.

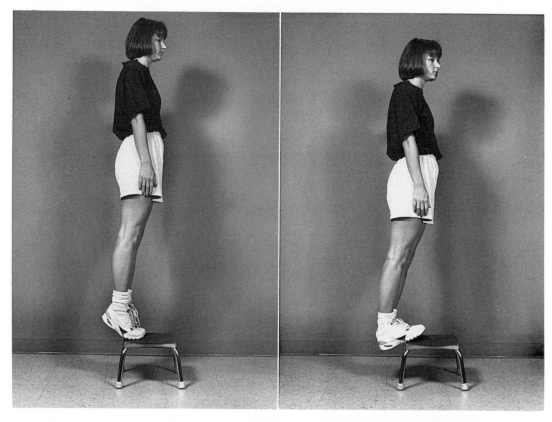

Fig. 14-30. Concentric and eccentric loading of the triceps surae is accomplished by heel raises.

however, physical therapy is an extremely important component to helping the patient return to a more functional status as healing occurs. Rehabilitation for hamstring pulls dictates the rate of return and helps to prevent recurrence.

In the initial phase of the injury, treatment consists of ice, elevation, a compression bandage, and partial weightbearing. After 24 to 48 hours, the patient can usually begin gentle active range of motion and treatment with oral anti-inflammatory medications. Crutches should be used until the patient is relatively pain-free and can walk normally with voluntary leg control. Weightbearing is progressive, as tolerated. Heat modalities may be added through the subacute phase, and active and passive stretching are started as discomfort decreases. Once range of motion is restored, increased muscle work is added. Bicycling is an excellent way to maintain endurance and range of motion of the knee, although the seat should be adjusted if the patient had discomfort in the proximal ischium. Friction massage and ultrasound can be beneficial, and it is important to continue stretching until full range of motion is achieved.

Full muscle strength with the proper ratio of hamstring to quadriceps should be achieved before the patient is allowed to return to more than minimal jogging. The tendency for reinjury is great with hamstring injuries, and athletes must be advised that healing usually takes a prolonged period. A program of controlled high-velocity and high-resistance isokinetic work must be completed to prevent reinjury with eccentric work that includes resisted work at the extremes of muscle activity.

Stretching techniques such as the hurdler's stretch (Fig. 14-29) and the double hamstring stretch are important to maintain flexibility. Taping can be used to maintain support around the thigh in the initial phases and also when returning to activity.

The major causes of reinjury are insufficient rehabilitation and insufficient timing for resumption of activity. Reinjuries usually occur within 2 months of the return to sports; in most injuries, the patient has demonstrated flexibility and power deficits because of inadequate rehabilitation.

Medial gastrocnemius strain

Tennis leg is the lay term for an avulsion of all or part of the medial or lateral head of the gastrocnemius muscle from its musculotendinous junction. Injury to the musculotendinous junction of the medial gastrocnemius muscle is often mistaken for rupture of the plantaris muscle.[18]

This injury occurs more frequently in people over the age of 40 years and in tennis players. The tears are usually produced by sudden dorsiflexion of the ankle or by sudden extension of the leg with the foot dorsiflexed. The patient often feels a sharp stabbing pain or pop in the posterior aspect of the calf wall while playing tennis. There is usually a rapid onset of swelling and discoloration in the posterior calf. The patient may be unable to stand on his or her tiptoes on the affected side. Radiographs are negative, and the

history and examination are straightforward for the diagnosis.

Initial treatment includes oral anti-inflammatory medications and the use of ice and a compression wrap to prevent further swelling. Protected weightbearing is continued until the foot can be placed down and the patient can walk plantar grade. A heel lift helps to prevent forced dorsiflexion of the ankle and restraining of the gastrocnemius muscle. Immobilization is usually not indicated unless the patient is toe-touch or partial weightbearing with crutches. The rate of recovery is much the same as with proximal hamstring ruptures.

Following the initial injury, long-term rehabilitation includes concentric and eccentric exercises, as well as extrinsic loading for both anterior and posterior lower leg musculature. It is important to regain flexibility of both the triceps surae (Fig. 14-30) and the Achilles tendon (Fig. 14-31) to prevent reinjury.

Taping and compression stockings may be useful when the patient initially returns to activity. Often, athletes continue to wear heel lifts while performing agility exercises to lessen the tendency for recurrence.

SYNOPSIS

Musculotendinous units about the knee are frequently the source of knee pain and disability, and a thorough under-

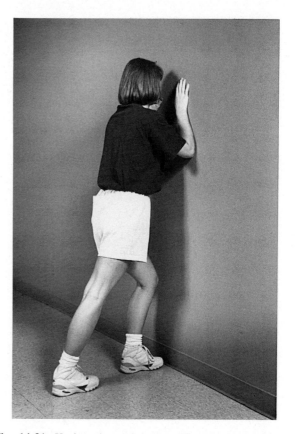

Fig. 14-31. Heel cord stretch helps athlete regain flexibility of Achilles tendon.

standing of the complex relationship between the anatomy and the biomechanics of the knee is necessary for the practitioner who is treating these injuries. Most soft tissue injuries about the knee are injuries to the musculotendinous structures. Pain is most often felt at the insertion of these structures and is related to tendonitis or bursitis. Often, correction of preexisting strength and flexibility deficits and maintenance of a good conditioning and flexibility program can help an athlete avoid disabling overuse knee injuries that can markedly inhibit participation. When they cannot be avoided, early recognition of the problem, early institution of treatment, and aggressive rehabilitation are the keys to returning the injured person to full participation in previous activities.

REFERENCES

1. *Dorland's illustrated medical dictionary,* ed 26, Philadelphia, 1981, WB Saunders.
2. American Academy of Orthopaedic Surgeons: *The knee.* In *Athletic Training and Sports Medicine,* ed 2, Park Ridge, Ill, 1991.
3. Ho G, Tice AD, Kaplan SR: Septic bursitis in the prepatellar and olecranon bursae: an analysis of 25 cases, *Ann Intern Med* 89:21–27, 1978.
4. Kerlan RK, Glousman RE: Tibial collateral ligament bursitis, *Am J Sports Med* 16:344–346, 1988.
5. Brantigan OC, Voshell AF: The tibial collateral ligament: its function, its bursae, and its relationship to the medial meniscus, *J Bone Joint Surg [Am]* 25:121–131, 1943.
6. Jones DC, James SL: Overuse injuries of the lower extremity: shin splints, iliotibial band friction syndrome, and exertional compartment syndrome, *Clin Sports Med* 6:273–290, 1987.
7. Noble CA: Iliotibial band friction syndrome in runners, *Am J Sports Med* 8:232–234, 1980.
8. Renne JW: The iliotibial band friction syndrome, *J Bone Joint Surg [Am]* 57:1110–1111, 1975.
9. Hughston JC, Baker CL, Mello W: Popliteal cyst: a surgical approach, *Orthopedics* 14:147–150, 1991.
10. Blazina ME, et al: Jumper's knee, *Orthop Clin North Am* 4:665–678, 1973.
11. Reid DC: *Sports injury assessment and rehabilitation,* New York, 1992, Churchill Livingstone.
12. Ray JM, Clancy WG, Lemon RA: Semimembranosus tendinitis: an overlooked cause of medial knee pain, *Am J Sports Med* 16:347–351, 1988.
13. Basmajian JV, Lovejoy JF: Functions of the popliteus muscle in man: a multi-factorial electromyographic study, *J Bone Joint Surg [Am]* 57:1110–1111, 1975.
14. Brody DM: Running injuries, *Clin Symp* 32: 1980.
15. Mayfield GW: Popliteus tendon tenosynovitis, *Am J Sports Med* 5:31–36, 1977.
16. Ryan JB, et al: Quadriceps contusions: West Point update, *Am J Sports Med* 19:299–304, 1991.
17. Jackson DW, Feagin JA: Quadriceps contusions in young athletes: relation of severity of injury to treatment and prognosis, *J Bone Joint Surg [Am]* 55:95–105, 1973.
18. Miller WA: Rupture of the musculotendinous juncture of the medial head of the gastrocnemius muscle, *Am J Sports Med* 5:191–193, 1977.

Chapter 15

PERIARTICULAR AND INTRA-ARTICULAR FRACTURES OF THE KNEE

Thomas J. Moore

In the past the emphasis of orthopedics has been on retrospective clinical studies (i.e., time to fracture healing). Recently, there has been an increasing trend in the United States for functional outcome studies to evaluate treatment modalities for various diseases.[1] Unlike retrospective clinical studies, functional outcome studies emphasize the patient's and society's perception of successful treatment (i.e., the rapidity of return to work following an injury). Although the current purpose of functional outcome studies is primarily informational, in the near future the results of functional outcome studies will be used to establish guidelines for selection of treatment modalities.[2]

Periarticular and intra-articular fractures of the knee have been successfully treated by both closed methods (functional cast brace) and by surgery (internal fixation and external fixation). In the past, it has been difficult to compare the outcomes of these different treatment modalities because of the different systems that have been used to classify fracture patterns. There are multiple fracture classifications for supracondylar femur fractures including the Neer classification,[3] the Seinsheimer classification,[4] and the Hall classification.[5] In addition, there is no conformity of opinion of what constitutes satisfactory range of motion following fracture healing of periarticular knee fractures. "Satisfactory" range of motion of the knee following treatment of supracondylar femur fractures has ranged from 65 degrees[5] in one study to 117 degrees in another study.[6]

The purpose of this chapter is to present guidelines for rehabilitation of the knee following periarticular and intra-articular fractures. Rather than discussing the benefits or disadvantages of different fracture management techniques, the emphasis is on enhancing postoperative management of periarticular and intra-articular fracture of the knee, in order to achieve the optimal functional outcome.

PERIARTICULAR FRACTURES OF THE KNEE
Femur fractures

Diaphyseal femur fractures have been successfully treated in the past with traction and functional braces[7] with satisfactory fracture healing. Plate fixation of diaphyseal femur fractures has been done with satisfactory clinical outcome.[8] In rare instances, primarily with contaminated open fractures, external fixation has been used in diaphyseal femur fractures,[9,10] but knee range of motion is often impaired secondary to quadriceps adhesions from transfixing external fixator pins. In the last several decades, intramedullary nailing has become the predominant procedure for internal fixation of diaphyseal femur fractures.[11-14]

Closed, statically locked intramedullary nailing allows stabilization of comminuted diaphyseal femur fractures that previously would have required either prolonged traction or cast immobilization. In a study comparing functional outcome in diaphyseal femur fractures treated by traction or locked intramedullary nailing, the group treated with the locked intramedullary nails had less malunion and shortening and better knee range of motion than the group treated with traction and functional braces.[15]

In the preinterlocking nail era, the end functional outcome of treatment following femur fractures was often unsatisfactory. Prolonged traction or cast immobilization resulted in decreased range of motion of the knee as well as thigh muscle atrophy. Mira et al.[16] in a study of 29 femoral fractures found that only 17% of patients had normal knee range of motion and quadriceps strength compared with the uninjured knee after fracture healing. Primary fracture management in this study consisted of spica casts in 10 patients, cast braces in 9, intramedullary nailing in 7, and plate fixation in 2. Two patients had combined treatment: One had plate fixation followed by spica cast, and one had intramedullary nailing followed by a cast brace. Moore et al.,[17] in a series of nine patients with severe femoral fractures, reported only an average of 30 degrees of knee flexion at the time of fracture healing. In these patients a quadricep-splasty was required to achieve acceptable motion for normal gait. In this series, initial fracture management consisted of external fixation in two patients, closed intramedullary nailing in three patients, open intramedullary nailing in three patients, plate fixation in three patients, and a spica cast in one patient (several patients required more than one procedure).

Locked intramedullary nailing of comminuted diaphyseal femur fractures results in sufficient stability to allow immediate active and passive range of motion of the knee. Despite this early range of motion, if knee function is objectively measured, knee function is often unsatisfactory. In a study of 25 patients with femoral fractures treated with locked intramedullary nails,[18] knee function was objectively measured once fracture healing had occurred. Clinical alignment and range of motion were satisfactory. A dynamic quadriceps and hamstring ratio was determined by isokinetic testing of maximal peak torque at 60 degrees per second of both limbs using an isokinetic dynamometer (Cybex II). A previous study demonstrated that the average quadriceps strength in both legs in normal subjects varied an average of 6% with a standard deviation of 4%.[16] In this study, a ratio of the involved fractured extremity to the uninjured extremity of less than 88% (12% less than the uninvolved limb) was considered abnormal. Seventeen of the 23 patients (73%) had a dynamic quadriceps ratio of less than 88% (average 53.4%, range 24% to 86%). Fourteen of the 23 patients (60%) had a hamstring dynamic ratio of less than 88% (average 57%, range 32% to 86%). In addition, 15 of the 23 patients (65%) had thigh atrophy of greater than 1 cm (average 2.5 cm, range 1 to 4 cm). In contrast to other studies, where associated ipsilateral ligamentous injuries to the knee after femoral fractures range from 33%[19] to 70%,[20] only 1 of the 23 patients had a clinically significant ligamentous injury to the knee.

Supracondylar femur fractures present special problems for knee function.[20a] Many different treatment modalities have been used for supracondylar femur fractures. Neer et al.[3] suggested a period of traction followed by a long leg cast. Several groups have advocated initial traction followed by a cast brace to allow early knee range of motion. Operative stabilization of supracondylar femur fractures have been successfully accomplished with blade plates,[21] Rush rods,[6] Zickel devices,[22] supracondylar plates,[23] compression screw apparatus, and intramedullary rods.[24,25] In rare instances, external fixation has been used for supracondylar femur fractures. It has been difficult to compare functional outcome of the different treatment modalities for supracondylar femur fractures. Different authors have used various classification systems including the Neer,[3] Hall,[5] Seinsheimer[4] classification or no classification at all. In ad-

dition, there is no consensus as to criteria for successful treatment. For example, acceptable knee motion after treatment ranged from 65 degrees[26] in one study to 117 degrees[6] in another study.

Knee motion is particularly limited in supracondylar femur fractures as the quadriceps tendon is primarily tendinous in the supracondylar region, and adhesions with fracture calluses occur commonly. Therefore, stable fracture stabilization and early range of motion improve the ultimate knee function.[20a,27-29]

In summary, the orthopedic management of femur fractures should not end with osseous union of the fracture. Once pain has subsided in stabilized femur fractures, active range of motion of the knee should begin. Clinical assessment of knee function should be monitored. If significant limitation of knee function occurs (limited range of motion or thigh atrophy), a formal physical therapy program should be initiated.

Tibial fractures

There is much less impairment of knee function with tibial fracture than with femoral fractures. In the past, management of tibial fractures involved prolonged immobilization with long leg casts. Modern fracture management of tibial diaphyseal fractures consists of early knee mobilization and weightbearing either with functional braces or with internal fixation. In long-term follow-up of patients with tibial diaphyseal fractures, more than 25% had decreased range of motion of the ankle in comparison with the uninjured ankle, whereas fewer than 3% had decreased range of motion of the knee.[30] In a study of patients with ipsilateral femoral and tibial fractures (floating knee), ankle range of motion was much more impaired than knee range of motion.[25]

There is controversy concerning criteria for adequate alignment in tibial fractures.[31] Satisfactory results in the literature have ranged from 10 degrees of varus or valgus malalignment and 20 degrees of malalignment in the anterior-posterior plane[32,33] to "anatomic" alignment.[34,35] Despite the multiple criteria for acceptable alignment of tibial fractures, there are few scientific data concerning the sequelae of malunited tibial fractures.

Ankle impairment, both clinically and experimentally, occurs more frequently with tibial malunion than knee impairment with tibial malunion.[32,36] Distal one-third tibial malunions increase the likelihood of ankle impairment.[36a,36b] Distal one-third tibial malunions decrease tibial-talar contact area and increase tibial talar contact pressure,[37] which theoretically leads to arthritis of the ankle joint. In contrast, posttraumatic degenerative arthritis of the knee occurs rarely with malunion of the tibia.

In summary, although there is no conclusive evidence that tibial malunion leads to degenerative arthritis of the knee,[30,38] it seems reasonable that maximal anatomic axial alignment is desirable following tibial fractures. In patients with knee pain and tibial malalignment, the source of the pain should be determined prior to operative intervention. In a retrospective study of healed tibial fractures with long follow-up (31 years),[39] there was little correlation between knee pain and radiographic tibial malalignment. However, if there is significant tibial malalignment in a healed tibial fracture and concomitant narrowing of either the medial or lateral compartment, then tibial osteotomy (similar to high tibial osteotomy for unicompartmental degenerative arthritis of the knee) has been successful in alleviating symptoms (Figs. 15-1 through 15-4).

INTRA-ARTICULAR FRACTURES

Intra-articular fractures of the knee present different problems than diaphyseal fractures of the knee. Nonunions occur relatively infrequently in intra-articular fractures of the knee, as the fractures occur in metaphyseal bone (distal femur in supracondylar femur fractures and proximal tibia in tibial plateau fractures). Axial malalignment in intra-articular fractures cause similar problems as axial malalignment in diaphyseal fractures.[40] Similar to the incidence of ipsilateral ligamentous injuries to the knee with femur fractures, there is a significant incidence of ligamentous injury and meniscal injuries in tibial plateau fractures.[41-43] The unique aspect of intra-articular fractures is injury to the hyaline cartilage of the joint.

In fractures involving hyaline cartilage, anatomic reduction is necessary to restore joint function,[44] as any joint incongruity increases the contact stress locally.[45] In addition, once an injury occurs to hyaline cartilage, Salter[46] has shown that continuous passive motion (CPM) of the joint induces repair tissue superior to the repair tissue that occurs with either immobilization or intermediate motion. CPM-mediated repair tissue in experimentally induced hyaline cartilage defects is superior in structural integrity, nature of repair tissue, and incidence of late degenerative changes to repair tissue after immobilization or intermediate motion.[47] The mechanism by which CPM enhances the repair tissue after injury to hyaline cartilage is not entirely known, but CPM apparently stimulates the biosynthesis of new chondrocytes and enhances the regenerative potential of injured chondrocytes. Unlike bone, which has both periosteal and endosteal circulation, hyaline cartilage is relatively avascular and receives its nutrition from synovial fluid. CPM

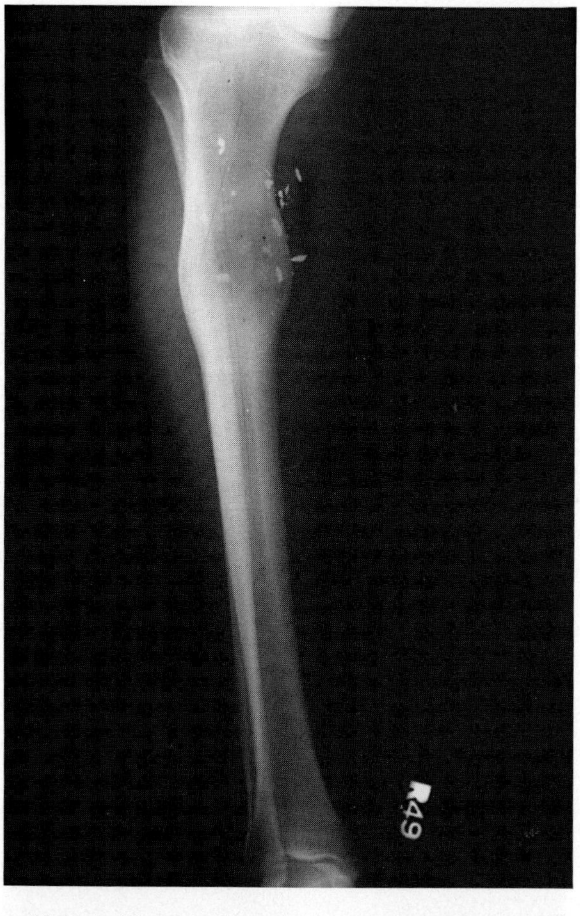

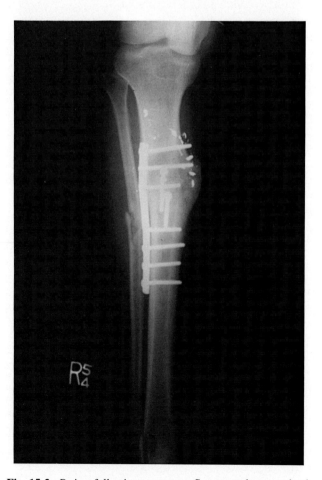

Fig. 15-1. A 25-year-old man with gunshot wound, 25-degree varus, and rotational malalignment. Patient's symptoms were medial compartment.

Fig. 15-2. Patient following osteotomy. Symptoms have resolved.

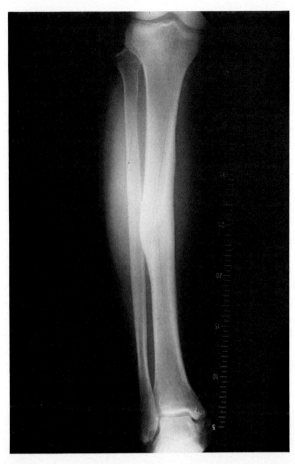

Fig. 15-3. A 27-year-old man with diaphyseal tibial fracture, 15-degree varus, and rotational malalignment. Patient's symptoms were medial compartment and ankle pain.

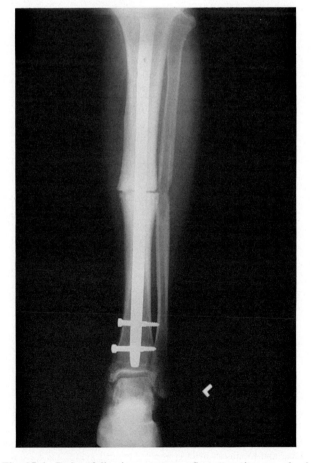

Fig. 15-4. Patient following osteotomy. Symptoms have resolved.

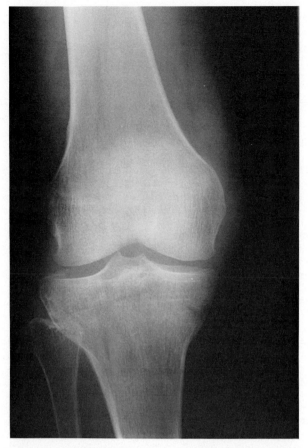

Fig. 15-5. A 52-year-old man who, as a pedestrian, was hit by an auto. Plain radiograph shows minimally displaced tibial plateau fracture.

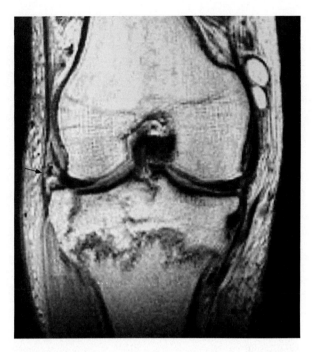

Fig. 15-6. Magnetic resonance image shows more extensive fracture. Arrow points to disruptions of lateral collateral ligament.

theoretically enhances the transport of nutrients from the synovial fluid to the injured hyaline cartilage.

In addition to the beneficial aspects of CPM in healing defects of hyaline cartilage, CPM also enhances tendon healing. In experimental[48,49] and clinical studies,[50] protected mobilization of repaired flexor tendons of the hand improves the gliding function of the tendon as well as increasing the tensile stiffness and strength of the repair. As mentioned previously, there is a small incidence of ligamentous injury to the knee following diaphyseal femur fractures.[51] Similarly, there are also associated ligamentous and meniscal injuries to the knee following tibial plateau fractures.[41,43,52] Although there have been no studies to show that CPM improves healing of knee ligamentous injuries, it is reasonable to expect that CPM will not only enhance hyaline cartilage healing in intra-articular fractures but also improve associated ligament injuries (Figs. 15-5 and 15-6).

In conclusion, management of intra-articular fractures, either supracondylar femur or tibial plateau fractures, requires anatomic reduction to achieve optimal results.[53] In general, rigid internal fixation of intra-articular fractures of the knee allows early range of motion and therefore de-

creases subsequent muscle atrophy and impaired motion.[6,23,28,53-58] Perioperative CPM in intra-articular fractures enhances hyaline cartilage repair and may improve associated ligamentous injury healing.

REFERENCES

1. Rineberg B: A call to leadership: the role of orthopaedic surgeons in musculoskeletal outcome research, *J Bone Joint Surg [Am]* 72:1439, 1990.
2. Epstein A: The outcome movement: will it get us to where we want to go? *N Engl J Med* 323:266, 1990.
3. Neer C, Granthano S, Shelton M: Supracondylar fracture of the adult femur, *J Bone Joint Surg [Am]* 49:591, 1967.
4. Seinsheimer F: Fractures of the distal femur, *Clin Orthop* 153:169, 1980.
5. Hall M: Two-plane fixation of acute supracondylar and intracondylar fractures of the femur, *South Med J* 71:1474, 1978.
6. Shelbourne K, Brueckmann F: Rush pin fixation of supracondylar and intercondylar fractures of the femur, *J Bone Joint Surg [Am]* 64:161, 1982.
7. Crotwell W: The thigh-lacer: ambulatory nonoperative treatment of femoral shaft fractures, *J Bone Joint Surg [Am]* 60:112, 1978.
8. Sanders R, et al: Double plating of comminuted unstable fractures of the distal part of the femur, *J Bone Joint Surg [Am]* 73:341, 1991.
9. Alonso J, Geissler W, Hughes J: External fixation of femoral fractures, indications and limitations, *Clin Orthop* 241:83, 1989.
10. Rooser B, et al: External fixation of femoral fractures, *J Orthop Trauma* 4:70, 1990.
11. Garland D, Rothi B, Waters R: Femoral fractures in head-injured adults, *Clin Orthop* 166:219, 1982.
12. Kempf I, Grosse A, Beck G: Closed locked intramedullary nailing: its application to comminuted fractures of the femur, *J Bone Joint Surg [Am]* 67:709, 1985.
13. Winquist R, Hansen S, Clawson D: Closed intramedullary nailing of femoral fractures: a report of five hundred and twenty cases, *J Bone Joint Surg [Am]* 66:529, 1984.

14. Zuckerman J, et al: Treatment of unstable femoral shaft fractures with closed intramedullary nailing, *J Orthop Trauma* 1:209, 1987.

15. Johnson K, Johnston D, Parker B: Comminuted femoral shaft fractures: treatment by roller traction, cerclage wires and an intramedullary nail, or an interlocking intramedullary nail, *J Bone Joint Surg [Am]* 66:1222, 1984.

16. Mira A, Markley K, Greer R: A critical analysis of quadriceps function after femoral shaft fractures in adults, *J Bone Joint Surg [Am]* 62:61, 1980.

17. Moore T, et al: The results of quadricepsplasty on knee motion following femoral fractures, *J Trauma* 27:49, 1987.

18. Moore T, et al: Knee function after complex femoral fractures treated with interlocking nails, *Clin Orthop* 261:238, 1990.

19. Walling A, Seradge H, Spiegel P: *Femur fracture with simultaneous knee ligament injuries.* In Spiegel P, editor: *Topics in orthopaedic trauma,* Baltimore, 1984, University Park Press.

20. Dunbar W, Coleman S: Occult knee injuries associated with ipsilateral femoral fractures: a prospective study, *Orthop Trans* 2:253, 1978.

20a. Moore T, et al: Complications of surgically treated supracondylar fractures of the femur, *J Trauma* 27:402, 1987.

21. Merchan E, Maestu P, Blanco R: Blade plating of closed displaced supracondylar fractures of the distal femur, *J Trauma* 32:174, 1992.

22. Zickel R, Hobeika P, Robbins D: Zickel supracondylar nails for fractures of the distal end of the femur, *Clin Orthop* 212:79, 1986.

23. Schatzker J, Lambert D: Supracondylar fractures of the femur, *Clin Orthop* 138:77, 1979.

24. Butler M, et al: Interlocking intramedullary nailing for ipsilateral fractures of the femoral shaft and distal part of the femur, *J Bone Joint Surg [Am]* 73:1492, 1991.

25. McAndrew M, Powtarelli W: The long-term follow-up of ipsilateral tibial and femoral diaphyseal fractures, *Clin Orthop* 232:190, 1988.

26. Brown B, D'Arcy W: Internal fixation for supracondylar fractures of the femur in the elderly patient, *J Bone Joint Surg [Br]* 53:420, 1971.

27. Egund N, Kolmert L: Deformities, gonarthrosis and function after distal femoral fractures, *Acta Orthop Scand* 53:963, 1982.

28. Siliski J, Mahring M, Hofer H: Supracondylar-intercondylar fractures of the femur: treatment by internal fixation, *J Bone Joint Surg [Am]* 71:95, 1989.

29. Pritchett J: Supracondylar fractures of the femur, *Clin Orthop* 184:173, 1984.

30. Merchant T, Dietz F: Long-term follow-up after fracture of the tibial and fibular shafts, *J Bone Joint Surg [Am]* 71:599, 1989.

31. Waddell J, Reardon G: Complications of tibial shaft fractures, *Clin Orthop* 178:173, 1983.

32. Nicoll E: Fractures of the tibial shaft: a survey of 705 cases, *J Bone Joint Surg [Br]* 46:373, 1964.

33. Puno R, et al: Critical analysis of results of treatment of 201 tibial shaft fractures, *Clin Orthop* 212:113, 1986.

34. Johnson K: Management of malunion and nonunion of the tibia, *Orthop Clin North Am* 18:157, 1987.

35. Olerud C: The pronation capacity of the foot: its consequences for axial deformity after tibial shaft fractures, *Arch Orthop Trauma Surg* 104:303, 1985.

36. Puno R, et al: Long-term effects of tibial angular malunion on the knee and ankle joints, *J Orthop Trauma* 5:247, 1991.

36a. Ting A, et al: The role of subtalar motion and ankle contact pressure changes from angular deformities of the tibia, *Foot Ankle* 7:290, 1987.

36b. Wagner K, Tarr R, Resnick C: The effect of simulated tibial deformities on the ankle joint during the gait cycle, *Foot Ankle* 5:131, 1984.

37. Tarr R, et al: Changes in tibiotalar joint contact area following experimentally induced tibial angular deformities, *Clin Orthop* 199:72, 1985.

38. Green S, Moore T, Spohn P: Nonunion of the tibial shaft, *Orthopedics* 2:1149, 1988.

39. Kettlekamp K, et al: Degenerative arthritis of the knee secondary to fracture malunion, *Clin Orthop* 234:159, 1988.

40. Zehntner M, et al: Alignment of supracondylar-intercondylar fractures of the femur after internal fixation by AO technique, *J Orthop Trauma* 3:318, 1992.

41. Reibel D, Wade P: Fractures of the tibial plateau, *J Trauma* 2:337, 1962.

42. Benirschke S, et al: Immediate internal fixation of open complex tibial plateau fractures, *J Orthop Trauma* 6:78, 1992.

43. Rasmussen P: Tibial condyle fractures: impairment of knee joint stability as an indication for surgical treatment, *J Bone Joint Surg [Am]* 56:1331, 1973.

44. DeCoster T, Nepola J, ElRhoury G: Cast brace treatment of proximal tibial fractures: a ten years follow up study, *Clin Orthop* 231:196, 1988.

45. Brown T, et al: Contact stress aberrations following imprecise reduction of simple tibial plateau fractures, *J Orthop Res* 6:851, 1988.

46. Salter R: The biological concept of continuous passive motion of synovial joints: the first 18 years of basic research and its clinical application, *Clin Orthop* 242:12, 1989.

47. Kim H, Moran M, Salter R: The potential for regeneration of articular cartilage in defects created by chondral shaving and subchondral abrasion, *J Bone Joint Surg [Am]* 73:1301, 1991.

48. Gelberman R, et al: The influence of protected passive mobilization on the healing of flexor tendons: a biomechanical and microangiographic study, *Hand* 13:120, 1981.

49. Takai S, et al: The effects of frequency and duration of controlled passive mobilization on tendon healing, *J Orthop Res* 9:705, 1991.

50. Gelberman R, et al: The excursion and deformation of repaired flexor tendons treatment with protected early motion, *J Hand Surg [Am]* 11:106, 1986.

51. Moore TM, Patzakis M, Harvey J: Ipsilateral diaphyseal femur fractures and knee ligament injuries, *Clin Orthop* 232:182, 1988.

52. Delamarter R, Hohl M, Hopp E: Ligament injuries associated with tibial plateau fractures, *Clin Orthop* 250:226, 1990.

53. Duvelius P, Connolly J: Closed reduction of tibial plateau fractures: a comparison of functional and roentgenographic end results, *Clin Orthop* 230:116, 1988.

54. Moore TM, Patzakis M, Harvey J: Tibial plateau fractures: definition, demographics, treatment rationale and long-term results of closed traction management or operative reduction, *J Trauma* 1:97, 1987.

55. Drennan D, Locker F: Fractures of the tibial plateau: treatment by closed reduction and spica cast, *J Bone Joint Surg [Am]* 61:989, 1979.

56. Tylman D, Siwek W: Long-term results of functional treatment in intra-articular knee fractures and multifragment fractures of the shaft of the femur, *Clin Orthop* 272:114, 1991.

57. Gausewitz S, Hohl M: The significance of early motion in the treatment of tibial plateau fractures, *Clin Orthop* 202:135, 1986.

58. Koval K, et al: Indirect reduction and percutaneous screw fixation of displaced tibial plateau fractures, *J Orthop Trauma* 3:340, 1992.

59. Leung K, et al: Interlocking intramedullary nailing for supracondylar and intercondylar fractures of the distal part of the femur, *J Bone Joint Surg [Am]* 73:332, 1991.

Part IV

SPORT-SPECIFIC KNEE REHABILITATION

Chapter 16

FOOTBALL

Robert Poole
Tim Uhl

The sport of football requires the athlete to run, cut, backpedal, accelerate, and decelerate, all within seconds. The goal of rehabilitation is to develop a controlled progression of these sport-specific skills, ending with the return of the player to full-speed and full-contact competition.

The purpose of this chapter is to describe advanced functional exercises used to condition an athlete to a full level of football competition after knee injury. The functional exercises and position-specific conditioning exercises (PSCE) described in this chapter are applicable to all levels of football from PeeWee to professional.

The average high school football game lasts 123 minutes. The average play lasts 5.5 seconds with a recovery time of 46.5 seconds between plays (unpublished data). As these data suggest, football is a highly anaerobic sport. The duplication of training activities for specific sports requirements is commonly known as the specific activity for imposed demand (SAID) principle. SAID means that for each position on a football team there are certain physiologic requirements that the athlete must meet to perform adequately.

Most football players need the same basic skills; therefore, many of the same exercises are applicable to all positions. For instance, because most plays are short in duration, all players need explosive power, which is developed by functional agility exercises. Following the SAID principle, the final level of rehabilitation prior to return to full participation is PSCE, which mimic skills used by the players to perform their particular assignments on the playing field. These exercises can be adapted in level of difficulty, to meet the athlete's capability. Therefore, the development of an advanced rehabilitation program needs to be specific not only to the sport but also to the position-imposed demand.

Other chapters have described injury-specific knee rehabilitation programs. This chapter concentrates on advanced sport- and position-specific knee rehabilitation for the football athlete. Prior to beginning this functional exercise program, athletes have reached an appropriate level through basic rehabilitation programs and met the following criteria:

1. Where tested isokinetically, the athlete would have 85% of quadriceps and hamstring strength as compared to the uninjured side. If isokinetic testing is unavailable, other objective criteria may be used, such as manual muscle test for quadriceps, hamstrings, gastrocnemius, and iliopsoas. A grade of good plus to normal strength is expected.

2. The athlete should be able to complete 30 minutes of exercise bicycling without difficulty.

3. When measured circumferentially, muscle bulk 3 inches and 7 inches above the joint line should be within ⅜ to ¼ inch or less of the uninjured leg.

4. Complete pain-free knee range of motion should be demonstrated. Pain tolerances differ, but minimal pain with activity may be accepted.

Knee bracing during sport-specific activities may be left to the discretion of the sports medicine team (i.e., physician, physical therapist, athletic trainer) training the athlete. Bracing is more common in football than in other sports and is more accepted by these athletes. It is quite common to use a functional rehabilitation brace after surgery during the early phases of the rehabilitation program. As the athlete moves through the functional phases, reassessment of the effectiveness of the brace is recommended.

GENERAL PROGRESSION

Initially, basic running skills are practiced and refined through form running and acceleration-deceleration zone running, progressing from half to three-quarter and then to full speed. When athletes can perform full-speed, straight-ahead running with no to minimal pain and swelling, they are ready to progress to functional agility exercises commonly used in rehabilitation of football knee injuries for all positions:

1. Acceleration-deceleration zone running
2. Side shuffle
3. Carioca
4. Wave drills
5. Bag drill

Acceleration-deceleration zone running

The athlete starts from a standstill and progresses from a walk to a jog over a 10-yard distance. At the 10-yard mark, the athlete breaks into a sprint for 40 yards. At the 40-yard mark the athlete gradually slows down from a sprint to a walk over a 10-yard distance. The idea is to avoid acceleration or deceleration stress on the rehabilitating knee. The 10-yard acceleration-deceleration zone prevents this occurrence. The athlete progresses from half- to three-quarter- to full-speed sprints as tolerated and may take 2 to 6 weeks. The difficulty of this exercise can be increased by shortening the acceleration-deceleration zones (Fig. 16-1).

Side shuffle

The athlete performs this drill over a 5- to 10-yard distance. The athlete faces the same direction during the entire drill and side shuffles his feet over the 10 yards as fast as possible without crossing his feet. The difficulty of this exercise can be increased by not letting the athlete stop at the end of each 10-yard distance. Instead, the athlete can be required to plant his foot and immediately start side shuffling in the opposite direction. It is important that the athlete is planting on the involved side to facilitate proprioception and increase eccentric and concentric strength of the involved leg (Fig. 16-2).

Carioca

Carioca exercise is performed in the same manner as the side shuffle, except the athlete alternately crosses one foot in front and then in back of the other foot. It is important that along with the crossover step the athlete swivel his hips while performing this exercise to avoid tripping. The difficulty is increased in the same manner as the side-shuffle exercise (Fig. 16-3).

Wave drill

The athlete starts this exercise in the "athlete ready position," with his feet shoulder width apart, knees flexed approximately 30 degrees, hands at waist level and slightly in front of the body, and head up. The athlete faces the leader of the exercise and responds to hand signals. The athlete runs in the direction the leader points. If the leader points to the right, the athlete runs in a straight line to the

right of the leader. If the leader points toward the athlete, he immediately stops running to the right and starts backpedaling. The leader randomly chooses the direction the athlete is to move in. The exercise generally lasts 15 to 30 seconds per repetition. If the athlete is unfamiliar with this exercise, it is started with a longer time period and fewer directional changes. As the athlete improves, the speed the athlete is moving is increased and more frequent directional changes are made (Fig. 16-4).

Bag drills

Five "bags" (The Agile One, Rogers Athletic, Claire, Michigan) blocking dummies, or cones (Wolverine Sports, Ann Arbor, Michigan) are lined up, approximately 1 yard apart. Four different exercises can be performed with the bags. The first exercise involves running straight over the bags and emphasizes lifting the knees high and pumping the arms (Fig. 16-5). The athlete is started out at half speed, progresses to full speed, and is instructed not to hit the bags with his feet. The second exercise is hopping over the bags with both feet together, again without touching the bags (Fig. 16-6). The athlete is instructed to lift the knees up so as to touch the chest while performing this exercise. In the third exercise, the "weave" or "snake," the athlete starts perpendicular to the bag, facing the same direction through the entire drill. The athlete runs around the front of the first bag and behind the second bag and continues to weave or snake around all the bags until he has reached the starting point (Fig. 16-7). The fourth exercise has the athlete sidestep over the bags as fast as possible without touching the bags (Fig. 16-8). Upon reaching the end of the bags, the athlete rests before returning. The difficulty of the side-stepping exercise can be increased by having the athlete respond to right or left hand signals for 10 to 30 seconds. Changing direction unexpectedly facilitates knee proprioception and increases lateral acceleration-deceleration capabilities.

Functional agility exercises are always started with acceleration-deceleration zone running. This assures that the athlete can tolerate straight-ahead, full-speed activities without guarding the knee or increasing in symptoms. When no problems with straight-ahead running are demonstrated, the other agility exercises are added. Generally 10 repetitions of all activities are performed with a 15- to 45-second rest between repetitions, thus mimicking a normal football game situation. These exercises can be made more difficult by throwing a football to the athlete during his performance of many of the exercises. For example, throwing a football to an athlete performing the wave drill increases the attention

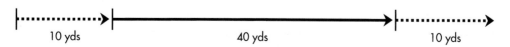

Fig. 16-1. Acceleration-deceleration zone running.

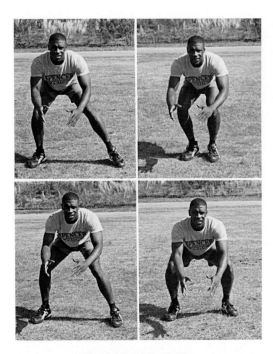

Fig. 16-2. Side shuffle.

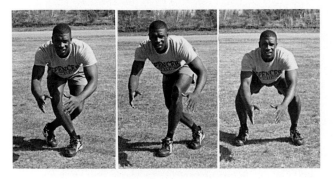

Fig. 16-3. Carioca.

the athlete is paying to the leader and distracts attention from protecting an involved knee. If the athlete happens to be a defensive back, this activity duplicates the athlete's primary responsibility on the football field, which is pass coverage. Upon successfully completing the functional agility exercises (which might take from 2 to 6 weeks), as long as no clinical symptoms of knee irritation are present such as pain, swelling, or giving way, the football player is ready to progress to position-specific conditioning exercises:

1. Four-cone exercise
2. Grass drill
3. Pass patterns
4. Dropbacks
5. Hole drill
6. First step drill
7. Breakdown drill
8. Sled drill

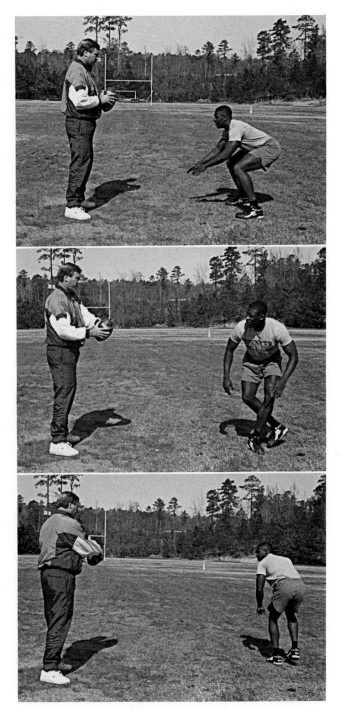

Fig. 16-4. Wave drill.

Four-cone exercise

This activity is performed on all fours (hands and feet) for linemen or the athlete ready position for backs. The athlete starts at one cone and crawls or runs forward for 10 yards to the next cone. He then sidesteps or shuffles for 10 yards to the next cone, facing the same direction. The athlete then crawls backward or backpedals 10 yards to the next cone. Then the athlete sidesteps on all fours or side shuffles

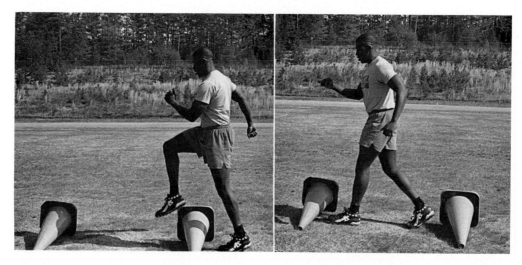

Fig. 16-5. Bag drill, high-stepping.

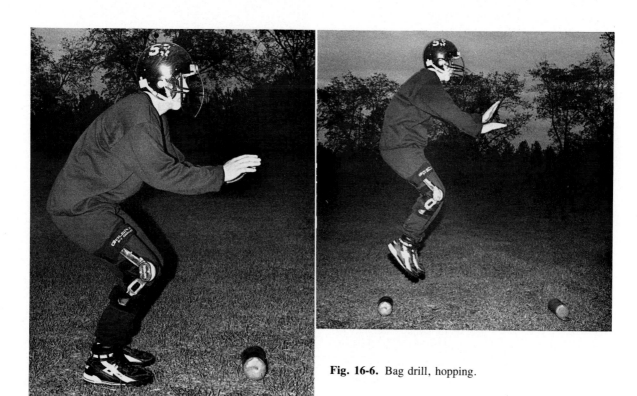

Fig. 16-6. Bag drill, hopping.

to the cone where he began. An alternation of this drill is to have the athlete stand up from crawling backward and sprint to the starting cone. This mimics "pulling," which is a common task for down linemen. The drill can be run clockwise or counterclockwise to add variety and place different stresses on the involved leg (Figs. 16-9 and 16-10).

Grass drill

The athlete runs in place with knees high and arms pumping. The athlete then falls forward, letting his chest and arms touch the ground, and then immediately pushes back up with his arms (Fig. 16-11). This is repeated 10 times. To increase the difficulty of this activity, the athlete can be

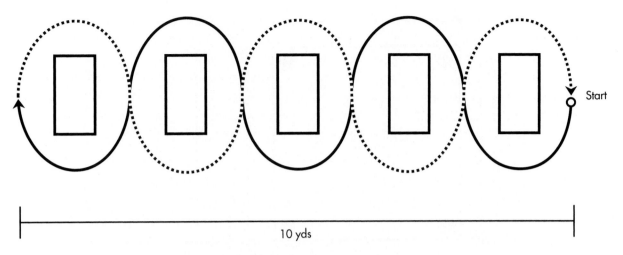

Fig. 16-7. Bag drill, the weave.

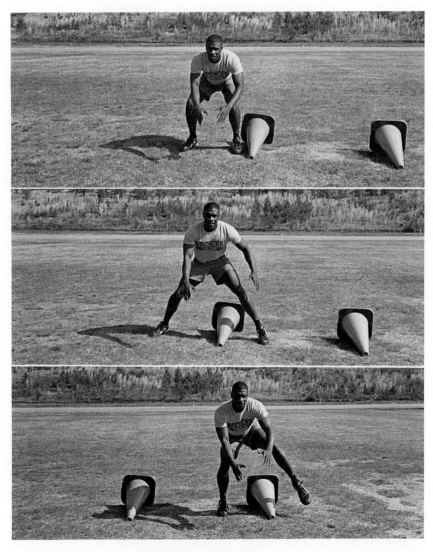

Fig. 16-8. Bag drill, sidestep over.

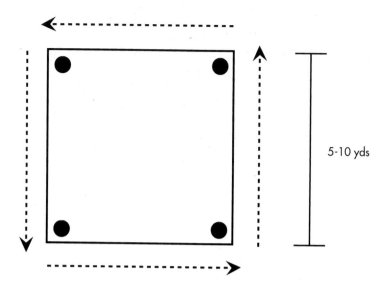

Fig. 16-9. Four cone exercise—layout.

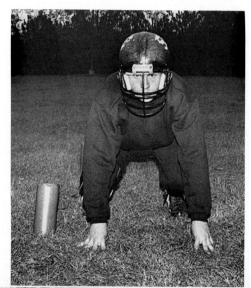

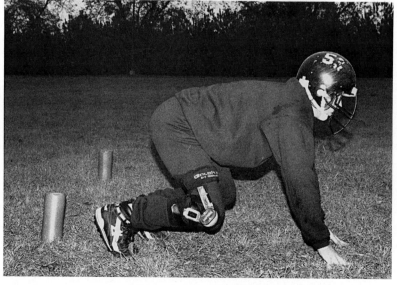

Fig. 16-10. Four cone exercise—performed.

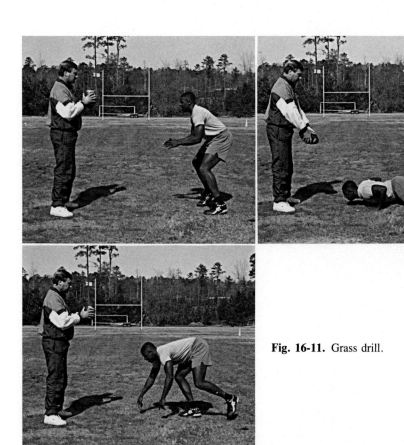

Fig. 16-11. Grass drill.

instructed to hit the ground and roll to the right or left as directed. The athlete should alternate the leg used for pushing up, so as not to protect the involved leg (Fig. 16-12).

Pass patterns

This exercise incorporates into PSCE standard patterns run by receivers. The athlete progresses from half to three-quarter to full speed as tolerated. The patterns are alternately run to the right and left. The difficulty of this exercise can be increased by requiring the athlete to catch a football as he performs the exercise (Figs. 16-13 and 16-14).

Dropbacks

This requires the athlete to start in the ready position while holding the football in both hands. In the first maneuver, the athlete runs backward 5 yards, stops, and then steps up to throw the ball. This is performed while running backward five times looking over the right shoulder and five times looking over the left shoulder. The second maneuver is to have the athlete take one step backward and run 5 to 10 yards in a helical pattern to the right and left. This is commonly called a *rollout* pattern. The athlete stops at the end of the rollout and sets up to throw the football. The difficulty of this exercise is increased by having the athlete actually throw the football after the setup. To increase the difficulty, the athlete throws the football without setting up while rolling out (Figs. 16-15 and 16-16).

Hole drill

The athlete starts at one end of the five bags lined up for the bag drill. The holes are numbered 1 through 5, with the five hole being outside the last bag. The athlete starts in the ready position 1 yard behind the bags facing the same direction as the bags. The athlete turns, runs to the first hole between the first two bags, makes a 90-degree cut, and runs through the hole 5 yards. This is repeated for each hole with the athlete starting on the right and the left side of the bags. The difficulty of this drill is increased by having the athlete run parallel to cones while the leader calls out a number; the athlete has to respond by running through the hole called. This duplicates the situation a running back might actually face when a play may be planned to be run between the tackle and end, but the hole opens between the guard and center (Figs. 16-17 and 16-18).

First step drill

The athlete lines up in a correct four-point stance in front of a sled and explodes straight ahead for three steps. This can also be performed with the athlete taking one step forward and then turning to the right or left for two more steps. In another variation, the athlete takes one step forward, then two steps backward, and positions himself in the athlete ready position. This drill can incorporate the upper arm motions used by a defensive lineman who sweeps his arm over his head as he steps and turns, thus mimicking

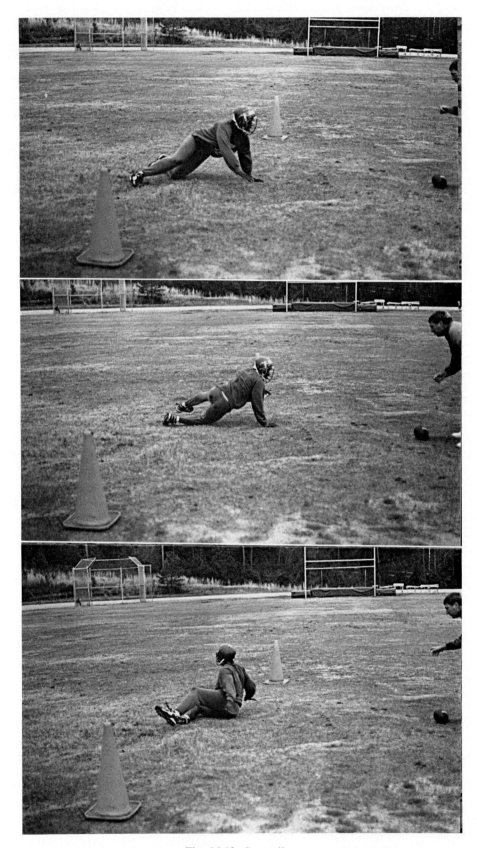

Fig. 16-12. Seat roll.

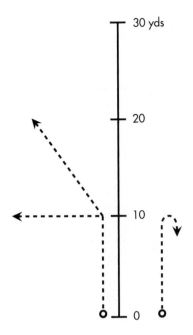

Fig. 16-13. Pass pattern—layout.

a penetration method known as the *swim technique* (Fig. 16-19).

Breakdown drill

This drill is run like the wave drill, except the athlete does not stop following hand signals. On the verbal order of "Breakdown," however, the athlete runs as fast as he can to the leader no matter where he is. The athlete must stop in the ready position as close to the leader as he can without touching the leader. To increase the difficulty of this exercise, the leader can run away from the athlete, making the athlete pursue the leader (Fig. 16-20).

Sled drill

The athlete lines up in front of a sled in a four-point stance. The athlete explodes and drives the sled straight back for 5 yards. A variation is to have the athlete drive the sled back 2 yards and then turn it 90 degrees to the right or left and drive it 3 more yards. The leader instructs the athlete to maintain and use a proper blocking technique, which is to stay low on the sled, keep the head up, keep a

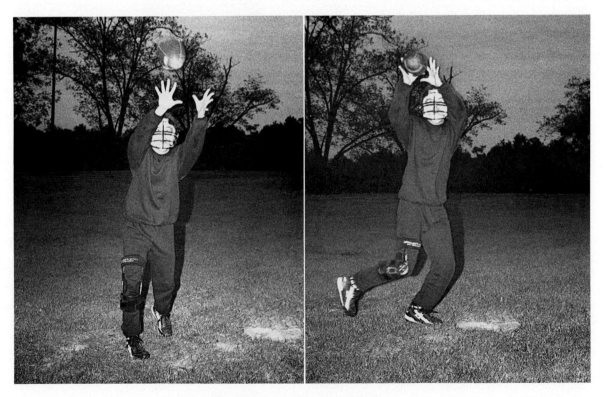

Fig. 16-14. Pass pattern—performed.

10 yds

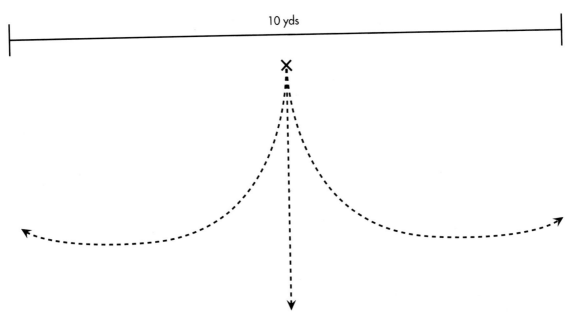

Fig. 16-15. Dropbacks—layout.

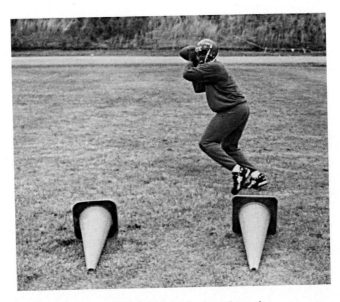

Fig. 16-16. Dropbacks—performed.

wide base of support with the feet, and drive the sled. To increase the difficulty of this exercise, add weight to the sled by having the leader of the drill standing on the sled (Fig. 16-21).

PSCEs are repeated 10 times, with a 15- to 45-second break between repetitions as needed. The exercises should be tailored for the particular athlete as much as possible.

Each player of the football team has a specific assignment, which requires specific skills. For simplicity and specificity and to assist the clinician in choosing the appropriate exercises, these players have been grouped here according to the required skills and position-specific conditioning exercises.

The offensive line is made up of the center, guards, and tackles. Their primary responsibility is blocking, which requires explosive straight-ahead movement and an occasional a quick step backward as, for example, in a pulling guard.

Specific exercises
Four-cone exercises
Grass drill
Sled drill

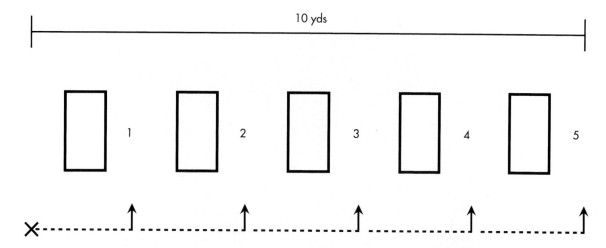

Fig. 16-17. Hole drill—layout.

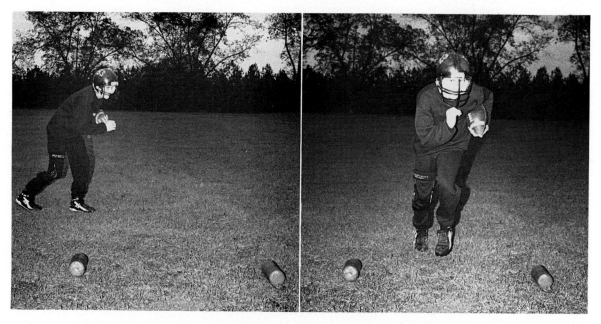

Fig. 16-18. Hole drill—performed.

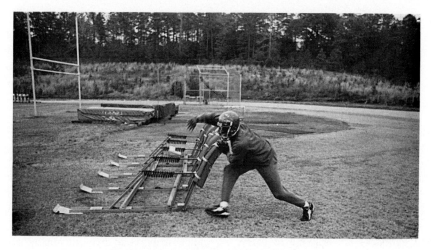

Fig. 16-19. First step drill, swim technique.

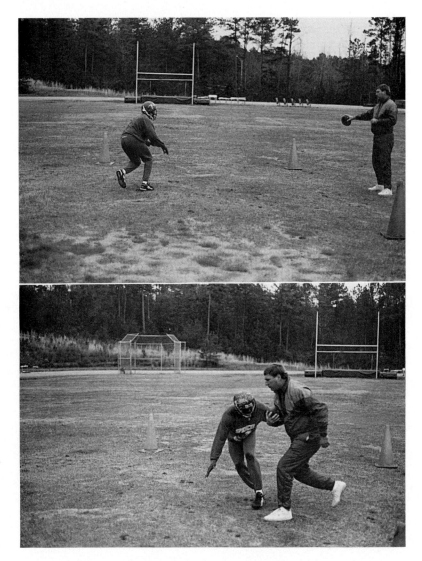

Fig. 16-20. Breakdown drill.

Receivers consist of wide receivers and tight ends. Their primary responsibility is running and catching the ball. This requires straight-ahead speed, cutting agility, and eye-hand coordination.

Specific exercises
Wave drill
Pass patterns
Bag drills

As the athlete's abilities improve, add catching the football to these exercises.

Offensive backs are the quarterback, halfbacks, and fullbacks. Their primary responsibility is to move the ball down the field. Fullbacks and halfbacks are required to carry, catch, and sometimes block. The quarterback receives the football from the center and hands off, throws, or carries the ball himself. The emphasis for this group of players is speed, agility, and hand-eye coordination.

Specific exercises
Dropbacks
Wave drill
Hole drill
Pass patterns

The defensive line is made up of nose guards, defensive tackles, and defensive ends. Their primary responsibility is to tackle the ball carrier and prevent forward movement of the football. Lateral movement, upper body strength, and quick reaction to ball movement are emphasized in this group.

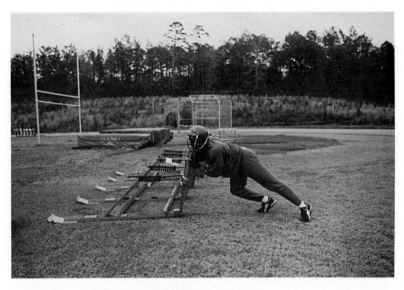

Fig. 16-21. Sled drill.

Specific exercises

Bag drill
First step drill
Four-cone drill

Defensive backs consist of linebackers, corner backs, and safeties. Their primary responsibility is pass defense, with emphasis on running defense for the linebackers. The emphasis is on backward and lateral movements, cutting, agility, and deceleration.

Specific exercises

Wave drill
Breakdown drill
Bag drill

SUMMARY

Sport-specific rehabilitation techniques have been used for years by clinicians to simulate the types of stress placed on an injured player performing his or her assignment during sports activity. This chapter outlines position-specific conditioning exercises that can be used to bring a football player with a knee injury from the basic rehabilitation exercises producing strength and range of motion, outlined in other chapters, to the skills and agility required to return to his position in full-contact football competition. These skills are essential if the player is to be able to perform his assignment properly while preventing reinjury of the involved knee. It is hoped these exercises will be helpful and fun for the clinician and athlete while producing results and satisfying the criteria for return to participation.

ACKNOWLEDGMENTS

The authors wish to thank Paul Schmidt, head athletic trainer at the University of Michigan, for his invaluable assistance and knowledge of football drills; Alonzo James, Spencer High School, for suffering through two photo sessions; and Marvin Smith, Smith Station High School, because we still did not get it right. To Coach Ellerbee, for his dedication to athletes—he's the only one of us still coaching—thanks for your knowledge and your crazy ways.

REFERENCE

1. McCluskey B, Howell M: Describing the aerobic & anaerobic components of high school football, 1991.

Chapter 17

BASKETBALL

Dale F. Blair

There are several programs described in the literature for the rehabilitation of the knee.[1-9]

There have also been many articles written regarding strengthening and conditioning for the sport of basketball.[10-15] This chapter combines the components of traditional knee rehabilitation with the functional elements of a basketball conditioning and training program. Because high stresses are applied to the knee in basketball, an incomplete or nonspecific rehabilitation program can lead to disastrous results when the player returns to the court.

BASKETBALL INJURIES

Knee injuries have been one of the most troublesome problems among basketball players. Chronic overuse injuries such as patellar tendonitis or patellofemoral arthralgia can cause persistent pain and hamper performance. However, intra-articular ligamentous disruptions often result in considerable down time for the athlete and have the potential to be career-threatening.

The cutting and pivoting associated with basketball are prime mechanisms for a severe knee ligament injury. In recent years, a number of professional, collegiate, and scholastic basketball athletes have suffered severe knee ligament ruptures, usually involving the anterior cruciate ligament (ACL).[13,14,16-18]

There have been several hypotheses as to etiology of severe ligament injuries in basketball:

1. Faster, stronger players who create more torque on the knee
2. Taller players with longer lever arms, which produce greater torque on the joint
3. Shoes that grip the floor better and create a fixed axis of knee rotation
4. Less than optimal quadriceps-hamstring strength ratio, that is, inadequate hamstring strength

The epidemic of basketball knee injuries among females

The rate of serious knee injuries in female basketball players has reached nearly epidemic proportions. Garrick

reported twice as many knee injuries in girls' basketball than in boys' basketball in a 2-year injury study in Seattle high schools.[19] Zelisko also found the injury rate for women to be twice that of men. His results were from a two-season comparison of male and female professional basketball players.[18] Wirtz reported significantly more knee injuries among female high school basketball players as compared with male players.[17] Chandy and Grana found the severity, rate, and incidence of knee injuries involving surgery among female basketball players significantly greater than males.[16] In their 3-year study, they found a significant difference in the injury rate between the sexes only in basketball.

Morrison and Boyd described a significant rise in the rate of "severe" knee injuries (player missed 2 weeks or more of the season) during a 3-year period among college basketball players.[14] The injury rate rose from 2.9 severe knee injuries per 100 participants in the 1985-86 season to 5.1 per 100 in 1987-1988. Fifty-nine percent of all "severe" knee injuries involved the anterior cruciate ligament.

Gray et al. found in a study of 76 female basketball-related injuries that the knee was involved in 72% of the cases.[20] The ACL rupture accounted for 25% of all basketball injuries. During the same 30-month period, 151 male basketball players were seen in their clinic. Only 4 of the 151 males were diagnosed with an ACL rupture, whereas 19 of 76 females had the same injury.

Moore and Wade found a ratio of 10 females to every male interscholastic athlete with ACL injury during a 2-year clinical investigation.[13] However, a program of hamstring strengthening and education in basketball fundamentals for female high school basketball teams in their area reduced the female injury rate dramatically.[21]

The difference in injury rates between male and female basketball players may be attributed to the following factors:[13,14]

1. Females have 12% to 16% less muscle mass than males.
2. Females generally have less strength than males. Moore and Wade found 30% less strength in the quadriceps and 35% in the hamstrings on three-speed (60,

---

208

180, and 300 degrees per second) isokinetic testing in a high school-age population.[13]

3. Females carry about 12% to 16% more body fat, which translates to inert weight.

4. Some adolescent girls may lead a less active life-style than adolescent boys, which may leave them less prepared to face the rigors of a ballistic contact sport like basketball.[14]

5. Some females may start playing basketball at a later age, and they may not have developed their fundamentals as well as their male counterparts.

Prevention of basketball knee injuries

Numerous articles have been written on the rehabilitation of knee injuries; however, less emphasis has been placed on prevention. The concepts of prevention and rehabilitation are similar. However, preventive exercises do not have the constraints and functional limitations of many rehabilitative exercises. Thus, it is easier to perform exercises in a preventive mode than in a rehabilitative fashion.

There are several general coaching and conditioning principles that should be employed in the prevention of knee injuries:[5,11-15,21,22]

1. Intensive strengthening for *all* lower extremity muscle groups.

2. Adequate quadriceps muscle strength is needed to maintain the flexed-knee position required of basketball players. As players fatigue, they tend to play in a more upright position, increasing injury risk. (See Table 17-1 for desired strength goals.)

3. Hamstring strengthening to prevent muscular imbalances. The sport of basketball tends to emphasize the quadriceps, and the hamstring muscle strength may be mediocre in comparison. (See Table 17-1 for desired strength goals.)

4. Sport-specific isokinetic training to adapt muscles to high-speed muscle contractions.

5. Conditioning and drills that utilize the SAID (specific adaption to imposed demands). The ligaments of the knee adapt (increase in strength) with regular, controlled cutting and pivoting.

6. Proprioceptive enhancement to increase awareness of knee movement and activity.

7. Practice cutting and deceleration activities with the knee slightly bent (rather than straight) to decrease ACL strain. This position also placed the hamstrings at a mechanical advantage in stabilizing the joint.

8. Cutting and deceleration activities with the feet under the hips.

9. Gradual deceleration with a two-step stop instead of a rapid, one-step stop.

BASKETBALL-SPECIFIC REHABILITATION

Knee rehabilitation programs vary greatly depending upon the specific pathology, surgical versus conservative treatment, and other factors. The program presented in this

Table 17-1. Isokinetic strength goals from male and female basketball players

	Centers	Forwards	Guards
60 degrees/second			
Knee extension goal	1.20	1.20	1.30
Knee flexion goal	0.70	0.70	0.70
180 degrees/second			
Knee extension goal	0.75	0.80	0.85
Knee flexion goal	0.83	0.83	0.83
300 degrees/second			
Knee extension goal	0.55	0.65 (M)	0.70 (M)
		0.60 (F)	0.65 (F)
Knee flexion goal	1.00	1.00	1.00

Adapted from Moore JR, Wade G: Prevention of the anterior cruciate ligament, *Natl Strength Conditioning Assoc J* 11:35–40, 1989.

Tested with Cybex, Division of Lumex, Ronkonkoma, NY.

The numbers in this table are multiplication factors by which to determine proper quadriceps and hamstring strength goals. (Knee extension factor multiplied by body weight, knee flexion factor multiplied by knee extension goal.)

Sample for 130-pound female basketball forward testing at 60 degrees per second:

Body weight (130) × 1.20 = 156 ft/lb (knee extension goal)
Knee extension goal (156) × 0.70 = 109 ft/lb (knee flexion goal)

section is a generic series of exercises that can be adapted for various knee injuries. This program includes the sport-specific exercises and drills that are implemented *after* full (or nearly full) range of motion has been obtained. The program should emphasize early motion and early weight-bearing to reap the benefits of a "rapid rehabilitation" protocol.[1,8] The neuromuscular pathways also must be functioning adequately to commence a basketball-specific program.

Strengthening

Strengthening of thigh musculature is extremely important to the basketball athlete. Closed kinetic chain exercise (with the distal body segment stabilized) provides specificity of training better than open-chain exercise (distal segment not stabilized). Open kinetic chain exercises may also stress ligamentous reconstructions and irritate the patellofemoral joint. Closed-chain exercises can also help train the "pseudo-isometric" response,[23] a cocontraction of the quadriceps and hamstrings that is utilized during functional activities and cannot be reproduced during open-chain exercise.

Heavy rubber tubing provides both concentric and eccentric resistance. It is vital to train and rehabilitate basketball athletes with both types of muscle contractions because they are used extensively in the sport. When using tubing or any strengthening exercise, the number of repetitions and amount of resistance vary, depending on the level of strength, severity of injury and/or surgery, and stage or recovery.

These exercises should be primarily closed chain; however, selected open-chain exercises can be employed as well. The rubbing tubing exercises can include the following.

Hip flexion, extension, abduction, and adduction. These exercises can be performed while the athlete is standing on the uninvolved leg and holding onto the back of a chair. The tubing is looped around the athlete's ankle. Painful or stressful exercises should be avoided for certain injuries. For example, straight leg hip flexion should be avoided following an anterior cruciate ligament injury or surgery. Hip adductions should not be performed in the early stages after a medial collateral ligament injury.

Seated hamstring pull. This exercise is performed with the athlete in a seated position with rubber tubing attached in front and around the ankle. The involved leg's foot slides posteriorly along the floor and then is *slowly* returned to the starting point for eccentric hamstring strengthening.

Closed-chain extensions. Closed kinetic chain terminal knee extensions provide functional strengthening of the quadriceps by placing the tubing above the knee (Fig. 17-1). With the foot fixed, the athlete moves from 30 degrees of flexion to full extension against the resistance of the tubing.

Quarter squats with tubing. While standing on a piece of tubing, the athlete performs a quarter-squat from full extension to approximately 30 degrees of flexion (Fig. 17-2). The key to this exercise is the eccentric (down) phase of the squat. The functional eccentric phase of exercise is of paramount importance in returning the thigh musculature to a competitive level of strength.

Other strengthening exercises

Step-ups. The athlete stands on a 2- to 6-inch block of wood. The heel of the involved leg touches the floor as the body is lowered in a slow, controlled fashion (Fig. 17-3). The body is then raised to the starting position. Step-ups help to promote muscle control through the improvement of proprioception and eccentric strengthening.

Leg press. The leg press, also classified as a closed-chain activity because the distal segment is stabilized, effectively strengthens the quadriceps. The range of motion should be limited to the final 30 degrees of extension to prevent patellofemoral pain.

Stair machine. A stair machine (such as the StairMaster 4000) provides effective closed-chain resistance to enhance thigh muscle strength and endurance.

Chair scoot. A chair with wheels can function as an effective strengthening modality[1] (Fig. 17-4). "Walking" the chair forward in a sitting position strengthens the hamstrings and, if it is done for extended periods, can also enhance hamstring endurance. A carpeted floor provides additional resistance.

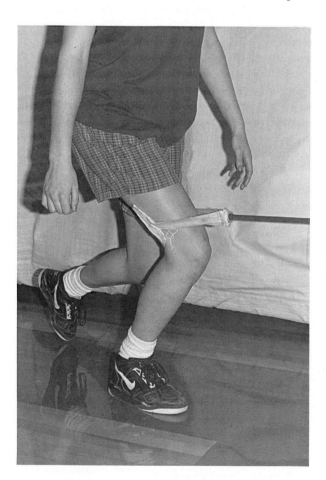

Fig. 17-1. Closed kinetic chain extensions.

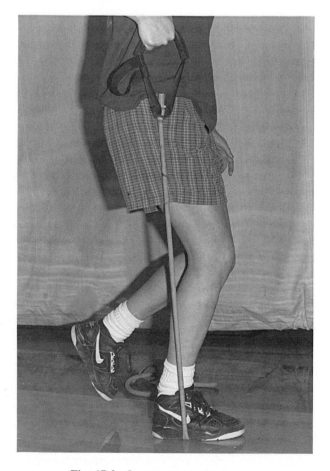

Fig. 17-2. Quarter-squats with tubing.

Stationary exercise bicycle. Cycling is excellent for regaining strength and endurance in the thigh musculature. Single-leg cycling isolates the involved leg and forces the hamstrings to pull the leg through the upswing of the cycling motion.[1]

Other isotonic exercises. A complete series of strengthening exercises (e.g., hamstring curls, squats, hip sled, standing toe raises, and seated toe raises) with traditional isotonic equipment can be added to the program.

Tibial internal-external rotations. Strengthening the tibial internal-external rotators can be accomplished through the use of surgical tubing or the Multi-Axial Ankle Exerciser (Multi-Axial, Lincoln, Rhode Island).[1]

Other activities

Swimming and pool activities. The buoyancy of the water allows the athlete to continue range-of-motion and strengthening exercises without placing undue stress on the knee. Pool activities are beneficial because the dynamic

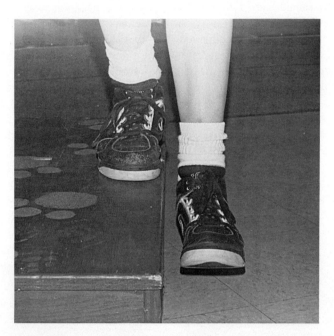

Fig. 17-3. Step-ups.

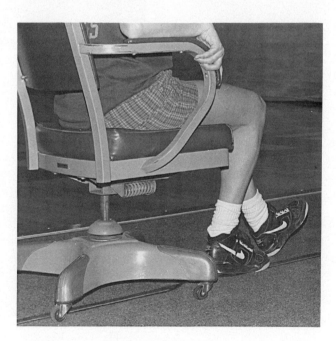

Fig. 17-4. Chair scoot.

resistance of the water aids in the strengthening of the supportive musculature. Flotation vests are valuable modalities for conducting pool activities, which can include walking, running, treading water, squats, tucks, front-back kicks, flutter kicks, and high steps.[24]

Proprioceptive exercises. Proprioceptive awareness is vital in the rehabilitation of basketball knee injuries. Barrack et al.[26] found that patients with instability following complete anterior cruciate ligament tears may experience a decrease in proprioceptive function of the knee.

The proprioceptive program should start with simpler activities and progress to more challenging exercises. A strong sport-specific component should also be added to many of the proprioceptive exercises. The following progression of proprioceptive-strengthening exercises can be started when the athlete can demonstrate functional readiness.[1,5]

- One-foot balancing with eyes open, then closed
- One-foot balancing with eyes open or closed while performing a quarter-squat (then adding rubber tubing resistance)
- One-foot balancing on minitrampoline
- One-foot balancing on minitrampoline while performing a quarter-squat (progressing to tubing) (Fig. 17-5)

- Two-foot unidirectional balance board
- Two-foot multidirectional balance board
- One-foot unidirectional balance board
- One-foot multidirectional balance board
- One- or two-foot multidirectional balance board with basketball-specific drills

These drills can include shooting, passing, and dribbling (Figs. 17-6 through 17-8). These basketball-specific drills should be performed to assure that proprioception becomes an "automatic" activity. Performing basketball drills helps to divert attention away from the balance component of the activity. Maintaining balance should take place without concentrated thought.

- Balance board walk: Walking across a series of balance boards helps to prepare the basketball player for coming down on other players' feet.

Additional functional exercises. As the rehabilitation program progresses, additional functional exercises may be instituted. However, functional testing should be performed before these drills are started. Muscular strength and power also should be objectively asssessed. This can be accomplished through high-speed isokinetic testing (180 degrees per second or faster). The criteria for initiating *controlled* functional drills may vary, depending on the type of injury

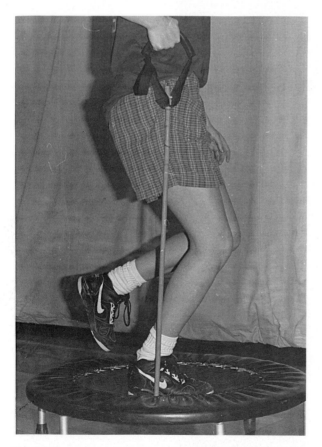

Fig. 17-5. One-foot balancing on minitrampoline with tubing quarter-squat.

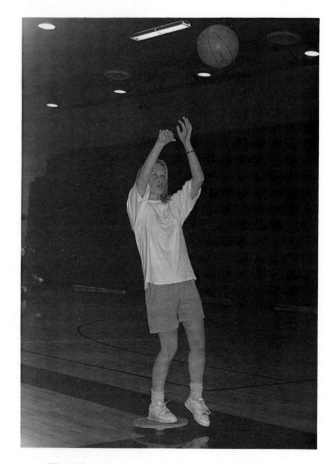

Fig. 17-6. Basketball shooting on balance board.

and length of time since the injury. The strength should be approximately 70% of uninvolved side.

Specific agility exercises

- Jumping rope: The athlete can start with two-foot jumping and progress to one-foot jumping. Other specialty patterns such as cross-overs and double jumps can be incorporated to add variety and increase difficulty.
- Slide board: Side-to-side movements, similar to a speed skater's motion, are effective for building eccentric control and lateral strengthening. These movements can be accomplished on one of several commercially available slide boards on the market today.
- Fitter (Fitter International, Calgary, Canada): This strengthening-proprioception device provides elastic cord resistance. Several different patterns can strengthen various components of the lower extremity musculature.
- Minitrampoline hops: Lateral strengthening can be achieved by hopping side to side between two minitrampolines.[5] This exercise can also be done between two foam-rubber high jump or pole vault pits.

Tubing agilities

- Side-to-side hops: Lateral agility hops can be performed while maintaining muscular control against the resistance of the heavy tubing (Fig. 17-9). The eccentric (return) phase of the exercise is critical in the execution of this activity.
- Backward running: Retro running can be performed with the tubing attached around the athlete's waist. The athlete then runs in place against the resistance of the tubing.
- Arc slides: The athlete slides in a shuffle fashion around the radius of an 8-foot semicircle with tubing attached around the athlete's waist (Fig. 17-10). This drill can also be used as a functional test.[25]

Sport-specific agilities and drills

- Forward and backward jogging and running: Start at approximately half-speed, progress to three-quarters speed, and then full speed. Backward running should not be neglected because it helps to strengthen the hamstrings.[6] In the later stages of rehabilitation, the line drill can be implemented. In the line drill, the athlete starts at the baseline, runs to the foul line, touches the line, and returns to the baseline. This procedure is repeated to the center court line, opposite foul line, and opposite baseline.
- Figure 8 running: A program of figure 8 running pro-

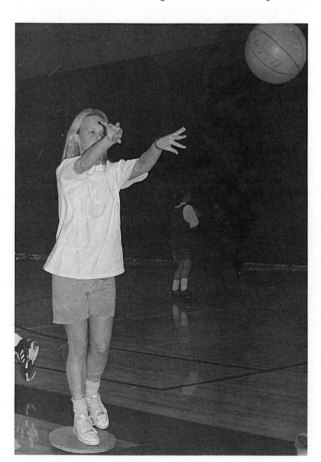

Fig. 17-7. Basketball passing on balance board.

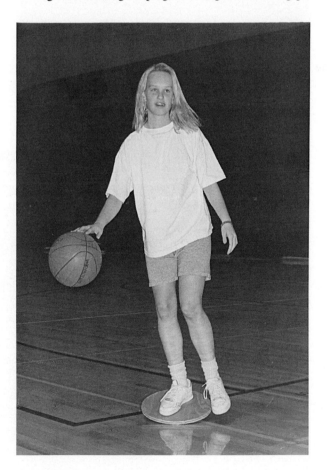

Fig. 17-8. Basketball dribbling on balance board.

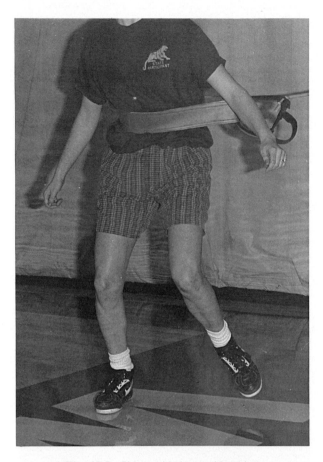

Fig. 17-9. Side-to-side hops with tubing.

vides functional, sport-specific conditioning and testing.[7] A progression begins with a lazy 8 pattern the length and width of a basketball court. The athlete starts at half-speed and gradually progresses to full speed. Once full speed is attained, the pattern can be downsized to half-court, then to the size of the key (Fig. 17-11).

• Progressive cutting on minitrampoline: These drills emphasize cutting, running, planting, and functional motor patterns with the minitrampoline.[1,5] The drill, viewed from above, should look like a wheel. The minitrampoline would be the hub and the run-throughs the spokes of the wheel. The wheel should be about 60 feet in diameter (Fig. 17-12). The athlete starts the drill by jogging or running at the desired speed and then cuts off the minitrampoline (Fig. 17-13). The minitramp provides a forgiving surface for the first step, then a change of surface for the plant off the trampoline. After coming off, the athlete continues to jog or run to the perimeter of the wheel, gradually decelerating to a stop. The athlete then laterally shuffles half the circumference of the wheel to the starting point of the next run-through. These start and stop points can be marked with tape on the floor.

Progression 1: Involved leg on minitrampoline, then uninvolved leg loaded with first step off the trampoline.

1. Straight ahead
2. 45-degree cut away from involved leg
3. 90-degree cut away from involved leg
4. 45-degree cut across involved leg
5. 45-degree cut across involved leg

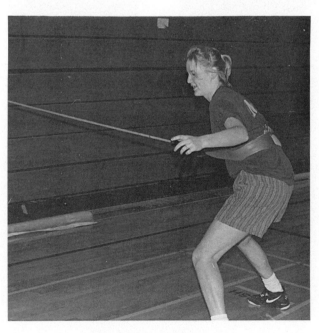

Fig. 17-10. Tubing arc slides.

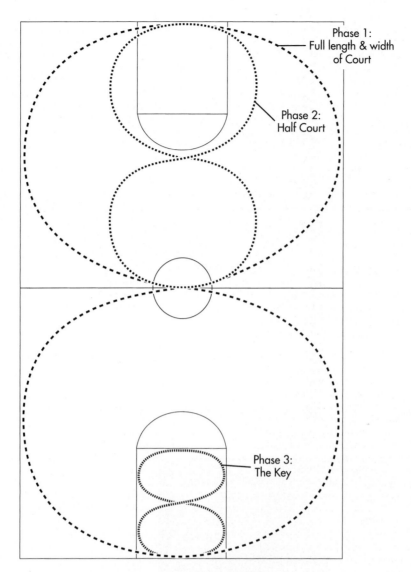

Fig. 17-11. Figure 8 jog/run drill.

Progression 2: Uninvolved leg on minitrampoline, then involved leg loaded with first step off the trampoline.

1. Straight ahead
2. 45-degree cut away from the uninvolved leg
3. 90-degree cut away from the uninvolved leg
4. 45-degree cut across uninvolved leg
5. 90-degree cut across uninvolved leg

- Basketball patterns: There are numerous sport-specific patterns that can be used in the functional rehabilitation of basketball knee injuries. Basketball coaches can be helpful in working with you on the specific drills. This type of drill should incorporate several basketball skills, including forward and backward running, lateral shuffles, carioca steps (cross-over steps alternating front and back), passing, and dribbling. Figure 17-14 illustrates a basketball-specific agility drill.

BASKETBALL-SPECIFIC CONDITIONING

Basketball is a sport requiring short bursts of anaerobic work, followed by varying degrees of recovery. It has been said that basketball is 85% to 90% anaerobic.[12,22] The basketball player also needs a limited degree of aerobic conditioning to maintain a high work output for a relatively prolonged period of time. Thus, aerobic (sustained energy system), anaerobic–adenosine triphosphate/creatine phosphate (short-burst energy system), and anaerobic–lactic acid (medium-burst energy system) all need to be addressed, in appropriate proportions, in a basketball-specific conditioning program.[22]

RETURN TO PLAY

The timing of return to full, competitive activity is highly variable among basketball players and is dependent upon

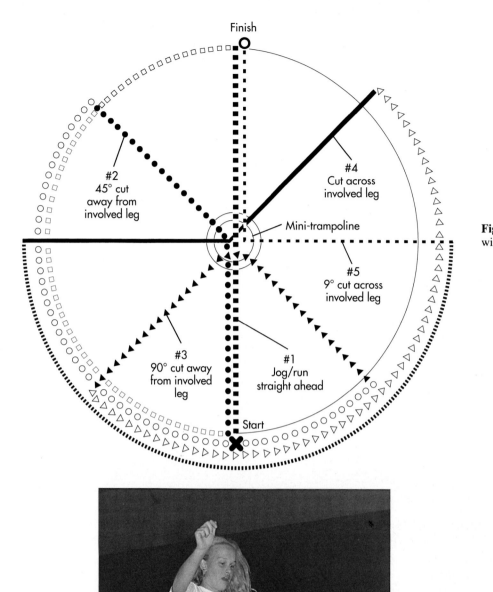

Finish

#2
45° cut
away from
involved leg

Mini-trampoline

#4
Cut across
involved leg

#5
9° cut across
involved leg

#3
90° cut away
from involved
leg

#1
Jog/run
straight ahead

Start

Fig. 17-12. Progressive cutting drills with minitrampoline.

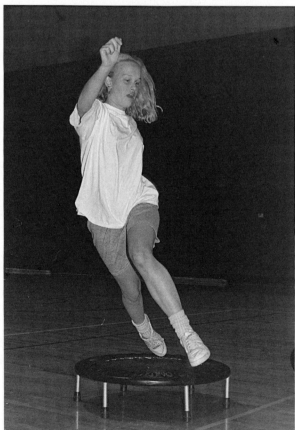

Fig. 17-13. Cutting off minitrampoline

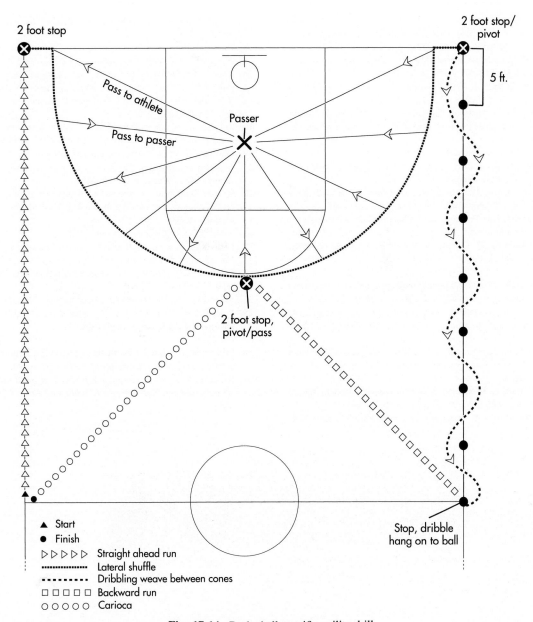

2 foot stop

2 foot stop/
pivot

5 ft.

Pass to athlete

Pass to passer

Passer

2 foot stop,
pivot/pass

Stop, dribble
hang on to ball

▲ Start
● Finish
▷ ▷ ▷ ▷ ▷ Straight ahead run
●●●●●●●●● Lateral shuffle
- - - - - - Dribbling weave between cones
□ □ □ □ □ Backward run
○ ○ ○ ○ ○ Carioca

Fig. 17-14. Basketball-specific agility drill.

many factors. Athletes can return to full activity when the following criteria have been met:[1]

1. Minimum strength level (quadriceps strength/body weight ratio) (see Table 17-1)
2. Better than 90% side-to-side strength on isokinetic testing
3. Adequate quadriceps/hamstring strength ratio (see Table 17-1)
4. Adequate proprioceptive awareness (tested by both subjective and objective means)
5. Adequate sport-specific agility
6. Functional in all basketball skills

This basketball-specific program emphasizes early motion, closed kinetic chain exercises, functional propriocep-

tive exercises, and sport-specific agility drills. As with any rehabilitation program, one cannot use a cookbook approach. This chapter serves only as a general outline for a basketball rehabilitation program, which may vary greatly from athlete to athlete. The protocols are athlete-driven and are designed to improve outcomes and, consequently, to enhance athlete satisfaction. The ultimate goal is to return basketball athletes to the court as quickly and safely as possible, without increasing the risk of reinjury.

ACKNOWLEDGMENT

Donni Reddington of the Wenatchee High School Photographics Department for her photography and darkroom work.

REFERENCES

1. Blair DF, Wills RP: Rapid rehabilitation following anterior cruciate ligament reconstruction, *Athletic Training* 26:32–43, 1991.
2. Caillouet H: Knee rehabilitation following anterior cruciate ligament injury, *Sports Med Update* 4:15–18, 1989.
3. Crochet DJ: Anterior cruciate ligament rehabilitation conceptual approach, *Sports Med Update* 4:11–14, 1989.
4. Fu FH, Woo SLY, Irrgang JJ: Current concepts for rehabilitation following anterior cruciate ligament reconstruction, *J Orthop Sports Phys Ther* 15:270–278, 1992.
5. Kola B: Personal communication, 1988.
6. Mangine RE, Noyes FR: Rehabilitation of the allograft reconstruction, *J Orthop Sports Phys Ther* 15:294–302, 1992.
7. Seto JL, et al: Rehabilitation of the knee after anterior cruciate ligament reconstruction, *J Orthop Sports Phys Ther* 11:8–18, 1989.
8. Shelbourne KD, Nitz P: Accelerated rehabilitation after anterior cruciate ligament reconstruction, *Am J Sports Med* 18:292–299, 1990.
9. Wilk KE, Andrews JR: Current concepts in the treatment of anterior cruciate ligament disruption, *J Orthop Sports Phys Ther* 15:279–293, 1992.
10. Hanrahan M: Preseason conditioning program using five-week station exercises, *Natl Strength Conditioning Assoc J* 10:26–29, 1988.
11. Hitchcock W: Individualized strength and conditioning program for women's basketball, *Natl Strength Conditioning Assoc J* 10:28–30, 1988.
12. Malone T: Team approach to care of basketball players. In Malone T, editor: *Basketball injuries and treatment,* Baltimore, 1988, Williams & Wilkins.
13. Moore JR, Wade G: Prevention of anterior cruciate ligament injuries, *Natl Strength Conditioning Assoc J* 11:35–40, 1989.
14. Morrison NL, Boyd LA: Proactively preventing knee injuries in women's basketball, *College Women's Basketball* November/December: 16–21, 1988.
15. Perry JE: Pre-season conditioning program for women's basketball, *Natl Strength Conditioning Assoc J* 7:62–63, 1985.
16. Chandy TA, Grana WA: Secondary school athlete injuries in boys and girls: a three-years comparison, *Phys Sportsmed* 13:106–111, 1985.
17. Wirtz PD: High school basketball knee ligament injuries, *J Iowa Med Soc* 72:105–106, 1982.
18. Zelisko JA: A comparison of men's and women's professional basketball injuries, *Am J Sports Med* 10:297–299, 1985.
19. Garrick JG: *Epidemiology of knee injuries in sports. In American Academy of Orthopedic Surgeons symposium on sports medicine,* Baltimore, 1985, Williams & Wilkins.
20. Gray J, Taunton JE, McKenzie DC: A survey of injuries to the anterior cruciate ligament of the knee in female basketball players, *Int J Sports Med* 6:314–316, 1985.
21. Koto T: Personal communication, 1988.
22. Chandler J: Goals and activities for athletic conditioning in basketball, *Natl Strength Conditioning Assoc J* 8:28–30, 1986.
23. Palmittier RA, et al: Kinetic chain exercise knee rehabilitation, *Sports Med* 11:402–413, 1991.
24. Kuland D: *The Injured Athlete,* Philadelphia, 1982, JB Lippincott.
25. Lephart SM, Perrin DH, Fu FH: Functional performance tests for the anterior cruciate ligament insufficient athlete, *Athletic Training* 26:44–49, 1991.
26. Barrack RL, Skinner HB, Buckley SL: Proprioception in the ACL deficient knee, *Am J Sports Med* 18:292–299, 1990.
27. Richardson T, et al: Improved rebounding performance through strength training, *Natl Strength Conditioning Assoc J* 5:6–7, 70–71, 1983.

Chapter 18

BASEBALL AND TENNIS

W. Ben Kibler
Jeff Chandler

Baseball and tennis are the two most prevalent "overhead throwing" or "upper body" sports. Most rehabilitation efforts have traditionally been directed toward functional restoration of the upper body injuries. However, knee injuries do occur and can have major implications for performance. This chapter addresses the local and distant effects of knee injuries; compares and contrasts the physiology, mechanics, and demands of the sports; and illustrates rehabilitation principles for functional restoration of the knee in these sports.

IMPORTANCE OF THE KNEE IN UPPER BODY SPORTS

The knee is of high importance in baseball and tennis, even though these sports are traditionally thought of as upper body sports. Injuries to the knee cause adverse effects locally at the joint but also may cause adverse effects at anatomic sites distant to the joint. Rehabilitation must be planned and implemented with both of these effects in mind.

Injury statistics are scarce in both sports (Table 18-1). A survey of the disabled list for major league baseball in 1990 and 1992 showed that knee injuries comprised 46, or 13.2%, of the 349 total injuries. It was the fifth-ranked anatomic areas, behind the shoulder, elbow, back, and thigh. Unlike the other anatomic areas, most of the knee injuries were due to macrotrauma. Knee sprains, meniscal tears, ligament tears, and direct contusions accounted for 31, or 67.4%, of the total. Patellar tendonitis, chondromalacia, or other tendonitis, all due to microtrauma, accounted for 15, or 32.6%, of the total. Statistics from the U.S. Tennis Association national teams show that knee injuries comprised 14, or 19.7%, of the 71 total injuries. It was the fourth most common anatomic area of injury, behind the shoulder, back, and ankle. Once again, macrotrauma injuries predominated, accounting for 10, or 71.4%, of the injuries.

Local adverse effects from an injured or incompletely rehabilitated knee in any sport relate to internal derangement, loss of stability, restriction of motion, loss of strength, or loss of quickness of reaction in the internal structures or external supporting structures around the joint. These effects are usually accompanied by pain, swelling, or both, which have their own effects on joint function. The sports of tennis and baseball place certain inherent demands on the knee, such as sprinting, jumping, bending, twisting, and start-stop movements. These demands require optimum flexibility, strength, strength balance, and agility from the knee structures. Rehabilitation must focus on how the adverse local effects interact with the inherent demands to compromise function.

In addition, however, the knee acts in each sport as an important link in the kinetic chain of throwing, serving, batting, or hitting ground strokes. Each of these chains represents a pattern of sequential events involving force generation, force transfer, and force absorption that allow the particular athletic movement to be performed with maximum efficiency. A typical kinetic chain for the tennis serving motion is shown in Figure 18-1. The characteristic parts of each link include a phase of force generation in the link *(A)* and a phase of force transfer to the next link *(B)*. Force absorption occurs in follow-through, mainly after the force has been applied. Abnormalities in the knee, which is located at the beginning of the kinetic chain, can have effects all along the rest of the chain.

In the kinetic chain of the tennis serve, force generation in the legs is by muscle contraction. The legs are fairly close together and move very little in the force-generation phase. Rotation of the body, mainly around the front leg, also contributes to force generation. The force is then transferred up through both legs to the torso and trunk. Force absorption in the legs is accomplished by jumping into the serve and by eccentric work of the knee muscles as the legs land in follow-through.

In the kinetic chain of the baseball pitch, force generation in the legs is mainly concentrated in the back or "push-off" leg. Rotation of the entire body around the back leg adds a significant amount to the generated force. The force is transferred not only to the torso and trunk for the arm but

Table 18-1. Injury statistics for baseball and tennis

	Baseball	Tennis
Total injuries	349	71
Knee injuries:	46 (13.2%)	14 (19.7%)
Macrotrauma	31 (67.4%)	10 (71.4%)
Microtrauma	15 (32.6%)	4 (28.6%)

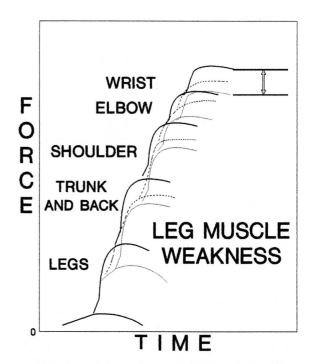

Fig. 18-2. Muscle weakness in the leg results in a net decrease in force produced in the serve or makes the smaller shoulder and arm muscles work more to produce the same force.

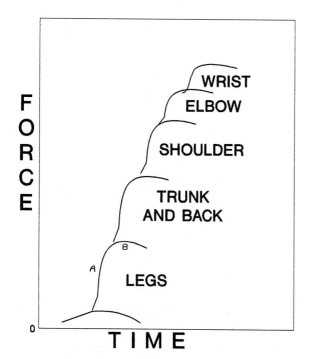

Fig. 18-1. The kinetic chain of the tennis serve. Each link serves to generate force and then stabilizes so the next link can work.

also to the front or "plant" leg by forward movement of the entire body. Force absorption in the legs is accomplished by eccentric work of the knee muscles in the front leg and by movement of the front knee into flexion.

Abnormalities of the knee can affect the kinetic chain in any of the phases of this process by "breaking" the normal sequence of the chain. If knee muscle strength is weak or imbalanced, insufficient force may be generated, as is shown in Figure 18-2. This could cause either decreased force delivered to the arm, with subsequent decreased pitch or serve velocity, or increased motor activity in other links, in an attempt to compensate for the force decrement. However, the laws of physics mitigate against this compensatory effort being safe or effective over a long period of time. Because the maximum force generated in a muscle is proportional to the cross-sectional area of that muscle, the smaller muscles of the kinetic chain links cephalad to the legs (closer

to the arm in the kinetic chain) have to work harder and closer to their maximum capacity to produce the extra needed force. This can lead to fatigue and overload. Also, the equations for the kinetic energy put into the athletic activity (K.E. = $\frac{1}{2}$ mass $\times$ velocity^2) and the force generated (F = mass $\times$ acceleration) are related to the mass of the object. Because all of the cephalad kinetic chain links have a smaller mass than the leg link, rotational velocities and accelerations have to increase in these links in the effort to provide more energy or force. These increases can enhance the tensile and torque stresses on the joints and muscles in the cephalad links, leading to possible injury.

Breaking the kinetic chain at the knee could also lead to alterations in force transfer. Internal derangement of the knee, such as torn menisci or ligament deficiency, by altering the movement of the instant center of motion would change the smoothness of knee motion. This would inhibit force transfer by rotation on the back leg in baseball or the front leg in tennis, and would not allow normal force transfer from the push-off leg to the plant leg in baseball. The athlete's usual response to this problem is to reduce the force generated caudad to the knee, which then causes decreased force to be passed cephalad. This pattern may also lead to reinjury of the knee if rotational forces are excessive, or to overload injury to the supporting structures of the knee as they try to accept the excessive loads.

Force absorption may also be altered in the plant leg in baseball or the front leg in the tennis serve or ground strokes.

Weak or imbalanced muscles or inflexible joints or muscles are not able to do the large amount of eccentric work necessary to smoothly absorb the high loads present in throwing or serving activity. The extra stresses are then applied to other areas of the kinetic chain, such as the calf, ankle, or back, or the athlete alters the athletic motion to decrease the load to the knee. These altered motions may increase stresses at the shoulder or back.

In summary, rehabilitation of the knee is important for the tennis and baseball player, not only because of the need to normalize the local effects of the injury but also to normalize the knee's role as a link in the kinetic chain of athletic activity.

DIFFERENCES BETWEEN BASEEBALL AND TENNIS: IMPLICATIONS FOR REHABILITATION

Baseball and tennis are usually considered together as "overhead throwing sports" and are treated virtually the same for rehabilitation purposes. A lot of the knee rehabilitation program content is the same for both sports. However, differences around the knee in these sports should be considered in the formulation of the sport-specific rehabilitation plan.

The differences in biomechanical demands between the two sports relate to the fact that there is much more movement in the knees, and more distance between the legs, in most kinetic chain patterns of baseball, compared with tennis.

In baseball the three main kinetic chains are for throwing, batting, and running (see box below). In throwing, as has been described, force generation is started through muscle contraction of the back leg, which then rotates and transfers force to the other leg. This leg moves forward and acutely flexes to absorb the force of the forward movement. Peak ground reaction forces on the push-off leg are reached in the early acceleration phase and are quickly passed up the chain to the arm and to the front leg (Table 18-2). In batting, once again, there is separation of the legs, with a striding or forward motion phase to transfer force from the back leg to the front leg. Smaller forces are present in batting as compared with pitching. Running in baseball is usually straight ahead, with a small amount of stop-start or pivoting action. The longest distance usually run is less than 150 feet, and there may be fairly long intervals between successive runs. The alactic anaerobic system is used almost exclusively as an energy source (Table 18-3).

In tennis, the four main kinetic chains are for serving, forehand, backhand, and running (see box this page). The service motion is carried out with both feet close together and no striding motion. Force generation is through contractions in both legs. There is some force transfer from the back to the front leg, and there is a larger rotational component to the force transfer, as the upper body rotates around the legs and trunk. Less knee flexion is noted on the front leg (Table 18-2). On the ground strokes, the legs are usually farther apart, but both legs are on the ground, and little striding is present. Running in tennis is characterized by many stop-start and pivoting movements. The longest distance run is less than 45 feet, but the running movements are repeated frequently with short intervals of rest. Once again, the alactic anaerobic system is the most commonly used energy source (Table 18-3).

In summary, there are differences in biomechanical and anatomic demands between the two sports that need to be considered when evaluating an athlete before initiating a rehabilitation program. There are more start-stop, pivoting, and rotational demands to the knee in tennis. This may account for the slightly higher incidence of macrotrauma injuries seen in tennis. Higher forces are generated in pitching compared with serving, and there is more need for leg-

---

Kinetic chains in baseball and tennis

Baseball kinetic chains

Pitching
Batting
Running

Tennis kinetic chains

Serving
Forehand
Backhand
Running

Table 18-2. Differences in leg activity in the kinetic chain of pitching and serving

	Pitching	Serving
Force generation	Back leg and leg rotation	Both legs
Foot placement	Apart	Together
Leg movement	Striding	Little
Ground reaction forces	Back leg	Both legs
Front leg	Flexion at knee, force absorption	Rotation at knee, force absorption

Table 18-3. Differences in leg activity in running between baseball and tennis

	Baseball	Tennis
Direction	Straight ahead	Start-stop, pivot, change of direction
Distance	30–180 feet	5–45 feet
Rest interval	Fairly long	Short
Frequency	Intermittent	Every point
Energy system	Alactic anaerobic	Alactic anaerobic

to-leg force transfer because of the striding motion. Knee injuries may play a large role in disrupting the kinetic chains of baseball and tennis and should be evaluated carefully with these effects in mind. How the injuries affect the chains depends on the sport, and rehabilitation should be implemented with this in mind.

Specific examples

There are no knee injuries or knee injury patterns that are unique to tennis or baseball. Treatment of the local effects of the knee pathology such as chondromalacia or torn menisci are the same as described in the chapters devoted to those entities. Emphasis in this chapter is on rehabilitation of these injuries in the context of the kinetic chain of tennis and baseball. The framework for evaluation outline in Chapter 8 is followed, and principles of rehabilitation are suggested. A complete and accurate diagnosis and an exercise prescription are formulated for two specific injuries. These are then used to implement a detailed rehabilitation plan.

Case I. A 24-year-old tennis player has a history of a twisting injury to the left knee, with clinical and arthroscopic diagnosis of a torn medial meniscus. It was repaired and immobilized for 4 weeks. The patient had good healing and resolution of the intra-articular injury and is ready to start formal rehabilitation.

Injury evaluation

Method of presentation	Acute macrotrauma injury
Clinical symptoms and signs	Negative McMurray's test
	No pain
	Slight swelling
	Generalized weakness in quadriceps, hamstrings, and gastrocnemius
	Generalized stiffness of knee joint, range of motion 0 to 40 degrees flexion
	Patella baja
Tissue injury	Meniscus, healed
Tissue overload	None
Biomechanical deficits	Quadriceps and iliotibial band inflexibility
	Quadriceps-hamstrings cocontraction deficit
	Muscle inhibition
	Patellar tightness
Subclinical adaptations	None

TENNIS-SPECIFIC REHABILITATION EXERCISE PRESCRIPTION

Initial phase. There is a lack of "acute" symptoms and signs at this stage of healing (see box on p. 223). However, all of the local effects resulting from treatment and subsequent immobilization have to be reversed to allow functional restoration. Medications and modalities may be helpful during this phase to relieve pain and inflammation. Release of the patella from any retinacular tightness should be done. Early restoration of normal neurologic control of muscle firing is important to retard atrophy and rebuild strength. A lightweight brace can aid in controlling swelling and giving support. The upper body and opposite leg should continue to be conditioned for strength and endurance. The two most important criteria for advancement to the next phase are the elimination of swelling and the ability to straight leg raise 8 lb. This indicates very little intra-articular abnormality and good neural control of motor neuron firing.

Recovery phase. Range of motion (ROM) should become normal in this phase. Vigorous, active ROM activities should be stressed. Likewise, vigorous strengthening can be pursued. Proprioceptive neuromuscular facilitation (PNF) techniques are excellent ways to challenge the muscles, but require individual attention by a skilled therapist. Single-plane strengthening is a prelude to multiple-plane patterns. Open-chain activities, in which the foot moves with a weight, can be used to isolate specific muscles. Closed-chain activities are thought to be more physiologic because the foot is fixed and muscle cocontractions are more common. This makes the muscles work as force couples to control the forces generated by the attached resistance. After muscle strength is obtained, tennis-specific arthrokinematic drills are instituted. Kinetic chain movement patterns that involve knee flexion and extension, hip and leg rotation around both legs, and gentle acceleration and deceleration movements such as lunges are started. These patterns start the integration of isolated muscles into purposeful tennis-specific activities. Other purposeful activities that may be started involve integrating the knee back into the kinetic chain. Easy ground strokes may be hit, and the service motion may be practiced. Both should be done with emphasis on smoothness of mechanics. Playing of points or matches should be delayed. Criteria for advancement include 75% normal strength, good quadriceps-hamstrings balance, and smooth arthrokinematic motion.

Maintenance phase. Tennis-specific muscle coordination patterns and tennis-specific functional progressions are the main goals of this phase. Multiple-plane motions, such as start and stop, slide lunges, and directional changes, simulate tennis movements. Plyometric drills, which employ relatively slow muscle lengthening followed by rapid muscle shortening, provide power and explosiveness for short bursts of activity. Examples of plyometric drills are "depth jumps," jumping off or over a platform at varying heights; "lunges," striding one leg forward, backward, or sideways, with rapid recovery to the starting point; repeated vertical jumps, with knee bends between jumps; and knee-chest or foot-butt drills, movement of the leg and hip so that the knee approaches the chest and the foot touches the buttock during running. Rope jumping and shuttle run agility drills also contain plyometric activity. Doing the agility and footwork drills with tennis racquet in hand simulates tennis-playing situations and improves neuromuscular control. Plyometric activities can achieve rapid and significant gains in power for performance, but are quite stressful to the muscle-tendon units. The potential for overload injury in these ac-

Exercise prescription for rehabilitation of acute macrotrauma meniscal injury—case I

I. Acute phase
  A. Goals
    1. Reduce effects of immobilization
    2. Retard muscle atrophy of entire lower extremity
    3. Neuromuscular control of the patella
    4. Maintain components of fitness
  B. *Effects of immobilization*
    1. NSAID 48-96 hours if needed
    2. Modalities 2-3 weeks
    3. Patellar mobilization
    4. Joint protection (brace/nonweightbearing)
    5. Range of motion
  C. *Muscle atrophy/neuromuscular control*
    1. Local
      a. Isometrics
      b. Straight leg raises (avoid adduction and abduction times 2 weeks)
      c. Biofeedback—patellar control
    2. Distant
      a. Open chain—nonpathologic areas (ankle, hip)
        1) Concentrics
        2) Eccentrics
  D. *Maintain components of fitness*
    1. Aerobic endurance for upper body
      a. Ergometer
    2. Strength for upper body and opposite leg
      a. Weights
      b. Machines
  E. *Criteria for advancement*
    1. Elimination of most swelling
    2. Level II pain
    3. Healing of injured tissue to allow mild tensile stress, ROM, weightbearing
    4. Straight leg raise 8 lb
II. Recovery phase
  A. Goals
    1. Reestablish nonpainful active and passive ROM
    2. Regain and improve lower extremity muscle strength
    3. Improve lower extremity neuromuscular control
    4. Normal arthrokinematics in single plane of motion
  B. *Range of Motion*
    1. Dependent
      a. Patellar mobilization
      b. Manual capsular stretch and cross-friction massage
    2. Independent
      a. Knee flexion and extension, active and passive
      b. Heel wall slides
      c. Bike and rowing machine
      d. Stretching—quadriceps, hamstring, iliotibial band, hip flexor, gastrocsoleus
  C. *Strengthening*
    1. Dependent
      a. PNF
    2. Independent single planes (avoid aggressive hamstring work after horn tear)

      a. Open chain
        1) Concentric and eccentric isotonics
        2) Isokinetics
        3) Tubing and free weights
      b. Closed chain
        1) Nautilus/Stairmaster
        2) Lifeline/tubing
        3) Free weights
  D. *Neuromuscular control*
    1. Balance board
    2. BAPS
    3. Fitter and slide board
    4. Minitrampoline
    5. Lifeline
  E. *Arthrokinematics*
    1. Joint mobilization
    2. Kinetic chain movement patterns, tennis-specific
      a. Flexion and extension
      b. Hip and leg rotation
      c. Acceleration and deceleration
  F. *Other activities*
    1. Practice service motion
    2. Hit ground strokes
    3. No intense play
  G. *Criteria for advancement*
    1. Nearly full active and passive nonpainful ROM equal to other side
    2. Quadriceps/hamstring ratio 66% and strength 75% of noninvolved side
    3. Static balance on one leg times 1 minute
    4. Normal and smooth arthrokinematics with single-plane motion
III. Maintenance phase
  A. Goals
    1. Increase power and endurance in lower extremity
    2. Increase normal multiple-plane neuromuscular control
    3. Tennis-specific activities
  B. *Power and Endurance* (avoid compressive and shear loads times 6–8 weeks)
    1. Multiple-plane motions
      a. Start and stop
      b. Side lunges
      c. Change of directions
    2. Plyometrics
    3. Anaerobic conditioning based on periodization
  C. *Neuromuscular control, multiple planes*
    1. Agility drills
    2. Footwork drills
  D. *Sport-specific training functional progression—tennis* Stage I
    1. Standing on one foot
    2. Jumping on two legs (forward, backward, sides)
    3. Jumping on a minitrampoline
    4. Jumping from stool, 40 cm (1 foot)
    5. Rope skipping on both feet

Continued.

Exercise prescription for rehabilitation of acute macrotrauma meniscal injury—case I—cont'd

 6. Balance board with both feet (forward, side to side, 45-degree angle)
 7. Balance board with both feet (catch tennis ball)

Stage II
 1. Rope skipping on one foot
 2. Jumping from stool, 40 cm, land one foot
 3. Jumping from stool, 80 cm, land two feet
 4. Hopping one foot (forward, backward, sides)
 5. Jogging in place
 6. Jogging around court
 7. Jog figure 8 (large and small)
 8. Jog figure 8 backward
 9. Balance board with one foot (forward, side to side)

Stage III
 1. Running with direction changes
 2. Carioca running
 3. Running 1 to 1½ miles
 4. Jumping: two-footed takeoff, land on one foot

Stage IV
 1. Anaerobic sprints with cutting on demand
 2. Split step
 3. Sport-specific training
　　 a. Motions
　　　　 1) Five-dot drill
　　　　 2) Hexagon drills
　　　　 3) Spider drills
　　 b. Skills
　　　　 1) Normal service
　　　　 2) Volleys
　　　　 3) Overheads
　　 c. Match conditions

IV. Criteria for return to play
　 A. Negative clinical exam
　 B. Normal ROM and flexibility equal to opposite side
　 C. Isokinetic strength 90% of normal side
　 D. Normal arthrokinematics in multiple plane
　 E. Pass functional exam—hop test, spider agility drill

---

tivities is quite high, especially if done when the musculoskeletal base is inadequate. Plyometric activity should be done only twice per week, should be done in the maintenance phase of rehabilitation, and is not recommended for athletes under 15 years of age. After muscle strength and coordination are optimized, functional progressions determine return-to-play suitability. Stages I and II can usually be mastered quickly. Stages III and IV require normal knee anatomy and physiology. Direction changes, repeated anaerobic sprints with cutting, and jumping and landing on the rehabbed leg should be done. Sport-specific training should emphasize the full spectrum of tennis strokes, and play conditions should be simulated.

Criteria for return to play. Normalization of all of the anatomic, physiologic, and mechanical alterations, with normal clinical exam, normal flexibility and strength, and normal running and hitting patterns.

Case II

A 30-year-old baseball pitcher with a 3-week history of pain, tenderness, and slight swelling at patellar insertion of patellar tendon on plant leg has symptoms that increase with running or in later innings of game. He had similar symptoms last season, but symptoms decreased after one injection and off-season rest. No therapy was done in the off-season. Symptoms returned in spring training and now interfere with pitching, with decreased velocity and inability to throw low strikes. The pitching coach notes that the player is pitching from a more upright position.

Injury evaluation	
Method of presentation	Acute exacerbation of chronic microtrauma injury
Clinical symptoms and signs	Pain
	Swelling
	Inflammation
	Abnormal performance, velocity, location, endurance
	Decreased knee flexion (0 to 100 degrees)
	Quadriceps weakness
Tissue injury	Proximal patellar tendon, tensile overload tendonosis with secondary inflammation
	Distal patella
	Fat pad
Tissue overload	Patellar tendon
	Quadriceps
	Iliotibial band
Biomechanical deficit	Quadriceps and iliotibial band inflexibility
	Quadriceps-hamstring strength imbalance
	Altered force couples
Subclinical adaptations	Shortened stride
	Higher ball release
	More wrist snap

Initial phase. The rather acute onset of this current problem, accompanied by signs of acute injury, suggests this injury may have resulted from macrotrauma (see box on p. 225). However, the history of previous similar injury, plus a detailed physical exam showing specific flexibility and strength alterations, reveals that this has resulted from a

Exercise prescription for rehabilitation of chronic microtrauma tendonosis—case II

I. Acute phase
  A. Goals
    1. Reduce pain and inflammation
    2. Reestablish nonpainful active and passive ROM
    3. Reverse muscle atrophy
    4. Maintain components of fitness
  B. *Pain and inflammation*
    1. NSAIDs for less than 2 weeks
    2. Modalities for 2–3 weeks
    3. Joint protection (braces and counterforce)
    4. Decrease activities
  C. *Range of motion*
    1. Dependent
      a. Cross-friction massage (end of acute stage or with chronic)
    2. Independent
      a. Stretching of quadriceps, hamstrings, and iliotibial band
      b. Knee flexion and extension, active and passive
  D. *Reverse muscle atrophy*
    1. Local
      a. Isometrics and gentle, pain-free straight leg raises
      b. Biofeedback patellar control
    2. Distant
      a. Open chain—nonpathologic areas (ankle, hip)
        1) Concentric
        2) Eccentric
  E. *Components of fitness*
    1. Aerobic endurance for upper body
      a. Ergometer
    2. Strength for upper body and opposite leg
      a. Weights
      b. Machines
  F. *Criteria for advancement*
    1. Eliminate most swelling
    2. Level II pain
    3. Healing of injured tissue to allow mild tensile stress
    4. Half-squat without pain, body weight only
II. Recovery phase
  A. Goals
    1. Regain and improve lower extremity muscle strength
    2. Improve lower extremity neuromuscular control
    3. Normal arthrokinematics in single plane of motion
  B. *Strengthening*
    1. Independent single planes
      a. Open chain
        1) Eccentric isotonics
        2) Isokinetic
      b. Closed chain
        1) Nautilus/Stairmaster
        2) Lifeline/tubing
        3) Free weights
  C. *Neuromuscular control*
    1. Balance board
    2. BAPS
    3. Fitter and slide board
    4. Minitrampoline
    5. Lifeline
  D. *Arthrokinematics*
    1. Kinetic chain movement patterns (baseball activities)
      a. Flexion and extension
      b. Striding and follow-through
    2. Protective bracing
  E. *Other activities*
    1. Short toss with stride—normal mechanics, no mound
    2. Batting
  F. *Criteria for advancement*
    1. Full active and passive ROM to other side
    2. Quadriceps/hamstring ratio 66% and strength 75% of noninvolved side
    3. One-leg squat 10 to 15 reps without pain
    4. Smooth arthrokinematics with single-plane motion
III. Maintenance phase
  A. Goals
    1. Increase eccentric power and endurance in lower extremity
    2. Increase normal multiple-plane neuromuscular control
    3. Baseball-specific activities
  B. *Power and endurance*
    1. Eccentric work
      a. Quadriceps
      b. Hamstrings
      c. Gastrocnemius
      d. Hips
    2. Plyometrics
    3. Backward walking against tubing
  C. *Neuromuscular control, multiple plane*
    1. Agility drills
    2. Footwork drills
  D. *Sport-specific training functional progression—baseball*
    Stage I
    1. Standing on one foot
    2. Jumping on two legs (forward, backward, sides)
    3. Jumping on a minitrampoline
    4. Jumping from stool, 40 cm (1 foot)
    5. Rope skipping on both feet
    6. Balance board with both feet (forward, side to side, 45-degree angle)
    7. Balance board with both feet (catch baseball)
    Stage II
    1. Rope skipping on one foot
    2. Jumping from stool, 40 cm, land on one foot
    3. Jumping from stool, 80 cm, land on two feet
    4. Hopping on one foot (forward, backward, sides)
    5. Jogging in place
    6. Jogging around field

Continued.

Exercise prescription for rehabilitation of chronic microtrauma tendonosis—case II—cont'd

7. Jog figure 8 (large and small)
8. Balance board with plant foot (forward, side to side)

Stage III
1. Running with no direction changes
2. Running 1 to 1½ miles

Stage IV
1. Sprint start, slow stop
2. Sprint start, fast stop
3. Jump on two feet, land on one foot
4. Sport-specific training
    a. Crow hop to the mound

    b. Crow hop from mound to half windup to full windup
    c. Stride on mound
    d. Full windup

IV. Criteria for return to play
    A. Negative clinical exam
    B. Normal ROM and flexibility equal to opposite side
    C. Isokinetic test 90% of normal and 65% quadriceps/hamstring ratio
    D. Normal arthrokinematics in multiple-plane motion
    E. Pass functional exam—hop test, normal stride

---

chronic microtrauma process. Symptom control is paramount early in the acute phase, with modalities of ice or other cold therapies, ultrasound, or electrogalvanic stimulation used with NSAID and protection by a lightweight brace. Painful activities, such as acute knee flexion or eccentric work, should be decreased. Range-of-motion activities should be started and maintained, to normalize quadriceps and iliotibial band (ITB) tightness. This is usually fairly easy to accomplish in this phase. As the pain subsides, gentle isometrics and biofeedback should be used to decrease quadriceps inhibition and gain control over patellar motion. Other anatomic areas should continue to be conditioned for strength and endurance. Important criteria for advancement include little pain and ability to half-squat with body weight.

Recovery phase. Achievement of adequate strength, power, and strength balance is the major goal of this phase. Because of long-standing quadriceps overload and inhibition, the neural firing patterns and motor unit recruitment patterns are disorganized, resulting in loss of force production and patellar control and decreased force absorption. Eccentric isotonics are emphasized in this process. This phase may be prolonged because of the slow return of muscle strength. Occasionally, muscle stimulation is necessary. Baseball-specific arthrokinematic movement patterns should be instituted carefully, for the movements of knee flexion and extension and leg striding and follow-through place tensile loading demands on the previously overloaded tissues of the quadriceps, and patellar tendon bracing with counterforce type braces may be beneficial in this stage. Low-velocity throwing for short distances up to 45 feet may be started, with emphasis on normal mechanics of weight transfer and arm motion. The pitches should not be from the mound. Batting, but no running, is allowed. Advancement is based on achievement of good quadriceps strength and normal quadriceps-hamstrings balance.

Maintenance phase. The front or plant leg in baseball pitching should have a better-than-average ability to do eccentric work in the acceleration and follow-through phases of throwing. Extra work in this area, along with the baseball

functional progression, is the main goal of this phase. Weightlifting, tubing exercises, and plyometrics should be directed toward eccentric emphasis. Stages I and II of the functional progression protocol are similar to those of tennis because they both emphasize control of balance and rapid alternating movements. The differences in the two sports show up in stages III and IV. The baseball program places more emphasis on straight-ahead sprinting and running and on landing on one foot. The sport-specific training would include "crow hopping," or taking short jumps on the back leg before throwing, and eventually striding off the mound with low-velocity throws. The final step of the progression would involve full windup, normal strides, and normal velocities.

Criteria for return to play. The criteria are the same as for case I: normal clinical exam, normal flexibility and strength, and normal running and throwing patterns.

SUMMARY

The knee is not often emphasized in rehabilitation of upper body sports such as tennis or baseball. However, knee injuries can have not only local but also distant effects on athletic performance in these sports because of the importance of the knee in the kinetic chains of upper body activities. Each sport exerts its own physiologic and biomechanical demands, and knee rehabilitation for that sport must be specific enough to address the differences and normalize the tissues to respond to the appropriate demands. The use of the injury evaluation framework can guide the evaluation process, help formulate an exercise prescription, and formulate a rehabilitation program.

REFERENCES

1. Kibler WB, editor: The kinetic chain of the throwing motion: a symposium, *Med Sci Sports Exerc,* in press.
2. Kibler WB, Chandler TJ: *Racquet sports.* In Fu F, Stone D, editors: *Sports injuries: mechanisms, prevention, and treatment,* Baltimore, Williams & Wilkins, in press.
3. Leach R: *Running injuries of the knee.* In Drez D, D'Ambrosia R, editors: *Prevention and treatment of running injuries,* Thorofare, N J, 1980, Slack.

Chapter 19

TRACK, CROSS-COUNTRY, AND LONG-DISTANCE RUNNING

David Apple

The running sports—track, cross-country, and long-distance running—are associated with a different spectrum of knee injuries than the contact sports. Knee injuries in running consist largely of inflammatory and overuse problems, in contrast to the grade II and III tendon and ligament injuries and the tears of menisci and other supportive structures seen in contact sports.

Common knee problems experienced by track and field or marathon runners in decreasing order of frequency are patellofemoral pain syndrome, iliotibial band syndrome, patella tendonitis, and popliteal tendonitis.[1] The most common cause of overuse injuries is reported to be increased training mileage. Shellock et al.[2] looked at the prevalence of meniscal abnormalities on magnetic resonance imaging (MRI) in asymptomatic runners. They found that 9% of asymptomatic runners had meniscal lesions on MRI, compared with 20% of asymptomatic nonrunners, and 16% in the general nonathletic population. Their conclusion was that running did not increase the likelihood of a meniscal problem. Two studies[3,4] have demonstrated no increased risk of developing osteoarthritis in runners versus nonrunners.

Fully understanding the rehabilitation of knee injuries in the running sports requires comprehending the changes that occur in the musculoskeletal system as the athlete attempts to improve aerobic functioning. Running aerobically strengthens the postaxial muscles more than the preaxial muscles. Selective strengthening of the hamstrings and the gastrosoleus group (the postaxial muscles) compared with the quadriceps and anterior tibial muscles (the preaxial muscles) causes a muscle imbalance that results in a shortening or tightening of the postaxial group, thereby decreasing the range of motion of the knee and the ankle. Eventually the loss of ankle flexibility may be sufficient to cause an athlete to run on a slightly flexed knee, thus creating unusual loading stresses on the ligamentous structures or the cartilaginous surfaces of the patella and femoral condyles.

Therefore, unless the athlete maintains flexibility and strength of the preaxial muscles equal to that of the postaxial muscles, a musculotendinous overuse injury may develop. An example of an inherent structural problem is an increased Q-angle, which affects tracking of the patella and can result in lateral patella facet problems. Another structural difficulty is malalignment syndrome, in which the hip has limited external rotation, the knee is externally rotated, the tibia is in varus, and the foot is pronated.

In order to understand how these muscle imbalances affect gait, it is necessary to review the gait cycle. With heel strike, the lower extremity is relatively externally rotated. As full weight is borne on the foot, the bulk of the weight is directed to the lateral border of the foot. With planting of the foot, weight is gradually shifted to the first metatarsal, and the tibia is internally rotated.

The subtalar joint must be in a locked position to provide stability for push-off; therefore, just prior to push-off, there is a transfer of weight to the midportion of the foot and a concomitant external rotation of the tibia. This repeated rotation during the gait cycle creates tension on the patella tendon, either distally on the tibial tubercle or proximally on the inferior pole of the patella. Some of these forces may be transferred through the patella to the quadriceps mechanism.

Therefore, in evaluating a runner's knee problem, the initial physical examination is very important, often more so than x-rays or other diagnostic studies. It is essential to observe the athlete for inflexibility and abnormal anatomic variants that may predispose her or him to injury.

For example, a common knee problem caused by loss of flexibility is the iliotibial band syndrome, in which the athlete typically complains of lateral knee pain toward the end of a run or when running downhill. Pain is produced when a tight iliotibial band moves from anterior to posterior in relation to the lateral epicondyle as knee flexion increases past 30 degrees. Treatment consists of stretching the iliotibial band as pictured in Figure 19-1.

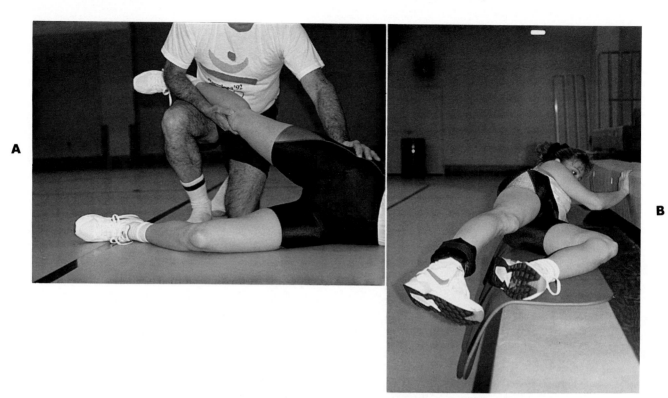

Fig. 19-1. Iliotibial band stretch. **A,** The iliotibial band is difficult to stretch without help. With the hip abducted, the helper fixes the hip, extends the leg, gradually adducts, at resistance holds for 10 to 20 seconds, and then repeats. **B,** The athlete can perform this stretch alone by lying with the back at the edge of a table in a similar position shown in Figure 19-6. The affected leg is allowed to adduct behind the leg resting on the table until the affected leg hangs below the table edge. This position is maintained for 10 to 20 seconds and relaxed. Repetition is done for 2 to 3 minutes.

Rehabilitation of the acutely symptomatic knee in a runner is similar to that of a nonrunner: RICE (rest, ice, compression, elevation), nonsteroidal anti-inflammatory agents, therapeutic modalities and exercises, and the judicious use of injectable steroids. In addition, muscle inflexibility or malalignment problems may also need to be identified and corrected before the injury resolves.

Unequal strength in the preaxial and postaxial muscles can, as mentioned earlier, result in inflexibility and create difficulties in the low back, knee, ankle, and foot, although the knee is most frequently affected. The inflexibility can be remedied by reducing the postaxial tightness and by strengthening the preaxial muscles (Figs. 19-2 through 19-5). The latter exercises should be done in the knee-sparing mode, that is, utilizing only the last 15 degrees of extension, as many of these athletes also have mild to moderate patellofemoral pain.

When performing stretching exercises, the athlete should hold the tension for 10 to 20 seconds, rest, and then repeat. Progression is obtained either by increasing the tension time to 30 to 45 seconds or by increasing the total stretch cycle beyond 2 to 3 minutes.

Strengthening activities can be done in various ways to achieve different results. If strength and endurance are desired, lighter weights and more repetitions are used. If strength and bulk are desired, heavier weights and fewer repetitions are used. To increase both endurance and bulk, heavier weights and more repetitions are used. Frequently, a period of rest from running is required to resolve the athlete's symptoms. Although running and stair-climbing should be avoided, the athlete may be able to participate in other forms of exercise such as walking, swimming, or using a stationary bicycle or rowing machine. In this way, the athlete can maintain strength and cardiovascular fitness without repetitive loading of the knee.

I have used the run-stretch program successfully for 15 years (see box on p. 232 and Figs. 19-6 and 19-7). It has been useful in the treatment of both mild and more significant knee injuries. The athlete begins by warming up with hamstring and gastrosoleus stretching exercises, walks 200 to 400 yards, and then jogs the same distance very slowly. A 30- to 45-second stretch of the hamstrings and gastrosoleus group follows, and then the cycle is repeated, at first for only 2 to 3 miles.

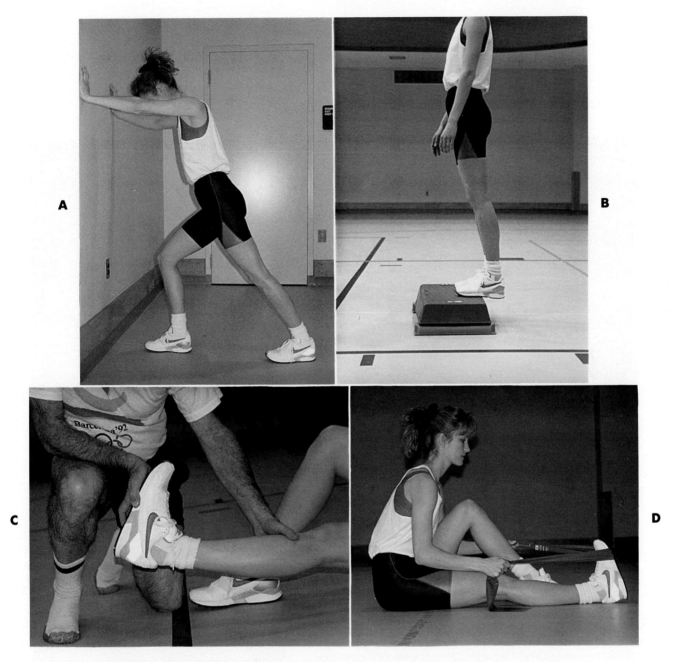

Fig. 19-2. Achilles tendon stretching. **A,** Wall lean. **B,** Standing step. Standing on a low stool or a step as if to do a back dive, allow body weight to dorsiflex foot to feel stretch in the gastrosoleus muscle. Hold for 10 to 20 seconds and release stretch by plantar flexing foot. Repeat for 2 to 3 minutes. **C,** Assisted stretch. Have another person dorsiflex foot with knee in extension until resistance is encountered, hold stretch for 10 to 20 seconds, and relax. Repeat for 2 to 3 minutes. **D,** Using rubber tubing or elastic strip, apply tension to dorsiflexed foot. Hold for 10 to 20 seconds and relax. Repeat for 2 to 3 minutes. This exercise may also be used to strengthen the anterior tibial muscles by plantar flexing the foot against the elasticity of the material.

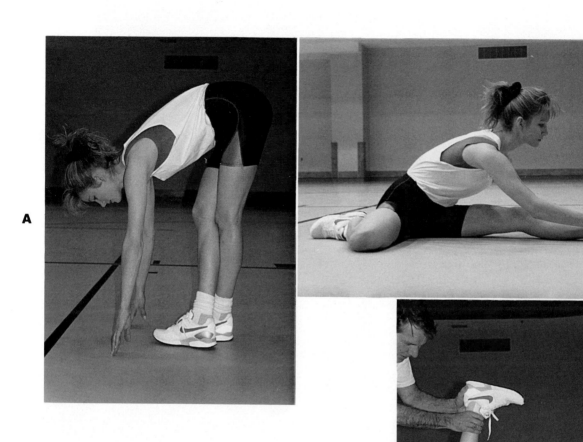

Fig. 19-3. Hamstring stretch. **A,** Cross-legged standing stretch. **B,** Hurdler's stretch. One leg is placed in full extension, and the opposite leg is abducted and externally rotated (or it may be abducted and internally rotated); the toes are touched or the nose is brought toward the knee until tension is felt in the hamstring. The tension is maintained for 10 to 20 seconds and relaxed. The procedure is repeated for 2 to 3 minutes; if the opposite hamstrings are tight, the leg positions are reversed. **C,** Assisted hamstring stretch. Another person grasps the athlete's ankle and, with the knee extended and the opposite leg extended on the floor, the hip is gradually flexed until hamstring tension occurs. Tension is maintained for 10 to 20 seconds, followed by relaxation. The process is repeated for 2 to 3 minutes.

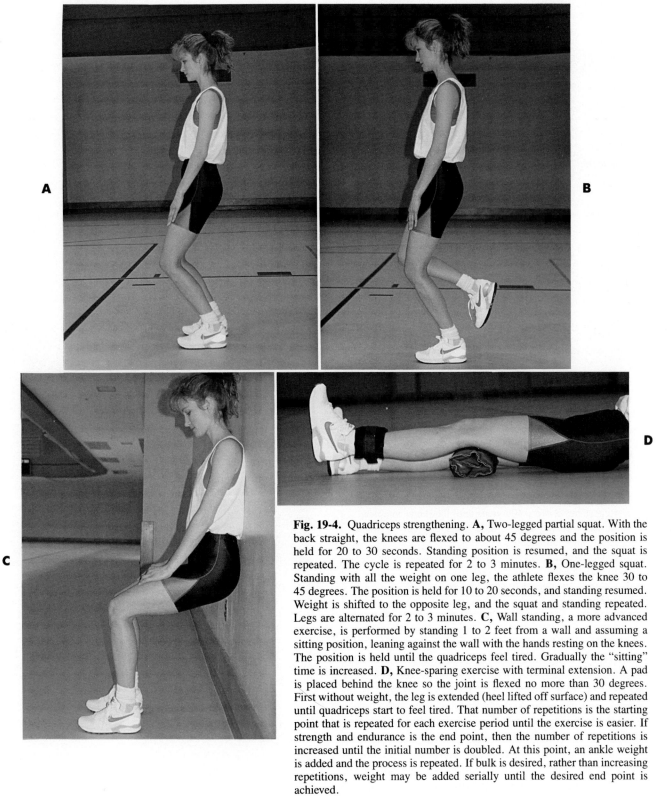

Fig. 19-4. Quadriceps strengthening. **A,** Two-legged partial squat. With the back straight, the knees are flexed to about 45 degrees and the position is held for 20 to 30 seconds. Standing position is resumed, and the squat is repeated. The cycle is repeated for 2 to 3 minutes. **B,** One-legged squat. Standing with all the weight on one leg, the athlete flexes the knee 30 to 45 degrees. The position is held for 10 to 20 seconds, and standing resumed. Weight is shifted to the opposite leg, and the squat and standing repeated. Legs are alternated for 2 to 3 minutes. **C,** Wall standing, a more advanced exercise, is performed by standing 1 to 2 feet from a wall and assuming a sitting position, leaning against the wall with the hands resting on the knees. The position is held until the quadriceps feel tired. Gradually the "sitting" time is increased. **D,** Knee-sparing exercise with terminal extension. A pad is placed behind the knee so the joint is flexed no more than 30 degrees. First without weight, the leg is extended (heel lifted off surface) and repeated until quadriceps start to feel tired. That number of repetitions is the starting point that is repeated for each exercise period until the exercise is easier. If strength and endurance is the end point, then the number of repetitions is increased until the initial number is doubled. At this point, an ankle weight is added and the process is repeated. If bulk is desired, rather than increasing repetitions, weight may be added serially until the desired end point is achieved.

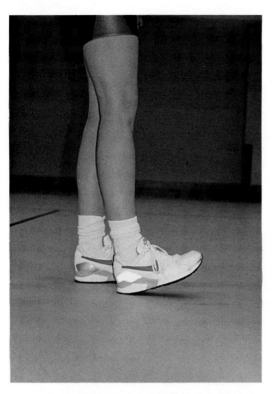

Fig. 19-5. Anterior tibial strengthening. Toe rises: dorsaflex foot and walk for 2 to 3 minutes on heels; repeat after rest period. Perform twice daily.

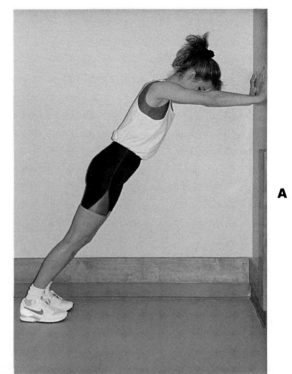

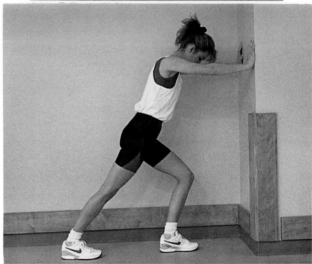

A

B

Fig. 19-6. A and **B,** Run-stretch program. Gastrosoleus stretch can be done with both legs on stretch or one at a time alternating. Stretch is performed by leaning toward the wall with the heel on the ground, the knee in extension, and the hip locked. When tension is felt in the gastrosoleus, the stretch is held for 10 to 15 seconds and then relaxed by pushing away from the wall. The exercise is repeated for 2 to 3 minutes and may be performed three times per day.

Run-stretch program

1. Prerun stretch of Achilles tendon using wall lean and of hamstrings using the crossed-leg stretch: 2 to 3 minutes total or 1 minute for each mile run, split evenly between Achilles and hamstrings.
2. Run 400 yards (one-quarter mile), stop, and repeat both stretches for 20-30 seconds each.
3. Repeat step 2 every 400 yards until the run is complete.
4. Stretch 1 minute for each mile run, split evenly between hamstrings and Achilles.
5. Every three or four runs, increase the distance by 200 to 300 yards.
6. Continue program until stretching only at the beginning and end of run.

As the athlete's conditioning improves, running is substituted for walking, and the distance is gradually increased; the athlete continues to perform stretching exercises every quarter of a mile. Every 5 to 7 days, the distance is increased, and the interval between stretching exercises is lengthened. Over a period of weeks, the athlete achieves the goal of stretching, completing the run, and finishing with stretching. This program has been very effective in alleviating the anxiety that many runners, especially long-distance and marathon runners, experience as they deal with musculoskeletal injuries.

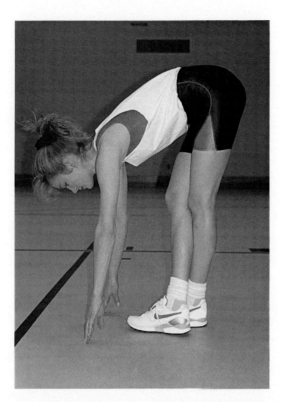

Fig. 19-7. Run-stretch program: hamstring stretch. The posterior leg is locked by the anterior leg. Forward bending is done until hamstring tension is felt. The stretch is maintained for 10 to 15 seconds and repeated for 2 to 3 minutes. Legs can be alternated, depending on which leg is tight or is symptomatic.

REFERENCES

1. Taunton JE, et al: Nonsurgical management of overuse knee injuries in runners, *Can J Sport Sci* 12:11–18, 1987.
2. Shellock FG, et al: Do asymptomatic marathon runners have an increased prevalence of meniscal abnormalities? An MRI study in the knees of twenty-three volunteers, *AJR Am J Roentgenol* 157:1239–1241, 1991.
3. Konladsu L, Kensen EM, Smderguard L: Long distance running and osteoarthritis, *Am J Sports Med* 18:379–381, 1990.
4. Lane NE, et al: Long distance running bone density and osteoarthritis, *JAMA* 255:1147–1151, 1986.

Chapter 20

GYMNASTICS

Mark E. Longacre
W. Michael Walsh

Rehabilitation of the gymnast's knee offers many challenges. In very few sports are loads so great on the knee. The gymnastic routine incorporates extreme twisting, impact loading, and explosive muscular contractions every few seconds. The length of the time spent practicing is much greater than for other sports. With the number of interscholastic gymnastics programs decreasing across the country (25,000 participants in high school and college in 1991), the number of participants in the National Gymnastics Federation continues to climb (48,821 competing and 87,123 noncompeting gymnasts in 1991). As the numbers become greater, so do the demands on the coaches and the risks for injury.

Multiple authors have documented the relationship between the length of time spent in the gym on a specific apparatus and knee injury.[1-4] Most injuries tend to occur between 30 minutes to 1 hour and 30 minutes into the workout and after 20 minutes on a single event.[1,4]

Multiple studies[1-5] have looked at which gymnastics routines tend to produce the greatest numbers of injuries; the floor exercise and balance beam are the top two. They did not specify which area of the body was injured. However, Linder and Caine[1] and Hunter and Torgan[5] have attempted to correlate which specific moves cause knee injuries. Garrick and Requa[3] stated that of 106 injuries studied, 10% involved the knee. Linder and Caine[1] stated that of 19 knee injuries encountered, 13 were acute and 6 were chronic. They go on to state that "tendinitis in the knee region was the single most frequently occurring overuse injury."

Andrish[6] in a review of records found 170 injuries related to gymnastics, of which 60% were related to the extensor mechanism and 17.6% related to ligament sprains of the knee.

The entire range of knee injuries is discussed throughout this book. It is not our intent to discuss the rehabilitation of each of these with respect to gymnastics. Suffice it to say that each of these injuries has occurred at some time in gymnastics. Instead, we use as prototypes (1) the most common ligament injury requiring postsurgical rehabilitation, anterior cruciate ligament (ACL) tear, and (2) the disorder most commonly treated in a nonsurgical fashion, patellofemoral problems. These principles can then be extended to any knee disorder in the gymnast.

ACL REHABILITATION

Many guidelines have been proposed for knee rehabilitation following ACL reconstruction.[7-10] Current rehabilitation focuses on the use of an accelerated protocol. This is especially beneficial to the athlete wishing to return to competition as early as possible. In many rehab protocols, return to sports-specific training occurs between 2 months[7] and 3 to 4 months,[9] with the return to activity phase at 5 to 6 months.[7,9]

It must be remembered that protocols based on time tables are only guidelines and often serve best as a motivational tool for the patient. The medical team (physician, therapist, trainer, coach) needs to use a criteria-based protocol that makes the patient meet specific outcomes prior to progressing.

Advanced functional exercises typically begin about 3 months after surgery. Prerequisites for entering this phase are (1) no patellofemoral irritation, (2) quadriceps recruitment to approximately 80% of the uninvolved side, and (3) control of effusion. Athletes begin with level running, advanced proprioceptive skills (i.e., BAPS, balance board with rebound thrower), two-legged rope jumping, half-squats and three-quarter squats, basic plyometrics encompassing the leg press, and box jumping. All plyometric exercises are discussed later in this chapter. Two-legged activities are then advanced to one leg. Special emphasis is placed on quality of performance. If proper control is not exhibited by the patient, he is not allowed to progress. During this phase, the gymnast can return to performing basic-level gymnastic skills. These sport-specific proprioceptive skills include arabesque (Fig. 20-1), side scale (Fig. 20-2), and lunges (Fig. 20-3). Again, emphasis is placed on the quality of the movements.

At approximately 5 months, provided (1) there is no increase in effusion, (2) lower extremity mechanics are appropriate with single-leg activities, (3) there is no patellofemoral irritation, and (4) the patient has advanced appropriately, the athlete is allowed to return to the gymnasium to begin apparatus work. Advanced plyometrics are also initiated at this time. Return needs to be in a safe, noncompetitive environment. Skills are practiced in a progressive format, and dismounts are not introduced until at least 9 months after surgery, provided vault and floor exercise skills are performed competently.

The uneven bars can begin at the earliest stages and involve all skills except the dismount. The balance beam begins with basic locomotive skills with minimal turns. The athlete needs to be able to perform arabesque turns, forward and backward swing turns (Fig. 20-4), and lunge and squat turns initially. Progression is then made into walkovers and cartwheels (Fig. 20-5) prior to performing handsprings. Advancement needs to be from the low beam (about 4 to 6 inches off the floor) on to the high beam with crash pads

underneath. Spotters must always be used initially to ensure safety and to restore confidence. Floor exercises should begin with locomotor skills (running, somersaults, leaps). Once they are mastered, advancement should proceed through round-offs, back handsprings, lay-out somersaults, and then a full twist, double twist, and double backs. The basic skill on the vault is the "punch" on the springboard (Fig. 20-6). Incorporating plyometric training prepares the knee for these stresses. Vault landings should be initiated into the pit, then onto soft mats, then to 4- to 8-inch firm mats, and finally onto a firm surface (Fig. 20-7). The Tsukahara maneuver is performed on the vault with either a quarter or half twist onto the horse, landing with the hands, with a back salto off the horse into the dismount. The Tsukahara maneuver should be attempted only after gymnasts are able to land on a firm surface with excellent control. Dismounts are the last skill attempted and progress from the pit to progressively firmer surfaces. They should be initiated from a handspring, adding in twists and flips if the patient is functionally able. Initial dismounts must always have the assistance of spotters. Hunter and Torgan[5] propose a need to reevaluate the scoring system for dismounts. Seven of 12 knee injuries they studied occurred during the dismount and

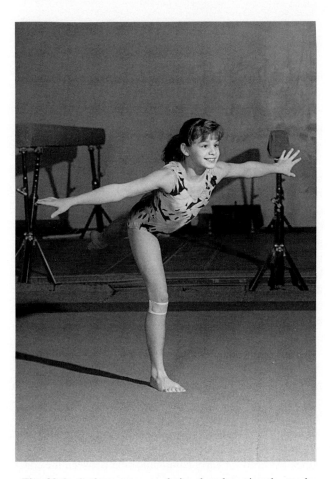

Fig. 20-1. Arabesque to a scale involves lowering the trunk.

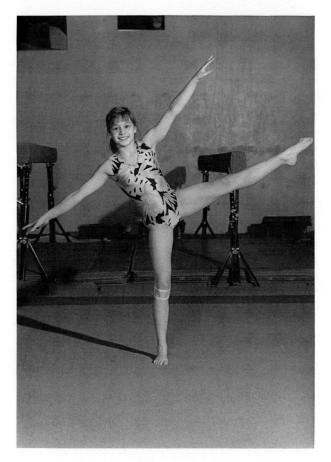

Fig. 20-2. Side scale.

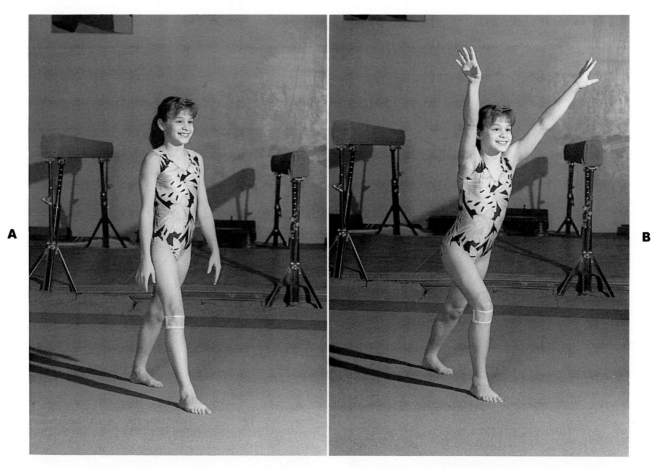

Fig. 20-3. Lunges.

all involved the ACL. Dismounts occur at the end of routines when fatigue is most evident. In an effort to reduce injuries, dismounts should be evaluated for accuracy rather than degree of difficulty.

It is standard practice following ACL reconstruction to place a patient in a functional, derotation brace. This is often done when athletes begin advanced functional exercises, more from the psychological aspect for the patient than actual biomechanical control. The role of the brace is to supplement the patient's neuromuscular efforts to control instability of the knee.[11] The effectiveness of these braces still remains controversial. In a study by Branch et al.,[12] comparison of two braces demonstrated that neither could control anterior tibial translation from a 20-lb force with the knee flexed to 90 degrees. Beck et al.[13] stated that as the force on the knee increased the effect of functional braces in controlling anterior tibial displacement decreased. Wojtys et al.[11] demonstrated that functional braces were better in controlling rotation than translation and results were better at 60 degrees of flexion than at 30 degrees. They felt that the brace provided a "restraining influence." Branch et al.[14] stated no significant differences in muscle timing were found between braced and unbraced subjects—suggesting that a

brace does not work by proprioceptively influencing the muscles to work sooner or harder.

Many studies exist regarding the biomechanical advantages of bracing; however, these studies continue to look at bracing under static conditions, use of ACL-deficient limbs, or the use of surrogate limbs. There is yet to be a study developed to look at ACL reconstructions undergoing dynamic stresses. There is no greater need for this information than for gymnasts desiring to return to their competitive levels. Subjective reports are currently being used to assess the role of the brace. Currently, functional braces cannot be expected to provide the necessary dynamic support to stabilize the knee during high loading activities. This further enhances the need for an appropriate rehabilitation program.

Concern exists on how many gymnasts, after undergoing ACL reconstruction, ever return to preinjury levels of competition. Often, the emotional demands of returning to such a stressful sport outweigh the physical demands. Investigation is needed into their rehabilitation program to find whether this is due to physical limitations or whether it is just lack of confidence by the gymnast. This further amplifies the need for early communication between the coach and the medical team in order to address these concerns.

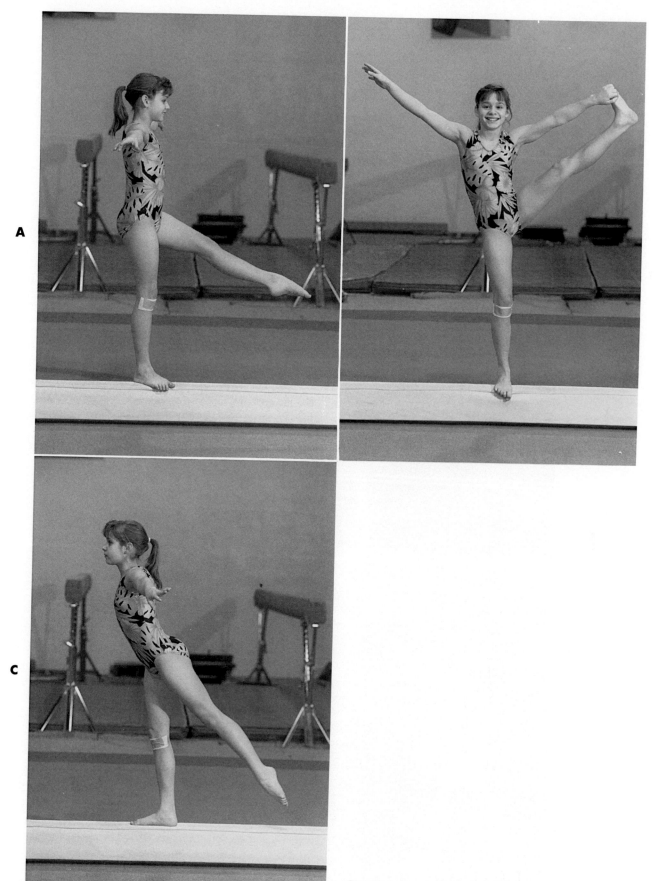

Fig. 20-4. Forward swing turn incorporating a Y-scale.

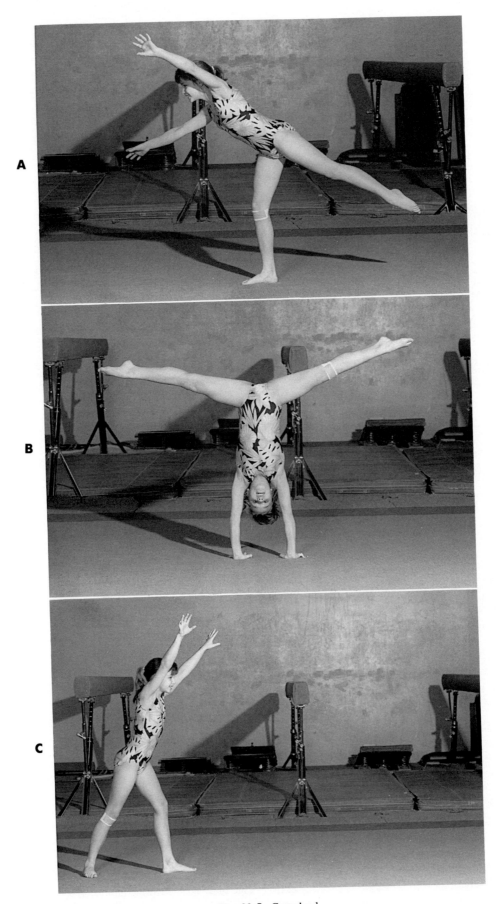

Fig. 20-5. Cartwheel.

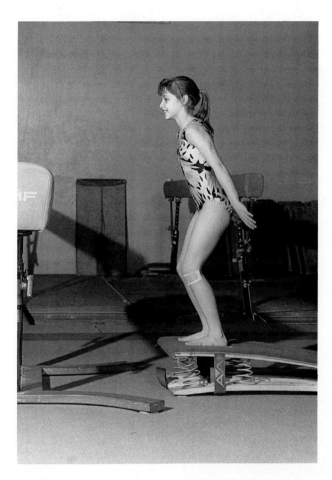

Fig. 20-6. The "punch" on the springboard, which must be performed for all vault routines.

PATELLOFEMORAL REHABILITATION

Although training for gymnastics can reach more than 20 hours per week[2] and is necessary to gain strength, stamina, and skills, it may be the cause of overuse and fatigue-related injuries. The most common overuse problem in the knee involves the extensor mechanism. Multiple structures and pathologies are encompassed under the term *extensor mechanism malalignment* (EMM), including the quadriceps musculature and tendon, patellar tendon, lateral retinaculum, patella, tibial tuberosity, synovium, plica, and infrapatellar fat pad. Abnormalities and pathologies in any of these anatomic structures can lead to patellar instability, Osgood-Schlatter's disease, fat pad impingement, tendonitis, chondromalacia, osteochondral fractures, or pathologic synovial plica.

The evaluation of EMM has been covered in great detail[15-17] and is outside the scope of this chapter. The treatment of these extensor mechanism problems has undergone drastic change in the past few years because of the advances made by Jenny McConnell, PT.[17] The McConnell program encompasses muscle reeducation through the use of biofeedback, lower extremity flexibility and strength, evaluation of lower extremity biomechanics with particular em-

phasis on the patellofemoral joint, and patellar-soft tissue taping. It is vital that biofeedback be used initially during rehab if muscle reeducation of the VMO/VL is necessary. Changing motor programs is difficult and often requires external feedback for the patient to master.

Flexibility, in general, is typically not a problem with gymnasts; however, patella mobility must be evaluated and incorporated into the treatment plan if necessary. Particular emphasis needs to be placed on evaluating hip external rotation strength. Weakness here tends to cause hip internal rotation upon weightbearing and a lateral pull on the patella, leading to abnormal tracking, abnormal alignment, and pressure on the patella. Foot biomechanics are often overlooked in the treatment of knee problems. Gymnasts with pes planus are harder patients to treat because they do not wear any footwear during training or competition. In their case, treatment typically involves taping of the arch. This has been quite successful in controlling foot biomechanics for short durations.

Taping plays a roll in breaking up the pain cycle, thus decreasing the inflammatory process and allowing athletes to remain in their sport. The role of taping has been proven to improve control subjectively and decrease pain from tendonitis, muscle imbalances (patella tracking), Osgood-Schlatter's disease, and fat pad irritation. Often, however, if a plica is present, it makes the symptoms worse. If taping has proven beneficial, the gymnast needs to use it as long as there are pain or control problems during activities. McConnell has proposed a series of closed kinetic chain functional strengthening exercises,[17] focusing on concentric-eccentric strengthening and control. The time for short arc quads and straight leg raises being the primary treatment has passed.

Typically, EMM disorders still allow for training and competition while patients are undergoing rehabilitation. Gymnasts are known to try to work through most chronic injuries, and it is important that these athletes be allowed to stay competitive without compromising their care. This is where the term *relative rest* comes in. By allowing them to exercise based on their symptoms, gymnasts may be more compliant with their rehabilitation.

With pain typically occurring in weightbearing positions with the knee moving from extension into flexion, an early return to uneven bars is not a concern. Dismounts should be held out of all routines, secondary to their high eccentric loading component, until gymnasts are pain-free with floor exercises.

Progression of weightbearing activities begins with basic gymnastic skills to evaluate muscular strength and control. Such activities include box jumping from various heights (Fig. 20-8), rolls with jumps, progressing stride leaps (Fig. 20-9), tuck jumps (Fig. 20-10), and squat turns from the ground onto the beam. For gymnasts to advance to the higher-level skills in their routines, these basic skills must not increase their symptoms.

Because of the demands placed on the soft tissue about

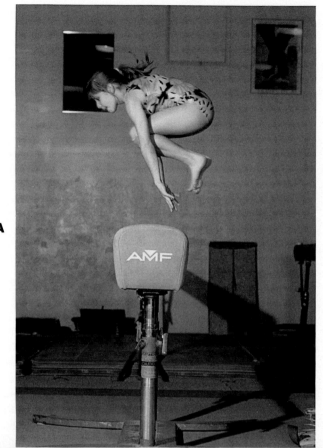

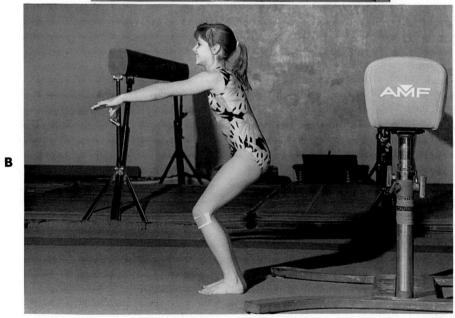

Fig. 20-7. The completion of the squat vault onto a firm surface.

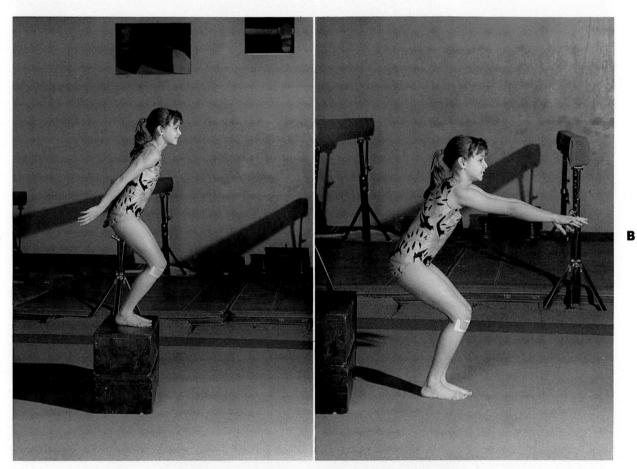

Fig. 20-8. Box jumping may be performed from various heights. Concentration is placed on the eccentric component upon landing.

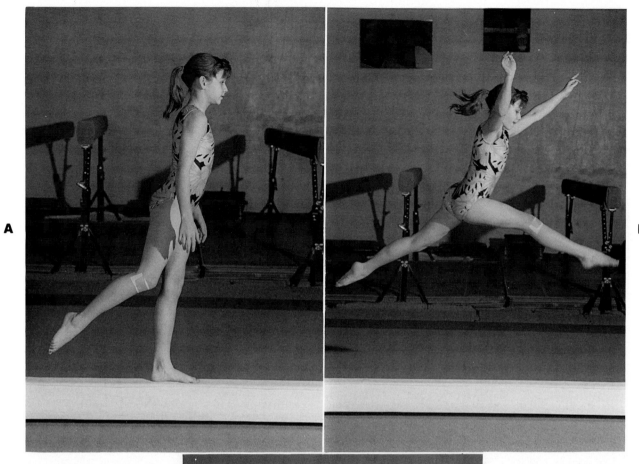

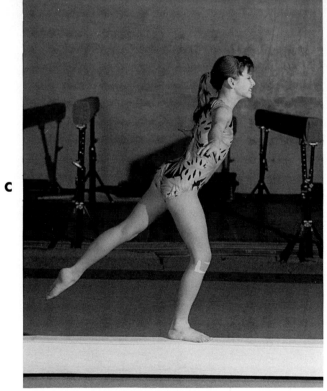

Fig. 20-9. Stride leaps.

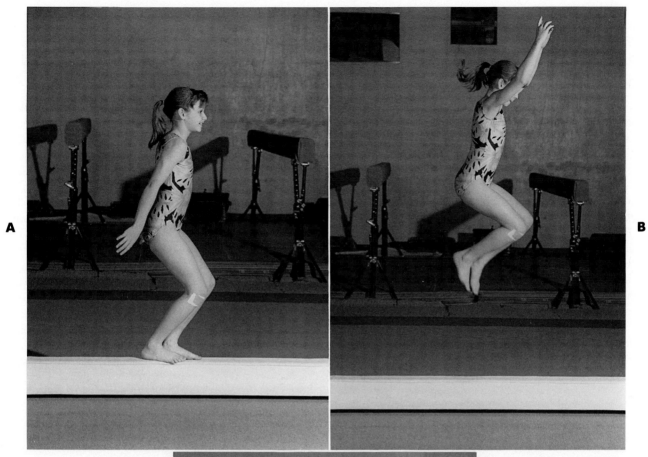

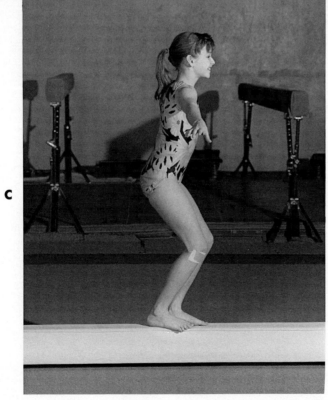

Fig. 20-10. Tuck jumps.

the knee, a portion of gymnasts' time needs to be spent on eccentric quadriceps strengthening such as lunges (Fig. 20-3), stepdowns (Fig. 20-11), and squats (Fig. 20-12), and plyometric training.

STRENGTH AND PLYOMETRIC TRAINING

Structured weight-training programs for gymnasts continue to gain popularity;[18-20] however, there is much controversy on how to conduct such a program. With most routines lasting from 5 seconds to 90 seconds, gymnastics is considered an anaerobic activity. Training needs to be based on overload principles, meaning high-intensity and short-duration exercises performed to fatigue. One consistent concept is the role of plyometrics for gymnasts.

Plyometrics theoretically bridges the gap between strength and speed and training muscles for explosive, powerful contractions. The control of movement is regulated by the central nervous system utilizing feedback from proprioceptors. The proprioceptors involved in plyometrics are the Golgi tendon organ (GTO) and the muscle spindle (MS). Their effects are to facilitate, reinforce, or inhibit muscle contraction.

The muscle spindle, located throughout muscle tissue,

is involved in the process termed *stretch reflex*. As the intrafusal (IF) muscle fibers are stretched (eccentric contraction), the muscle begins to contract with a corresponding inhibition of the antagonist muscle. The more rapid the stretch is applied, the stronger the muscle spindle fires with a corresponding contraction.

Because the GTO has an inhibitory effect on muscle, it is less sensitive to stretch. During a muscle contraction, the MS does not fire. The GTO is stimulated and has an effect of inhibition to prevent too much tension within the muscle.

Certain activities (e.g., depth jumps), however, can be used to raise the firing threshold of the GTO, thus improving the tolerance for increased stretch loads in the muscle. This provides better use of the elastic energy stored, resulting in a more powerful concentric muscle contraction.

There needs to be minimal rest between the eccentric and concentric phases of the motion to ensure full use of the elastic energy stored during the amortization phase (time spent between eccentric and concentric phases). Plyometric training appears to increase the possibility of storing greater amounts of elastic energy within muscles during eccentric work.

The specific drills can simulate the large ground reaction

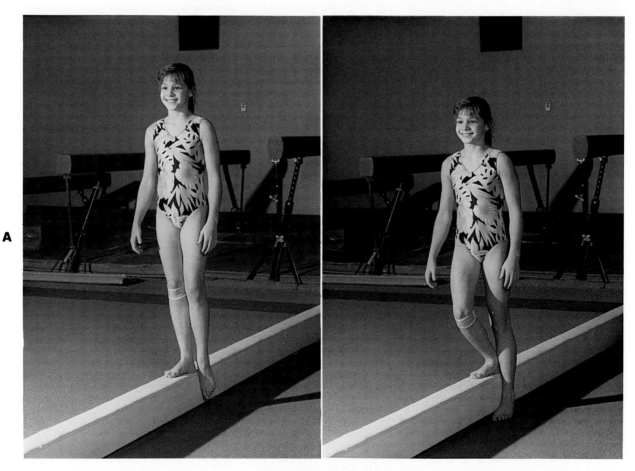

A   B

Fig. 20-11. Stepdowns may be performed off the low beam early in the rehab process.

forces that occur in gymnastics and improve the body's neuromuscular response to these forces.[18]

Plyometrics should not be done more than three times per week.[21] Repetitions should be kept at 8 to 10 but controversy ranges from doing 3 to 10 sets. Studies show drills are being done from a height of 0.5 to 3.2 m.[22,23] There appears to be no need to go over 48 inches in height. The potential for injury at the greater height outweighs the gains. The gymnasts get the greater heights with their activities.

Plyometrics are best performed during the preseason and off-season.[18,24] Sport-specific strengthening is still of greatest benefit, and gymnasts obtain increased loading forces during the season from the hours of practice on specific events.

Chu[24] describes a progression of plyometric exercises: jumping in place, standing jumps, multiple jumps and hops, in-depth jumps and box drills, and bounding exercises.

Jumping in place

1. *Squat jumps:* Athlete stands with feet a shoulder-width apart. Athlete squats to 110-degree knee flexion and explodes vertically. Upon landing, the process is then repeated as rapidly as possible.

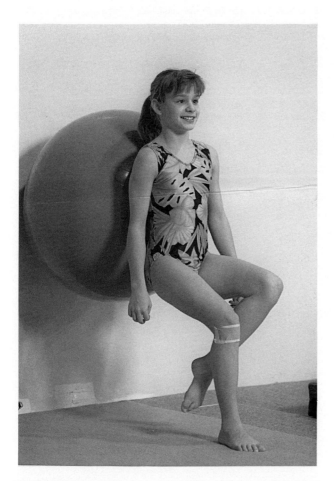

Fig. 20-12. Squats are used to simulate the high eccentric demands on the quadriceps muscles in a protective situation.

2. *Double-leg and single-leg tuck jumps:* The athlete springs from the ground until thigh or thighs are parallel with the ground, grasps the knee(s) with both hands, extends the legs to the ground surface, and repeats the movement.
3. *Cone jumping:* This activity requires use of 12-inch cones. The athlete stands with both feet together facing the cone, jumps vertically and forward over, and upon landing moves in the opposite direction.

Standing jumps

1. *Standing long jump:* Stand in place and plan to use arms to assist motion. The athlete squats down to achieve some elastic strength and leaps as far as possible.
2. *Cone jumping:* The athlete stands facing a cone approximately 18 inches away. Movement involves squatting, jumping, and landing.

Eccentric landing jumps

1. Athlete starts at a specified height above a landing surface, steps or jumps off onto the ground, squats to a predetermined depth, and maintains the contraction for approximately 3 seconds.

In-depth jumps

1. The athlete stands on both legs on top of a specified height, steps off with one foot leading, and lands on both feet, exploding immediately from the ground as rapidly as possible. Variations include, upon landings, jumping vertically onto another box; and jumping linearly out as far as possible.
2. The athlete stands as in the previous jump, but landing contact is with one foot. Then an immediate change of direction is made. Variations include stepping backward and then jumping back onto the same box; and, upon landing, jumping onto another box.
3. The athlete runs a few feet on a surface higher than the landing surface, drops down to the lower surface, and propels himself into single-leg hops.

Box drills

This exercise requires the use of five or six sets of low (12 to 18 inches) boxes spaced equally to allow for forward movement, landing, and transition.

1. The athlete performs an in-depth jump onto each subsequent box, repeating until all boxes are covered and ending with an explosive vertical jump.

Bounding

1. Bounding is performed with a running start in which the athlete bounds on a single leg over a specified distance and then initiates successive bounds when able.
2. Combinations: The athlete performs a rhythmic coordination of alternate and/or single-leg bounds (e.g., L-L-R, R-R-L patterns)

Plyometrics are vital following an injury that has required a prolonged relative rest period. They help to provide the proprioceptive input necessary for a return to gymnastics activities.

Basic plyometric exercises for both ACL and EMM patients should include the leg press, progressing from straight jumping to four corners to diagonals, box jumping and eccentric landing jumps at a 4- to 8-inch height, and jumping (such as the exercises described by Chu[24]).

Advanced plyometrics incorporate the in-depth jumps, bounding exercise, eccentric landing jumps, box drills (forward and backward), with height and intensity of the drill as symptoms and control allow.

CONCLUSION

Injuries are a natural part of gymnastics, and the knee is commonly affected. Most knee injuries are to the ACL and the extensor mechanism; however, with proper rehabilitation, gymnasts should be able to return to preinjury levels of competition. The gymnast's response to progressive treatment is the basis of return to activity. At no point should a time table be the basis for that return. Communication among the gymnast, coach, therapist, and physician is vital for recovery. Prevention, the key to injury management, includes using more spotters, having high-quality equipment, altering the amount of concurrent time spent on an apparatus, and, most important, altering dismount routines.

REFERENCES

1. Lindner KJ, Caine DJ: Injury patterns of female competitive club gymnasts, *Can J Sport Sci* 15:254–261, 1982.
2. Pettrone FA, Ricciardelli E: Gymnastic injuries: the Virginia experience, 1982–1983, *Am J Sports Med* 15:59–62, 1987.
3. Garrick JG, Requa RK: Epidemiology of women's gymnastic injuries, *Am J Sports Med* 8:261–264, 1980.
4. Weiker GG: Injuries in club gymnastics, *Physician Sports Med* 13:63–66, 1985.
5. Hunter LY, Torgan C: Dismounts in gymnastics: should scoring be reevaluated? *Am J Sports Med* 11:208–210, 1983.
6. Andrish JT: Knee injuries in gymnastics clinics in sports medicine, *Am J Sports Med* 4:111–121, 1985.
7. Shelbourne KD, Klootwyk TE, DeCarlo MS: Update on accelerated rehabilitation after ACL reconstruction, *JOSPT* 15:303–308, 1992.
8. Shelbourne KD, Nitz P: Accelerated rehabilitation after ACL reconstruction, *JOSPT* 15:256–264, 1992.
9. Wilk KE, Andrews JR: Current concepts in the treatment of ACL disruption, *JOSPT* 15:279–293, 1992.
10. DeCarlo MS, et al: Traditional versus accelerated rehabilitation following ACL reconstruction: a one-year follow-up, *JOSPT* 5:309–316, 1992.
11. Wojtys EM, et al: Use of a knee brace for control of tibial translation and rotation, *J Bone Joint Surg [Am]* 72:1323–1329, 1990.
12. Branch T, Hunter R, Reynolds P: Controlling anterior tibial displacement under static load: a comparison of two braces, *Orthopedics* 2:1249–1252, 1988.
13. Beck C, et al: Instrumented testing of functional knee braces, *Am J Sports Med* 14:253–256, 1986.
14. Branch TP, Hunter R, Donath M: Dynamic EMG analysis of anterior cruciate deficient legs with and without bracing during cutting, *Am J Sports Med* 17:35–41, 1989.
15. Walsh WM, Helzer-Julin M: Patellar tracking problems in athletes, *Sports Medicine: Musculoskeletal Problems—Primary Care* 19:303–330, 1992.
16. Walsh WM, Huurman WW, Shelton GL: Overuse injuries of the knee and spine in girls' gymnastics, *Orthop Clin North Am* 16:329–391, 1985.
17. McConnell J: *The advanced McConnell patellofemoral treatment plan course notes*, 1991.
18. O'Shea P, O'Shea K: Power endurance training for the female gymnasts, *NSCA J* 7:47–50, 1985.
19. Stern WH: Weight training for men's gymnastics, *NSCA J* 8:50–51, 1986.
20. Trifonov AG, Yessis M: Gymnasts also need slow strength, *NSCA J* 8:43–50, 1986.
21. DuVillard S, et al: Plyometrics for speed and explosiveness, *Scholastic Coach* 59:80–81, 1990.
22. Brzycki M: Plyometrics: a giant step backwards, *Athletic J* 66:22–23, 1986.
23. Lundin P, Berg W: A review of plyometric training, *NSCA J* 8:22–30, 1991.
24. Chu DA: Plyometric exercise, *NSCA J* 9:6–11, 1984.

Chapter 21

SWIMMING AND DIVING

Brian Gastaldi
Peter J. Fowler

In aquatic sports, knee injuries are commonly the result of overuse and muscle imbalance rather than trauma, which differentiates them from injuries in sports such as football, hockey, and basketball, where changes in direction, rapid deceleration, and impact expose the knee to ligamentous, capsular, or meniscal trauma. Despite the differing injury mechanisms, the principles of treatment are those that apply to the symptomatology of all soft tissue injuries, including absolute or relative rest (depending on the severity of the injury), topical application of ice to reduce local cellular metabolic activity, electrotherapy, nonsteroidal anti-inflammatory medication, transverse friction massage, acupuncture or acupressure, and massage. These modalities, which mitigate inflammation and promote tissue healing and regeneration, have been discussed in previous chapters, along with methods of planning and guiding effective rehabilitation programs. This chapter describes stretching and strengthening activities to restore muscle balance and allow a return to preinjury levels.

In aquatic sports, knee function is particularly influenced by remote anatomic structures. Evaluation of the degree of their involvement in the mechanism of injury should precede any rehabilitation regimen. Analysis of strength and flexibility ensures that appropriate muscle groups are treated.

CAUSES OF INJURY DISTAL TO THE KNEE

In diving, the activity is initiated by a ballistic, closed-chain event in the lower extremity as the athlete springs from the board or platform. Stiffness of the hindfoot, particularly the subtalar joint, defines the limits of calcaneal valgus (foot-flat position) and calcaneal varus (toe-raised position). A decrease in range of ankle motion can produce shortening of the triceps surae muscle complex and necessitate slightly increased knee flexion, which, in turn, increases the patellofemoral compressive force. Subtalar mobilization (Figs. 21-1 and 21-2), as well as a stretching program for both gastrocnemius and soleus muscles (Figs. 21-3 and 21-4), helps to restore full range of ankle motion,

lengthen the triceps surae, and reduce patellofemoral compressive forces.

CAUSES OF INJURY PROXIMAL TO THE KNEE

Tightness of the hip flexors, tensor fascia lata, iliopsoas, and rectus femoris is often a result of postural and functional patterns and may contribute to patellofemoral pain. Sahrmann's two-joint hip flexor test (Fig. 21-5) is a valuable clinical tool that identifies the involved muscle. Tightness of tensor fascia lata increases the tension of the iliotibial band, which may result in a lateral patellar tilt through lateral retinacular tightness. Tensor fascia lata or iliotibial band tightness may also cause iliotibial band friction syndrome. Symptoms of this are felt lateral to the patellofemoral joint. Iliopsoas tightness may cause an anterior rotation of the pelvis, resulting in passive lengthening of the hamstrings. If the knee remains in a minimally flexed position, patellofemoral compressive forces are often increased. In the springing stage of diving or the start or kick turn in swimming, the quadriceps, because of the anterior pelvic rotation caused by the tight iliopsoas, must work harder to produce full extension of the knee. This muscle imbalance may also adversely affect the patellofemoral articulation in sports such as water polo or synchronized swimming, where full knee extension is necessary. Rectus femoris tightness contributes to overall increased tension of the quadriceps, a synergistic group. This, in turn, can produce an increased patellofemoral compressive force.

In these situations, alleviating hip flexor tightness relieves knee pain. Figures 21-6 through 21-8 demonstrate proper clinical stretching techniques for tensor fascia latae, iliopsoas, and rectus femoris. Figures 21-9 through 21-11 demonstrate practical home stretching techniques for the same muscles. Patient compliance is essential to the effectiveness of such a program.

Several other tests may be used to complement and confirm the two-joint hip flexor tests.

- Ely's test (Fig. 21-12) for rectus femoris tightness

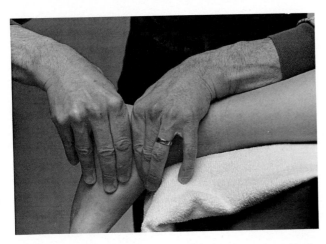

Fig. 21-1. Subtalar traction mobilization. The lower leg and talus are fixed against the treatment table by a steady downward pressure. The calcaneus is grasped from the side and behind and then moved distally in relation to the talus to produce traction in the subtalar joint.

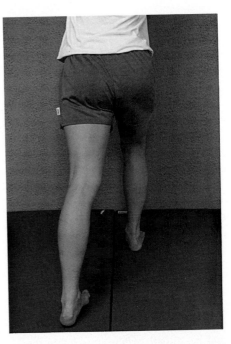

Fig. 21-3. Proper stretching for the gastrocnemius muscle. Because the gastrocnemius is a two-joint muscle, the knee is fully extended. The foot is slightly internally rotated to facilitate optimal stretch of the gastrocnemius. It is imperative that the heel remain in full contact with the floor. This stretching should be done in bare feet.

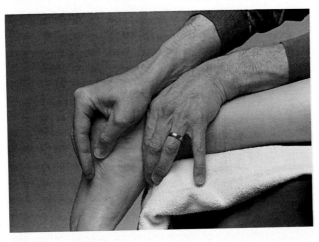

Fig. 21-2. Subtalar glide. The patient lies in a prone position with the leg resting against the therapist's hand on the table. A sandbag or foam wedge may be used to help support the foot and ankle. The lower leg and talus are fixed against the treatment table by a steady downward pressure. The calcaneus is gripped and moved distally in relation to the talus to produce traction of the subtalar joint.

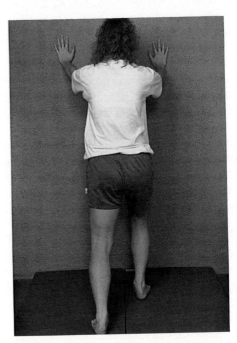

Fig. 21-4. Proper stretching of the soleus muscle. The soleus muscle is a one-joint muscle. The foot position is the same as for stretching the gastrocnemius, but the knee is bent.

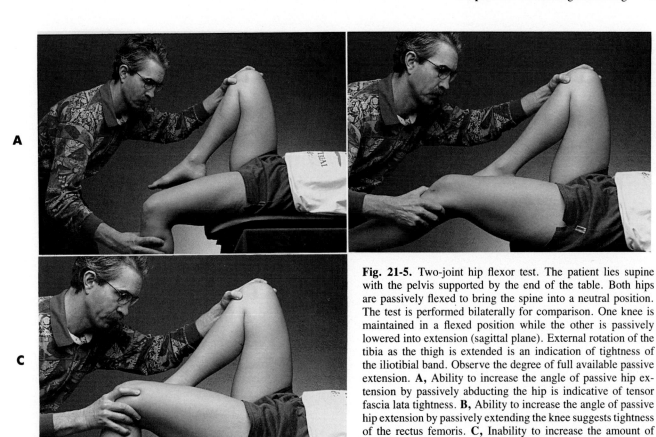

Fig. 21-5. Two-joint hip flexor test. The patient lies supine with the pelvis supported by the end of the table. Both hips are passively flexed to bring the spine into a neutral position. The test is performed bilaterally for comparison. One knee is maintained in a flexed position while the other is passively lowered into extension (sagittal plane). External rotation of the tibia as the thigh is extended is an indication of tightness of the iliotibial band. Observe the degree of full available passive extension. **A,** Ability to increase the angle of passive hip extension by passively abducting the hip is indicative of tensor fascia lata tightness. **B,** Ability to increase the angle of passive hip extension by passively extending the knee suggests tightness of the rectus femoris. **C,** Inability to increase the amount of passive hip extension is indicative of tightness of the iliopsoas.

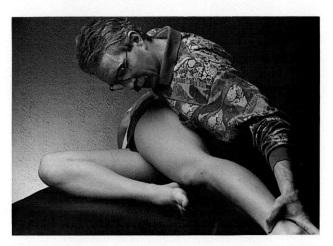

Fig. 21-6. Proper clinical stretching for the tensor fascia lata. The therapist stabilizes the pelvis and lifts the leg to passively extend the hip.

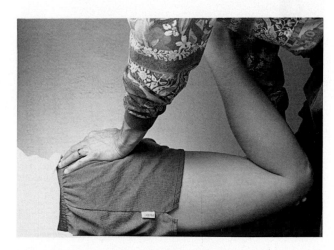

Fig. 21-7. Proper clinical stretching for the iliopsoas. The pelvis is stabilized and the knee is passively flexed.

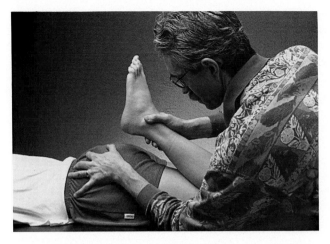

Fig. 21-8. Proper clinical stretching for the rectus femoris.

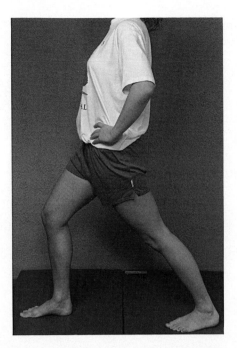

Fig. 21-10. Home stretching for the iliopsoas. This stretch is called the *fencer's lunge*. To achieve optimal iliopsoas stretching, the pelvis is tilted posteriorly.

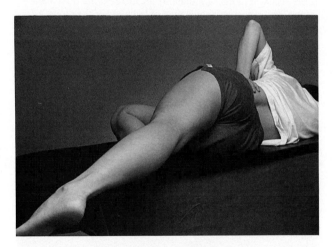

Fig. 21-9. Correct home stretching of the tensor fascia lata. The abdominal muscles must be contracted to stabilize the pelvis. The lower extremity then hangs passively in adduction, extension, and external rotation to stretch the tensor fascia lata.

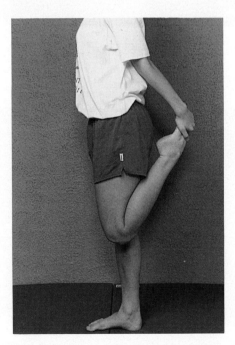

Fig. 21-11. Correct home stretching for the rectus femoris. Alternatively, the foot of the affected leg can be hooked on a bed or table. The thigh must remain vertical and the trunk upright.

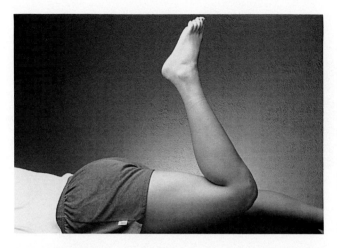

Fig. 21-12. Ely's test for rectus femoris tightness is positive if the patient has to arch the pelvis when actively bringing the heel towards the buttock.

- Ober's test (Fig. 21-13) for iliotibial band tightness
- The gluteal strength test (Fig. 21-14) for hip extensor positional strength
- The side-lying hip rotation test (Fig. 21-15) to determine or confirm tightness of the tensor fascia lata

Figure 21-16 demonstrates a supine pretzel stretch for patients who require stretching of the gluteal origin to relieve iliotibial band tightness. Figure 21-17 demonstrates a seated pretzel stretch and a standing pretzel stretch. Figure 21-18 demonstrates the proper technique for a self-administered stretch for the iliotibial band. As a result of hip flexor tightness, the short hip extensors become lengthened and consequently weak (stretch weakness). It is important to assess positional strength of the gluteal muscles.

In addition to stretching specific muscles to help restore flexibility to the lower kinetic chain, it is necessary to prescribe specific strengthening exercises. Strengthening for the gluteals has been demonstrated. The other specific muscle that is often weak and requires strengthening is the vastus medialis "oblique portion." The particular weightbearing

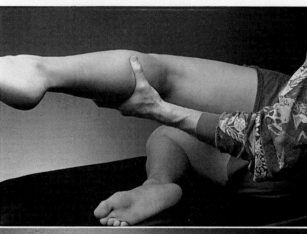

A

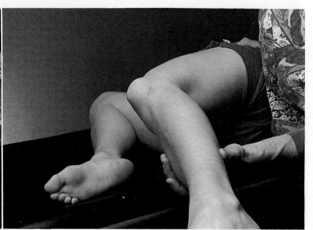

B

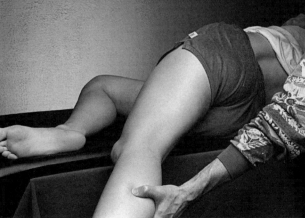

C

Fig. 21-13. The starting test for Ober's position, with the patient in the side-lying position, is demonstrated. The pelvis is stabilized to prevent compensatory lumbar side bending. The leg is brought into flexion followed by abduction (**A**), extension (**B**), and finally adduction. Inability to reach the horizontal passively demonstrates iliotibial band tightness. **C,** The most common error in using Ober's test is demonstrated. Trunk side bending of the lumbar spine is used to approach horizontal with the affected leg.

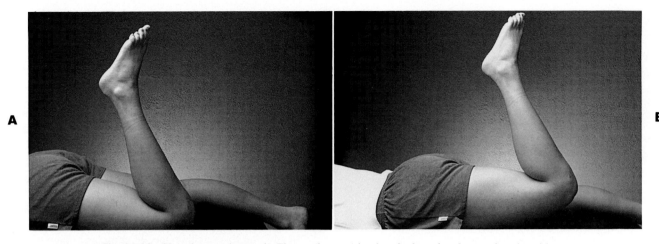

Fig. 21-14. Gluteal strength test. **A,** The starting position has the knee in a bent, relaxed position. **B,** Gluteals are used to lift the hip into extension without the use of the hamstrings. Side-to-side comparison should reveal weakness.

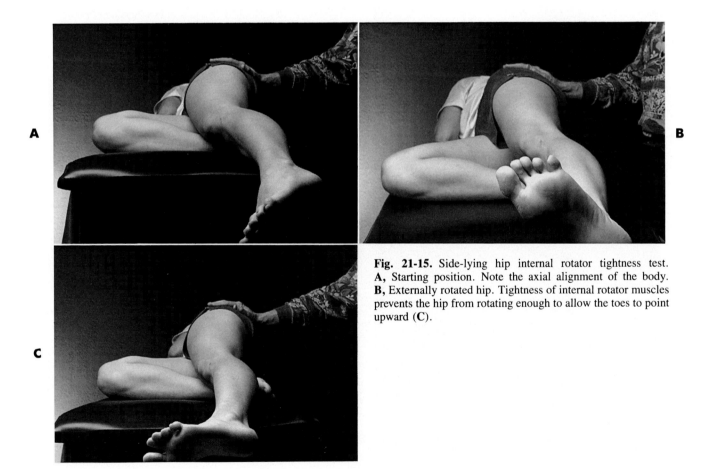

Fig. 21-15. Side-lying hip internal rotator tightness test. **A,** Starting position. Note the axial alignment of the body. **B,** Externally rotated hip. Tightness of internal rotator muscles prevents the hip from rotating enough to allow the toes to point upward (**C**).

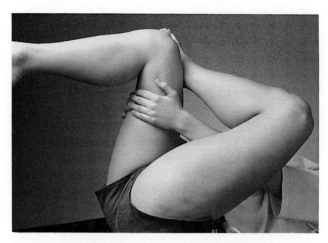

Fig. 21-16. Supine pretzel stretch for stretching the gluteal origin of the iliotibial band.

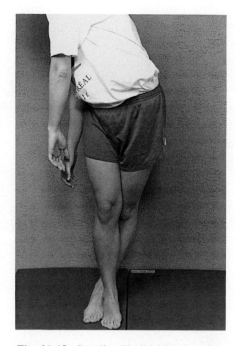

Fig. 21-18. Standing iliotibial band stretch.

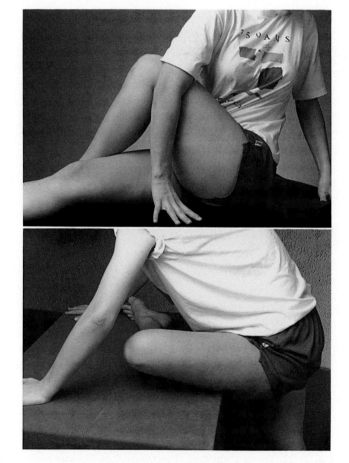

Fig. 21-17. Seated and standing pretzel stretches.

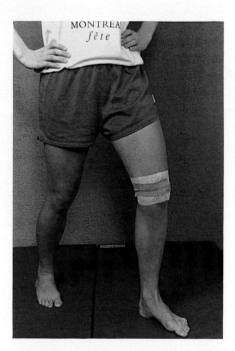

Fig. 21-19. Correct position for selectively strengthening the oblique portion of the vastus medialis. The foot is supine and fully weightbearing. The knee is bent so that the midpoint of the patella lines up vertically above the interspace between the second and third toes. The knee is flexed to where the view of the toes is just blocked by the knee. A McConnell taping may be necessary to reduce lateral patellar tilt and correct patellar alignment.

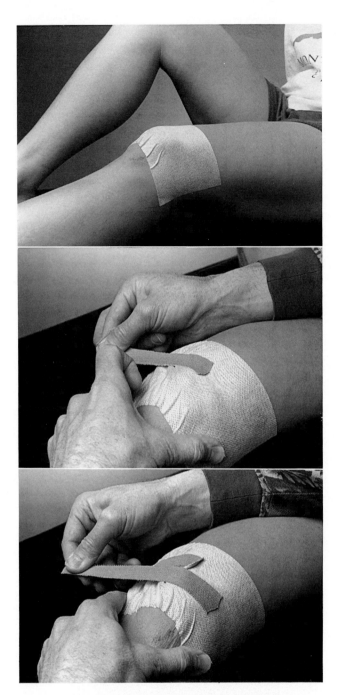

Fig. 21-20. Correct application of the McConnell taping to correct patellar tilt.

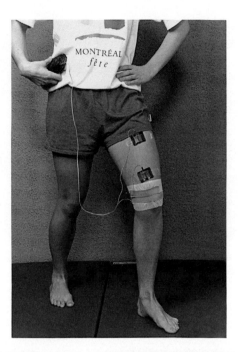

Fig. 21-21. Electrical muscle stimulation to augment vastus medialis contraction when performing quadriceps-strengthening exercise for patellar pain.

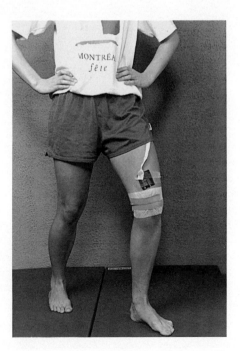

Fig. 21-22. Proper positioning of biofeedback to facilitate vastus medialis oblique contraction during quadriceps strengthening.

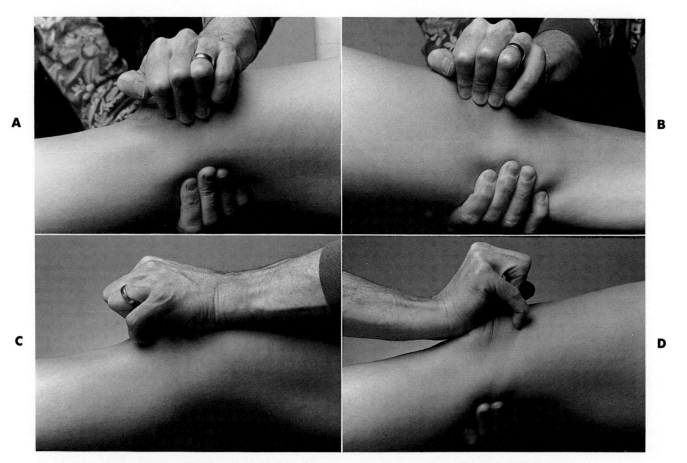

Fig. 21-23. Patellar mobilization for reducing soft tissue stiffness that may ensue following traumatic patellar injury or longstanding chronic problems: **A,** lateral glide; **B,** medial glide; **C,** caudal glide; **D,** cranial glide.

technique illustrated in Figure 21-19 demonstrates the synchronous function of the foot-ankle, knee, and hip-pelvic joints. This strengthening exercise helps to correct maltracking of the patella caused by poor quadriceps muscle balance. In a patient whose patella demonstrates marked lateral tilt, it may be necessary to use McConnell taping (Fig. 21-20) in addition to the vastus medialis strengthening exercises to help correct the tilt. Electrical stimulation may be used to augment the contraction of the vastus medialis (Fig. 21-21). Biofeedback can be effective in specifically training the vastus medialis (Fig. 21-22).

Stretching of the lateral retinaculum and ligamentum patellae can be achieved by specific patellar mobilization (Fig. 21-23). Quadriceps reeducation, strengthening, or both should be carried out immediately following the patellar mobilization. This will help to facilitate proper muscle balance and appropriate patellar mobility.

SUGGESTED READING

1. Evjenth O, Hamberg J: *Muscle stretching in manual therapy,* Alfta Rehab, 1980.
2. Gould J, Davies G: *Orthopedic and sports physiotherapy,* St Louis, 1985, Mosby–Year Book.
3. Hunter L, Funk J: *Rehabilitation of the injured knee,* St Louis, 1984, Mosby–Year Book.
4. Kaltenborn F: *Manual mobilization of the extremity joints,* ed 4, Oslo, 1989, Olaf Norlis Bokhandel.
5. Kapjandi IA: *The physiology of the joints,* vol 2, ed 5, Edinburgh, 1987, Churchill-Livingstone.
6. Maitland G: *Peripheral manipulation,* ed 3, London, 1991, Butterwork-Heinemann.
7. McConnell J: *McConnell patello-femoral treatment plan,* 1989.
8. Sahrmann S: *Imbalances and musculo-skeletal pain syndromes,* 1992.

SOCCER: PART I— CHARACTERISTIC KNEE INJURIES AND REHABILITATION

J. Andy Sullivan

Soccer, known as *football* throughout most of the world, is the most popular game in the world.[1] It is a sport that can be enjoyed by participants of almost all ages and levels of ability and can be played with a minimum of equipment and cost. It is an excellent activity for cardiovascular fitness and a recreational sport that can be carried over into adult life. Injuries are infrequent at most ages. The laws of the game are such that, although contact is possible under selected circumstances, intentional collision is strictly limited.

Supervision of rehabilitation of the knee and return to play requires that the physician have an understanding of the demands placed upon the players. Smodlaka has reviewed several of the articles concerning the cardiovascular aspects of soccer.[2] A typical game involves 90 minutes of nonstop play requiring high levels of cardiovascular fitness and endurance. It has been estimated by various studies that the players can run up to 15 k. This involves running at a slow pace interspersed with sprinting and walking. To head the ball requires leaping. Players are required to dribble the ball with their feet and to kick repetitively throughout a game. Heart rates can range from 150 to 190 beats per minute. The player must maintain or regain a high level of cardiovascular fitness to resume competition and be able to compete effectively.[2,3]

CHARACTERISTICS OF INJURIES IN SOCCER

Injuries among players at all levels of play, at all ages, and in both sexes have certain characteristics in common. The incidence of injury increases with age approaching that of senior players around 15 to 18 years of age.[4,5] Of all injuries, 50% to 84% involve the extremity.[4-8] In youth soccer players, 70% were in the lower extremity, particularly the knee (26%), and the ankle (23%).[8] For Danish players at all levels of play, the lower extremities were involved in 84% of injuries, with ankle sprain the most common (23%).[4] In a study of insurance claims made for high school soccer injuries, the lower extremity accounted for more than half, with minor strains accounting for 75%, and 49% of all costs. Knee injuries represented 11.7% of all injuries and 28.2% of medical costs paid by the insurance company.[7]

In a study of elite female players, there were 12 major injuries, of which 7 (58%) were knee ligament or meniscal injuries.[6] Seventeen percent of the players sustained a knee injury during the year while running, cutting, or kicking or in player contact.

In a study from Denmark, more than 20% of the knee injuries were caused by tackling.[4] *Tackling* in soccer is defined as regaining possession of the ball. The player tackles by challenging an opposing player to take away the ball. If this is performed correctly, the timing should enable the player to knock the ball away from the other player with minimal contact. At times, however, both players simultaneously contact the ball, which can result in a variety of knee injuries including sprains of the medial collateral and anterior cruciate ligaments. Another circumstance is that the tackle is less than perfectly performed so that the player attempting to tackle the ball goes above the ball and contacts the shin of the opposing player, which can cause strain to the knee or fracture to the tibia. The player possessing the ball can also trip over the tackling player and sustain a variety of injuries to the knee and ankle. Many anterior cruciate ligament tears occur in noncontact situations because of sudden force placed on the knee when the player plants a foot to pivot or change direction.

Engstrom et al analyzed three Swedish elite soccer teams to determine the significance of injuries and in particular whether they sidelined an elite soccer player.[9] A total of 49 of 60 players sustained 85 injuries. These were more likely to occur during the game than during training. Only 20% of the injuries required hospital facilities. One third of all injuries occurred in the knee, with overuse accounting for 35%, usually early in the season. Traumatic injuries were equally distributed between the first and second half with a predominance toward the ends of the halves, suggesting a potential fatigue factor. Roughly 28% of the traumatic injuries were a result of violation of the rules of the game. Eleven of these injuries required surgical intervention (7 ruptured anterior cruciate ligaments). At follow-up, 4 of 12 players with major knee injuries had returned to play at the elite level, with others transferred to lower divisions or still in rehabilitation.

Soccer players have been found in general to be less flexible than a group of nonplayers at the same age. No correlation is demonstrated between past injuries and existing muscle tightness.[1]

KNEE INJURY PREVENTION

In a study on the efficacy of injury prevention, there was a randomized trial of 12 teams, 1 team being given a prophylactic prevention program and the others serving as a control.[10] The prevention program consisted of the following principles:
1. Correction of training
2. Provision of optimal equipment
3. Prophylactic ankle taping
4. Controlled rehabilitation
5. Exclusion of players with knee instability
6. Information about the importance of disciplined play and the risk and prevention of injury
7. Supervision by a physician and a physiotherapist
There were 75% fewer injuries in the prophylactically treated team than in the control group.

PRINCIPLE OF REHABILITATION

Specific injuries require specific principles of rehabilitation, which vary not only from injury to injury but also from treating physician to treating physician. One need only peruse the literature regarding different rationales for postoperative management of anterior cruciate ligament or medial collateral ligament injuries to understand that this chapter could not begin to cover all of the various injuries and the patients' return to soccer.[11,12] The general principles are the most that can be covered.[3,13,14] Any rehabilitation program for return to soccer must emphasize the following:
1. The injury must be recognized early and appropriately managed.
2. The patient must maintain cardiovascular fitness.
3. The player should not return to sport until the involved extremity has regained full strength, full motion, and return of muscle bulk or loss of atrophy.
4. This requires the patient have near-normal or normal strength and sufficient cardiovascular fitness and endurance of the muscle group to achieve the power necessary to run and kick the ball.

5. The player requires sufficient return of function and proprioception, including agility in cutting, leaping to head the ball, sprinting, and knee control necessary for kicking and stopping in order to return to participation in the sport.
6. Last, these skills should be achieved in a pain-free manner with all signs of irritation and inflammation abated.

As with all injuries, rehabilitation begins with early recognition and proper management of the injury.[13] Significant injuries, when recognized, should be treated with rest, ice, compression, and elevation to prevent additional swelling and pain. Knee injuries comprise one of the most serious threats to soccer players. They should be evaluated early by an experienced physician so that an appropriate treatment and rehabilitation program can be instituted. This evaluation may prevent unnecessary damage that could occur if a player returned too quickly to practice or competition.

The second stage is maintenance of function to the greatest extent possible, both of the knee and of the cardiovascular system, in order to return to soccer. Cardiovascular endurance and rehabilitation from knee injury can be maintained by low-impact exercises such as swimming, cycling, or jogging in a pool with a buoyant vest. As weightbearing and motion return, the player can proceed to cycling, cross-country skiing, or using a cross-country simulator to promote a limited arc of motion while maintaining cardiovascular fitness and rehabilitation of hamstrings and quadriceps.

Minimizing immobilization with cast braces and orthotic devices can be beneficial in maintaining range of motion and muscle activity.[13] Early after injury, return to motion can be achieved by allowing the player to move the joint passively through a range of pain-free motion. This can be achieved with assistance or with gravity. The next stage is for the player to begin to move the joint actively through its full range of motion.

After return of motion, the player should be allowed to swim or jog in place in a pool with a buoyant vest or to use a stationary bicycle, rowing machine, stair-stepper, or other aerobic device. This activity promotes return of motion in the knee, return of strength, and maintenance of cardiovascular fitness.

The next stage is to progress to strengthening exercises. Immediately after the injury, the player should be taught isometric quadriceps and hamstring exercises to begin doing as soon as pain allows. Resisted motion is added to achieve return of strength, power, and endurance. Isotonic and isokinetic exercises should be added last, using the SAID principle (specific adaptation to imposed demands), with exercises to strengthen the athlete and allow a return to soccer. The principles of these various modalities and types of exercises are described in earlier chapters. Isokinetic techniques and exercises can be used at this stage to measure progress and for diagnostic testing. This quantifies the status of the program. Prior to return to play, plyometric exercises involving leaping can be initiated in that plyometric activity is involved in soccer in leaping, sprinting, and, at times, tackling the ball.

Running should not be begun until the injured extremity has regained two thirds the strength of the untreated leg, and pain and swelling have subsided. This should be confirmed by isokinetic testing. The earliest running should be either walking or slow jogging straight ahead. Only after this has been achieved and cardiovascular fitness has returned should cutting be allowed. Early kicking exercises should concentrate on touch of the ball and at very short distances against a wall with almost no power. Side dribbling, dribbling with the instep and outside of the foot, should be delayed until there is full knee control and adequate strength. Shots on goal should be prohibited until the program is nearing release of the athlete to return to practice and play. Power kicks and shots on goal require tremendous quadriceps power equivalent to leaping for rebounds in basketball. In one study, shots on goal were prohibited prior to warm-up because of the high association of injury.[10] Specific ball exercises should be given to strengthen the leg and improve agility.

Prophylactic bracing is discussed in another chapter. The only variation in soccer may be that no player is allowed to wear a device during a game that may be injurious to another player; therefore, the brace frequently has to be padded or covered to prevent any sharp edges from injuring an opponent.

REFERENCES

1. Ekstrand J, Gillquist J: The frequency of muscle tightness and injuries in soccer players, *Am J Sports Med* 10:75–78, 1982.
2. Smodlaka VN: Cardiovascular aspects of soccer, *Physician Sports Med* 7:59–67, 1979.
3. Smodlaka VN: Rehabilitation of injured soccer players, *Physician Sports Med* July:66–107, 1978.
4. Nielsen AB, Yde J: Epidemiology and traumatology of injuries in soccer, *Am J Sports Med* 17:803–807, 1989.
5. Sullivan JA, et al: Evaluation of injuries in youth soccer, *Am J Sports Med* 8:325–327, 1980.
6. Engstrom B, Johansson C, Tornkvist H: Soccer injuries among elite female players, *Am J Sports Med* 19:372–375, 1991.
7. Pritchett JW: Cost of high school soccer injuries, *Am J Sports Med* 9:64–66, 1981.
8. Schmidt-Olen S, et al: Injuries among young soccer players, *Am J Sports Med* 19:273–275, 1991.
9. Engstrom B, et al: Does a major knee injury definitely sideline an elite soccer player? *Am J Sports Med* 18:101–105, 1990.
10. Ekstrand J, Gillquist J, Liljedahl S: Prevention of soccer injuries: supervision by doctor and physiotherapist, *Am J Sports Med* 11:116–120, 1983.
11. Indelicato P, Hermansdorfer J, Huegel M: Nonoperative management of complete tears of the medial collateral ligament of the knee in intercollegiate football players, *Clin Orthop* 256:174–177, 1990.
12. Podesta L, et al: Rationale and protocol for postoperative anterior cruciate ligament rehabilitation, *Clin Orthop* 257:262–273, 1990.
13. Eriksson E: Sports injuries of the knee ligaments: their diagnosis, treatment, rehabilitation, and prevention, *Med Sci Sports* 8:133–144, 1976.
14. Larson RL, Grana WA: *The knee: form, function, pathology and treatment,* Philadelphia, 1993, WB Saunders.

SOCCER: PART II–FUNCTIONAL KNEE REHABILITATION

Troy McIntosh
Laurie Tis

One of the most challenging aspects of the rehabilitation process, the final phase of rehabilitation, is preparing an athlete for return to competition. The athlete must be ready both physically and psychologically before returning to competition. In addition to regaining range of motion, strength, and proprioceptive skills, a complete rehabilitation program also allows the athlete to regain confidence in the injured limb and progressively increase training and sport-specific skills.

The beginning stages of the rehabilitation process have been outlined in a previous chapter. By the final stage of rehabilitation, we assume the athlete has no present or recurring swelling, has achieved full range of motion, and has 75% of strength compared with the uninvolved extremity. The athlete has begun a slow progression of jogging to light running and is able to achieve 50% to 60% intensity over a distance of 2 to 3 miles without increasing symptoms or aggravating the injury.

The rehabilitation process at this point is much like building a pyramid. It begins with a strong base and progresses to more intricate additions until the final block is added and the pyramid is complete (Fig. 22-1). By following this basic format, the athletic trainer or physical therapist allows the athlete ample time to adapt to new training loads and intensities, to prepare mentally for return to competition, and to gain confidence in the injured limb. This process makes the transition to competition smooth and atraumatic.

Creativity and knowledge of soccer skills are necessary for both the physician and the athletic trainer or physical therapist who prepare the athlete for return to competition. There are many ways to adapt the rehabilitation process for the injured player. Maintaining an open mind and being as creative as facilities and equipment allow help to maximize the athlete's success.

This chapter discusses the basic principles of a functional rehabilitation pyramid (Fig. 22-1) as they apply to the soccer player who sustains a knee injury. *Functional rehabilitation* is defined as those aspects of the total rehabilitation process that most directly relate to preparing the athlete for return to competition. Throughout the chapter, there are figures and tables describing exercises related to each stage, as well as hints to aid in progressing the athlete safely up the pyramid.

STAGE I: BUILDING THE FOUNDATION

At the foundation, the emphasis is on building the player's chief allies in the defense against injury and reinjury, that is, on increasing muscular strength, increasing or maintaining cardiovascular fitness, and regaining proper running mechanics and proprioceptive skills. Begin the rehabilitation protocol by establishing base strength levels in all body parts, while striving to achieve a 1:1 ratio of strength between the injured and noninjured lower extremities. (See the first box on page 260 for examples of specific lower extremity strengthening exercises.)

The progression and intensity of these exercises should be such that maximal recovery time can take place both between sets and between individual workouts. The time between individual sets should range from 30 seconds to 1 minute, depending upon the intensity of the exercise; recovery time between workouts depends upon the type of program used for strengthening. Examples of workout schedules are (1) 2 days on, 1 day off; (2) 3 days on, 1 day off; and (3) every other day. Schedules like these allow the athlete not only to avoid overtraining the injured limb but also to increase the total benefit of each and every repetition. Intensities should be progressive in nature, allowing the athlete to work with increasing loads. There are several ways to monitor the load and intensity factors, such as the DAPRE (daily adjusted progressive resistance exercise) and DeLorme techniques (Table 22-1 and the second box on page 260). The advantages to these progressive resistance pro-

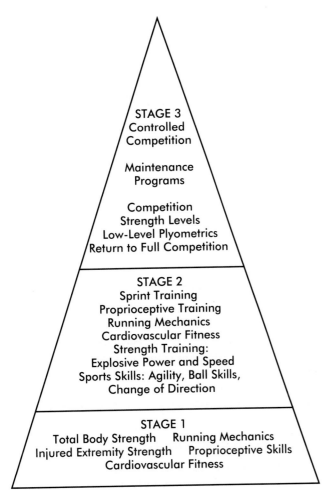

Fig. 22-1. Functional rehabilitation pyramid.

Examples of specific rehabilitation exercises for the knee

Straight leg raises (weighted, resistive tubing, or manually performed) for hip flexion, hip abduction, and hip adduction

Wall squats (add resistive tubing or dumbbells and a medium-sized ball such as a basketball for increased resistance and intensity)

Box step-ups (add weight in athlete's hands *or* increase step height for increased resistance and intensity)

Knee flexion and extension (machines, weighted, resistive tubing, or manually performed)

Hip sleds or leg press machines

Squat machines (hack squat, safety squat bars, etc.)

Standing and seated calf-strengthening machines

Lunges (free weight or machine)

Other conventional lower body strengthening machines can be utilized to emphasize a single leg

---

Table 22-1. DAPRE (Daily Adjustable Progressive Exercise) technique[1,2]

Set #3: total repetitions performed	Adjusted working weight for set #4: initial working weight for next workout
0–2	Decrease 5–10 lb
3–4	Decrease 0–5 lb
5–6	No change necessary
7–10	Increase 5–10 lb
11	Increase 10–15 lb

Step 1. Determine the six repetition maximum = initial working weight
Step 2. Set #1: 10 repetitions at half the working weight
Step 3. Set #2: six repetitions at three quarters of the working weight
Step 4. Set #3: as many repetitions as possible with the working weight
Step 5. Set #4: as many repetitions as possible with the *adjusted working weight;* this will be the initial working weight for the next workout

---

DeLorme technique[1,3]

Step 1: Determine the 10-repetition maximum
Step 2: Set #1 = half the 10-repetition maximum for 10 repetitions
Step 3: Set #2 = three quarters the 10-repetition maximum for 10 repetitions
Step 4: Set #3 = 10 repetitions of the full 10-repetition maximum
Step 5: The 10-repetition maximum is increased each week as strength increases

---

tocols are that load and intensity are carefully monitored and that progression to higher weights is efficiently and safely accomplished.

A common mistake in this early stage is to change the total training load and intensity of the uninvolved extremity to match that of the injured extremity. It is very important that normal training of the uninvolved limb continue. If the unaffected lower extremity is allowed to decondition because of less activity, the data gathered by comparison testing for strength increases in the injured limb will be inaccurate. The athlete will then be progressed in rehabilitation too quickly, decreasing the overall effectiveness of the program and possibly leading to reinjury or a new injury. Of course, the nature of the injury will dictate some constraints, but this is where creativity is important. Many strength-training exercises and conditioning modalities can be utilized or modified to accommodate unilateral training. Manual resistance exercise is an excellent alternative strengthening tool for this stage, as is the use of Theraband or surgical or bicycle tubing.

To maintain or regain cardiovascular endurance, conditioning modalities such as bicycles or ergometers, rowing machines, upper body ergometers, and swimming pools can be used for training as the athletic injury allows. Aerobic fitness is especially important for soccer field players; by contrast, soccer goalies require less aerobic conditioning, but more anaerobic power training. Anaerobic power training can be performed on the training modalities previously mentioned by using interval types of training.

During the early functional stage of training, distance running as well as a reintroduction to running form (see box at right) can begin as soon as the injury allows. Form running exercises should be initially executed at approximately 50% to 60% intensity for three to six sets, three to five times per week. The intensity can be increased by changing the speed, varying the distance, and increasing the number of repetitions per workout to create overload and cause adaptation. The emphasis in these exercises should not be conditioning, but rather proper running mechanics.

Proprioceptive skills are defined as those motor skills that create a three-dimensional awareness of the body and its positioning in space. The athlete relies on sensory input from the muscles, tendons, and joints for proprioceptive feedback.[4-6] Therefore, proprioceptive skills begin to deteriorate with prolonged inactivity. Proprioceptive drills using balance boards and single-leg balancing drills on different surfaces (mats, minitrampolines, pillows, uneven surfaces) allow the athlete to begin regaining those motor skills that have been lost or slowed because of the inactivity created by the injury. Another excellent proprioceptive training modality is a progressive routine of sand pit training done by initially walking in sand and then progressing to jogging and running in the sand.

The final component to the initial functional phase is sport-specific activities. Sport-specific drills should be limited initially to dribbling the soccer ball while walking to allow the athlete to regain some feel for the foot-to-ball contact. Cones and other marking devices to create predetermined patterns work well to deter boredom. As the athlete's running skills and endurance begin to increase, dribbling at a slow jog may progress to dribbling at moderate running speeds. Drills should be done three to five times per week, initially covering short distances of 30 to 50 yards for three to six sets. Increasing the distance covered and decreasing the amount of time taken to cover a set distance are the best ways to create overload. At this stage, sharp changes of direction should not be emphasized, although large figure-of-eight patterns or other large patterns with a low degree of cutting can be used as the athlete's skill levels begin to increase.

In summary, the initial stage of functional rehabilitation should create a strong base for more intensive rehabilitation and increasing levels of sport-specific skills to be reintroduced in the following stages. Total body strength, as well as strength within the injured limb, should be addressed. Cardiovascular fitness should be regained or increased, and proper running mechanics should be relearned. Sport-specific drills should be limited to basic ball dribbling. At all times during the rehabilitation process, the athlete should be monitored for any increase in pain or swelling or decrease in range of motion. Increases in symptoms indicate overly aggressive progression in this phase. When this occurs, the

---

> **Examples of form running exercises (to be performed at 20- to 40-yard distances)**
>
> High knees (emphasis on knee drive and hip flexion)
> Hip extension kicks (emphasis on knee flexion)
> Straight leg kicks (emphasis on hip flexion)
> Overstrides (exaggeration of the entire running cycle, especially stride length)
> Mountain climbers (emphasis on knee drive and hip flexion)
> Backwards running (emphasis on reaching back with leg as far as possible)

athlete's progress should be slowed or the total amount of training lessened; progression should begin again at the point before symptoms began.

STAGE 2: INCREASED INTENSITY AND INTRODUCTION TO SPORT-SPECIFIC SKILLS

The criterion for movement into the second stage is a score of 85% to 90% strength when compared with the uninvolved extremity. The athlete should be able to carry out stage 1 tasks with confidence and skill. Goals in the second stage include the beginning of strength training for increasing explosive power and speed, progressive sprint training, and a gradual reintroduction to sport-specific skills, including change of direction, agility, ball skills, and proprioceptive training.

Strength training should now emphasize multijoint exercises. Table 22-2 describes categories that relate to the knowledge levels of both the athlete and the supervising athletic trainer or physical therapist. Level 1 exercises are those that are easily taught by the athletic trainer or physical therapist and are easily understood by the athlete. The athlete need not have preinjury experience with these exercises. Level 2 exercises require more knowledge about proper teaching and instruction techniques by the athletic trainer or physical therapist, as well as an existing knowledge of basic technique by the athlete. Level 3 exercises require extensive knowledge on the part of the athletic trainer or physical therapist and preinjury knowledge of proper technique and execution by the athlete. Because minimizing the teaching period helps to maximize the effect of each individual exercise, the athlete should perform low- and medium-level exercises unless he or she was instructed in the proper technique of the high-level exercises before the injury occurred. Because level 3 exercises create a higher level of adaptation and a more sport-specific strength training environment, they are recommended if the athlete has some previous skill experience with them.

Remember that these strengthening exercises are in addition to the single-leg exercises implemented in stage 1. Multijoint exercises are executed at maximum tolerated intensity two to four times per week for four to six sets each.

A periodization program is the suggested method to mon-

Table 22-2. Exercises to develop lower body strength and power

Level 1	Level 2	Level 3
Leg press	Free bar squat	Power cleans
Squat machines	Straight leg deadlift	Deadlift
Knee flexion machines	Dumbbell squats	Hang cleans
Knee extension machines	Push press	Front squat–push press combination
Hip sleds	Glute-hamstring raise machine	Power clean–front squat combination
Other conventional weight-training machines for the lower body	Front squats	

Table 22-3. Six-week periodization model

Week 1			
Workout 1	70% × 2 reps	75% × 2 reps	80% × 2 reps × 4 sets
2	70% × 2 reps	75% × 2 reps	80% × 3 reps × 4 sets
3	70% × 2 reps	75% × 2 reps	80% × 2 reps × 4 sets
Week 2			
Workout 1	70% × 2 reps	75% × 2 reps	80% × 4 reps × 4 sets
2	70% × 2 reps	75% × 2 reps	80% × 2 reps × 4 sets
3	70% × 2 reps	75% × 2 reps	80% × 5 reps × 4 sets
Week 3			
Workout 1	70% × 2 reps	75% × 2 reps	80% × 2 reps × 4 sets
2	70% × 2 reps	75% × 2 reps	80% × 6 reps × 4 sets
3	70% × 2 reps	75% × 2 reps	80% × 2 reps × 4 sets
Week 4			
Workout 1	70% × 2 reps	75% × 2 reps	85% × 5 reps × 4 sets
2	70% × 2 reps	75% × 2 reps	80% × 2 reps × 4 sets
3	70% × 2 reps	75% × 2 reps	90% × 4 reps × 4 sets
Week 5			
Workout 1	70% × 2 reps	75% × 2 reps	80% × 2 reps × 4 sets
2	70% × 2 reps	75% × 2 reps	95% × 3 reps × 4 sets
3	70% × 2 reps	75% × 2 reps	80% × 2 reps × 4 sets
Week 6			
Workout 1	70% × 2 reps	75% × 2 reps	100% × 2 reps × 4 sets
2	70% × 2 reps	75% × 2 reps	80% × 2 reps × 4 sets
3	70% × 2 reps	75% × 2 reps	105% × 1 rep × 4 sets

Percentages are based on a one-repetition maximum.

itor the athlete's training regimen to avoid overtraining and to maximize strength gains. Table 22-3 shows an example of a 6-week periodization program. This program may require modification of the single-leg exercises.

Once proper running form is established, a slow introduction to sprint running can begin with training at medium distances (100 to 200 m) at training intensities of 60% to 80% of maximum sprint speed. As the athlete becomes more comfortable within this training zone, distances can be decreased and intensity increased with the goal of achieving maximum speed. Adding longer training distances at medium intensity (60% to 80%) facilitates training of the lactic acid system[7] for anaerobic muscular endurance. The athletic trainer or physical therapist should place less emphasis on the form running exercises of the previous stage (use these as part of a complete warm-up prior to sprint training) and address mechanical flaws during the actual sprint training sessions.

Sport-specific skill training now commences. A good working relationship with the coach to understand the techniques favored is helpful when developing drills and activities for the athlete. For example, one coach may want the athlete to use a certain cross-over dribble step, another coach may teach this technique differently, and still another may not want it as part of the athlete's repertoire at all. Adhering to the coach's biases speeds the transitional period in stage

3 where the athlete is advanced into team practice.

During middle to late stage 2, changes in direction, agility, and ball skills should be stressed. Change in direction and agility drills, such as those shown in Figures 22-2 and 22-3 and described in Table 22-4, should first be done at moderate speeds (60% to 80% intensity) and increased slowly with the athlete's skill level. As soon as the athlete is able to carry out these skills at 100% intensity, the soccer ball should be introduced and the progression repeated. At the time these drills are added to the protocol, forward speed should be well established (95% to 100% intensity). This is also an appropriate time to begin low-intensity jumping and bounding. Four-square drills (Fig. 22-4), low-intensity single-leg vertical and horizontal jumps, and single-leg bounding increase the athlete's lower body power and also aid in further increasing proprioception and confidence in the injured extremity. Begin with light loads, such as two to three sets of five to eight jumps at a moderate intensity (60% to 80%), and progress as the athlete shows signs of confidence and skill. Surfaces for these activities should be shock-absorbing (e.g., aerobic mats) so as not to cause further trauma to the injured knee. Goalies benefit greatly from these types of exercises, as many of their movements are explosive jumps, hops, and bounds.

The athletic trainer or physical therapist should be skilled at monitoring the athlete's progress and determining the appropriate time frame of progressions based on the individual athlete's proven abilities. Just as in the sprint and strength training, the criteria for moving to a higher skill level or increasing the intensity of the activity are the athlete's ability to recover from one exercise session to the next and to show mastery of the given task.

At this point in the athlete's rehabilitation, emphasis should be on speed and variety of movement using the ball (e.g., toe touches, cross-over step dribbling, backwards dribbling, and start-stops with the ball). Once basic ball skills have been reestablished, a training partner (the athletic trainer or physical therapist may double in this role if no partner is available) should begin to work with the athlete on teamwork drills such as passing and receiving. Kicking intensities should start out low (50%) at short distances (15 to 20 m) and progress to increasing intensities and distances as the athlete demonstrates ability and tolerance. Goalies should be working on these drills, as well as on throws and nondiving saves. When working with goalies, the training partner should attempt goal shots at 75% of maximum intensity within the athlete's grasp. This allows the goalkeeper to gain confidence without executing explosive movements prematurely.

Proprioceptive activities, begun in stage 1, should be continued, with the focus on maintaining skills, but there is no need to increase once they have reached a satisfactory skill level as determined by the athletic trainer or physical therapist. This level should be based on the athlete's preinjury abilities and will differ among athletes.

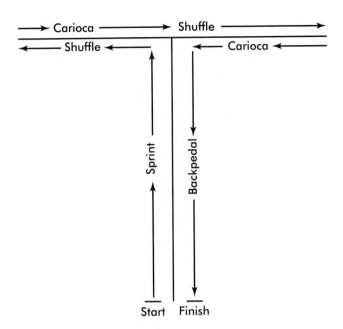

Fig. 22-2. The T-drill. Begin with a **T** of 15 m vertical and 30 m horizontal. Increase this distance proportionally as the athlete is able, and increase speeds. Three to eight sets are adequate to create overload and cause adaptation. Pay close attention to the athlete's footwork when changing directions; watch for hesitation, slowing down too soon, or stumbling, which indicate that the athlete has progressed too rapidly.

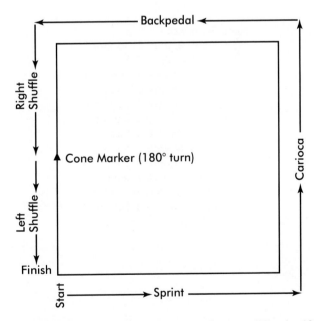

Fig. 22-3. The square. Begin with a small square (10 m by 10 m) and progress to larger squares and increasing speeds. Three to eight sets are adequate to create overload and cause adaptation. Pay close attention to the athlete's footwork. Stumbling, hesitation, and slowing down too soon are signs that the athlete has progressed too rapidly.

Table 22-4. Signal calls

Signals	Reaction to signal by athlete
Both hands overhead	Forward run
Pointing straight ahead	Backwards run
Right hand pointing right	Carioca or shuffle step to athlete's left
Left hand pointing left	Carioca or shuffle step to athlete's right
Either hand pointing at a 45-degree angle	Angled running away from signal caller in direction of the point (right or left)

The purpose of this drill is to train the athlete to begin processing visual cues into reactions. The athlete is instructed to react to certain hand signals, such as those listed here, given by the athletic trainer/physical therapist that relate to specific movements.

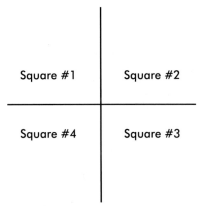

Jump Sequence:
Square 1–Square 2–Square 1
Square 1–Square 3–Square 1
Square 1–Square 4–Square 1
Square 2–Square 3–Square 2
Square 2–Square 4–Square 2
Square 2–Square 1–Square 2
Square 3–Square 4–Square 3
Square 3–Square 1–Square 3
Square 3–Square 2–Square 3
Square 4–Square 1–Square 4
Square 4–Square 2–Square 4
Square 4–Square 3–Square 4
Repeat as Necessary

Fig. 22-4. Four square drill. Begin with three sets of one time through the cycle and increase to sets of 30 or more seconds in duration.

The athlete, nearing the end of stage 2 rehabilitation, should be showing increasing confidence in the injured extremity and desire to resume normal activity. If this behavior is not apparent, now is an appropriate time for psychological intervention to determine the athlete's state of mind relating to both the injury and returning to participation. The athlete must be both physically and mentally ready to move into stage 3 of the rehabilitation process. The athlete who lacks confidence and fears reinjury is at an increased risk for injury with reintroduction to controlled play in stage 3.

STAGE 3: TRANSITION TO LIMITED AND CONTROLLED LEVELS OF PARTICIPATION

Stage 3 involves bringing together the components of stages 1 and 2 as the athlete progresses toward resumption of normal competition. Movement into stage 3 is based on a score of 95% or better muscular strength when compared with the uninvolved extremity. Also, as previously stated, the athlete must show confidence in the injured limb while performing all exercises from the previous two stages. Throughout stage 3, it is important to maintain the skills the athlete has acquired up to this point. Strength training, proper running form, sprint speed, and proprioceptive skills, as well as actual sport-specific skills (dribbling, passing, shooting) need to be maintained or progressed. (It is up to the supervising athletic trainer or physical therapist to determine whether the skills need to be simply maintained or progressed.) The goals in this stage are to create a controlled atmosphere of competition, to complete the strengthening process, and to allow for fine-tuning the highly demanding components of the game.

Strength training should continue as in stage 2, with increasing emphasis on powerful explosive movement while maintaining a schedule of specific strengthening for the injured limb. Dribbling and passing skills should be refined and brought up to 100% intensity. Athletes should continue practicing goal shots, progressively increasing the distance and intensity to maximum. Distance running and long and short sprint training should now make up the majority of the conditioning regimen in conjunction with practicing ball skills.

Power training with the use of cutting and explosive movements such as jumping and bounding should be continued with increasing intensity. Cutting and agility drills addressing change of direction with and without the ball should be carried on as in stage 2, but should now be at or approaching 100% intensity. Also, low-intensity plyometric drills may now be introduced to aid in fine-tuning the athlete's ability to react powerfully and gracefully. Plyometric exercises such as double leg bounds, 100% effort vertical and horizontal jumping, and jumps and bounds followed by changes in direction and sprinting should be introduced.[8] The intensity of these exercises should be high, with an emphasis on quality and not quantity. Sets and repetitions should range from 3 to 8 and 4 to 15, respectively, allowing for maximal recovery both between sets and between workouts.

Once the athlete has achieved the ability to participate at or near 100% intensity, reintroduction to controlled levels of play is the next step. Initial play consists of one-on-one play with the training partner. Tackling and being tackled at 90% speed and intensity should be introduced, gradually progressing to full speed as the athlete grows more confident and skillful. Progression through two-on-two, three-on-three, and three-on-two games with close supervision by the athletic trainer or physical therapist is an excellent way for the athlete to begin bringing together all aspects of the game. These controlled games should initially be short in length (10 to 15 minutes) and then progress to increasing lengths. As training partners are added, it is advisable to decrease the time initially and then progress to longer periods of time.

When the athlete shows mastery of all phases of the game in these controlled situations, it is time to reintroduce the athlete to full practice. Begin first by allowing the athlete only one third to one half the total practice time, and increase daily as tolerated. Slowly allowing the athlete to readjust to the intensity of full practice situations under the supervision of the athletic trainer or physical therapist minimizes the risks of injury and reinjury. It is advisable, first, to allow the athlete to participate in practice drills and conditioning, followed by gradual introduction to controlled team scrimmages only when the athlete has adjusted to the practice schedule.

Once the athlete has been reintroduced to the flow of practice, a maintenance program should be instituted. The maintenance program will depend upon the type of training in which the team is involved. Many collegiate soccer teams follow a year-long periodized strengthening program. Under these circumstances, a minimal rehabilitation program would need to be followed, utilizing single-leg exercises (stage 1). If the team is not involved in a strength training program, the rehabilitation program should be modified to include a mixture of single-leg exercises and multijoint exercises (stage 2). It is important to emphasize to the athlete the need to maintain a strengthening program for as long as the athlete continues to participate in competitive sports to deter reinjury to the involved structures.

The first actual competition or game situation should also be controlled. Game situations cannot be fully simulated in practice scrimmages; therefore, the athlete should also be slowly reintroduced to actual game situations, just as with introduction to practice drills, conditioning, and scrimmages. These reintroductions should come only after the athlete has had ample time to bring together all facets of the game in practice. How this is done depends on rules governing substitutions during games, the level of play, and the time of the year this phase of rehabilitation occurs. The athletic trainer or physical therapist and the head coach should work together to devise a plan according to the time of year (preseason, midseason, offseason) that will best benefit both the individual athlete and the team. The amount of time taken to reach this point in the rehabilitation process, as with all phases of rehabilitation, depends upon the severity of the injury, the structures that were injured, and the total amount of time the athlete has been away from competition.

CONCLUSION

This chapter has presented general guidelines for the functional rehabilitation of the soccer player with a knee injury. The amount of time for total rehabilitation depends upon the severity and nature of the injury and on the individual athlete. The ideas presented in the previous pages are meant to provide a basic understanding of the rehabilitation process as it applies to the sport of soccer. The three distinct phases and the individual components within those phases have been discussed. When designing any rehabilitation plan, allow room for creative thinking by both the athletic trainer or physical therapist and the athlete.

Always remember to take into account the differences among athletes and to allow for flexibility and individuality. The functional rehabilitation process should be an exciting and challenging part of the total rehabilitation process for both the athlete and athletic trainer or physical therapist. The design of an individual rehabilitation protocol is a result of borrowing ideas from others, formulating an individual philosophy, implementing one's own ideas, and then making changes and adjustments as they are needed. With these guidelines, a successful rehabilitative approach can be developed and instituted.

References 1 to 17 provide further information.

REFERENCES

1. Kisner C, Colby LA: *Therapeutic exercise: foundations and techniques,* ed 2. Philadelphia, 1990, FA Davis.
2. Knight KL: Knee rehabilitation by the daily adjustable progressive resistance exercise technique, *Am J Sports Med* 7:336, 1979.
3. Blair DF, Wills RP: Rapid rehabilitation following anterior cruciate ligament reconstruction, *JNATA* 26:32–43, 1991.
4. DeLorme TL, Watkins AL: *Progressive resistance exercise,* New York, 1951, Appleton-Century.
5. Case JG, et al: Knee rehabilitation following anterior cruciate ligament reconstruction/repair: an update, *JNATA* 26:22–31, 1991.
6. American Academy of Orthopaedic Surgeons: *Athletic training and sports medicine,* ed 2. 1991, American Academy of Orthopaedic Surgeons.
7. Arnheim DD: *Modern principles of athletic training,* ed 7, St Louis, 1989, Mosby–Year Book.
8. Fahey TD: *Athletic training: principles and practice,* Mountain View, Calif., 1986, Mayfield.
9. Hatfield FC: *Power: a scientific approach,* Chicago, 1989, Contemporary Books.
10. Powers SK, Howley ET: *Exercise physiology: theory and application to fitness and performance,* 1990, Wm C Brown pp. 448, 452.
11. Radcliff JC: *Plyometrics: explosive power training,* Champaign, Ill., 1985, Human Kinetics Publishers.
12. Orosz P: *Year-round planning of preparation in soccer,* 1989, National Strength and Conditioning Association.
13. Pronk NP: Sports performance series: the soccer push pass, NSCAJ 13:6–8, 77–81, 1991.
14. Roundtable: athletic rehabilitation: part 1, *NSCAJ* 14:10–18, 1992.
15. Roundtable: athletic rehabilitation: part 2, *NSCAJ* 14:10–19, 1992.
16. Torg JS, et al: *Rehabilitation of athletic injuries: an atlas of therapeutic exercise,* St Louis, 1987, Mosby–Year Book.
17. Wardle H: Resistance training: strength training for soccer, *NSCAJ* 14:72–74, 1992.

Chapter 23

WRESTLING

Robert M. Barnette
George Cernansky

Following an athletic injury, an essential aspect of the rehabilitative process is redeveloping functional skills needed for the eventual return to competition. This step, and its extension—that of the eventual return to contact or pivotal sports—should be approached carefully. There are many areas of consideration for athletes as they prepare themselves both physically and mentally for their return to competition, including adequate healing time, full strength, good endurance, excellent flexibility, agility, and psychological well-being.

In wrestling, as in many other sports, there is a need for both aerobic and anaerobic conditioning. Although many injuries associated with wrestling involve the upper extremity and trunk, injuries to the knee joint and lower extremity are also commonly encountered. These injuries include minor knee sprains, patellofemoral dysfunction, contusions, and significant ligament and cartilage injuries. Because of the demands placed on the knee joint during wrestling, an insufficiency in range of motion, strength, or proprioception may predispose an athlete to injury or reinjury.

Once a fundamental rehabilitation program has restored the wrestler's full range of motion to the injured joint, as well as at least 75% to 80% of the injured extremity's strength, the wrestler should be ready to begin specific drills to enable him to return to competitive wrestling. These drills should address lateral movement, changes of direction, and close contact drills in both the neutral position and the referee's position. Following are some of the most commonly used basic skill and conditioning drills that can be used to accomplish these goals.

GENERAL CONDITIONING DRILLS

When a 75% to 80% strength and functionality base has been achieved through the initial rehabilitation program, the wrestler may begin work on jogging and neutral (upright) position skills. These drills may be progressed in intensity and difficulty as long as the wrestler remains pain-free and no swelling occurs in the injured extremity. The drills should emphasize a gradual increase in explosive power and speed, as well as proprioceptive awareness.

Jogging and short sprints

Gradual increased jogging on a track or in a gymnasium that incorporates changes in direction of laps is one way to reestablish cardiovascular conditioning. This routine should incorporate long, slow runs, as well as brief, short bursts of activity. The therapist or trainer should monitor frequency and intensity as well as surface type. Too much, too soon may lead to overuse problems.

Short sprint drills of 20 to 30 yards should follow circular jogging. These sprints should initially be straight ahead with no change of direction. As the athlete progresses, the length of the sprints can be increased, followed by increased intensity.

Once the athlete can perform straight-ahead, long, slow activities as well as short, rapid bursts of activity, the therapist or trainer may incorporate numerous drills to work on changes in direction, acceleration, and deceleration skills. The shuttle run, cross-over running, carioca drills, and figure 8 running all address changes in direction and changes in speed. Gradual progression should be emphasized in all drills as the level of performance increases. The therapist or trainer should closely guide the athlete through a progression beginning at 60% to 70% effort until the athlete reaches a 100% intensity level. As the sprinting and jogging programs progress, the wrestler may begin specific work on the mat with a partner.

Shooting drills

The ability of a wrestler to penetrate and gain control of the opponent is a fundamental skill in wrestling. In order to score points or pin his opponent, he must be on the offensive or counteroffensive. A "shot" or "shooting maneuver" usually begins with both wrestlers in the upright position. The offensive or shooting wrestler may then pick from a number of maneuvers to gain control of his opponent's legs or upper body. This attempt to gain control while in the offensive mode is called a *shot*. Once the offensive wrestler has gained control of his opponent, he is awarded points and may then begin his offensive work for a pin. Shooting drills allow the wrestler to fine-tune proprioceptive awareness, as well as give the wrestler a safe practice tool to regain confidence following injury.

Initial shooting drills should involve only the injured wrestler to decrease any outside chances of injury, as well as give the wrestler a chance to relearn basic awareness and skill. Place emphasis on the quality of shots with each session. An increase in intensity and repetitions may follow

initial practice sessions. A normal shooting session may involve the following: The wrestler begins on either side of the mat. Begin with a good stance and proper positioning. The wrestler should try to achieve four to six individual shots for each length of the mat. The right and left legs should be alternated to ensure that the injured knee is used as both lead leg and drive leg. Instruct the wrestler to be aware of body positioning and upper body control, which will become important for later drills and practice. Figures 23–1 through 23–4 show a shooting drill with no partner. Figure 23–1 shows the wrestler in an offensive stance position prior to his penetration or drive step. (Back leg is

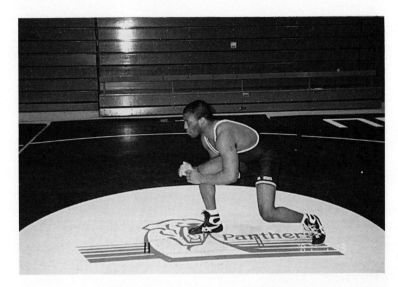

Fig. 23-1. Shooting drill: initial stance.

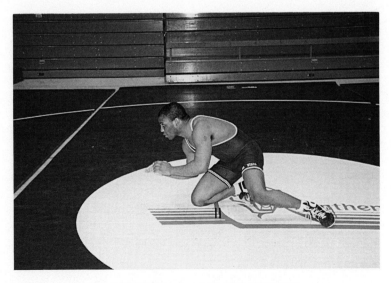

Fig. 23-2. Shooting drill: push-off/drive.

drive leg.) Figure 23–2 shows the wrestler moving toward his opponent. Notice the upright head position and hand placement. Figure 23–3 shows the wrestler regaining his base or positioning. Figure 23–4 shows the wrestler returning to his upright stance position, ready to return to an offensive position. Frequently during this time of early development of functional skills, bracing may be used to increase the athlete's awareness of the injured extremity, as well as to provide some mechanical support. As function, ability, and confidence increase, the wrestler advances to performing shooting drills with a passive partner. The main focus of the drill should emphasize body positioning and leg drive (penetration). Upper body control and the use of both legs for a proper base are important, so that further

injury may be avoided. Figures 23–5 and 23–6 demonstrate shooting with a passive partner. Figure 23–5 shows the offensive wrestler attempting to gain control of his opponent's lower body with no resistance from opponent. Figure 23–6 shows the situation reversed; the injured wrestler is now on the defensive.

Lateral movement and change of direction drills

Lateral movements and quick directional changes are very important in all sports. Following a knee injury, initial rehabilitative skills are conducted in a somewhat controlled, linear fashion and generally consist of jogging, sprint drills, figure 8 running, and the like. Once the wrestler has moved on to mat-oriented drills, the use of shuffle, or lateral move-

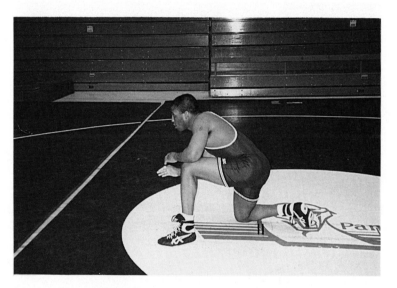

Fig. 23-3. Shooting drill: penetration step.

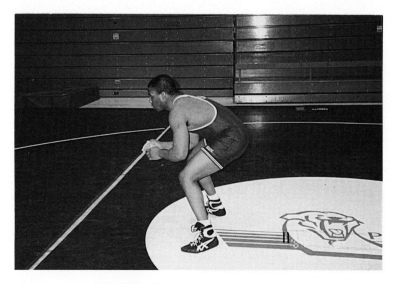

Fig. 23-4. Shooting drill: follow-through.

ment drills coupled with shooting drills, may be used. This should begin initially with a semipassive partner in order to allow the injured wrestler to concentrate on proper form and technique.

Begin the drill with the injured wrestler in stance position at the outer edge of the circle. The passive partner should be in the center of the circle and also in stance position facing his opponent (Fig. 23–7, *A*). The drill begins when the therapist or trainer gives one whistle blast. The injured wrestler (outside circle) then begins a lateral shuffle clockwise around the outer circle or designated area while being careful not to use cross-over steps. The passive opponent rotates with the injured wrestler to maintain face-to-face

contact. If the next whistle blast is one burst, the injured wrestler (outside circle) then changes his direction of movement to counterclockwise. If the next whistle blast is two short bursts, the outer wrestler (injured wrestler) then attempts to shoot and gain position and penetrate on his opponent (Fig. 23–7, *B*). Initially, simple single-leg or double-leg takedowns are best. The center wrestler or passive partner should present minimal defense or resistance by using sprawls or upper body defense. Once control and position have been achieved, the wrestlers resume neutral positions and begin again on whistle cues (Fig. 23–7, *C*). A minimum of 12 shots should be taken for each man. The wrestlers may then change positions to allow the injured

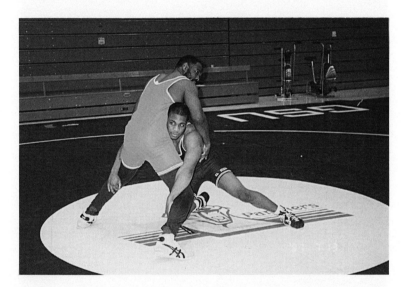

Fig. 23-5. Injured wrestler *(right)* in an offensive position with a passive partner.

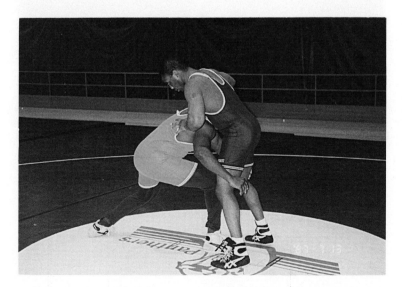

Fig. 23-6. Injured wrestler *(right)* in a defensive position with a passive partner.

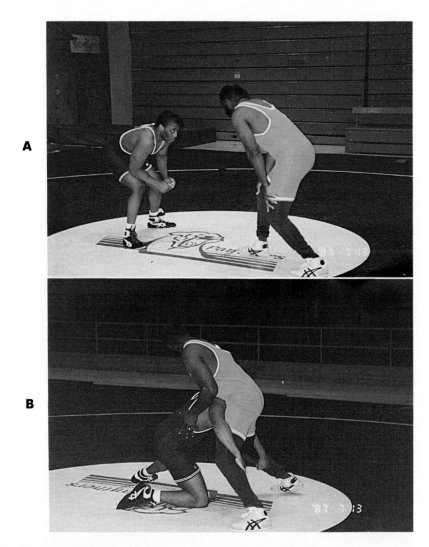

Fig. 23-7. Circle drill. **A,** Injured wrestler *(left)* with a passive partner. **B,** Injured wrestler *(left)* in an offensive position. **C,** Once control has been achieved by injured wrestler, resume neutral position. **D,** Injured wrestler *(left)* in a defensive position.

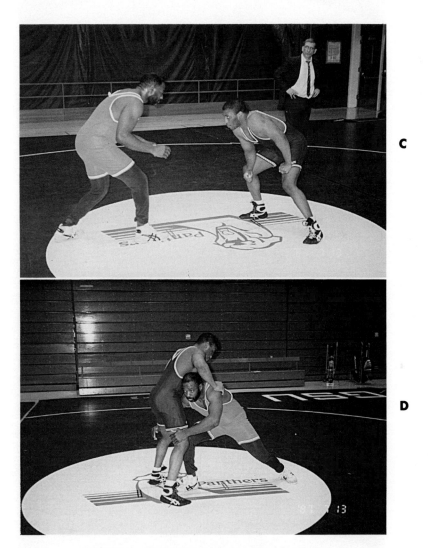

C

D

Fig. 23-7, cont'd. For legend see opposite page.

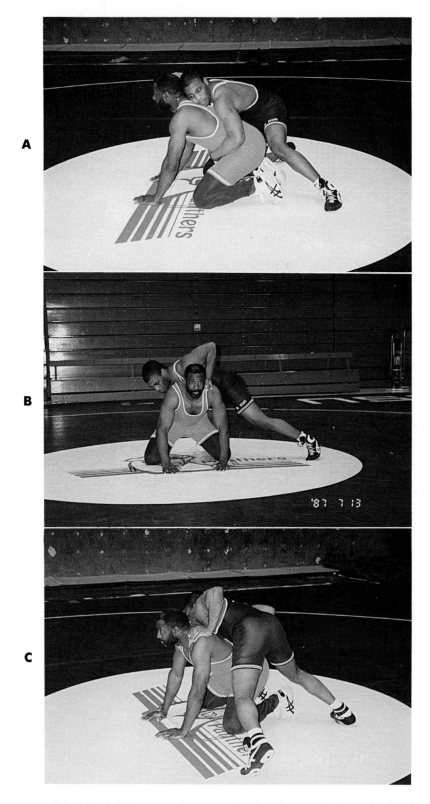

Fig. 23-8. Spin drill. **A,** Injured wrestler on top. **B,** Note chest and hands resting lightly on mid-back. **C,** Note wide base of foot placement.

wrestler to work on reaction skills and defensive moves (Fig. 23–7, *D*). As the wrestler progresses, the intensity as well as the duration of both takedowns and counter or defensive moves may increase.

Spin drills

Once the wrestler is comfortable with drills in the upright position, spin drills may allow the wrestler to regain awareness and proprioceptive skills while in the down or referee's position. Quick and powerful movement is very important in both the neutral position and the referee's position. While in the referee's position or wrestling in the down position, it is important to obtain a feeling of position in relation to the opponent. The spin drill not only increases endurance but also utilizes the proprioceptive abilities of the trunk and lower extremity.

Begin the drill with the wrestlers in the referee's position: the injured wrestler in the up position and the partner in the down position (Fig. 23–8, *A*). At the whistle cue, the top man (injured wrestler) takes his position on his partner's back with his chest and hands in contact with partner's midback. At the same time, the top man positions his feet away from the partner to achieve a wide base (Fig. 23–8, *B* and *C*). Once the top man achieves proper positioning, he immediately begins a clockwise shuffle around his partner. Again, avoid cross-over shuffle steps. Emphasize short shuffle steps, keeping poised on toes with knees slightly flexed. At the next whistle cue, the top wrestler changes to counterclockwise spins. In performing these drills, begin with 15- to 20-second sessions and progress to 1-minute sessions.

Return to competition

Once the injured wrestler has regained competency in performing fundamental wrestling skills, controlled sparring and competitive practice may begin. These practices should address all aspects of the sport. Begin sessions in controlled situations for both neutral and referee's positions. Emphasize technique and awareness for such moves as escapes, reversals, stand-ups, and pinning. This helps the wrestler regain his confidence as he returns to active participation in his sport.

The wrestler progresses from short practice sparring sessions to sparring periods, as in a regulation match. These periods should be 30 to 45 seconds initially, with a gradual progression to the regulation time of the three periods in a regulation match. Utilize both neutral position and referee's position for each period. The therapist-trainer or coach should try to utilize as many situations as possible for each practice session.

It is also extremely important to emphasize that the wrestler should continue to perform strength and flexibility exercises, as well as maintain his overall cardiovascular fitness level, while he is regaining his functional skills. Frequently, athletes neglect overall conditioning as the excitement of competition returns. Trainers and therapists need to be aware of this potential problem and ensure that the wrestler's workout sessions are balanced.

SUGGESTED READINGS

Fisher AC: Adherence to sports injury rehabilitation programmes, *J Sports Med* 9:151–158, 1990.

Lorish TR, et al: Injuries in adolescent and preadolescent boys at two large wrestling tournaments, *Am J Sports Med* 20:199–202, 1992.

McInerney VK, Mailly KH, Paonessa KJ: Rehabilitation of the sports-injured patient, *Orthop Clin North Am* 19:725–735, 1988.

Rovere GD, Curl WW, Browning DG: Bracing and taping in an office sports medicine practice, *Clin Sports Med* 8:497–510, 1989.

Valentine T: *Inside wrestling,* Chicago, 1972, Henry Regnery.

Walsh WM, Helzer-Julin M: Patellar tracking problems in athletes, *Prim Care* 19:303–330, 1992.

Chapter 24

DANCE

Carol Teitz

Few knee injuries are unique to dance, although many common knee injuries have unique dance-related etiologies. Regardless of the etiology of injury, returning the injured patient to dance activities requires dance-specific rehabilitation. This rehabilitation includes treating the initial injury, returning the injured structure and patient to normal function, and preventing recurrence. In order to understand dancers' needs, we must consider the milieu in which the dancer lives and works.

THE DANCE ENVIRONMENT

Dance disciplines include aerobic, ballet, ballroom, folk, jazz, modern, and tap. Each of these has specific requirements and types of movements. To a certain extent, different injuries are seen as a function of the specific dance discipline, although no musculoskeletal injury occurs exclusively in any dance form. Many dancers are multidisciplinary. Discussing all dancers together is a bit like discussing together all athletes whose sport involves a ball. Therefore, the reader must realize that, although we are discussing dancers as a group, the group is not homogeneous.

Ballet demands pointe work (dancing on the tips of the toes) for the female dancers and extreme external rotation of the hips. Folk dancing often includes percussive squats. Modern dance choreography may involve falling to the knees or rotating on the floor while on the knees.

All dancers require a combination of athletic ability, creativity, and artistic expression. Flexibility, strength, coordination, rhythm, balance, and timing are critical. The greatest flexibility is required in the spine, ankles, and hips. When flexibility is lacking in the hips and ankles, abnormal stresses are placed on the knees. Female dancers generally are more flexible than males. Few dancers are truly hypermobile.[1] The amount of flexibility present is not only a function of heredity, which plays a major role, but also the age at onset of training. The fact that male dancers begin their dance training at an older age than their female counterparts may account for the difference in flexibility. Lack of flexibility is a particular problem during adolescence,

when overgrowth of the skeleton relative to the soft tissues occurs.[2,3] Injuries in this age group are commonly associated with inadequate flexibility.

Generally dancers tend to be more supple than strong. Kirkendall and Calabrese found that relative isokinetic quadriceps muscle strength in male dancers is approximately equal to that of a variety of male athletes, whereas isokinetic quadriceps torque in female dancers was quite low compared with other female athletes.[4] Trunk strength is particularly important for centering body weight, especially during various maneuvers in which the dancer balances on one leg.

Aerobic dance obviously requires endurance. Dance performance often demands speed as well. Performance pieces run from 3 to 15 minutes. Whereas any one piece might be anaerobic, requiring spurts of high intensity and power, the need for a series of these pieces in performance demands endurance. Nevertheless, studies of performance dancers' oxygen-carrying capacity reveal values equal to those in nonendurance athletes.[5]

Aesthetics are a major issue for performing dancers. Dancing must appear effortless. In addition, because all but folk dancing demand a thin body habitus, nutritional problems are rampant. Poor nutrition can interfere with the ability to perform, concentrate and learn, and heal what would otherwise be minor injuries. Aesthetic demands also prevent dancers from using knee or ankle braces during performances, and dance footwear can make the use of orthotics in the treatment of knee problems difficult if not impossible. Aerobic shoes have improved markedly since their introduction, with better shock-absorbing material, control of the heel and forefoot, arch support, and room in the shoe for accommodative and supportive devices. Ballet shoes, by contrast, have not changed in centuries. Dancers need to "feel the floor" to increase their critically important kinesthetic sense. Hence they desire the least amount of material possible between foot and performing surface. Ballet and jazz shoes are soft slippers in which there is no shock absorption and no room for orthotics or other accommodative devices. Pointe shoes, in which the toe box is made of satin and cardboard, also have no shock absorbency or arch support. "Character" shoes worn in ballroom and folk dance often can accommodate a custom-made orthotic, but not an over-the-counter orthotic. Modern dancers often dance barefooted.

Finding a time during which to rehabilitate an injury is difficult because dancers, like other athletes, do not want to stop dancing, and dance is not a seasonal "sport." Dancers attend classes year round. Aerobic dance instructors teach, on average, 3 hours per day, 3 days per week.[6] Professional dancers often train 4 to 5 hours daily and perform three or four times in a given week. Finally, most dancers are not on fixed salaries and are not covered by either health or industrial insurance. Therefore, time lost due to injury is also a financial burden on the dancer. Financial constraints must be considered in return-to-sport decision making.

TYPES OF INJURY

Most of the epidemiologic studies on dancers' injuries have been of professional dancers or instructors and have not included the vast number of children and adults dancing recreationally, so true incidence is really unknown. Nevertheless, knee injuries average about 15% of all injuries reported during various types of dance activities.[7]

Overuse injuries are more prevalent than traumatic injuries in dancers.[8-11] Risk factors associated with overuse injuries include training errors (intensity, duration, or frequency), musculoskeletal imbalance (strength and flexibility), anatomic malalignment of the lower extremity (including leg length discrepancy, abnormal rotation, angular deformity, and flat feet), shoe wear, and floor surface. Technique (appropriate positioning and muscle use) is also a factor in many of the overuse injuries seen.[12-14] Lack of efficiency in movement, due to poor instruction, lack of readiness (flexibility, strength, experience), or both, leads to unnecessary overuse of certain muscle groups and strains of poorly positioned joints.[15]

Dancers, with the exception of aerobic dancers, typically do not engage in adjunctive training. Unlike other athletes whose training may include weightlifting or running, dancers dance to train. This repeated use of certain body parts in the same way, day after day, produces overuse injuries. In aerobic dance students, Garrick et al. found that the injury rate of 138 students who listed aerobics as their only fitness activity was nearly three times greater than that seen in students involved in multiple fitness activities.[8] In professional dancers, many injuries occur in the weeks immediately preceding performances. During this time the training schedule increases and dancers may repeat the same movements for up to 8 hours per day. In addition, for a professional dancer in a small company there is often no backup person to perform a given role. Fatigue and stress can interact negatively to increase the chances not only of overuse injuries but also of traumatic injuries.

Overuse injuries in dancers include patellofemoral pain,

patellar tendonitis, and medial knee strain. Common traumatic injuries are patellar subluxation and dislocation and torn menisci. Ligament tears are rare.[16] Patellofemoral problems are extremely common in aerobic dancers because of constant jumping, use of the step (bench), and the prevalence of lower extremity malalignment in these recreational dancers. Aerobic dancers must take care to position their knees over their feet to avoid patellofemoral problems; that is, a plumb line dropped from the flexed knee should land over the second or third toe. This positioning also is emphasized in ballet, in which patellofemoral problems are due to poor technique, too many grand plies (deep kneebends), or increased femoral anteversion, which makes the required 90 degrees of lower extremity external rotation difficult to achieve through the hips.[17] When external rotation of the hips is lacking, some ballet dancers attempt to achieve the expected lower extremity positions by rotating through the knee. Whereas significant malalignment is unlikely in the professional dancer, it is certainly common at the student level.

Patellar tendonitis, jumper's knee, is commonly seen in aerobic dancers and in male ballet dancers who jump and lift more than their female counterparts. Excessive use of the quadriceps during plie also produces patellar tendonitis and can aggravate patellofemoral problems.[18]

Medial knee strain is common in student dancers and presents as pain along the medial side of the knee with no history of specific injury. Pain is usually worse after class and gradually decreases when there is a day or two hiatus between ballet classes. There is no history of swelling or locking. Physical exam often reveals some tenderness along the medial aspect of the knee but not specifically over the joint line or over the medial collateral ligament. No effusion is present. Ligamentous laxity, meniscal signs, and patellar tenderness are lacking. One can confirm the suspicion of medial knee strain by asking the dancer to do a plie. An imaginary plumb line dropped from the knee should land over the second toe. If the plumb line falls medial to the foot during plie, then the medial capsule of the knee is seeing increased strain and is the likely source of pain.

Patellar subluxation or dislocation usually occurs during a turn initiated by pivoting off one foot. In Quirk's study of professional ballet dancers, patellar subluxation accounted for 0.3% of knee injuries.[9] Patellar subluxation is more common in those dancers trying to force turnout through the knee. In the ideal turned out position, the weight should fall from the body through the thigh and the center of the knee and ankle. This distribution of weight can be achieved if 90 degrees of external rotation occurs at the hip. Most commonly, because external rotation of the hip is lacking, and because of poor instruction, a dancer assumes what he or she perceives to be the desired amount of rotation by "turning out" the feet and then attempting to adjust from the floor upward by "screwing" the knee. Foot placement heel to heel on a straight line is easy when knees are flexed

(Fig. 24-1). However, if external hip rotation is limited, when the dancer tries to straighten the knees, they are forced to rotate abnormally and create a lateral force vector that can produce patellar subluxation. This screwing of the knee can also tear menisci.

Torn menisci are less common in dance than they are in sports.[10] This may be because the dancer is usually performing rehearsed movements in a controlled fashion, whereas the athlete may be starting or stopping or rotating in an unpredictable fashion as called for by the movements of an opponent. Torn menisci are seen most commonly in male theatrical dancers and in some folk dancers.[11] The lateral mensicus is at particular risk during Russian folk dancing involving a great deal of forced hyperflexion movements. In other dancers, the most common mechanism for tearing a meniscus is screwing the knee to increase turnout. In Quirk's study of professional ballet dancers, meniscal problems accounted for 16% of knee injuries.[9]

Anterior cruciate ligament (ACL) tears most often occur in dancers who land a jump on a hyperextended knee. Derotational braces, which are especially useful in returning athletes to sports after anterior cruciate ligament injury and reconstruction, are too cumbersome for dancers. Furthermore, they can be worn only during class and rehearsal and cannot be worn during performance. Therefore, reconstruc-

tion is usually indicated but fraught with problems. The patellar tendon should not be used because of potential problems with the quadriceps mechanism. Moreover, many reconstructions result in 5-degree flexion contractures, which are unacceptable in dancers.

REHABILITATION

Rehabilitation principles for injured dancers are not unique. However, as for other athletes, how they are put into practice can be tailored for the dancer. The principles we follow are

1. The injured structure must be protected while it is healing.
2. Range of motion about the injured joint should be maintained or regained.
3. Total body endurance, flexibility, and strength must be maintained while avoiding stress of the injured area.
4. During a period of activity restriction, keeping the injured dancer in his or her normal practice environment minimizes the psychosocial and economic stresses that occur following injury.
5. Any technical problems that led to the original injury must be corrected.
6. Before returning to full activity, rehabilitation must be activity-specific so that the patient will be able to return to preinjury performance levels.
7. During the rehabilitation period, a great deal of cooperation among the patient, the physician, the physical therapist, and the dance administrator is required if the goals of optimal healing, return to maximal performance levels, and prevention of additional injury are to be achieved.[19]

First, we must protect the injured structure. The knee may be braced, and activities may need to be limited for a certain period of time. During this time, if at all possible, return the dancer to class to work on the rest of the body, the arms, and the uninjured leg. In a typical class, dancers begin at the barre and then move to "center floor," where there is no support. Barre exercises are a fairly specific routine of movements done facing one way and then the other, while keeping one hand on the barre (railing). They are designed to stretch and strengthen the muscles and joints, as well as to work on the fine points of technique. Center floor work includes movement across the room, turns, jumps, and combinations thereof. Although center floor work is prohibited in the early postinjury period, barre work often is safe, particularly with a few adaptations. Extra support can be obtained from the barre. Often the injured leg can be the "gesture" leg rather than the support leg (Fig. 24-2). Barre exercises are useful even for nonballet dancers.

Second, retain and regain range of motion. The dancer requires full flexion to land jumps and full extension of the knee for aesthetics and, in ballet, for pointe work. Therefore, particular care must be taken to avoid even small

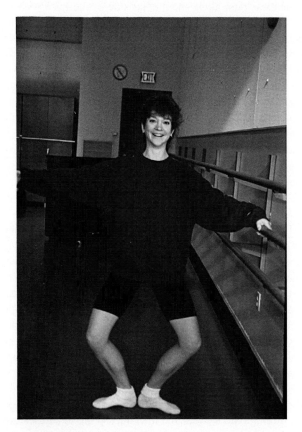

Fig. 24-1. When the knees are flexed, it is relatively easy to position the feet at a 180-degree angle.

flexion contractures. Especially after ACL reconstruction, full passive extension must be emphasized from the beginning. A physical therapist can help the dancer with range of motion. The dancer can also work the knee by moving it actively in warm water. Swimming is encouraged early, but avoiding the breast stroke with whip kick because of its angular and torsional forces on both the menisci and the patella.

Third, maintain total body endurance, as well as flexibility and strength in the uninjured parts. Endurance can be maintained by swimming, bicycling, or walking. Adaptations can be made in each, depending on the degree of functional impairment. During swimming, a Styrofoam float can be tied to the injured leg to allow it to trail along in the water while the rest of the body works. A bicycle seat can be raised (especially on a stationary bike) to compensate for limited knee flexion.

Before beginning flexibility work, assess, in particular, the tightness of the Achilles tendons, the quadriceps, the hamstrings, the hip rotators, and the lateral patellar retinacular structures. Most dancers have greater than average hamstrings flexibility. They need to be asked if their hamstrings seem tight. Hamstrings stretching using a partner for proprioceptive neuromuscular facilitation (PNF) techniques is effective in dancers[20] (Fig. 24-3). If the iliotibial band is tight, iliotibial stretching should be added to the rehabilitation program (Fig. 24-4). Stretching of the hip into external rotation is useful in ballet dancers[21] (Fig. 24-5). Myofascial massage often loosens a tight lateral patellar retinaculum.

Lifting weights is a concept often foreign and even repulsive to dancers, although this is changing. Cybex-testing quadriceps and hamstring muscles for strength and power is useful for pointing out deficiencies, setting goals, and assessing progress during the rehabilitation period. Rehabilitation of the knee always includes quadriceps strengthening to prevent the atrophy that occurs whenever pain or swelling is present in the knee. Vastus medialis obliquus strength is the key to patellar control. Quadriceps setting exercises should be initiated as soon as possible, progressing to straight leg lifts with the leg in external rotation to overwork the vastus medialis and to strengthen the adductors. Once the dancer can lift the weight of the leg repeatedly without fatigue, weights are applied to the leg, first just below the knee. These weights are gradually moved down the leg to the ankle, increasing their leverage. Short-arc isotonic exercises follow because the vastus medialis obliquus is known to be electrically most active during the terminal 30 degrees of extension. Finally, isokinetic exercises are added. Full-arc isotonic quadriceps exercises are recommended only if the patient has no preexisting patellar problems. We never recommend full-arc isotonic exercises to patients with malalignment or patellar injury as these exercises are poorly tolerated in those patients. In patients who are unable to recruit their vastus medialis muscles or

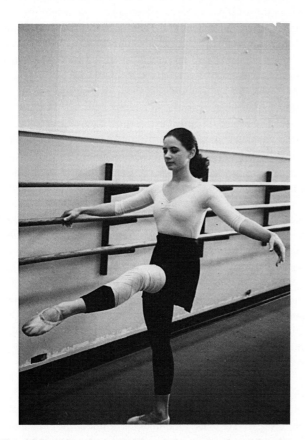

Fig. 24-2. Using the injured leg as the gesture leg rather than as the support leg.

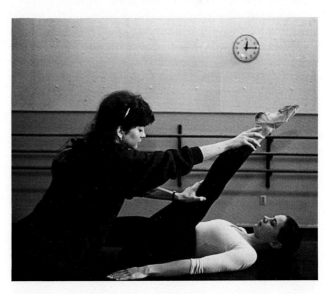

Fig. 24-3. Proprioceptive neuromuscular facilitation used to stretch the hamstring muscles. The dancer first tightens her quadriceps muscles, pushing her leg down against her partner. She then relaxes her quadriceps while her partner pushes upward on her leg, stretching her hamstrings. The contraction of the quadriceps automatically induces reciprocal relaxation of the hamstrings to allow greater stretch.

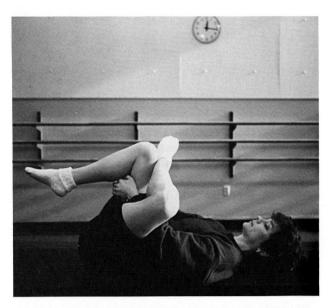

Fig. 24-4. An iliotibial stretch designed to stretch the tensor fasciae latae (muscle of origin).

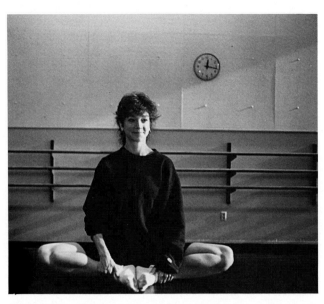

Fig. 24-5. Stretching adductors and internal rotators of the hip.

who have pain when trying to do quadriceps setting exercises, we have had a great deal of success with electrogalvanic stimulation of the quadriceps muscles.[22] We start with electrical muscle stimulation alone and then add self-initiated contractions simultaneously with the electrically-induced contractions. Gradually we wean the patient off electrical stimulation to isometric quadriceps strengthening exercises and then proceed as described previously.

Hamstrings strengthening also is recommended. Dancers tend to have strong quadriceps and gastrocsoleus muscles and weaker hamstrings and anterior tibial muscles. Pointe work, in particular, causes Achilles tightness and recurvatum at the knee with resultant laxity of the posterior structures in the knee. Hyperextension of the knee also increases the risk of patellar subluxation or dislocation. Hamstrings strengthening is usually done isotonically with gradually increasing weights and isokinetically with gradually increasing speeds.

During all of these exercises, the knee should be warmed up prior to activity, wrapped during activity, and iced down after activity. In addition to traditional methods, Pilates' work can be used to strengthen and stretch multiple body parts in positions that simulate dance.[23] Prior to the dancer's return to full activity, the strength of the injured knee should at least equal and preferably exceed that of the uninjured knee.

Fourth, keep the dancer in his or her usual environment. In a performing company, when a company member has been injured and no longer attends class, not only does the individual suffer but the other "team members" suffer as well. They have to increase their workload under the additional threat of knowing that injuries occur in their en-

vironment. Choreography can be learned by an injured dancer who is sitting in and watching the class.

Nurture the psyche of the dancer. Teaching the dancer relaxation skills increases endurance and improves aesthetics. A good teacher, in addition to providing audio, visual, and kinetic presentations of each skill, must be aware of fears, doubts, and anxieties on the part of the trainee. Disability also produces financial problems for most dancers, who are uninsured and have no income while injured.

Fifth, correct technical errors that contributed to the injury. We must make sure not only that the patient is fully rehabilitated but also that there are no technical faults or correctable anatomic problems that will produce another similar injury. First, analyze a few commonly used movement patterns, such as plié in first position (heels lift off the floor) and second position (heels stay down), and look to see if the knees line up over the feet or if the knee falls "inside" the foot, causing pronation. The thigh should externally rotate during the descent phase of plié, and the adductors should be working during the ascent phase of plié. If positioning is incorrect, screwing the knee is likely and may increase the likelihood of lateral patellar subluxation or dislocation. When quadriceps muscles are used during ascent from plié, increased patellofemoral forces are created, causing anterior knee pain.

In the usual ballet class, approximately one half to two thirds of class time is spent at barre exercises, most of which include pliés with the feet in various positions. Proper pliés are critical. They are fundamental to initiating turns and to initiating and landing jumps. If one's plié technique is incorrect, musculoskeletal problems are likely to follow. Plié technique is usually, although not always, correct in the professional dancer.

Common technical problems include errors in positioning and in muscle use. The best way for finding proper position using external rotation of the hip is to have the dancer stand with legs straight and feet together "in parallel" (pointing forward). Instruct the dancer to move his or her legs from parallel to a position of comfortable external rotation, keeping the back straight and head up. The turnout achieved is a function of the dancer's femoral neck-shaft angle. Keeping the knee straight ensures that the rotation occurs at the hips. Once in this position the dancer can assume the various ballet positions with the feet at this angle (Fig. 24-6). While performing pliés in these positions, the knees should fall directly over the feet. Most good ballet instructors accept this variation in positioning of their students and realize that not all students can achieve a 180-degree angle of their feet. In addition, good instructors teach the young dancer to obtain more external rotation by using the short external rotators of the hip rather than by cheating with lordosis of the lumbar spine or twisting the knee. Other dance forms do not require 90 degrees of external rotation, so turnout can be deemphasized.

When excessive use of the quadriceps during plié is noted as a technical error, we recommend practicing the usual sequence of barre exercises lying supine on the floor. The elimination of gravity allows concentration on appropriate muscle use. For example, instead of lowering the trunk during plié, the knees are bent by placing the feet heel to heel and drawing them toward the trunk. Hip external rotators should control the legs during the knee flexion phase of the plié, and adductors should control the leg during knee extension. Learning to flex the hip with the iliopsoas instead of the rectus femoris is also easier when supine and is critical for centering weight and good pelvic alignment. Although abdominal muscle and spine muscle strengthening are important, using the iliopsoas is most important in the dancer. Because of its anatomic position, originating posteriorly and inserting anteriorly, the iliopsoas is uniquely able to center body weight through the pelvis without excessively increasing or decreasing lumbar lordosis.[24] In order for the iliopsoas to function properly to position the pelvis, the rectus femoris, anterior hip capsule, and lumbodorsal fascia must be flexible.

Once positioning and muscle use have been mastered in the supine position, the dancer moves to the upright position. If bearing weight produces pain, proceed first to barre exercises in the shallow end of a pool prior to trying them in a dance studio. Barre exercises in the pool keep the dancer's psyche and general physical condition relatively intact while unloading the lower extremities.

Once back in the studio, we begin with barre work only. The injured dancer can initially "mark" steps in place, maintaining the support of the barre rather than performing the steps in center floor. *Marking* the steps means practicing

the choreography in place without traveling across the floor. Gradually, increasingly difficult movements are added. The dancer moves to center floor without turns or jumps and adds one at a time when strength and range of motion are normal. Jumping is restricted until full quadriceps strength has returned.

For aerobic dancers, one can start with aqua aerobics, then low impact (avoiding lunges), and then step and traditional aerobics. Ballroom, jazz, and folk dancers can mark steps, initially avoiding jumps and turns other than step turns. Tap, at the basic level, puts little stress on the knees as long as the feet are kept close to the ground while weight is shifted from one leg to the other.

Other anatomic problems include muscular imbalance of agonists and antagonists. Examples mentioned previously include quadriceps-hamstrings, gastrocsoleus–anterior tibial muscle, and hip abductors-adductors. Correcting these imbalances improves dance technique. Small felt arch supports taped to the foot can be used in place of orthotics. In addition to proprioceptive neuromuscular facilitation, visualization (ideokinesis) techniques work well in dancers because typically they have excellent body awareness.[25] These techniques are especially useful for repatterning muscle use. Certified movement analysts can help assess and correct poor mechanics that contributed to the injury.[24]

Sixth, assure proper completion of rehabilitation prior to returning to full activities. Although all patients with knee injuries may start with a general rehabilitation program, the rehabilitation program must incorporate motions that are required of the dancer. When full range of motion and strength have returned and limited participation has resulted in no aggravation of knee pain or swelling, the dancer can return to full dance activities. Patellar restraining braces, double upright braces, and derotational braces, although useful in providing additional support to the returning athlete, can be used by the dancer only during class or rehearsal but usually cannot be worn during performance.

Seventh, make rehabilitation a team effort. Usually if the physician or therapist explains the rationale of the treatment program to those involved, they cooperate in trying to meet the ultimate goal of returning the dancer to full activity. Make everyone aware of the initial restrictions as well as advances in the rehabilitation program as they occur. Ultimately, if each dancer is evaluated, trained, and treated as an individual, and if reasons for the injury are considered and changed when possible, recurrent injury should be avoided.

INJURY PREVENTION

Conditioning should include flexibility training, strength training, and cardiovascular endurance exercises. Flexibility training, especially of the ankle, anterior hip, and spine, prevents chronic excessive torque at the knee. Flexibility exercises are particularly important in adolescents. Hypermobile dancers need more emphasis on strengthening than

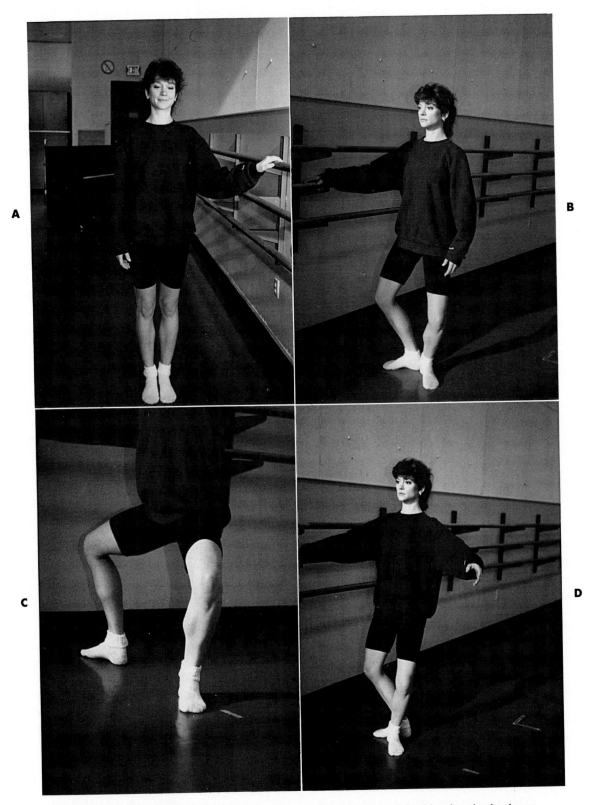

Fig. 24-6. The dancer begins with feet parallel (**A**). She then turns out her hips, keeping her knees extended. First position for this dancer places her feet at an angle of 140 degrees (**B**). Her feet stay at this angle while she is changing to second position (**C**), third position (**D**), fourth position (**E**), and fifth position (**F**).

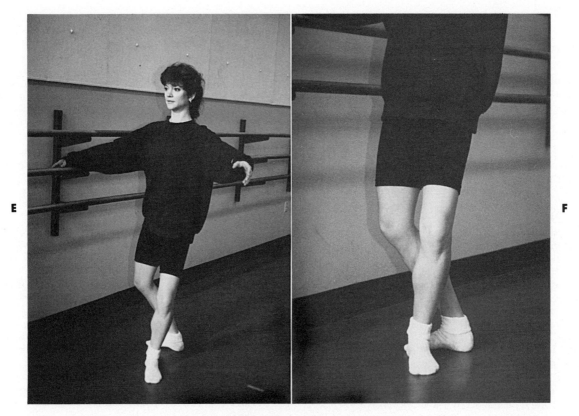

Fig. 24-6, cont'd. For legend see opposite page.

on flexibility. Therefore, each dancer must be evaluated and conditioned as an individual.

Strength conditioning is usually frowned on by dancers but is quite helpful in both prevention and treatment of injury. Lower extremity strength training outside the dance studio is needed for muscles that are infrequently used while dancing, such as anterior leg and posterior thigh. Upper extremity and trunk strengthening are important, too. Specifically, one should strengthen at least the iliopsoas and erector spinae, anterior and posterior tibial muscles, adductors, and hip abductors.

Fatigue is often noted as a factor associated with injury in dancers. The inclusion of aerobic exercise in the conditioning program might help to avoid fatigue and thereby decrease the number of injuries. In addition to increasing endurance, aerobic exercise increases the capillarization of muscles, thereby theoretically making them less subject to injury. Having a well-conditioned cardiopulmonary system allows the dancer to concentrate on technique rather than worry about making it to the end of the performance. Aerobic conditioning also is useful for the problem of weight control and is less likely to produce problems with amenorrhea and bone mineral density than is decreasing caloric intake for weight control.[26] The treating physician should be aware of signs of anorectic behavior so that proper counseling can be recommended. Amenorrheic athletes appear

to be at greater risk for musculoskeletal injury.[27,28] Therefore, the menstrual status of the female dancer needs to be taken into account.

Training must include attention to the frequency, duration, intensity, and specificity of activity. If at all possible, activities should be varied on alternate days to eliminate repetitive stress in any one part and avoid overuse injuries. In the professional dancer or aerobics teacher, encourage working on different routines or pieces on different days, even though the warm-up and warm-down may be the same. Warm-down is a new concept for nonaerobic dancers. This is a good time for stretching to produce permanent changes in flexibility. Proper technical training also is critical. The dancer must have the physical abilities, strength, body awareness, and flexibility needed to perform a given skill. Instruction in technique should follow a logical and systematic progression.

Because of the anatomic requirements for dance, a child who has limited flexibility, significant lower limb rotational abnormalities, or increased lumbar lordosis should be discouraged from a career in dance.[15] Marked genu valgum is a relative contraindication for participating in dance. Other lower limb alignment variations such as excessive femoral anteversion, internal tibial torsion, or metatarsus adductus may present technical problems, depending on the dance form.

SUMMARY

Dancers have many of the same physical and emotional demands as other athletes in addition to aesthetic demands and the need for artistic expression and musicality. Dance deals intimately with the relationships of body parts to the whole and can be useful in rehabilitating the nondance athlete as well.

REFERENCES

1. Klemp P, Stevens JE, Isaacs S: A hypermobility study in ballet dancers, *J Rheumatol* 11:692, 1984.
2. Kendall HO, Kendall FP: Normal flexibility according to age groups, *J Bone Joint Surg [Am]* 30:690–694, 1948.
3. Micheli LJ: Overuse injuries in children's sports, *Orthop Clin North Am* 14:337, 1983.
4. Kirkendall DT, Calabrese LH: Physiological aspects of dance, *Clin Sports Med* 2:525, 1983.
5. Cohen JL: *The cardiovascular and metabolic demands of classical dance.* In Ryan AJ, Stephens RE, editors: *Dance medicine: a comprehensive guide,* Chicago, 1987, Pluribus.
6. Teitz CC: Unpublished data.
7. Teitz CC: *Dance, gymnastics, and skating injuries in athletic females.* In Pearl A, editor: *The athletic female,* Champaign, Ill, 1992, Human Kinetics.
8. Garrick JG, Gillien DM, Whiteside P: The epidemiology of aerobic dance injuries, *Am J Sports Med* 14:67–72, 1986.
9. Quirk R: Ballet injuries: the Australian experience, *Clin Sports Med* 2:507–514, 1983.
10. Rovere GD, et al: Musculoskeletal injuries in theatrical dance students, *Am J Sports Med* 11:195–199, 1983.
11. Washington EL: Musculoskeletal injuries in theatrical dancers: site, frequency, and severity, *Am J Sports Med* 6:75–98, 1978.
12. Micheli LJ, Solomon RL: *Training the young dancer.* In Ryan AJ, Stephens RE, editors: *Dance medicine: a comprehensive guide,* Chicago, 1987, Pluribus.
13. Solomon RL, Micheli LJ: Technique as a consideration in modern dance injuries, *Phys Sportsmed* 14:83–92, 1986.
14. Solomon RL: *In search of more efficient dance training.* In Solomon RL, et al, editors: *Preventing dance injuries: an interdisciplinary perspective,* Reston, Va, 1990, AAHPERD.
15. Teitz CC: Sports medicine concerns in dance and gymnastics, *Pediatr Clin North Am* 29:1399–1421, 1982.
16. Teitz CC: *Knee problems in dancers.* In Solomon RL, et al, editors: *Preventing dance injuries: an interdisciplinary perspective,* Reston, Va, 1990, AAHPERD.
17. Teitz CC: *Gymnastic and dance athletes.* In Mueller F, editor: *Prevention of athletic injuries,* Philadelphia, 1991, FA Davis.
18. Clippinger-Robertson KS, et al: *Mechanical and anatomical factors relating to the incidence and etiology of patellofemoral pain in dancers.* In Shell CG, editor: *The dancer as athlete: Olympic Scientific Congress proceedings,* Champaign, Ill, 1986, Human Kinetics.
19. Teitz CC: *First aid, immediate care and rehabilitation of knee and ankle injuries in dancers and athletes.* In Shell CG, editor: *The dancer as athlete: Olympic Scientific Congress proceedings,* Champaign, Ill, 1986, Human Kinetics.
20. Molnar M: *Rehabilitation of the injured dancer.* In Ryan AJ, Stephens RE, editors: *Dance medicine: a comprehensive guide,* Chicago, 1987, Pluribus.
21. Stephens RE: *The neuroanatomical and biochemical basis of flexibility exercise in dance.* In Solomon RL, et al, editors: *Preventing dance injuries: an interdisciplinary perspective,* Reston, Va, 1990, AAHPERD.
22. Laughman RK, et al: Strength changes in the normal quadriceps femoris muscle as a result of electrical stimulation, *Phys Ther* 63:494, 1983.
23. Holmes J, Fitzsimons C, and Larkam E: *The dancer's knee: ACL injury rehabilitation using Pilates-based techniques.* Presented at the first annual meeting of the International Association for Dance Medicine and Science, Baltimore, June 1991.
24. Lauffenburger SK: *Bartenieff fundamentals: early detection of potential dance injuries.* In Solomon RL, et al, editors: *Preventing dance injuries: an interdisciplinary perspective,* Reston, Va, 1990, AAHPERD.
25. Sweigard LE: *Human movement potential: its ideokinetic facilitation,* New York, 1974, Harper & Row.
26. Brooks-Gunn J, Warren MP, Hamilton LH: The relation of eating problems and amenorrhea in ballet dancers, *Med Sci Sports Exerc* 19:41, 1987.
27. Drinkwater BL, et al: Bone mineral content of amenorrheic and eumenorrheic athletes, *N Engl J Med* 311:277–281, 1984.
28. Kadel NJ, Teitz CC: Stress factors in ballet dancers, *Am J Sports Med* 20:445, 1992.

Chapter 25

SKIING

Jack Harvey
Suzanne Tanner

The knee is commonly the most seriously injured site in skiers, with approximately 1 to 2 knee injuries per 1000 skiing days.[1] An estimated 5 to 10 million people ski an average of 14 times per year in the United States[2] and sustain at least 50,000 knee injuries.

Although improved bindings, machine-groomed slopes, better ski area management, and widespread ski instruction[3,4] may have contributed to a 60% decline in the overall rate of lower extremity injuries from 1972 to 1987,[3] an astronomic increase in complete tears of the anterior cruciate ligament (ACL) was found during this 15-year span[3] (Table 25-1). Improved diagnostic tests, higher and stiffer boots that transmit greater force to the knee, and tight bindings with no upward release at the toe piece may account for this dramatic jump in ACL injuries. Bindings with an upward release of the toe piece have recently been devised and ought to help protect the ACL.

Although contusions, dislocations, fractures, and overuse injuries such as patellofemoral pain are evident from ski injury statistics, knee ligamentous injuries are the most common acute injuries. Knee ligament sprains account for 20% of alpine (downhill) skiing injuries, with 85% of these sprains involving the medial collateral ligament.[5] Knee sprains account for 25% of cross-country skiing injuries.[5] Knee injuries from snowboarding are less common than knee injuries from alpine skiing,[6] but the recent development of higher, stiffer boots may place the knee at more risk. Only 2% of knee injuries involve torn menisci[5] as an isolated injury.

All injured skiers, whether treated operatively or conservatively, deserve a well-designed rehabilitation program to expedite their return to skiing and decrease their risk of reinjury. An effective rehabilitation program designed to mimic the strength, agility, and endurance demands of skiing involves closed-chain kinetic exercises, eccentric strengthening, and the use of ski-specific training devices. An added challenge is providing a seminomadic ski racer with portable rehabilitation equipment or designing a re-habilitation program for a skier who lives in a small community with no physical therapy facilities (Fig. 25-1).

FIRST AID AND INITIAL CARE

Following the RICE mnemonic as soon as the injured skier is transported off the slope greatly reduces swelling and expedites return of function. For an injured skier, the RICE mnemonic consists of *r*esting the knee by using crutches if walking is painful and applying a posterior splint for severe injuries; applying *i*ce for approximately 20 minutes several times per day until swelling lessens; *c*ompressing the knee with an elastic bandage; and *e*levating the injured knee above the level of the heart.

Physicians should think twice before placing an injured knee in the standard straight-leg immobilizer. Although the immobilizer may stabilize some fractures, it promotes atrophy and stiffness. Patients with ligamentous and meniscal injuries are often uncomfortable in an immobilizer.

Although anti-inflammatory medication may be prescribed, good adherence to the RICE mnemonic probably reduces swelling in an acutely injured knee more effectively than medications.

ACUTE KNEE INJURIES
Medial collateral ligament sprains

Medial collateral ligament (MCL) sprains often are caused by catching the inside edge of the ski, creating sudden flexion, lower leg external rotation, and valgus stress on the knee.[5] Slow, twisting falls may sprain the MCL because it is difficult, if not impossible, to adjust the toe piece of bindings at a tension that allows the binding to release during a slow, twisting fall, but not prematurely release while skiing aggressively.

If there is a question regarding whether a skier's medial collateral ligament may be injured, an on-slope assessment may be done by asking the skier to lift the ski of the injured leg off the slope and quickly twist it back and forth through internal and external rotation. This maneuver should not be performed, of course, if the knee is obviously injured. Apprehension or failure to tolerate this windshield-wiper-like motion requires cessation of skiing and obtaining assistance in descending the hill.

Patients with grade I MCL sprains may require an elastic knee wrap or simple knee sleeve to reduce swelling and provide slight support. Knee sleeves with medial and lateral hinges prevent valgus stress and reduce swelling while allowing motion in patients with grade II MCL sprains.

Proper treatment of third-grade MCL sprains (complete tears) is controversial. Nonsurgical treatment has recently been advocated[7] and is gaining acceptance nationally. Patients with grade III MCL sprains are usually most comfortable in a knee sleeve with medial and lateral hinges locked at 20 or 30 degress of flexion. Brace settings may be gradually advanced after the first 5 to 7 days to a range of 20 to 60 degrees. In any patient with an MCL sprain, extremes of flexion and extension and external rotation of

Table 25-1. Skiing injury trends over 15 years (1972–1987)

	Trend	Percentage
Overall injury rate	Declined	50%
Lower extremity injuries	Declined	60
Injuries below the knee	Declined	78
Tibia fractures	Declined	88
Ankle sprains	Declined	86
Knee injuries	Declined	36
Third-degree ACL sprains	Increased	172

From Johnson RJ, Ettlinger CF, Shealy JE: *Skier injury trends*. Presented at the Seventh Annual Symposia on Skiing Trauma and Safety, France, 1989.

the tibia on the femur[8] should be avoided early because these positions may stretch the ligament, cause pain, and delay healing. For all MCL sprains, the knee brace may be removed when pain-free motion is present between 5 and 100 degrees and the athlete can walk with minimal or no limp.[9]

Anterior cruciate ligament sprains

McConkey[4] has outlined four mechanisms that may injure the ACL while skiing.

1. Catching the inside edge of a ski produces sudden or prolonged external rotation of the lower leg and valgus stress. The ACL alone, or both the ACL and MCL, may tear.[4]

2. Hyperextension may produce an isolated tear of the ACL. "Hyperextension at the knee is caused by sudden arrest or slowing of forward progress of the ski under heavy snow. The ski boot and leg become relatively fixed in relation to the upper body, which progresses forward. Forces on the ACL are accentuated by internal rotation and varus (force)," explains McConkey.[4]

3. The term "boot-induced ACL rupture" has been coined by Johnson. This typically occurs when a ski racer lands on the tails of the skis after "taking air" off a bump. With the skier's weight back and the skis and boots rotating forward, boot force is transmitted to the calf,[4] forcing the tibia forward and tearing the ACL.

4. The fourth mechanism occurs only in advanced skiers. While falling backwards, an aggressive skier may try to regain balance by violently contracting the quadriceps. An anterior drawer force is applied to the

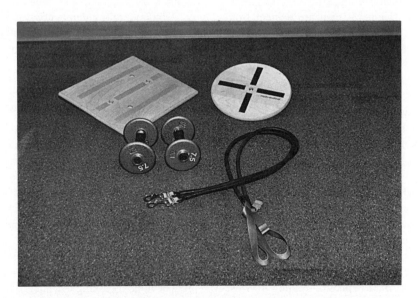

Fig. 25-1. Inexpensive, portable rehabilitation equipment includes hand-held weights for upper body strengthening, balance boards, and elastic tubing.

knee.[4] Failure of the binding toe piece to release vertically allows transmission of force to the ACL.

Conservative and postoperative rehabilitation programs for patients with ACL sprains are outlined in Chapters 10 and 13. Pool therapy is a valuable adjunct in the early phases of ACL rehabilitation for skiers. The buoyancy of water limits weightbearing and allows the initiation of ski-specific exercises, such as lateral hops, and proprioceptive drills soon after an operation.

During the later stages of ACL rehabilitation, strength, balance, and agility may be enhanced by performing exercises using elastic tubing as advocated by Steadman et al.[14] (box below and Figs. 25-2 through 25-7). These exercises may be designed to mimic skiing motions.

Avulsion fracture of the tibial eminence

An interstitial tear of the anterior cruciate ligament is less common in children than in adults. A child's ligament may tear at the tibial insertion. In both children and adults, an avulsion fracture of the tibial eminence may occur.[11]

There are two treatment options for avulsion fractures of the tibial eminence: (1) casting with the knee extended if anatomic reduction can be confirmed; the intercondylar notch presses against the tibial eminence in full extension and maintains reduction; and (2) open, or arthroscopic, reduction.[11] A postoperative rehabilitation program has been outlined by Rosenburg et al.[1] (Table 25-2).

Patellar trauma

A patellar contusion, patella fracture, or quadriceps tendon laceration can occur in telemark skiers. The telemark style of downhill skiing requires extreme flexion of the rear leg, with the rear patella near the snow. Blows to the patella occur when the rear knee strikes the tail of the forward ski during mogul skiing. Hitting a rock or tree stump hidden under the snow while skiing in the back country can also traumatize the patella. Knee pads are therefore strongly recommended for telemark skiers.

Exercises for skiers using elastic tubing

Hip flexion (standing)
Hip extension (standing)
Hamstring curls (supine or seated)
Leg press (seated)
Squats: single one-third knee bends (standing)
       double knee bends (standing)
Walking forward (standing, with band around waist)
Walking backward (standing, with band around waist)
Hip abduction (standing)
Hip adduction (standing)
Side-to-side jumping (standing, with band around waist)

From Steadman JR, Forster RS, Silferskiold JP: Rehabilitation of the knee, *Clin Sports Med* 8:605–627, 1989.

OVERUSE INJURIES
Patellofemoral pain

Patellofemoral pain is not unusual in alpine skiers from repetitive flexion while skiing moguls or from telemark skiing. Preparation for the ski season by running, use of Stairmaster machines, and participating in aerobics can also elicit patellofemoral pain. Patellofemoral pain may manifest itself as aching in the anterior aspect of the knee, especially during or after skiing the moguls, or it may present as a dull ache during the ski lift ride that requires use of the footrest for comfort.

Treatment for patellofemoral pain includes temporary rest, application of ice, anti-inflammatory medications, application of physical therapy modalities, and a therapy program as outlined in Chapter 11. Straight leg raises to strengthen the quadriceps may be performed initially. Leg press resistance exercises, as well as one-leg minisquats performed from full extension to 30 to 45 degrees of flexion (Fig. 25-2) are more sport-specific for skiers and load the patellofemoral joint less than open-chain (foot is not weight-

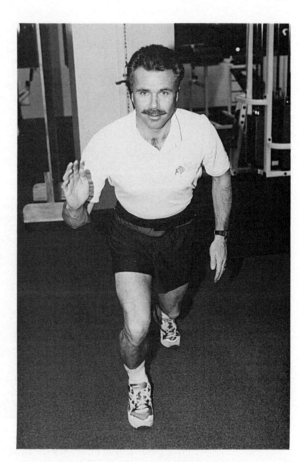

Fig. 25-2. Placing around the waist a belt attached to elastic tubing allows resistance to be applied during forward running, walking forwards and backwards, and jumping from side to side.[9]

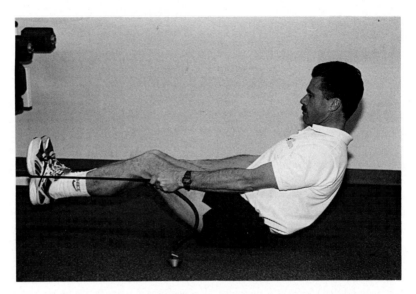

Fig. 25-3. Leg presses using elastic tubing allow quadriceps strengthening with low ACL stress.

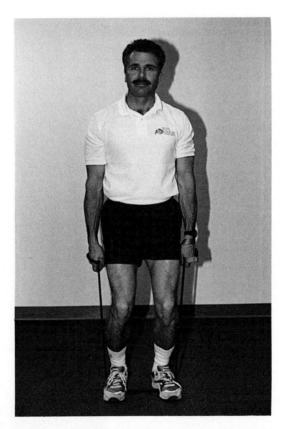

Fig. 25-4. Minisquats with elastic tubing. Quadriceps and gluteal strength can be improved by performing one-legged or two-legged squats, while minimizing ACL stress.[9] One-third squats may initially be done from full knee extension to 30 degrees of flexion.

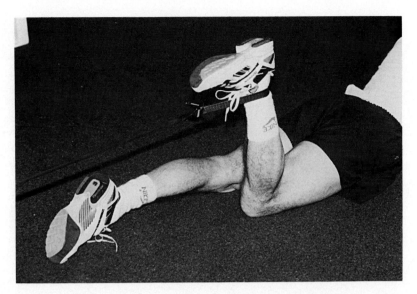

Fig. 25-5. Strengthening hamstrings is an important component of ACL rehabilitation. By securing elastic tubing to a fixed object, hamstring curls can be performed while the skier is seated or prone.

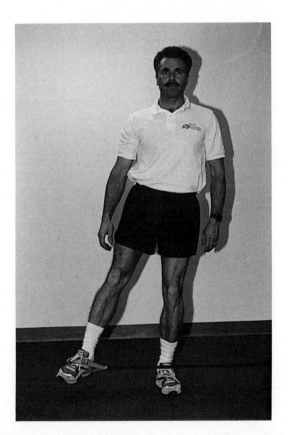

Fig. 25-6. Hip abduction strength is required for the skating technique used by cross-country skiers and to accelerate from the starting gate in alpine ski races. Hip adduction can be strengthened by placing the end of the elastic tubing around the medial side of the foot.

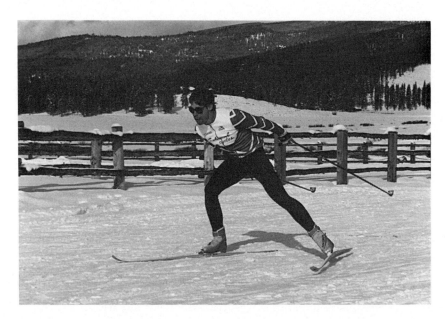

Fig. 25-7. Cross-country skating technique. Note the hip abduction required for effective push-off.

Table 25-2. Rosenburg's rehabilitation program for tibial spine avulsion fractures

Time post injury	Rehabilitation program
0–4 Weeks	Immobilization with knee extended Isometric exercises Straight leg lifts
4 Weeks	0 To 60 degrees of motion, and increase flexion by 10 degrees each week
6 Weeks	Partial weightbearing (depending upon type of graft and fixation)
8 Weeks	Full weightbearing
3 Months	Bicycling, swimming Leg press Elastic tubing exercises
4 Months	Jogging

From Rosenburg TD, Franklin JL, Paulos LE: Skiing. In Reider B, editor: *Sports medicine: the school-age athlete,* Philadelphia, 1991, WB Saunders.

bearing) leg extension resistance exercises. Because alpine skiing usually does not require knee flexion beyond 60 degrees of flexion, performing exercises with more flexion may not enhance skiing performance and may aggravate the patellofemoral joint. Skiers should also continue to strengthen the quadriceps during the ski season.

Patellar taping or a knee sleeve with a central patellar hole and buttresses surrounding the patella may reduce pain in skiers with clinically or radiologically identified patellar hypermobility or malalignment. Wearing the knee sleeve or patellar tape during strengthening exercises and while skiing may reduce pain.

Custom-made orthotics for ski boots and cross-country skiing shoes may reduce anterior knee pain in skiers in whom pronation or supination contributes to patellofemoral irritation.

Modification of skiing by avoiding the moguls and stopping skiing earlier in the day also reduces patellofemoral pain. The old adage "practice makes perfect" is correctly stated as "perfect practice makes perfect" and applies to patellofemoral problems.

Patellar tendonitis

Infrapatellar tendonitis develops from increased eccentric loading of the tendon while the athlete is skiing the moguls or landing from jumps. Treatment and rehabilitation are similar to those for patellofemoral irritation. Patellar taping may stabilize the tendon and apply compression to reduce swelling.

Iliotibial band irritation

The Skating technique used by cross-country skiers is the main cause of iliotibial band irritation. Repetitive knee flexion and extension by mogul and telemark skiers, and also conditioning for skiing by running, may also aggravate the iliotibial band. When symptoms first occur, the skier should temporarily avoid aggravating activity, take anti-inflammatory medications, apply ice, and use appropriate physical therapy modalities. As acute symptoms subside, iliotibial band stretching exercises should be instituted.

ADVANCED REHABILITATION AND TRAINING PROGRAM

A thorough rehabilitation program should include skiing-specific exercises to ensure that a skier can return to skiing safely and with good coordination. A thorough conditioning program should include exercises to improve strength, flexibility, anaerobic capability, aerobic endurance, and agility.

Before activities with high demands on the knee are performed, the athlete should be able to flex the knee actively from 0 to 120 degrees, walk without a limp, and exhibit good control while slowly descending an 18-inch step.[11]

Strengthening exercises

Alpine ski racing requires high isokinetic leg strength.[12] Isokinetic leg strength in alpine skiers and snowboarders can be enhanced by performing closed-chain exercises via leg press (Fig. 25-3) and squats (Fig. 25-4). Hamstring strength is particularly important in a patient with an ACL injury and can be gained by hamstring curl resistance exercises (Fig. 25-5). Performing abduction and adduction resistance exercises may enhance alpine ski racing and cross-country skating performance (Figs. 25-6 and 25-7). Abdominal and back musculature helps stabilize the trunk and allows a skier to maintain balance. Strengthening these areas can be accomplished with abdominal curls and back extension exercises.

Alpine downhill racers require high isometric leg strength to maintain the tuck, or crouched, position. Isometric strength may be enhanced by maintaining a "wall sit" position (Fig. 25-8) or tuck position (Fig. 25-9) for 1 to 2 minutes.

Good strength of the rhomboids, latissimus dorsi, and serratus anterior allows transfer of force from the upper back to arms at the start of an alpine ski race and while poling during uphill sections of cross-country courses. Upper back, deltoid, and triceps strength can be improved with free weights, resistance exercises, and elastic tubing.

Flexibility exercises

Pain around the patellofemoral joint and from patellar tendonitis or iliotibial band irritation may be alleviated with hamstring, quadriceps, and iliotibial band stretching. Good back, hip flexor, and hamstrings flexibility is required for efficient classical cross-country skiing. Cross-country skiers utilizing the skating technique also require good flexibility of the hip adductor muscles. Hip flexibility of the hamstrings and Achilles tendons is not required in downhill skiing because the ski boot holds the knee in slight flexion and limits dorsiflexion of the ankle. Lower extremity flexibility, however, may help prevent overuse injuries in alpine skiers during their conditioning by running and other activities.

Anaerobic conditioning

Alpine ski racing is mainly anaerobically demanding because the longest race, downhill, is performed in less than

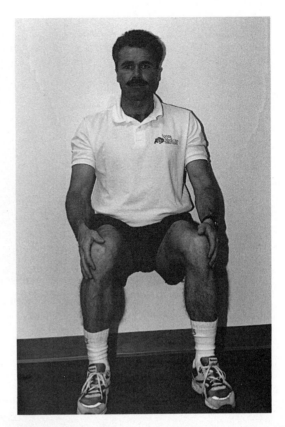

Fig. 25-8. Isometric wall sit exercise. Maintaining this position for 1 to 2 minutes improves quadriceps isometric strength required for alpine turns.

3 minutes. The high altitude of ski areas contributes to hypoxia in elite and recreational skiers. Anaerobic capacity can be improved by performing sprints while running or bicycling, running up stairs, and performing high-repetition, low-resistance exercises on equipment such as the leg press machine.

Aerobic conditioning

Endurance is especially important for cross-country skiers and may be enhanced by long-distance running, bicycling, and training on Stairmaster-type machines. Although a Nordic Track machine (Fig. 25-10) may help recreational cross-country skiers build endurance, cross-country racers often avoid this machine for fear of practicing inefficient technique. Ideal timing and body position differ between skiing on classical cross-country skis and on the Nordic Track.

Elite alpine skiers often have superior aerobic capacity, but greater maximal oxygen consumption does not correlate consistently with actual performance.[13] The high maximum oxygen uptake seen in elite alpine skiers may reflect the training program of the athletes rather than the actual demands of the sport.[12]

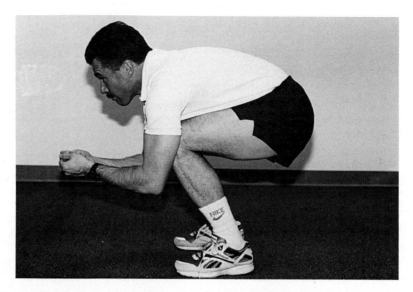

Fig. 25-9. Maintaining a tuck position during a downhill ski requires isometric quadriceps strength, which can be developed by holding this crouched position for 1 to 2 minutes.

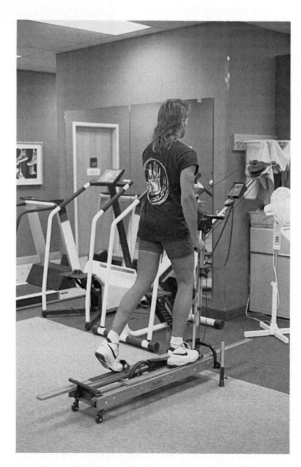

Fig. 25-10. Sport-specific training for diagonal stride cross-country skiing can be obtained on a Nordic Track.

Agility drills

Quickness and proprioception of alpine skiers may be enhanced by playing soccer, hopping through tires set up in the shape of a slalom course, running through an obstacle course of plastic cones, running down ski slopes during the summer, using balance boards (Fig. 25-11), roller blading around poles or plastic cones set up as a slalom course, jumping rope, training on a slide board (Fig. 25-12), using skiing simulators (Fig. 25-13), and jumping on a trampoline.

RETURN TO SKIING

To safely return to downhill skiing, an injured skier should ideally have good graft strength and fixation post-operatively, full range of knee motion, good strength, adequate aerobic conditioning, and psychological readiness. Strength of the involved leg should be at least 85% of that of the uninjured leg. An isokinetic machine may be utilized to measure quadriceps and hamstrings strength, or the maximum weight that can be moved for 8 to 10 repetitions with each leg may be compared on a leg press machine. If resistance equipment is not available, the height of one-legged vertical jumps and the length of one-legged horizontal jumps can be measured. Another functional test is to help decide whether the athlete has regained the strength and agility to ski moguls or a slalom course is to determine if the athlete can jump at least 15 times on one leg laterally, back and forth, over an object the size of a shoebox.

Healing time varies among individuals, but skiers with grade I MCL sprains may often return to the slopes within as little as 2 weeks after the injury. Grade II MCL sprains typically require at least 6 weeks before the skier can return to the slopes safely. It is not unusual for patients with grade III MCL sprains to require at least 2 months before healing.

Aerobic fitness makes skiing safer. A higher percentage of skiing injuries occur in the afternoon, suggesting that fatigue contributes to falling, predisposing a skier to injury.[14]

A ski binding check and adjustment at a reputable ski shop should precede a drive to the ski slope. Standardized tables guide adjusting the binding according to the skier's weight and ability.

Ski racers may regain coordination and confidence by limiting skiing to smooth slopes for several days and focusing on proper technique. After several days, if the knee is pain-free, they may advance to skiing steeper slopes and moguls. Following a ski racer of similar ability down the slopes may foster confidence before returning to practice on race courses.

The recommendation that a recreational skier with an incompletely healed injury return to skiing while "taking it easy on the green (easy) slopes" may be foolhardy because even expert skiers realize that any skier, of any ability, may fall on any slope and risk reinjury. Also, the presence of pain, stiffness, swelling, or inability to perform lateral hops

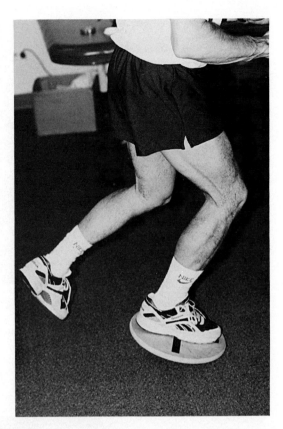

Fig. 25-11. The balance board exercise enhances the balance and proprioception required in alpine skiing and in skiing the downhill portions of cross-country courses.

well after skiing suggests the skier returned to the slopes too soon.

A high-level competitor who insists on returning to skiing before complete healing and rehabilitation have occurred should be warned of the risk of reinjury. Prescribing a brace if ligaments have been damaged and loosening ski binding settings may minimize risk. Analgesics and local anesthetics are contraindicated as they merely mask pain, placing the weakened extremity at even more risk. Taking trial runs initially on easy slopes, then on more difficult terrain, and finally on practice courses may convince even an impatient competitor that good performance is not possible and efforts would best be spent on recovery.

The release mechanism of ski bindings may function best if skiers avoiding walking on cement or gravel while wearing ski boots. These surfaces may erode the sole of the boot surface and alter the binding-to-boot interface. Wiping the snow off the sole of the ski boot before putting it into the binding may decrease friction between the boot and binding, allowing the binding to release properly. Bindings with an upwardly releasing toe piece may protect the ACL during backward falls. The skiers' responsibility code of the National Ski Area Association stresses skiing under control,

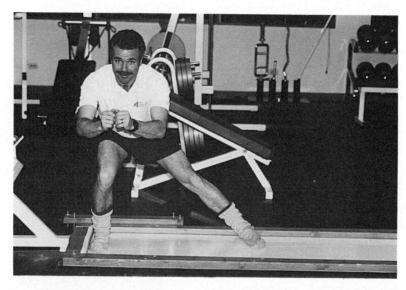

Fig. 25-12. A slide board may be constructed with an 8-foot-long sheet of Formica countertop surrounded by a padded wood frame. Forcefully gliding from side to side while wearing socks improves the balance and lower body strength necessary for alpine skiing and for skating while cross-country skiing.

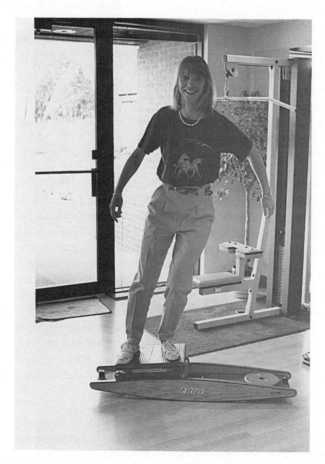

Fig. 25-13. The fitter helps provide aerobic and strength endurance training for alpine skiing.

stopping only at the edge of ski slopes, avoiding stopping in a position on the slope not visible from above, yielding appropriately to other skiers, using devices to prevent runaway skis, and obeying posted signs.[1] Drinking alcohol before, or during, skiing should also be avoided.

FUNCTIONAL BRACES

Knee braces seem to signify the "red badge of courage" among the ski crowd and may be seen on injured skiers of all levels. Studies assessing their functional and protective value during skiing, unfortunately, are lacking.

If a brace is prescribed to limit valgus force, such as with a medial collateral ligament sprain, the brace should at least have a hinge medially and laterally. Valgus and varus stress to the knee may be further minimized if the brace is constructed with a rigid shell for firm fixation to the thigh and lower leg.

Functional braces may prevent hyperextension injuries, but rotational forces are more difficult to control. Under low-load conditions, most functional braces prevent excessive anterior tibial translation to some degree, but as the load increases these braces provide little or no resistance to anterior translation of the tibia.[15] Functional braces may, therefore, be beneficial for a skier with a partially torn ACL or for a slow skier. The ability of a brace to provide stability for a ski racer or aggressive mogul skier with a torn ACL may be inadequate (see Chapter 10).

SUMMARY

A rehabilitation program that allows a skier with an injured knee to return to skiing safely and effectively includes following the RICE mnemonic as soon as the skier is brought off the ski slope, allowing limited motion initially, and gradually advancing activity to improve strength, flexibility, anaerobic capacity, and aerobic endurance. Agility and skiing performance are enhanced through skiing-specific exercises.

REFERENCES

1. Rosenburg TD, Franklin JL, Paulos LE: Skiing. In Reider B, editor: *Sports medicine: the school-age athlete,* Philadelphia, 1991, WB Saunders.
2. Moreland MS: Skiing injuries in children, *Clin Sports Med* 1:241–251, 1982.
3. Johnson RJ, Ettlinger CF, Shealy JE: *Skier injury trends.* Presented at the seventh international symposia on skiing trauma and safety, France, 1989.
4. McConkey JP: Anterior cruciate ligament rupture in skiing: a new mechanism of injury, *Am J Sports Med* 14:160–164, 1986.
5. Howe J, Johnson RJ: Knee injuries in skiing, *Orthop Clin North Am* 12:303–313, 1985.
6. Pino EC, Colville MR: Snowboard injuries, *Am J Sports Med* 17:778–781.
7. Noyes FR, et al: Advances in understanding of knee ligament injury repairs and rehabilitation, *Med Sci Sports Exerc* 16:427–443, 1984.
8. Davis JM: *Rehabilitation of knee injuries.* In Prentice WE, editor: *Rehabilitation techniques in sports medicine,* St Louis, 1990, Mosby–Year Book.
9. Garrick JG, Webb DR: *Sports injuries: diagnosis and management,* Philadelphia, 1990, WB Saunders.
10. Steadman JR, Forster RS, Silferskiold JP: Rehabilitation of the knee, *Clin Sports Med* 8:605–627, 1989.
11. Delitto A, Lehman RC: Rehabilitation of the athlete with a knee injury, *Clin Sports Med* 8:805–840, 1989.
12. Anderson RE, Montgomery DL: Physiology of alpine skiing, *Sports Med* 2:210–221, 1988.
13. White AT, Johnson SC: Physiological comparison of international, national, and regional alpine skiers, *Int J Sports Med* 12:374–378, 1991.
14. Steadman JR, et al: Training for alpine skiing, *Clin Orthop* 216:34–38, 1987.
15. Millet CW, Drez DJ: Principles of bracing for the anterior cruciate ligament deficient, *Clin Sports Med* 7:827–833, 1988.

Part **V**

SPECIAL CONSIDERATIONS

Chapter 26

WOMEN

Mary Lloyd Ireland
Mark R. Hutchinson

Medical research has traditionally focused on males more than females. Reasons cited included the easy accessibility of male subjects in the medical schools of the past and the increased risks and added variables associated with studying females of childbearing age. Similarly, because men participated in athletics in greater numbers than women and because they dominated the high-visibility sports, the focus of sports medicine research has been on the male athlete.

However, in the last decade as women have become increasingly active in both competitive and recreational sports, more research attention is being directed at female athletes, for whom anatomic, physiologic, and psychological gender differences create unique situations and concerns in the diagnosis and treatment of illnesses and injuries. In order to provide optimal care for female athletes, members of the sports medicine team must not only appreciate these gender differences but also understand how they affect injury patterns involving the knee as seen in various sports.

HISTORICAL PERSPECTIVE OF WOMEN IN SPORTS

Although women have participated in sports for more than 1000 years, only recently has the number of females participating in structured, competitive, and recreational athletics skyrocketed. There were no female participants in the first modern Olympic Games in 1896, and in 1932 only 4% of all participating athletes were female.[44] By 1968, however, the number of female participants had risen to 14%. Helen Wills Moody, "Babe" Didrikson Zaharias, and Althea Gibson were among the first well-known female athletes.

In the United States, the enactment and enforcement of the Title IX Educational Assistance Act of 1972 was a major impetus for the expansion of women's opportunities in athletics. Title IX mandated that all institutions receiving federal funds provide equal opportunities to women for all programs, including athletics.

With this added accessibility and encouragement, as well as the greater focus on fitness during the past two decades, the participation of women in sport has increased dramatically. Along with this increase in sports participation has come an associated increase in the incidence of sport-related injuries in women,[44,85,100] particularly those about the knee.

ANATOMY

The sports medicine professional must have a fundamental knowledge of knee anatomy in order to understand and implement a rehabilitation program that will permit the athlete to return to sport safely and effectively. The complex and intricate anatomy of the knee is discussed in Chapter 2. When compared with males, female athletes have certain anatomic differences that place them at greater risk for particular types of knee injuries.

Women: not just smaller men

Just as children are not adults in little packages, women are not just men in different packages. Most females have a lower center of gravity, wider pelvis, shorter legs, and greater genu valgum than males.[8,53] Women have less muscle mass and a greater percentage of body fat per body weight than men.[7,63]

However, during gait and normal running movements, muscle activity is the same for men and women by electromyographic (EMG) analysis.[77] There is no difference in EMG activity of the quadriceps muscle in women runners with and without patellofemoral pain,[77] but increased isokinetic and isometric torque production in men compared with women has been reported.[57] When corrected for weight, lower extremity strength in women is almost equal to that in men, but shoulder and upper extremity strength is less.[95]

With regard to injuries, the probability of injury increases with the weight of the participants.[39] Because women are smaller,[15,18,39] the likelihood of serious injury on the basis of total body weight is less than in men. However, in contact sports with participants of mismatched size, the smaller or less skilled participant is more likely to be injured, putting the female athlete at risk.

Alignment

Bony alignment contributes directly to the forces and strain on the knee compartments, ligaments, and musculotendinous structures. Therefore, anatomic gender differences are especially significant about the knee. In addition to the previously mentioned greater genu valgum, females often have increased femoral anteversion, less development of the vastus medialis obliquus (VMO), greater flexibility, and differences in femoral notch shape and width compared to males (Fig. 26-1). The genu valgum, VMO hypoplasia, and femoral anteversion enhance the laterally directed forces on the patellofemoral joint and intensify stresses on the medial compartment and the medial collateral ligament.[51]

The normal valgus alignment of the lower extremity creates a natural tendency for the mobile structures crossing the knee joint to be displaced laterally during gait.[6,29,32,51] The usual Q-angle, a measurement of the angle created by the intersection of the line from the anterior superior iliac spine to the center of the patella and the line from the center of the patella to the center of the tibial tubercle, is 12 degrees or less (Fig. 26-2). Increased Q-angles magnify the lateral vector and create asymmetry in the quadriceps force. These excessive lateral forces on the quadriceps mechanism, along with patella alta and rotatory limb malalignment, contribute to the destabilization of the patellofemoral joint and enhanced lateral patellar tracking (Fig. 26-3). Retropatellar pain or "miserable malalignment syndrome" is often seen in women who have femoral anteversion, genu valgum, vastus medialis hypoplasia, external tibial torsion, and/or foot pronation (Fig. 26-4).

Ligamentous laxity

Multiple factors contribute to an increased incidence of patellar subluxations and ligament sprains in the female athlete, including ligamentous laxity, flexibility, and strength.[37,98] Cyclic hormonal changes and pregnancy have been shown to increase connective tissue laxity in females, but studies have failed to demonstrate a relationship between knee laxity and injury.[30,62]

Although females tend to have more laxity than their male counterparts, athletic females have less laxity than their nonathletic counterparts.[62] Thus, laxity may be a function of conditioning rather than genetics.[6] Others argue that because patellofemoral conditions are often unilateral, anatomy alone cannot account for the increased incidence of knee injuries in the female athlete.[6] Further research and comparative studies will help to shed light on this complex issue.

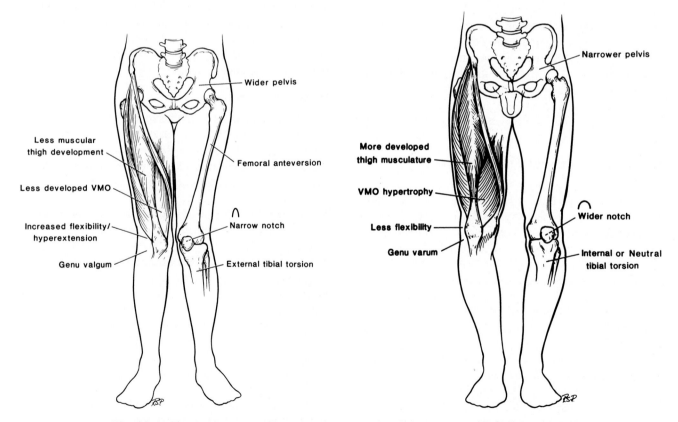

Fig. 26–1. Female alignment *(left)* is diagrammatically shown with wider pelvis, femoral anteversion, genu valgum, hyperflexibility, external tibial torsion, and narrow notch. Male alignment *(right)* demonstrates a narrower pelvis, more developed thigh musculature, genu varum, internal or neutral tibial torsion, and wider notch.

Role of the anterior cruciate ligament in knee stability

When compared with the male, the female may be more dependent on ligaments than muscles for knee stability. Because women are less muscular, they cannot as easily use strength to compensate for patellofemoral problems or rotatory instability. Where men rely on their strong quadriceps mechanism, strong hamstrings, and ability to maintain a relatively flexed position of the knee to prevent functional instability, women have less muscular power, often greater knee hyperextension, and increased laxity and are more dependence on the anterior cruciate ligament (ACL) for knee stability.

According to the NCAA surveillance survey,[91] females are at increased risk of ACL injury in a variety of sports, including gymnastics, soccer, and basketball. Contributing to this increased incidence may be the reduced femoral notch width and variable shape seen in some female knees when compared with male knees (Fig. 26-5).[95,130] Various authors have noted the relatively increased risk of ACL injury with reduced notch size.[68,115]

CONDITIONING

The baseline level of conditioning in most females is significantly lower than that of their male counterparts,[18,20,34,127,130] and this lower level of conditioning is thought to be related to the higher incidence of knee injuries in the female athlete.[8,53] This is not to imply that all women are in poor condition or that women athletes cannot benefit from conditioning; in fact, the opposite is true. Perhaps as a result of their lower level of fitness initially, women demonstrate more improvement with training, resulting in significant increases in strength, power, and muscular endurance.[9] Adequate conditioning is important in enhancing performance and reducing risk of injury.[42] Excellent comparative studies have been done in the military setting. Compared to men, women naval midshipmen improve their fitness more rapidly in aerobic and resistive training.[20] Athletic women in the Navy were found to have more success than their nonathletic female counterparts in the areas of stamina, strength, and self-discipline.[40] Women were capable of efficiency and aerobic metabolism on a par with men.[101]

Stress-related injuries, including those involving the knee, have long been known to be associated with poor conditioning.[6] A random review of 74 female and 74 male cadets demonstrated an increased incidence of stress fractures in the women.[95] In other studies at the Naval Academy, stress-related injuries were seen more frequently in women; however, as the women became acclimated to the rigors of training, their levels of serious injuries decreased to the level of the men's serious injuries.[67,101]

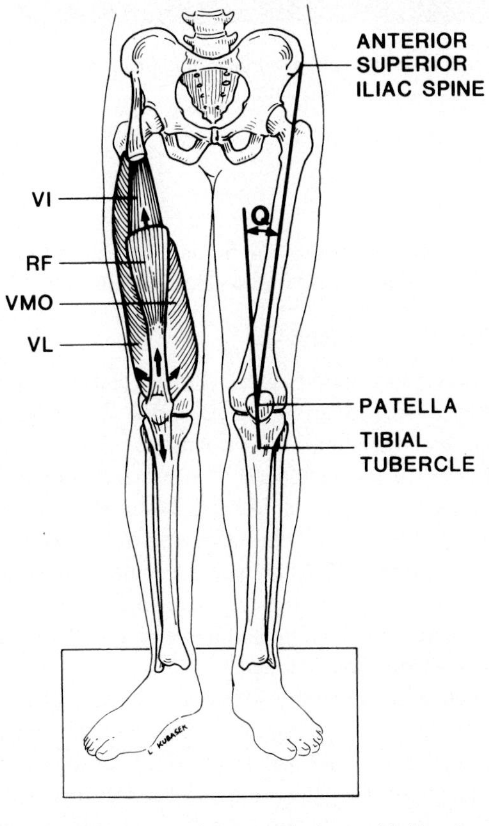

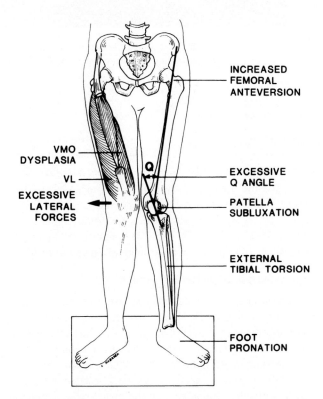

Fig. 26–2. Measurement of Q-angle is done with line drawn from ASIS to patella and patella to tibial tubercle. Normal Q-angle is less than 12 degrees.

Fig. 26–3. *Miserable malalignment syndrome* is a term coined to describe patients who have increased femoral anteversion, genu valgum, vastus medialis obliquus dysplasia, external tibial torsion, and forefoot pronation. These factors create excessive lateral forces and contribute to patellofemoral dysfunction.

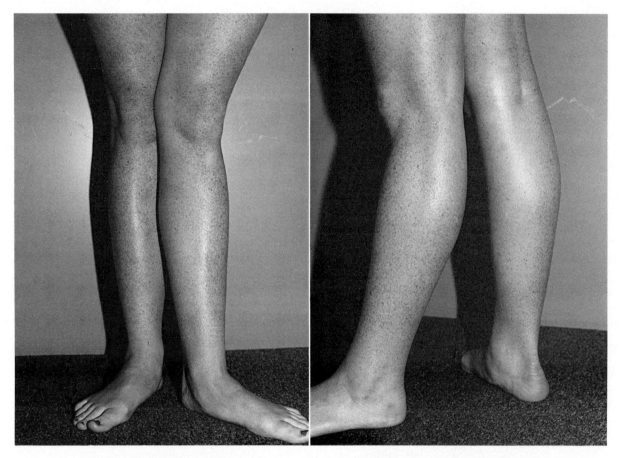

Fig. 26–4. Clinical view from the front and side of miserable malalignment syndrome alignment demonstrating knee hyperextension, VMO dysplasia, genu valgum, and pes planus.

Rehabilitation expectations and performance goals should be based on the athlete's preinjury level of conditioning. Often it is the poorly conditioned athlete who can make the greatest early strides in improving performance compared with the preinjury status of conditioning.[6,49,69,85,126] By increasing levels of conditioning in all athletic females, it may be possible to reduce the incidence and severity of injuries and associated time away from sport.

Injury-specific concerns for women

Certain specific injuries and injury patterns are seen more frequently in the female knee. Most injuries, however, are sport-specific, not gender-specific. Males sustain more injury by direct contact, whereas females are vulnerable to overuse syndromes and noncontact ligament sprains of the knee.[6] The increased incidence of contact-related injuries in males is directly correlated with the male predominance in certain sports, especially football and ice hockey.

Females are more likely to sustain noncontact injuries because of differences in anatomy, conditioning, and sport participation. Their injury rate is also influenced by the fact

that they may not acquire the fundamental motor skills necessary for sports during the developmental years.[6]

STRESS FRACTURES

As previously mentioned, women, and especially unconditioned women, are at increased risk of sustaining overuse injuries, including stress fractures.[95] The major factor contributing to the incidence of stress fractures in female military recruits is the rapid onset of training, which fails to allow for progressive exposure to stress and the development of tolerance.[67] Many stress fractures can be avoided with a progressive training regimen; in fact, as female recruits became more acclimated to the rigors of training, the incidence of injuries declined.[101]

Women with relatively low bone density, amenorrhea, and poor diets—for example, female runners with menstrual irregularities and ballerinas with poor diets and menstrual irregularities—are more susceptible to stress fractures.* A detailed nutritional history should be obtained

*References 31, 48, 72, 81, 89, 120.

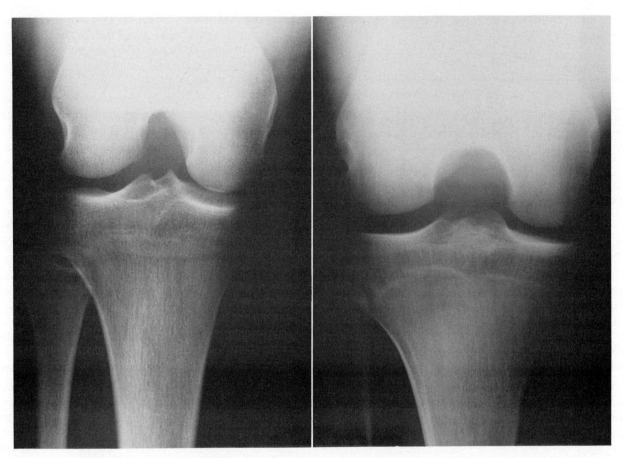

Fig. 26-5. Radiographs of notch views showing a narrow **A** shape of a female *(left)* and wide **C** shape of a male *(right)*. Smaller notch to femoral width ratios are contributing factors to ACL injury.

from these individuals so that nutritional deficiencies or eating disorders may be identified and treatment instituted. Obtaining a gynecologic history is also important; it may be possible to reduce the risk of stress fractures in some amenorrheic athletes by placing them on cyclic estrogens.

PATELLOFEMORAL STRESS SYNDROME

Patellofemoral joint problems are more common in female athletes than in male athletes.[6,24,53,62,127] Patellofemoral stress syndrome, or anterior knee pain, describes a vast array of disorders that may be categorized as inflammatory, mechanical, or miscellaneous (Table 26-1).[33] Patellofemoral stress syndrome is a clinical diagnosis that may be present with such concurrent pathologic processes as chondromalacia patella, symptomatic plica, lateral subluxation of the patella, and early degenerative disease. In addition, Ficat and Hungerford have described the "excessive lateral pressure syndrome," present in both males and females,[28] that has subtle abnormalities and symptoms unrelated to instability or significant malalignment.

Symptomatic plicas appear to be more common in women. The increased valgus alignment of the female knee increases the likelihood that the plica (a redundant flap of synovium[50,94]) will come in contact with the medial femoral condyle and become irritated and inflamed, causing anterior knee pain.

Most athletes with patellofemoral stress syndrome improve on a regimen of oral nonsteroidal anti-inflammatory medications, hamstring stretching, and quadriceps strengthening with particular emphasis on the vastus medialis obliquus (VMO). The VMO, the primary compensating factor for lateral patellar instability,[6,24,29,96] is the chief structure that provides an active medial vector to counterbalance the valgus force. VMO activity is not significantly different in symptomatic and asymptomatic individuals,[104] but patients with patellar subluxation exhibit decreased VMO activity.[79] The VMO is the first muscle to demonstrate atrophy in the injured knee,[29] and it is the most difficult part of the quadriceps to rehabilitate following injury.[6,29,111,128] VMO hypoplasia is more common in females and may be genetically

Table 26-1. Differential diagnosis of anterior knee pain

Inflammatory	Mechanical	Miscellaneous
Bursitis	Hypermobility	Reflex sympathetic
Prepatellar	Subluxation	dystrophy
Retropatellar	Dislocation	Osteochondritis
Pes anserinus	Patellofemoral	dissecans
Tendonitis	stress syndrome	Fat-pad syndrome
Pes anserinus	Pathologic plica	Systemic arthritides
Semimembranosus	syndrome	Muscle strain
Patellar	Osteochondral	Stress fracture
Synovitis	Arthrosis	Meniscal tear
		Iliotibial band syndrome

linked, making rehabilitation of the entire quadriceps, but particularly the VMO, especially important in these individuals.

OSGOOD-SCHLATTER'S DISEASE AND JUMPER'S KNEE

Osgood-Schlatter's disease, or tibial tubercle apophysitis, occurs more rarely in women than in men, which is probably related to sports played, intensity of participation, growth phases, and earlier maturation and physeal closure in females. Jumper's knee, or patellar tendonitis, is another condition seen less frequently in women, which may be a function of the reduced knee torque produced by females compared with males.

REHABILITATION CONSIDERATIONS IN WOMEN

In comparison with male athletes, the average female athlete has less experience in sports and less access to good coaching, athletic trainers, and facilities.* She may be subject to knee injury due to errors in the performance of sport-specific and rehabilitative skills.[6] Female athletes may not have access to or previous experience with the weight room. The coach, physical therapist, athletic trainer, or physician should provide thorough instruction in exercise and rehabilitation techniques, as well as monitor the athlete's progress.

For example, certain exercises are contraindicated in the athlete with patellofemoral pain. They include high-resistance exercises of the quadriceps in an arc of motion between 90 degrees and full extension.[52] The reason for this is the increase in patellofemoral contact area as knee flexion increases (Fig. 26-6),[2] which elevates the forces directed posteriorly, exacerbating pain and reducing the effectiveness of the exercise.

Another potential problem for these athletes is the extension machine (Fig. 26-7),[43,70,103] the use of which loads the anterior tibia, and as knee flexion increases, excessive patellofemoral joint pressures are created. Research has shown that loading the patellofemoral joint from above, as

in squats, and from the foot, as in leg presses, produces fewer patellofemoral joint forces than loading the anterior tibia.[28,50,103] However, squats or leg presses at 90 degrees or down to parallel should be avoided because they generate maximal patellofemoral joint reaction forces.[103]

A more focused approach of quadriceps rehabilitation for an athlete with patellofemoral stress syndrome might include terminal extension exercises and straight leg raising. Closed kinetic chain exercises, such as squats performed with the feet apart to shoulder width and involving low loads, multiple repetitions, and limited flexion, minimize patellofemoral forces and improve quadriceps strength and relieve pain.[8] Squats are performed with feet neutral and externally rotated, which accelerates VMO strengthening (Fig. 26-8). Leg presses executed in a pain-free range of motion also help to restore quadriceps function (Fig. 26-9). Stationary bicycling (with low to moderate resistance and an elevated seat) and swimming are usually well tolerated.[58] In all of these activities, maintaining proper body mechanics is essential.

Selective VMO strengthening improves patellar tracking, but simple straight leg raising or terminal extension exercises are not the optimal way to rehabilitate the VMO.[84] Instead, the femur should be externally rotated to reduce the lateral pull of the tensor fascia lata and to stretch the VMO. Hip adduction should be performed with the knee in extension to optimize the firing of the VMO, which originates in part from the adductor magnus. Electrical stimulation of the VMO, modalities, and biofeedback may also be beneficial.

PSYCHOLOGICAL CONSIDERATIONS IN THE REHABILITATION OF THE FEMALE ATHLETE

In the past, competitive or aggressive females were felt to be unladylike; those who participated in sports were likely to have their womanhood or femininity questioned.[10] Some girls feared being called tomboys or becoming musclebound if they exercised, and so they were forced by social pressures into more sedentary roles.

With the advent of Title IX of the Educational Assistance Act of 1972, the participation of females in sports as administrators, coaches, and athletes has increased dramatically. More women are learning about the benefits of sports and are using participation and success in athletics as a springboard to deal with the stress, competition, and challenges of professional life.[92] Young females participating in athletics have demonstrated improvements in self-confidence and overall performance.[19,95,117]

Positive reinforcement by a respected coach or athletic trainer can further enhance the self-confidence of female athletes.[19] Negative feedback, however, erodes the self-confidence of women more quickly than men. Three factors may affect female athletes' susceptibility to situational vulnerability and reduced self-confidence.[19] First, they tend to

*References 6, 24, 30, 36, 49, 62, 85.

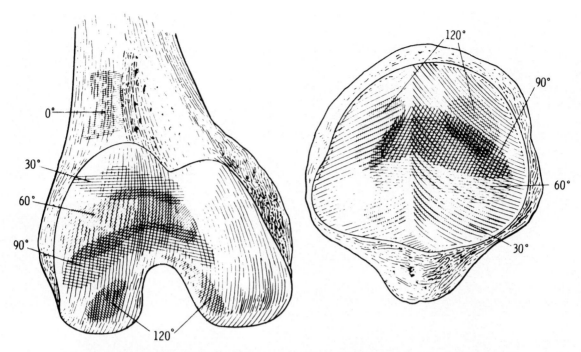

Fig. 26–6. Patellofemoral contact surface area increases with increasing degrees of flexion. The shaded areas match the respective angles of flexion at 0 degrees, 30 degrees, 60 degrees, maximal at 90 degrees, and 120 degrees. On femur, lateral is left; on patella, lateral is right. (From Aglietti P, Insall JN, Walker PS: A new patellar prosthesis, *Clin Orthop* 107:175, 1975.)

do poorly in sex-typed tasks considered to be masculine or sex-role inappropriate. Athletic trainers and physical therapists can counter this trend by emphasizing the appropriateness of the task—be it weight training or another rehabilitative technique—regardless of gender. Second, females are more sensitive to social evaluation than males. Women do not react as well as men when they are compared to other athletes or when they perceive themselves to be battling social pressures. Therefore, when rehabilitating a female athlete, it may be more effective to emphasize the individual's personal gains rather than comparing her progress with that of other athletes. Finally, women appear to be more effective in improving their performance when they receive objective, immediate, and accurate feedback. Without meaningful feedback, females tend to disparage their own performance, establishing a downward performance-confidence spiral.[19] Women may benefit from more frequent supervised rehabilitation sessions and more frequent objective evaluations (such as isokinetic studies) that can provide additional documentation and feedback regarding progress. Rehabilitation should be designed with a series of incremental realistic and attainable goals so the female athlete can see improvement.

Hormonal balance may also affect behavior. For example, menstruation may have a major impact on mood,[82] as demonstrated in one study, which showed that 60% of the athletes investigated noted mood changes with the menstrual cycle. However, only 25% detected a negative effect on

their performance, and a small percentage perceived a positive change.[82]

Various authors have performed psychological assessments comparing female and male athletes.[56,90,117] Using the Bem Sex Role Inventory, which assesses feminine, masculine, and androgynous traits, female athletes tend to be more androgynous and male athletes tend to be more masculine than their nonathletic, same-sex counterparts.[90]

Women are inclined to view athletics as a social outlet, whereas men are intensely focused on winning.[44] As it becomes more socially acceptable for women to strive for success and desire victory, this difference may disappear. At the elite level, it is highly unlikely that there is any difference in the wish to succeed based solely on gender. Similarly, it is doubtful that the female athlete has any less interest in rehabilitation than the male athlete.

REHABILITATION OF THE PREGNANT FEMALE

When working with athletic females in training and rehabilitation, the clinician will undoubtedly be confronted with the issue of pregnancy. Various authors have outlined special considerations for exercise in the pregnant female.* Physically fit women with normal pregnancies who exercise regularly may have larger babies, shorter labor, and decreased incidence of complications compared with those without planned exercise programs.[129] Older studies from

*References 41, 45, 61, 75, 87, 108.

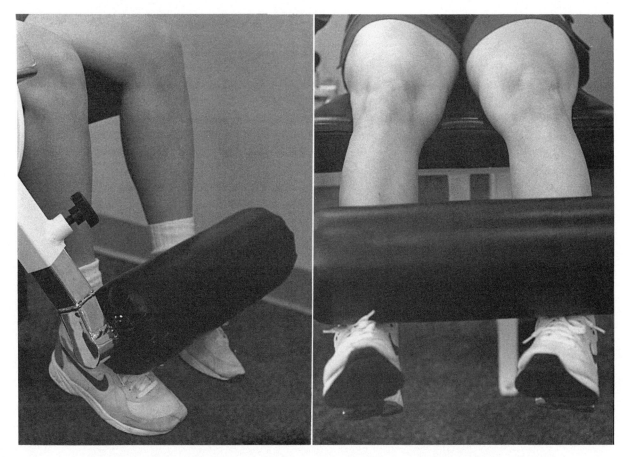

Fig. 26–7. Patient performing quadriceps strengthening exercises with knee extension machine generating excessive patellofemoral pressures with free distal movement and resistive forces on the anterior tibia.

Eastern Europe appear to confirm this.[26,27] Jogging during pregnancy may also improve the overall outcome.[60]

High-intensity exercise or change in the baseline level of exercise may, however, not always be in the best interests of the mother or the fetus. With strenuous exercise, maternal heart rates can rise as high as 200 beats per minute with an associated increase in blood pressure by 30 to 40 torr without apparent benefit to the fetus.[41] In fact, even in uncomplicated pregnancies, uterine blood flow is decreased during strenuous exercise and even more severely compromised in complicated pregnancies. There is concern that sustained exercise in pregnant women may elevate core body temperature, with possible teratogenic effects.[93,113]

Mild to moderate exercise, however, in the low-risk pregnant female is not deleterious to the fetus and may be beneficial in maintaining fitness and easing labor. A general rule of thumb is that if the athlete can carry on a conversation during her workout, then she has not exceeded her maximal physical effort.[41] The American College of Obstetricians and Gynecologists has created a set of guidelines for exercise during pregnancy and the postpartum period:[1,125]

1. Regular exercise (at least three times per week) is preferable to intermittent activities. (Competitive activities should be discouraged.)
2. Vigorous activities should not be performed in hot or humid weather or during a period of febrile illness.
3. Ballistic movements should be avoided. Deep flexion and extension of joints should be avoided because of connective tissue laxity. Activities that require jumping, jarring motions, or quick changes in direction should be avoided because of relatively increased joint instability.
4. Vigorous exercise should be preceded by a period of muscle warm-up and followed by a gradual decline in activity and cool-down.
5. Care should be taken when rising from the floor to avoid orthostatic hypotension.
6. During pregnancy, the maternal heart rate should not exceed 140 beats per minute.
7. During pregnancy, strenuous exercise should not exceed 15 minutes in length.

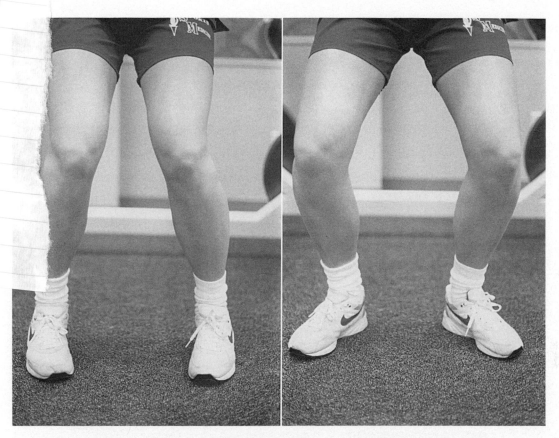

Fig. 26–8. Proper squat technique with feet apart at shoulder width *(left)* and with feet externally rotated *(right);* VMO stimulation is accentuated.

8. No exercises should be performed in the supine position after 4 months of gestation.
9. Liquid should be taken liberally and caloric intake should be adequate for the pregnancy and the exercise undertaken.
10. Maternal core temperature should not exceed 38°C.

High-intensity or prolonged endurance activities may be deleterious to the fetus, and the athlete and fetus may best be served if she refocuses her energies on shorter-duration aerobic activities. For moderate- to high-risk pregnancies, additional rest and reduced levels of exercise are indicated. Fortunately, the majority of pregnant athletic females can undergo rehabilitation for most knee injuries without added risk or difficulty.

EPIDEMIOLOGY OF KNEE INJURIES IN SPECIFIC SPORTS

The National Collegiate Athletic Association (NCAA) and Olympic competition include sports that are male and female combined, male only, and female only. In NCAA competition, female-only sports are field hockey and softball. Male-only NCAA sports include water polo, baseball,

football, ice hockey, and wrestling. Olympic sports limited to females are rhythmic gymnastics and synchronized swimming. Male-only Olympic sports include baseball, bobsled, boxing, ice hockey, modern pentathlon, ski jumping, Nordic combined skiing, soccer, water polo, weight lifting, and wrestling (see box on p. 307). The first women's Olympic marathon was run in 1984 at the Los Angeles games.

About the knee, sprains and strains are the most common type of injury for both males and females. However, females tend to have a higher concentration of injuries about the knee than their male counterparts.[23] This conclusion is confirmed by the findings of the NCAA Injury Surveillance System, which has collected data on injuries in collegiate sports since 1982.[91] Knee injuries were rated as involving the patella, menisci, anterior cruciate ligament (ACL), or collateral ligaments in 1000 athletic exposures in 16 sports. In all women's sports, female gymnasts, soccer players, and basketball players had not only the highest incidence of injury but the most ACL injuries as well (Table 26-2).

Four sports—gymnastics, soccer, basketball, and lacrosse—can be compared for gender differences in rates of ACL injuries. With the exception of lacrosse, women ath-

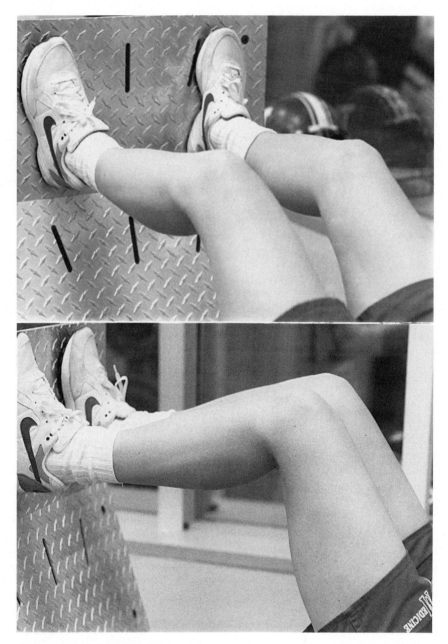

Fig. 26–9. Leg press is very effective for quadriceps strengthening with forces distal on plantar surface of feet through painless arc of knee motion.

Olympic and NCAA sports that are male or female, male only, female only, and combined

Olympic Sports

MALE AND FEMALE

Archery	Equestrian	Rowing	Table tennis
Athletics	Fencing	Shooting	Tennis
Basketball	Artistic gymnastics	Figure skating	Volleyball
Biathlon	Team handball	Speed skating	Yachting
Canoe/kayak	Field hockey	Alpine skiing	
Cycling	Judo	Nordic skiing	
Diving	Luge	Swimming	

MALE ONLY

Baseball	Nordic combined skiing
Bobsled	Soccer
Boxing	Water polo
Ice hockey	Weightlifting
Modern pentathlon	Wrestling
Ski jumping	

FEMALE ONLY

Rhythmic gymnastics
Synchronized swimming

NCAA Sports

COMBINED

	MALE ONLY
Fencing	Water polo
Rifle	Baseball
Skiing	Football
MALE AND FEMALE	Ice hockey
Gymnastics	Wrestling
Volleyball	FEMALE ONLY
Basketball	Field hockey
Cross-country	Softball
Lacrosse	
Soccer	
Swimming/diving	
Tennis	
Indoor/outdoor track	
Golf	

Table 26-2. Knee injury rates from the NCAA surveillance survey, 1991–1992

Sport	Athletic exposures	Total injuries	Rate per 1000 athletic exposures				
			Knee	ACL	Collateral	Meniscus	Patella
Women's							
Gymnastics	36,570	340	9.3	0.44	0.41	0.36	0.16
Soccer	75,064	595	7.93	0.27	0.39	0.29	0.17
Basketball	150,617	764	5.07	0.25	0.32	0.29	0.19
Field hockey	50,921	237	4.65	0.08	0.08	0.06	0.14
Lacrosse	33,315	156	4.68	0.12	0.15	0.09	0.18
Volleyball	120,258	492	4.09	0.11	0.12	0.14	0.2
Softball	71,179	255	3.58	0.13	0.11	0.08	0.11
Men's							
Spring football	39,894	378	9.48	0.18	1.03	0.18	0.28
Wrestling	108,990	977	8.96	0.11	0.86	0.29	0.19
Soccer	148,959	1221	8.2	0.13	0.53	0.19	0.23
Football	744,698	4853	6.52	0.21	0.69	0.25	0.14
Basketball	175,023	1055	6.03	0.07	0.21	0.14	0.24
Lacrosse	71,032	411	5.79	0.21	0.32	0.13	0.11
Gymnastics	10,046	54	5.37	0	0.1	0	0
Ice hockey	99,863	502	5.03	0.08	0.69	0.06	0.03
Baseball	176,702	602	3.41	0.02	0.08	0.06	0.07

letes sustained ACL injuries several times more frequently than men in the same sports.

The NCAA surveillance system has also documented injury rates in practices and games (Table 26-3). Men's spring football had the highest injury rate, followed by men's wrestling and women's gymnastics practices.[91] In women's athletics, gymnastics practice had the highest rate of injury, followed by soccer, basketball, volleyball, lacrosse, and softball practices.

Basketball

In the sport of basketball, females are at increased risk of knee injuries compared with their male counterparts.[130] Women have more patellofemoral disorders and noncontact ligament sprains, whereas men have more meniscal tears and direct contact ligament sprains.[6] An epidemiologic survey of athletes invited to the 1988 U.S. Olympic basketball trials showed that knee injuries occurred more frequently in females than males, and that females were more likely to require surgery.[57] As noted previously, the female basketball player is at increased risk for ACL injury not only over her male counterpart in basketball but also over female athletes in volleyball, lacrosse, and softball.[91]

Soccer

Female youth soccer athletes sustained injuries twice as frequently as their male counterparts, which may be attributed to less skill, conditioning, and training in the female athlete.[92,121] However, even elite female soccer athletes experienced a higher rate of injury (12 per 1000 hours of exposure) than a comparable group of male soccer players (5 per 1000 hours of exposure).[25] In soccer, knee injuries

consistently represented 12% to 20% of all injuries,[64] and approximately one in six injuries to female soccer athletes involved a tear of a meniscus or major knee ligament.[25] In addition, the rate of ACL injuries in female soccer and female basketball athletes was similar.[91]

Field hockey

In field hockey, the knee injury rate was similar regardless of gender (32% for females, 27% for males).[16] For both male and female field hockey athletes, the most common type of knee injury was ligament sprain, followed by muscle strain.[16]

Softball

The incidence of lower extremity injuries in women increases with the need for cutting activities in that sport. Hence, there is a lower incidence of serious knee injuries in softball than in soccer or basketball. In fact, 82% of the injuries associated with significant time lost from sport involved the upper extremity.[22,74] Another study revealed that 19% of all injuries sustained by female softball athletes, but only 7% of those experienced by their male counterparts, affected the knee.[16]

American-style, noncontact football

Because of differences in size and weight, as well as social pressures, only a few women have participated in men's American-style, contact football at the high school and college level. Instead, women are more often involved in intramural, noncontact touch or flag football. As might be expected, different injury patterns are seen in tackle football and flag football.[18] In tackle football, the most com-

Table 26-3. All sports summary injury rates and percentage in practice versus game from NCAA surveillance system, 1992-1993

Sport	Injury rate*	Percentage practice	Percentage game
Spring football	9.59	94	6
Wrestling	9.41	66	34
Women's gymnastics	8.59	78	22
Women's soccer	7.90	51	49
Men's soccer	7.87	47	53
Football	6.57	58	42
Men's lacrosse	6.05	54	46
Men's ice hockey	5.70	32	68
Men's basketball	5.61	65	35
Women's basketball	5.13	61	39
Men's gymnastics	5.06	81	19
Field hockey	5.00	59	41
Women's volleyball	4.76	65	35
Women's lacrosse	4.25	68	32
Women's softball	3.90	52	48
Baseball	3.37	44	56

*Per 1000 athletic exposures including practices and games. From National Collegiate Athletic Association: *NCAA Injury Surveillance System,* Overland Park, Kansas, 1992-1993 NCAA.

monly injured part of the body is the knee.[14,21,67] In women's intramural flag football, the fingers are most commonly injured (39%), followed by the knee (16%).[18]

Track and field

At the collegiate level, there appears to be no difference in the knee injury rates of male and female track athletes.[16] At the elite level, however, female runners have been found to be more susceptible than males to stress fractures.[12] In addition, menstrual irregularity and stress fractures in collegiate female distance runners have been shown to be related.[5]

Volleyball

Knee injuries in volleyball constitute anywhere from 7% to 60 percent of all injuries; there is no significant gender difference.[112] Data from the NCAA surveillance system indicates that in female volleyball players the knee is the second most commonly injured body part (8% to 19%) behind the ankle (26% to 33%).[91] The risk of knee injury in female volleyball players is similar to that of male basketball players and female track and field athletes, which is significantly less than that of female basketball or gymnastics participants.[16,19]

Gymnastics

Both men and women take part in gymnastics as a sport, but they participate in different events. Women participate in balance beam, uneven parallel bars, vault, and floor exercise. Men participate in pommel horse, horizontal bar, still rings, parallel bars, vault, and floor exercise.

Women's gymnastics has the second-highest injury rate of all sports, including contact sports.[59] The greatest number of injuries are associated with the floor exercise, followed by the balance beam, uneven parallel bars, and vault, respectively.[35,36,47,83] Most injuries that occur during competition involve the upper extremity;[16,97,110] the usual mechanism for knee injuries is twisting or a difficult dismount.[53]

Knee pain is reported to affect 14% to 24% of all women gymnasts. Most such knee pain is overuse in nature, associated with intrinsic or extrinsic factors such as patellar malposition, limb deformity, muscular imbalance, malalignment, symptomatic plica, and muscle tightness.[124]

According to NCAA data, in 1991–1992 female gymnasts had the highest incidence of ACL injuries (0.44 per 1000 athletic exposures) of all sports. No male gymnast sustained an ACL injury that year. In addition, female gymnasts experienced significantly more sprains and lower extremity injuries, particularly of the knee, than male gymnasts.[16]

Cheerleading

Although male athletes do participate in cheerleading at the collegiate level, at the high school level cheerleading is primarily a female sport. Because competitive cheerleading involves the routine and precision of dance and the athleticism of gymnastics, one would expect that the numbers and types of injuries seen in cheerleading would be similar to those seen in dance and gymnastics. To date, however, few articles on cheerleaders' injuries have been published.[3,114,122,126] It has been noted that cheerleading injuries in females tended to be more severe, with an average of 7.8 days lost from sport, compared to 6.6 days for males.[3] In a separate study of 23 sports, high school cheerleading had the highest average number of days lost per injury (28.8 days).[3]

A 2-year retrospective chart review in an active orthopedic sports medicine practice revealed more than 70 injuries to cheerleaders.[55] Sprains were the most common types of injuries (30%), and the knee was the most frequently injured body part (nearly 50%). Knee injuries consisted of ligament sprains (34%), inflammation or plica irritation (31%), and patella subluxation or dislocation (26%).[55]

Ballet and dance

Ballet and dance athletes require both flexibility and finesse to perform well in their sport. A primary goal of the ballet dancer is to obtain external rotation of the hips, or turnout.[86] If external rotation of the hips is not achieved, the dancer is at increased risk for knee injuries.[86] Sammarco felt that dancers attempt to make up for poor turnout by flexing the hips and the knee, "screwing the knee,"[109] and increasing the likelihood of meniscal tears, as well as of patellofemoral strain and subluxation, particularly in the inexperienced dancer.[86,109]

Hip and knee injuries constitute 40% of the injuries to classical ballet dancers.[102] Ballet dancers also tend to have a high incidence of tibial fatigue (stress) fractures.[86] Proper technique, adequate flexibility, and sufficient strength can reduce or prevent many of these injuries. However, a dancer with multiple fatigue fractures also deserves an evaluation of her gynecologic and nutritional status.

In aerobic dance, 60% of the injuries were to the lower extremity, and 9.2% involved the knee. Shin splints were the most common injury (24.5%).[106] There were no significant gender differences in frequency, incidence, or severity of injury.[106]

Swimming

Knee injuries in swimming are closely related to the biomechanics of the stroke and the kick. For example, breaststroker's knee may be secondary to collateral ligament sprain or patellofemoral stress syndrome.[65,80,119,123] Reports indicate no significant differences in the incidence of injury between male and female swimmers.[123] However, breaststroker's knee in the female typically involves the medial patellar facet, whereas the same condition in the male often affects the tibial collateral ligament.[119]

CONCLUSIONS

General recommendations for rehabilitation of the injured knee in the male and female athlete are similar, consisting of initial treatment with rest, ice, compression, and elevation, followed by injury-specific rehabilitation. Women experience the same physiologic response to injury that men do and they respond to comparable rehabilitation techniques and modalities.

It is important, however, to identify and appreciate factors such as anatomic and physiologic differences and the baseline level of conditioning, all of which should be considered when setting goals and expectations in the rehabilitation of the female athlete. In addition, the female athlete should be educated regarding the common mechanisms and types of injuries in her chosen sport so that she may optimally condition and train to prevent future injury.

The informed clinician, therefore, is not only able to accurately diagnose and treat the female athlete's injured knee but is also cognizant of psychosocial gender differences and associated medical issues (e.g., eating disorders, menstrual irregularities, pregnancy) that may influence the rehabilitation process.

REFERENCES

1. ACOG Home Exercise Programs: *Exercise during pregnancy and the postnatal period,* Washington, DC, 1985, American College of Obstetricians and Gynecologists.
2. Aglietti P, Insall JN, Walker PS: A new patellar prosthesis, *Clin Orthop* 179:175–187, 1975.
3. Axe MJ, Newcomb WA, Warner D: Sports injuries and adolescent athletes, *Del Med J* 63:359–363, 1991.
4. Baechle TR: Women in resistance training, *Clin Sports Med* 3:791–880, 1984.
5. Barrow GW, Saha S: Menstrual irregularity and stress fractures in collegiate female distance runners, *Am J Sports Med* 16:209–215, 1988.
6. Beck JL, Wildermuth BP: The female athlete's knee, *Clin Sports Med* 4:345–366, 1985.
7. Behnke AR, Royce J: Body size, shape, and comparison of several types of athletes, *J Sports Med Phys Fitness* 6:75–88, 1966.
8. Benas D: *Special considerations in women's rehabilitation programs.* In Hunter LY, Funk FJ, editors: *Rehabilitation of the injured knee,* St Louis, 1985, Mosby–Year Book.
9. Berg K: Aerobic function in female athletes, *Clin Sports Med* 3:779–789, 1984.
10. Berlin P: The woman athlete. In Gerber EW, et al, editors: *The American woman in sport,* Reading, Mass, 1974, Addison-Wesley.
11. Borges O: Isometric and isokinetic knee extension and flexion torque in men and women aged 20–70, *Scand J Rehabil Med* 21:45–53, 1989.
12. Brunet ME, et al: A survey of running injuries in 1505 competitive and recreational runners, *J Sports Med Phys Fitness* 30:307–315, 1990.
13. Butts NK, Gushiken TT, Zarins B, editors: *The elite athlete,* New York, 1985, Spectrum.
14. Canale ST, et al: A chronicle of injuries of an American intercollegiate football team, *Am J Sports Med* 9:384–389, 1981.
15. Carter JEL, et al: Anthropometry of Montreal olympic athletes. In Carter JEL, editor: *Medicine and sport,* vol 16, Basel, 1982, S Karger.
16. Clarke KS, Buckley WE: Women's injuries in collegiate sports, *Am J Sports Med* 8:187–191, 1980.
17. Colisimo AJ, Ireland ML: Isokinetic peak torque and knee laxity comparison in female basketball and volleyball college athletes, *Med Sci Sports Exerc* 23(suppl 4):135, 1991 (abstract).
18. Collins RK: Injury patterns in women's flag football, *Am J Sports Med* 15:238–242, 1987.
19. Corbin CB: Self confidence of females in sport and physical activity, *Clin Sports Med* 3:895–908, 1984.
20. Cox JS, Lenz HW: Women midshipmen in sports, *Am J Sports Med* 12:241–243, 1984.
21. Culpepper MI, Niemann KMW: High school football injuries in Birmingham, Alabama, *South Med J* 76:873–878, 1983.
22. DeGroot H, Mass DP: Hand injury patterns in softball players using a sixteen inch ball, *Am J Sports Med* 16:260–265, 1988.
23. DeHaven KE, Lintner DM: Athletic injuries: comparison by age, sport, and gender, *Am J Sports Med* 14:218–224, 1986.
24. Eisenberg I, Allen WC: Injuries in a women's varsity athletic program, *Phys Sportsmed* 5:112–120, 1978.
25. Engstrom B, Johansson C, Tornkvist H: Soccer injuries among elite female players, *Am J Sports Med* 19:372–375, 1991.
26. Erdelyi GJ: Gynecological survey of female athletes, *J Sports Med Phys Fitness* 2:174, 1962.
27. Erkkola R: The influence of physical training during pregnancy on physical work capacity and circulatory parameters, *Scand J Clin Lab Invest* 36:747, 1976.
28. Ficat RP, Hungerford DS: *Disorders of the patellofemoral joint,* Baltimore, 1977, Williams & Wilkins.
29. Fox TA: Dysplasia of the quadriceps mechanism, *Surg Clin North Am* 55:199–226, 1975.
30. Franklin BA, Lussier L, Buskirk ER: Injury rates in women joggers, *Phys Sportsmed* 7:104–112, 1979.
31. Frusztajer N, et al: Nutrition and the incidence of stress fractures in the ballet dancers, *Am J Clin Nutr* 51:779–783, 1990.
32. Fulkerson JP, Hungerford DS: *Disorders of the patellofemoral joint,* ed 2, Baltimore, 1990, Williams & Wilkins.
33. Fulkerson JP, Shea KP: Current concepts review: disorders of patellofemoral alignment, *J Bone Joint Surg [Am]* 72:1424–1429, 1990.
34. Garrick JG, Requa RK: Girl's sports injuries in high school athletics, *JAMA* 239:2245–2248, 1978.

35. Garrick JG, Requa RK: Epidemiology of women's gymnastics injuries, *Am J Sports Med* 8:261–264, 1980.

36. Gillette J: When and where women are injured in sports, *Phys Sportsmed* 2:61–63, 1975.

37. Glick JM: The female knee in athletics, *Phys Sportsmed* 1:35–37, 1973.

38. Goldberg MJ: Gymnastic injuries, *Orthop Clin North Am* 11:717–726, 1980.

39. Goldberg B, Rosenthall PP, Nicholas JA: Injuries in youth football, *Phys Sportsmed* 12:112–120, 1978.

40. Good JE, Klein KM: Women in the military academies: US Navy, *Phys Sportsmed* 17:99–106, 1989.

41. Goodlin RC, Buckley KK: Maternal exercise, *Clin Sports Med* 3:881–893, 1984.

42. Griffin LY: The female as a sports participant, *J Med Assoc Ga* 81:285–287, 1992.

43. Grood ES, et al: Biomechanics of knee extension exercise, *J Bone Joint Surg [Am]* 66:725–734, 1984.

44. Hale RW, editor: *Caring for exercising women,* New York, 1991, Elsevier.

45. Hall DC, Kaufman DA: Effects of aerobic and strength conditioning on the pregnancy outcomes, *Am J Obstet Gynecol* 157:1199–1203, 1987.

46. Haycock CE: *Sports medicine for the athletic female,* Oradell, NJ, 1980, Medical Economics.

47. Haycock CE, Gillette JV: Susceptibility of women athletes to injury: myths versus reality, *JAMA* 236:163–165, 1976.

48. Hershman EB, Mailly T: Stress fractures, *Clin Sports Med* 9:183–214, 1990.

49. Highgenboten CL: Children's knee problems, *Orthop Rev* 10:37–48, 1981.

50. Hughston J, Andrews J: The suprapatellar plica and internal derangement, *J Bone Joint Surg [Am]* 55:1318, 1973.

51. Hungerford DS, Barry M: Biomechanics of the patellofemoral joint, *Clin Orthop* 144:9–15, 1979.

52. Hungerford DS, Lennox DW: Rehabilitation of the knee in disorders of the patellofemoral joint: relevant biomechanics, *Orthop Clin North Am* 14:397–402, 1983.

53. Hunter LY, et al: Common orthopaedic problems of female athletes. In Frankel VH, editor: *Instructional course lectures XXXI,* St Louis, 1982, Mosby–Year Book.

54. Hunter LY, Torgan C: Dismounts in gymnastics: should scoring be reevaluated? *Am J Sports Med* 11:208–210, 1983.

55. Hutchinson MR, Ireland ML, Jacobs DC: *Injuries in cheerleaders,* 1992 (unpublished).

56. Ikponmwosa O: Influence of sex role standards in sport competition anxiety, *Int J Sport Psychol* 12:289–292, 1957.

57. Ireland ML, Wall C: Epidemiology and comparison of knee injuries in elite male and female United States basketball athletes, *Med Sci Sports Exerc* 14, 1990 (abstract).

58. Ireland ML: Patellofemoral disease in runners and bicyclists, *Ann Sports Med* 3:77–84, 1987.

59. Jackson DS, Furman WK, Berson BL: Patterns of injuries in collegiate athletes: a retrospective study of injuries sustained in intercollegiate athletics in two colleges over a two year period, *Mt Sinai J Med* 47:423–426, 1980.

60. Jarrett R, Spellacy W: Jogging during pregnancy, *Obstet Gynecol* 61:705, 1983.

61. Jarski RW, Trippett DL: The risks and benefits of exercise during pregnancy, *J Fam Pract* 30:185–189, 1990.

62. Jones RE: Common athletic injuries in women, *Compr Ther* 6:47–49, 1980.

63. Katch VL, et al: Contribution of breast volume and weight to body fat distribution in the female, *Am J Phys Anthropol* 53:93–100, 1980.

64. Keller CS, Noyes FR, Buncher CR: The medical aspects of soccer epidemiology, *Am J Sports Med* 15:230–236, 1987.

65. Kennedy JC, Hawkins R, Krissoff WB: Orthopaedic manifestations of swimming, *Am J Sports Med* 6:309–322, 1978.

66. Kirby RL, et al: Flexibility and musculoskeletal symptomatology in female gymnasts and aged matched controls, *Am J Sports Med* 9:160–164, 1981.

67. Kowal DM: Nature and causes of injuries in women resulting from an endurance training program, *Am J Sports Med* 8:265–269, 1980.

68. LaPrade RF, Burnett QM: Femoral intercondylar notch stenosis and correlation to anterior cruciate ligament injuries: a prospective study, *Am J Sport Med,* 1993 (in press).

69. Levine J: Chondromalacia patellae, *Phys Sportsmed* 7:41–49, 1979.

70. Lieb FJ, Perry J: Quadriceps function: anatomical and mechanical study using amputated limbs, *J Bone Joint Surg [Am]* 50:1535–1548, 1968.

71. Lindner KJ, Caine DJ: Injury patterns of female competitive club gymnasts, *Can J Sport Sci* 15:254–261, 1990.

72. Lloyd T, et al: Interrelationship of diet, athletic activity, menstrual status, and bone density in collegiate women, *Am J Clin Nutr* 46:681–684, 1987.

73. Lockey MW: The sport of cheerleading, *J Miss State Med Assoc* 32:375, 1991 (letter).

74. Loosli AR, et al: Injuries to pitchers in women's collegiate softball, *Am J Sports Med* 20:35–37, 1992.

75. Lotgering FK, Gilbert RD, Longo LD: The interactions of exercise and pregnancy: a review, *Am J Obstet Gynecol* 149:560, 1984.

76. Lysens R, et al: The predictability of sports injuries, *Sports Med* 1:6–10, 1984.

77. MacIntyre DL, Robertson DG: Quadriceps muscle activity in women runners with and without patellofemoral pain syndrome, *Arch Phys Med Rehabil* 73:10–14, 1992.

78. Malone TR, et al: *Relationship of gender to anterior cruciate ligament injuries in intercollegiate basketball participants,* Durham, NC, 1991, Duke University, Dept of Physical Therapy and Occupational Therapy and Dept of Surgery, Division of Orthopaedics.

79. Mariani P, Caruso I: An electromyographic investigation of subluxation of the patella, *J Bone Joint Surg [Br]* 61:169–171, 1979.

80. Marino M: Profiling swimmers, *Clin Sports Med* 3:211–228, 1984.

81. Matheson GO, et al: Stress fractures in athletes: a study of 320 cases, *Am J Sports Med* 15:43–58, 1987.

82. May JR, et al: *A preliminary study of elite adolescent women athletes and their attitudes toward training and femininity.* In Butts NK, Gushiken TT, Zarins B, editors: *The elite athlete,* New York, 1985, Spectrum.

83. McAuley E, et al: Injuries in women's gymnastics: the state of the art, *Am J Sports Med* 15:558–565, 1987.

84. McConnell J: The management of chondromalacia patellae: a long term solution, *Aus J Phys Ther* 32:215–223, 1986.

85. Micheli L: *Female runners.* In D'Ambrosia R, Drez D, editors: *Prevention and treatment of running injuries,* Thorofare, NJ, 1982, Slack.

86. Micheli LJ, Gillespie WJ, Walaszek A: Physiologic profiles of female professional ballerinas, *Clin Sports Med* 3:199–209, 1984.

87. Mullinax KM, Dale E: Some considerations of exercise during pregnancy, *Clin Sports Med* 5:559–570, 1986.

88. Murphy RJ, et al: Five year football injury survey, *Phys Sportsmed* 6:95–102, 1978.

89. Myburgh KH, et al: Low bone density is an etiologic factor for stress fractures in athletes, *Ann Intern Med* 113:754–759, 1990.

90. Myers AM, Lips HM: Participation in competitive amateur sports as a function of psychological androgyny, *Sec Roles* 4:571–578, 1978.

91. National Collegiate Athletic Association: *NCAA injury surveillance system,* Overland Park, Kansas, 1991-1992, 1992-1993, NCAA.

92. Nilsson S, Roass AA: Soccer injuries in adolescents, *Am J Sports Med* 6:358–361, 1978.

93. Orseli RC: Possible teratogenic hyperthermia and marathon running, *JAMA* 243:332, 1980 (letter).

94. Patel D: Plica as a cause of anterior knee pain, *Orthop Clin North Am* 17:273, 1986.
95. Pearl A: *The Athletic Female,* Champaign, Ill, 1992, Human Kinetics.
96. Perry J: Function of the quadriceps, *J Can Physiother Assoc,* 1972.
97. Pettrone FA, Ricciardeli E: Gymnastic injuries: the Virginia experience, *Am J Sports Med* 15:59–62, 1987.
98. Powers JA: Characteristic features of injuries in the knee of women, *Clin Orthop* 143:120–124, 1979.
99. Protzman RR: Physiologic performance of women compared to men, *Am J Sports Med* 7:191–194, 1979.
100. Protzman RR, Bodnari LM: Women athletes, *Am J Sports Med* 8:53–55, 1980.
101. Protzman RR, Griffis C: Stress fractures in men and women undergoing military training, *J Bone Joint Surg [Am]* 59:825, 1977.
102. Reid DC, et al: Lower extremity flexibility patterns in classical ballet dancers and their correlation to lateral hip and knee injuries, *Am J Sports Med* 15:347–352, 1987.
103. Reilly DJ, Martens M: Experimental analysis of quadriceps muscle force and patellofemoral joint reaction force for various activities, *Acta Orthop Scand* 43:126–137, 1972.
104. Reynolds L, et al: EMG analysis of the vastus medialis obliquus and the vastus lateralis in their role in patellar alignment, *Am J Phys Med* 62:61–71, 1983.
105. Robinson SJ, Hoeltzel LE, editors: The injured athlete, Philadelphia, 1982, JB Lippincott.
106. Rothenberger LA, Chang JI, Cable TA: Prevalence and types of injuries in aerobic dancers, *Am J Sports Med* 16:403–407, 1988.
107. Ryan AJ, Allman JR, editors: *Sports medicine,* ed 2, New York, 1989, Harcourt Brace Jovanovich.
108. Sady SP, Carpenter MW: Aerobic exercise during pregnancy: special considerations, *Sports Med* 7:357–375, 1989.
109. Sammarco GJ: *Dance injuries.* In Nicholas JA, Hershman EB, editors: *The lower extremity and spine in sports medicine,* St Louis, 1986, Mosby–Year Book.
110. Sands W: Competition injury study: a preliminary report on female gymnasts, *USGF Technical Journal,* 1981, p 7.
111. Santavirta S: Integrated electromyography of the vastus medialis muscle after meniscectomy, *Am J Sports Med* 7:40–42, 1979.
112. Schafle MD, et al: Injuries in the 1987 national amateur volleyball tournament, *Am J Sports Med* 18:624–631, 1990.
113. Schaeffer CF: Possible teratogenic hyperthermia and marathon running, *JAMA* 241:1892, 1979 (letter).
114. Shields RW, Jacobs IB: Median palmar neuropathy in a cheerleader, *Arch Phys Med Rehabil* 67:824–826, 1986.
115. Souryal TO, Moore HA, Evans JP: Bilaterality in anterior cruciate ligament injuries: associated intercondylar notch stenosis, *Am J Sports Med* 16:449–454, 1988.
116. Snyder ED, Spreiter E: *Social aspects of sports,* Englewood Cliffs, N J, 1978, Prentice Hall.
117. Stark JA, Toulesse A: The young female athlete: psychological considerations, *Clin Sports Med* 3:909–920, 1984.
118. Strauss RH, editor: *Sports medicine,* Philadelphia, 1984, WB Saunders.
119. Stulberg SD, et al: Breaststroker's knee: pathology, etiology and treatment, *Am J Sports Med* 8:164–171, 1980.
120. Sullivan D, et al: Stress fractures in 51 runners, *Clin Orthop* 187:188–192, 1984.
121. Sullivan JA, et al: Evaluation of injuries in youth soccer, *Am J Sports Med* 8:325–327, 1980.
122. Tehranzadeh J, Labosky DA, Gabriele OF: Ganglion cysts and tears of triangular fibrocartilages of both wrists in a cheerleader, *Am J Sports Med* 11:357–359, 1983.
123. Vizsolyi P, et al: Breaststroker's knee: an analysis of epidemiological and biomechanical factors, *Am J Sports Med* 15:63–71, 1987.
124. Walsh WM, Hurman WW, Shelton GL: Overuse injuries of the knee and spine in girls' gymnastics, *Clin Sports Med* 3:829–850, 1984.
125. White J: Exercising for two: what's safe for the active pregnant woman, *Phys Sportsmed* 20:179–186, 1992.
126. Whiteside JA, Fleagle JA, Kalenak A: Fractures and refractures in intercollegiate athletes, *Am J Sports Med* 9:369–377, 1981.
127. Whiteside PA: Men's and women's injuries in comparable sports, *Phys Sportsmed* 8:130–140, 1980.
128. Wild JJ, Franklin TD, Woods GW: Patellar pain and quadriceps rehabilitation, *Am J Sports Med* 10:12–15, 1982.
129. Woodward SL: How does strenuous maternal exercise affect the fetus: a review, *Birth* 8:17, 1981.
130. Zelisko JA, Noble HB, Porter M: A comparison of men's and women's professional basketball injuries, *Am J Sports Med* 10:297–299, 1982.

Chapter 27

CHILDREN

James L. Sarni
Lyle J. Micheli

Systemic rehabilitation of the injured child following injury or surgery is to be strongly advised. The rationale for this rehabilitation is the same as for the adult: the return to full function as rapidly as possible, the avoidance of reinjury at the same site, and the prevention of muscle imbalances or joint contractions that can predispose the child to injury at other sites. The medical dictum that states that pediatrics is not merely the study of small adults is especially true when rehabilitating a child after injury, particularly an injury to the musculoskeletal system. The dynamic process of growth with all its physiologic consequences places the skeletally immature athlete in a unique situation that merits special consideration. These considerations and the basis behind them are reviewed here.

GROWTH PATTERNS

Although children are quite active during the early school years, early and mid-adolescence is generally the time they begin to emphasize a particular sport. Middle adolescence is the period of most dramatic growth and change. It is the phase in which the bulk of the fat is deposited in females and the muscle in males.[1] Growth, however, is not proportional: "There is an orderly pattern of progression of skeletal growth from distal to proximal parts of the body, beginning with growth of the feet. This is followed approximately six months later by growth of the calf and then the thigh."[1]

This sort of uneven growth places certain muscles at a mechanical advantage and results in unequal strength and flexibility patterns. The resulting unequal forces across the joints can lead to an increased risk of injury. Several studies have elucidated this principle.[2–6]

These studies have involved female college athletes,[3] adolescent males and females,[5] and young males playing soccer.[2] The fact that these studies include very different patient populations yet all reached the same conclusion further supports the importance of balanced flexibility and strength.

As a result of this uneven growth, a growth-related tendency to tightness must also be borne in mind in managing rehabilitation of the injured child. Specifically, tight lumbodorsal fascia and hamstring muscles are associated factors in low back disorders in the child and adolescent. These become particularly evident during the growth spurt.[7]

This overgrowth tendency and its resultant tightening effect can influence the management and rehabilitation of childhood injuries, especially regarding immobilization of the extremities. This tightening tendency can be particularly exacerbated following injury. A sprained ankle in a child may be complicated by rapid tightening of the heel cord. Immobilization in such injury can help prevent this tightening.

SKELETAL GROWTH

It should be remembered that during growth spurts the physis is a region of tremendous physiologic activity. Growth hormone most likely acts on bone growth directly by stimulating the differentiation of epiphyseal growth plate precursor cells and indirectly by the increased responsiveness to somatomedins, for instance, growth factors[8] (Fig. 27–1). Mechanical stress to the growth plate during this dynamic process can alter cellular activity, resulting in structural changes[9] (Fig. 27–2). Recently, wrist pain in adolescent gymnasts has received a significant amount of attention. Some authors have found growth plate widening,[10,11] premature growth plate closure,[12] and fractures.[13]

Osgood-Schlatter's disease

Osgood-Schlatter's disease represents the perfect example of the overgrowth phenomenon. It is generally agreed that it is the result of repetitive microtrauma, avulsion stress being applied to the distal tibial tubercle in an actively growing child.[5,13–15] Active adolescence can generate forceful repetitive contractions of the quadriceps muscles during the apophyseal stage.[14] The tibial tubercle is susceptible to injury and micro-avulsions can occur through the bone and the cartilage of the secondary ossification center in that it

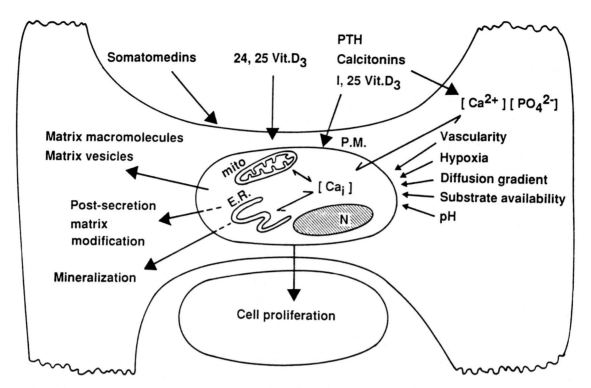

Fig. 27-1. Factors influencing growth plate chondrocyte function and matrix mineralization. (From Iannotti JP: Growth plate physiology and pathology, *Orthop Clin North Am* 21:1–17, 1990.)

is weaker than the distal fibrous tissue adjacent bone.[15] Because the trauma is repetitive, a local inflammatory action occurs at the site, in a continuum from acute to chronic, inflammatory changes can be found.[16]

The treatment and rehabilitation then must keep the etiology in mind. The goal is initial rest and reduction of the inflammation, which is done by decreasing or stopping the activity that precipitated the pain. In addition, a knee immobilizer can sometimes be used and, for severe cases, nonweightbearing on the involved limb. When the patient is able to painlessly walk up the stairs and there is minimal or no tenderness of the tibial tubercle, the rehabilitation program is started.

This is directed at decreasing the forces that contributed to the condition initially, namely, reducing the resisting pull on the tibial tubercle by stretching the hamstring muscles and decreasing traction on the tibial tubercle by stretching the quadriceps muscles.

Quadriceps muscles stretching is done without hyperflexion of the knee. This is accomplished by performing the classic Thomas test over the side of the table with the knee flexed no more than 90 degrees, or by lying prone and hyperextending the hip with the knee once again flexed no more than 90 degrees.

In addition to stretching, progressive resistive straight leg raising with three sets of 10 repetitions with each leg should also be performed. This should not be painful. Resistance

can be increased to a level of 12 lb performed with three sets of 10 repetitions.[17]

KNEE REHABILITATION PRINCIPLES

There are general principles of knee rehabilitation that relate to children as well as adults in regard to muscle strengthening about the knee joint. The goal is to strengthen the muscles about the knee in a manner that provides maximum strength gains while placing a minimal stress on the patellofemoral joints. Also, the exercise used should strengthen the muscles in a functional or sport-specific fashion. The biomechanics of the knee joint must be understood to appreciate the reasoning behind the rehabilitation program.

Biomechanics

Moment is defined as the torque necessary to angularly accelerate a body. *Torque* is equal to the force applied multiplied by the *perpendicular* distance of force from the center of rotation of the lever (T = ⊥ (d) × F).[17] Therefore, if an individual is sitting on a bench with a weight attached to the ankle while dangling the foot directly below the knee, the torque, or force, to cause an angular acceleration about the knee joint is 0 because the *perpendicular* distance from the center of rotation to the point of force application is 0.

However, as the knee is extended, the *perpendicular* distance from the point of force of application increases,

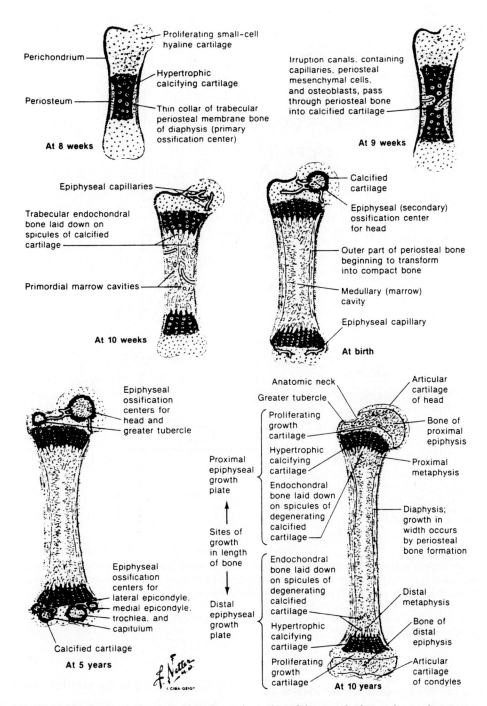

Fig. 27-2. Development of a typical long bone: formation of the growth plate and secondary center of ossification. (From the CIBA Collection of Medical Illustrations, CIBA-Geigy, copyright 1987.)

reaching a maximum at terminal extension. It follows from this that the quadriceps muscle force generated is greatest in terminal extension.[18,19]

The opposite occurs during standing because the point of force application is the ground reaction force pushing up upon the foot; therefore, the more the knee is bent, the further is the *perpendicular* distance from the line of force to the axis of rotation at the knee. Thus, the greater the knee

is bent, the greater the *perpendicular* force from the axis of rotation, the greater the force to cause rotation or flexion moment at the knee, and the greater the quadriceps force needed to resist such flexion (Fig. 27-3).

To summarize: (1) In the sitting position with a weight attached to the foot, the greater the knee is extended, the greater is the flexion moment about the knee, and, therefore, the greater the quadriceps force generated to resist such a

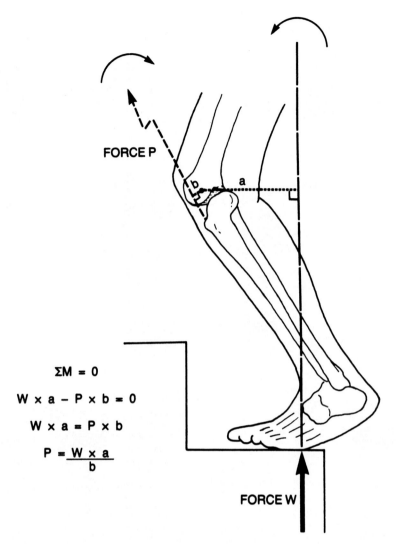

FORCE P

a
b

$$\Sigma M = 0$$

$$W \times a - P \times b = 0$$

$$W \times a = P \times b$$

$$P = \frac{W \times a}{b}$$

FORCE W

Fig. 27-3. The two main moments acting around the center of motion of the tibiofemoral joint *(solid dot)* are designated on the free body diagram of the lower leg during stair climbing. Because the lower leg is in equilibrium, the extending moment produced by the patellar tendon force *P* times its lever arm *(b)* counterbalances the flexing moment produced by the ground reaction force *W* times its lever arm *(a)*. The weight of the lower leg is disregarded. (From Nordin M, Frankel VH: *Basic biomechanics of the musculoskeletal system,* ed 2, Philadelphia, 1989, Lea & Febiger. Used with permission.)

flexion force. (2) In the standing position, the greater the knee is bent, the greater the flexion moment and thus the greater the quadriceps force generated to resist the flexion moment.

Patellofemoral joint reaction forces. It generally follows that the position that causes the greatest quadriceps force will cause the greatest force on the patellofemoral joint, the exception being in total knee extension because of several reasons. First, when the knee is locked in total extension, the hip and not the knee is the center of rotation; therefore, there are no rotatory forces about the knee. Second, there is little, if any, patellofemoral contact in 0 degrees of extension.[20]

Strength training in the growing athlete

Progressive resistance strength training has been shown to be effective and safe in producing increases in strength in prepubertal males[21] and females.[22] Strength gains have been found in the use of high repetition[21] as well as lower repetition with heavier weight use.[22]

Increases in torque production have been positively correlated with increases in integrated EMG (IEMG) activity.[23-26] Some investigators have noticed that these increases in IEMG occurred in the first 8 weeks of training.[25,27] This has led to the theory that the initial increases in strength development are due to motor units firing in a more coordinated, but not synchronized, manner. After the initial 8 weeks, strength gains are believed to be due to changes within the muscle fiber itself.

Such studies have not been performed on children to date. As children are still growing and developing neuromuscularly, it should not be assumed that their patterns of strength development are exactly those of adults.

SUMMARY

In devising a rehabilitation program for the skeletally immature athlete, one must take into account the dynamic process of growth and its consequences. Among these, patterns of growth and the ossification process are of prime importance. One must understand the biomechanics of the knee in order to plan a rehabilitation program that takes these factors into account. Although training by progressive routine exercises has proven effective in prepubescent children, neuromuscular adaptations to strength training in children are still unknown.

REFERENCES

1. Nelson WE, Vaughn VC: *Textbook of pediatrics,* ed 14, Philadelphia, 1992, WB Saunders.
2. Backous DD, et al: Sock injuries and their relation to physical maturity, *Am J Dis Child* 142:834–839, 1988.
3. Knapik JJ, et al: Preseason strength and flexibility imbalances associated with athletic injuries in female collegiate athletes, *Am J Sports Med* 19:76–81, 1991.
4. Micheli LJ: Overuse injuries in children's sports: the growth factor, *Orthop Clin North Am* 14:337–360, 1983.
5. Micheli LJ, et al: Patella alta in the adolescent growth spurt, *Clin Orthop* 213:159–162, 1986.
6. Taimela S, Kujala UM, Osterman K: Intrinsic risk factors and athletic injuries, *Sports Med* 9:205–215, 1990.
7. Micheli LJ: Low back pain in the adolescent: differential diagnosis, *Am J Sports Med* 7:362–364, 1979.
8. Isaksson OGP, et al: Action of growth hormone: current views, *Acta Paediatr Scand Suppl* 343:12–18, 1988.
9. Iannotti JP: Growth plate physiology and pathology, *Orthop Clin North Am* 21:1–17, 1990.
10. Caine D, et al: Stress changes of the distal radial growth plate, *Am J Sports Med* 20:290–298, 1992.
11. Roy S, Cain D, Singer KM: Stress changes in the distal radial epiphysis in young gymnasts: a report of twenty-one cases and a review of the literature, *Am J Sports Med* 13:301–308, 1985.
12. Albanese SA, Frankel VH: Wrist pain in distal growth plate closure of the radius in gymnasts, *J Pediatr Orthop* 9:23–28, 1989.
13. Micheli LJ: The traction apophysitises, *Clin Sports Med* 6:389–404, 1987.
14. Ogden JA, Southwick WO: Osgood-Schlatter's disease and tibial tuberosity development, *Clin Orthop* 116:180–189, 1976.
15. Reider B: *Sports medicine: the school age athlete,* Philadelphia, 1991, WB Saunders.
16. Ehrenborg G, Engfeldt B: Histologic changes in the Osgood-Schlatter's lesion, *Acta Chir Scand* 121:328–337, 1961.
17. Nordin M, Frankel VH: *Basic biomechanics of the musculoskeletal system,* ed 2, Philadelphia, 1989, Lea & Febiger.
18. Lieb FL, Perry AJ: Quadriceps function, *J Bone Joint Surg [AM]* 50:1535–1548, 1968.
19. Reilly DT, Martens M: Experimental analysis of the quadriceps muscle force and patellofemoral joint reaction force for various activities, *Acta Orthop Scand* 43:126–137, 1972.
20. Goodfellow J, Hungerford DS, Zindel M: Patellofemoral joint mechanics and pathology, *J Bone Joint Surg [BR]* 58:287–290, 1976.
21. Weltman A, et al: The effects of hydraulic resistance strength training in pre-pubertal males, *Med Sci Sports Exerc* 18:629–638, 1986.
22. Sewall S, Micheli LJ: Strength training for children, *Pediatr Orthop* 6:143–146, 1986.
23. Hakkinen K, Alen M, Komi PV: Changes in isometric force and relaxation time: electromyographic and muscle fiber characteristics of human skeletal muscle during strength training and detraining, *Acta Physiol Scand* 126:573–585, 1985.
24. Hakkinen K, Komi PV: Training induced changes in neuromuscular performance under voluntary and reflex conditions, *Eur J Appl Physiol* 55:147–155, 1986.
25. Hakkinen K, Komi PV: Electromyographic changes during strength training and detraining, *Med Sci Sports Exerc* 15:455–460, 1983.
26. Komi PV, et al: Effect of isometric strength training on mechanical, electrical, and metabolic aspects of muscle functioning, *Eur J Appl Physiol* 40:45–55, 1978.
27. Moritani T, DeVries HA: Neurofactors versus hypertrophy in the time course of muscle strength gain, *Am J Phys Med* 58:115–130, 1979.

Chapter 28

REHABILITATION OF THE ARTHRITIC KNEE

Frederic C. McDuffie
Moya Hambridge

Although damage to the knee from mechanical injury is the primary subject of this book, injury may occur from other causes such as infection, calcium pyrophosphate crystals, and autoimmune inflammation. Frequently, mechanical injury may precipitate an underlying systemic process, for example, an acute torsion strain causing an initial attack of gout in a young football player. Furthermore, mechanical injury resulting in a torn meniscus or anterior cruciate ligament may contribute 15 years later to the premature onset of osteoarthritis.[1]

TYPES OF ARTHRITIS AND DIAGNOSIS

Clinically significant (i.e., painful) osteoarthritis of the knee affects approximately 2 million people in the United States, and another 3 million have radiographic evidence of the disease without symptoms.[2] In recent years it has become evident that osteoarthritis represents the end result of a number of etiologic factors, the importance of which varies among individual patients. Heredity has long been known to be the primary cause of osteoarthritis of the hands.[3] The evolution of molecular genetics as a research tool in recent years has already demonstrated how an amino acid substitution in one portion of the collagen chain can lead to a familial form of severe generalized osteoarthritis.[4] In clinical practice one is most impressed by the importance of biomechanical factors in producing osteoarthritis of the knee. These biomechanical factors include congenital or acquired deformities such as genu valgus or varus, occupational stresses involving heavy lifting[5] or frequent squatting,[6] and, above all, obesity. An analysis of HANES (Health and Nutritional Epidemiologic Survey) data by Felson[7] indicates that the risk of developing osteoarthritis of the knees is 1.5 to 2 times normal in significantly overweight men and women. Additional risk factors for osteoarthritis of the knee are female gender, chondrocalcinosis, and probably ethnic background.[8]

Many other forms of arthritis including rheumatoid arthritis, systemic lupus, gout, calcium pyrophosphate deposition disease (RPPD), and juvenile rheumatoid arthritis may affect the knee. Although usually affecting several other joints as well, they may cause isolated arthritis of the knee at onset. In this respect, note should be made of the so-called Milwaukee shoulder-knee syndrome and of HLA-B27-associated spondyloarthropathy. These syndromes have attracted much recent attention as important causes of inflammatory arthritis of the knee. The former, originally described by Neer as cuff tear arthropathy,[9] is characterized by a destructive arthritis of the shoulder and progressive damage to the knee, which radiologically represents an osteoarthritis involving primarily the lateral compartment and the patellofemoral joints.[10] Hydroxyapatite, pyrophosphate, and sometimes calcium pyrophosphate are commonly found in the synovial fluid. Their role in the pathogenesis of the disorder continues to be debated. The HLA-B27 gene is present in more than 95% of whites with ankylosing spondylitis and in 50% of those with Reiter's syndrome.[11] In the last few years it has become apparent that a number of individuals with inflammatory pauciarthritis, usually of the lower extremity without associated spondylitis or extraarticular manifestations of Reiter's syndrome, may have a B27 arthropathy.[12]

Patients with acute or chronic knee pain whose x-rays are normal with or without demonstrated evidence of effusion and in whom the diagnosis is not straightforward should undergo a basic rheumatologic investigation, including serum uric acid, rheumatoid factor, antinuclear antibody, HLA-B27, and sedimentation rate. If an effusion is present, however small, it should be aspirated and sent for differential white count and examination for crystals. In our experience, failure to perform this latter test is the most common reason for missing a readily treatable disorder, either gout or calcium pyrophosphate deposition disease.

WEIGHT LOSS

Probably the most important measure that most individuals with chronic arthritis of the knee can carry out for themselves is losing enough weight to reach the normal level for height, sex, and age. As already pointed out, obesity is seldom the result of chronic arthritis of the knee but more often an etiologic factor. Whether cause or effect, however, reduction of the mechanical load on the knee can significantly reduce pain, enhance mobility, and delay the often inevitable day of total knee arthroplasty. Weight loss is, of course, difficult to achieve because it is so often the result of ingrained behavior that in turn reflects an underlying personality pattern. Effective weight loss is ideally achieved by a combination of diet and exercise, but most forms of exercise put demands on the legs that cannot be met by people with chronic arthritis of the knee. In our experience, aerobic pool exercises and the regular use of a stationary bicycle are the best tolerated, readily available forms of exercise, in spite of the relatively low caloric expenditure they require. Many people are willing to enter a commercial weight loss program such as Jenny Craig or Weight Watchers. These do help provide the motivation and reinforcement essential to successful weight loss but are often expensive and may require buying special low-calorie foods and drinks promoted by the operators. Furthermore, they often emphasize rapid initial weight loss, which is of little value to the person who needs to maintain reduced weight for the rest of his or her life. It is most important to be sure that the person understands the fundamental principles of nutrition and weight loss, and for the physician and other health professionals to continue to emphasize the importance of weight control and to monitor weight carefully. The use of such appetite suppressants as diethylpropion (Tenuate), fenfluramine (Pondimin), and benzphetamine (Didrex) are sometimes helpful, although chronic dependence may become a problem.

PHARMACOLOGIC MANAGEMENT

Nonsteroidal anti-inflammatory drugs (NSAIDs) are usually the mainstay of treatment of arthritis involving the knee. All of these drugs act primarily by inhibition of cyclooxygenase, an enzyme that catalyzes a key step in the production of prostaglandins from their common precursor, arachidonic acid. Aspirin is the oldest drug of this class, but because of its brief duration of action, its propensity to cause gastric ulceration, and the necessity to consume a large number of tablets (10 to 15 a day) to achieve therapeutic blood levels, it has fallen out of favor. The primary side effect of these drugs, gastritis and peptic ulceration, results from inhibition of the natural devices of the gastric epithelium that protect it from the harmful effects of pepsin and hydrochloric acid. Gastric prostaglandins inhibit secretion of acid and pepsin and promote secretion of protective mucus.[13] Other side effects of these drugs such as allergic hepatitis, interstitial nephritis, and azotemia secondary to

shutting off renal prostaglandin secretion are relatively uncommon but need to be kept in mind. Although patients who either fail to respond initially or later lose their response to a given NSAID may benefit from substitution of another drug of this class, most rheumatologists believe there is little to choose among them except on the basis of duration of action or therapeutic-toxic ratio. Short-acting drugs such as ibuprofen can be more readily manipulated and disappear from the body more rapidly when discontinued because of side effects. Longer-acting drugs such as piroxicam (Feldene) taken once or twice a day are easier for the patient to take regularly, but blood levels decline more slowly when they are discontinued. Most of them are usually administered twice a day. Phenylbutazone (Butazolidin), indomethacin (Indocin), and meclofenamate (Meclomen) are probably the most potent NSAIDs and are usually well tolerated by young individuals in good health. Naproxen (Naprosyn), sulindac (Clinoril), diclofenac (Voltaren), ketoprofen (Orudis), and flurbiprofen (Ansaid) appear to have intermediate therapeutic ratios. The nonacetylated salicylates such as magnesium trisalicylate (Trilisate), salsalate (Disalcid), and diflunisal (Dolobid) appear to be better tolerated by the stomach but may be somewhat less efficacious. Addition of a synthetic prostaglandin, misoprostol (Cytotec), has been shown to reduce the frequency of gastric erosions as detected by endoscopy[14] but does not affect the incidence of the dyspepsia and indigestion that are the most frequent reasons to discontinue these drugs. The use of an H_2-blocker, either ranitidine (Zantac), cimetidine (Tagamet), or famotidine (Pepcid), once a day often reduces or prevents these symptoms. Patients with elevated or borderline serum creatinine levels need to be watched carefully to be sure the use of these drugs does not precipitate renal failure. Many physicians believe that concurrent use of anticoagulants is an absolute contraindication to the use of NSAIDs not only because of the risk of gastrointestinal bleeding but also because they increase the effective blood level of warfarin (coumadin).

The most effective treatment of acute gouty arthritis of the knee is intra-articular injection of a crystalline corticosteroid. Intravenous colchicine, 2 mg, in patients not already taking the drug works almost as well. The traditional regimen of one 0.6-mg colchicine tablet an hour until relief or diarrhea occurs is too strenuous for most patients. A short-acting NSAID such as indomethacin given early in the attack is usually successful. Treatment for acute gout needs to be continued for 2 or 3 days after the attack is over to prevent recurrence. Long-term prevention of gouty attacks is beyond the scope of this chapter. A good discussion of the subject is that by Kelley.[15]

Individuals who have rheumatoid arthritis, psoriatic arthritis, Reiter's syndrome, or other forms of chronic inflammatory arthritis are best managed by a rheumatologist or internist with special interest or experience in these diseases. Several potent long-acting drugs such as methotrexate, sulfasalazine, azathioprine, and cyclosporine are now being used with increasing frequency. All can have significant side effects, and their use needs to be monitored by careful laboratory and clinical follow-up.

INJECTION THERAPY

The knee is the easiest joint of the body to aspirate. Fluid can sometimes be aspirated when even the most sensitive indicator, the bulge sign, is negative. This test can detect amounts of fluid in the order of 10 cc or so, much less than can be ascertained by classical ballottement of the patella. This test should be performed in any patient with knee pain who does not have evident swelling (Fig. 28-1).

Intra-articular corticosteroid therapy was introduced by Hollander and associates in 1951.[16] In Hollander's opinion, "no other form of treatment for arthritis has given such consistent local symptomatic relief to so many for so long with so few harmful effects."[17] The primary complications are a transient, crystal-induced flare seldom lasting more

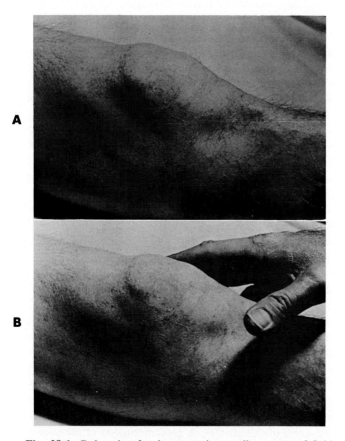

Fig. 28-1. Bulge sign for demonstrating small amounts of fluid in the knee. **A,** Medial side of knee after manual compression to displace any fluid laterally. **B,** Appearance of "bulge" below patella as lateral pressure with the hand displaces fluid into medial compartment. (From Polley HF, Hunder GG: *Rheumatologic interviewing and physical examination of the joints,* Philadelphia, 1978, WB Saunders, p. 227.)

than 24 hours and infection. Infection occurred 19 times after 12,000 injections performed by Hollander and his associates. Joint instability due to weakened capsular ligaments and possibly osteonecrosis has been occasionally seen, and thus most orthopedists and rheumatologists restrict the frequency of injections to no more than once every 3 months. In patients with progressive osteoarthritis or rheumatoid arthritis, the main reason for stopping injections is lack of efficacy as the knee deteriorates. Fortunately, for most patients total knee arthroplasty turns out to be a successful solution. A number of corticosteroid preparations are available for intra-articular injection. Following the experience of McCarty,[18] we believe that triamcinolone hexacetonide (Aristospan) is the most effective in a dose of 20 mg. It can cause subcutaneous atrophy if it leaks out into surrounding tissue.

The technique for injection or aspiration of the knee is relatively simple, using either a medial or lateral approach, inserting the needle just posterior to the patella at the tibial-femoral joint line. Sometimes obviously present fluid cannot be aspirated, probably because of impingement of synovial folds or inclusion bodies on the point of the needle. Partial withdrawal and redirection of the needle plus forceful injection of a small amount of anesthetic solution usually solves the problem. Techniques for injection and aspiration of other joints are described by Hollander.[17] For difficult joints, especially the hip, we usually perform the procedure under fluoroscopy or by use of x-ray and a lead marker taped to the skin.

A recently advocated intra-articular technique primarily for knee osteoarthritis of moderate severity is tidal joint irrigation. Installation of 800 to 1000 cc of saline in several 50- to 80-cc doses through a wide-bore (#11) perforated needle, followed each time by removal of the fluid, has been claimed to remove small particulate matter that may be promoting synovial inflammation. A controlled study of 77 patients with osteoarthritis undergoing either this procedure or standard medical management showed significant improvement in pain, although not in range of motion, walk time, or morning stiffness.[19] A commercial kit is available for performing this procedure.* In our experience the procedure is difficult to perform either with or without the commercial kit because of inability to consistently remove the major proportion of the fluid instilled each time. The same procedure can be performed more efficiently via arthroscopy, but the effort and expense then become considerable.

Another intra-articular injection technique that has been reported to be effective in rheumatoid arthritis is radiation synovectomy. As reported by Sledge and associates, the installation of a short-half-life, β-emitting isotope, dyspropium-105, in the form of ferric hydroxide macroaggregates, can be effective in controlling active synovitis for a year or

*Abbott Home Care, Lake Bluff, Illinois.

more.[20] Because of the short half-life of the isotope (139 minutes) and the necessity of obtaining it from a nearby cyclotron, the logistics of the procedure, and the limited benefit it can produce, it is unlikely to become widely available.

PHYSICAL THERAPY

Physical therapy plays a relatively minor role in acute arthritis of the knee such as that due to gout or calcium pyrophosphate crystal disease. Icepacks may be helpful in reducing pain until anti-inflammatory drug therapy has done its job. In order to prevent deformity, positioning instruction is necessary, and joint protection education should be given. A careful, daily, one- to three-repetition range-of-motion check in the comfortable range helps to offset limitations. Once the inflammatory response has been controlled by the anti-inflammatory medication and swelling is minimal, the physical therapist should work aggressively to prevent deformity and regain normal range of motion, functional strength, and exercise tolerance. Range-of-motion, gentle stretching exercises, and splinting (if necessary) should be the primary focus. Thermal agents help achieve the optimal range more quickly and comfortably.

In a carefully monitored program using a stationary bicycle, Harkcome et al.[21] demonstrated that brief exercise programs improved overall conditioning and exercise tolerance without exacerbation in inflammation. Therapeutic programs of exercise in water also suggest similar benefits.[22] Joint protection through reduction of weightbearing stress should be encouraged: sitting rather than standing for activities, and use of a walk aid for long distances.

In chronic arthritis of the knee, physical therapy plays a major and, in fact, essential role. The primary aims of physical therapy directed toward chronic arthritis of the knee are reduction of pain; maintenance and, if possible, improvement of range of motion; prevention of further stress and deformity; improvement in muscle strength and endurance; and increase in overall conditioning and mobility.

Following initial assessment to establish baseline measures, the thermal modalities of heat or cold may be used to prepare the patient for exercise. The aquatic medium is a useful option that provides warmth and support in a non-weightbearing environment. A program of range-of-motion, stretching, and strengthening exercises and walking, which the patient can perform at home to achieve some verbalized goals, is the foundation of management.

Instruction in joint protection techniques, transfer, and gait training (with an appropriate walk aid to relieve stress on the joint) also help the person regain a greater degree of mobility and exercise tolerance. This, in turn, provides greater independence in daily functioning. Because a downward spiral in muscle weakness characteristically develops, it is essential to teach a progressive program of simple muscle strengthening and endurance, preferably using such resistances as gravity or Theraband-type elastic devices (Fig.

28-2). Dead weight may create too much sudden joint stress on weakened soft tissue structures. These individuals must also be educated in guidelines for exercise to prevent adverse reactions. Studies by Kovar et al.[23] and Fisher et al.[24] both showed good correlations between exercise and various improved daily functioning parameters. Individuals with chronic arthritis of the knee need to understand clearly the need for a specific, daily exercise program until a maintenance level is reached, when twice a week is adequate.[25] Because most insurance companies cover only a brief course of therapy, self-management is the ultimate and early goal. For this to be achieved, the individual must come to recognize the relationship between performing specific exercises and regaining functional capacity.

Once the maintenance level is approached or reached, the Arthritis Foundation's basic and advanced recreational aquatic program, offered at many YMCAs and other community centers, can provide an enjoyable way of exercising for the whole body. In addition, a walking program that can be carried out within a person's capability can help maintain this essential function while helping to avoid the long-term complication of osteoporosis.

ACTIVITIES OF DAILY LIVING

Many of the limitations of ordinary living can be managed by intelligent planning and the use of certain aids and devices. Difficulty in climbing stairs can be decreased by installation of rails or ramps at appropriate points (Fig. 28-3). Getting in and out of the tub can present a serious obstacle, but grab bars and a tub bench can ease this transfer and prevent falls (Fig. 28-4). Because sitting and exercising in a hot tub can be so beneficial, the purchase of a whirlpool device or, if one can afford it, even a tub lift can do wonders. Physical therapists and occupational therapists can help provide many ingenious solutions to such common problems as getting up from a toilet seat or a low chair, driving, and getting in and out of a car.

OCCUPATION

Younger individuals with arthritis of the knee usually suffer from a generalized form of arthritis such as rheumatoid arthritis, although premature osteoarthritis secondary to torn menisci and ligaments may occur. Data obtained by Yelin et al.[26] indicate that the factors limiting employment for individuals with arthritis are not disease-dependent (e.g., number of joints involved, x-ray changes, type of drug therapy) but relate more to the conditions of work and the individual's background. The most important single factor influencing ability to continue working in spite of arthritis is the amount of control the person has over working conditions. The individual with flexible hours who is not necessarily tied down to a single workplace is more likely to continue to work than the individual tied to an assembly line whose income depends on piecework. Other factors influencing employment are educational background, length

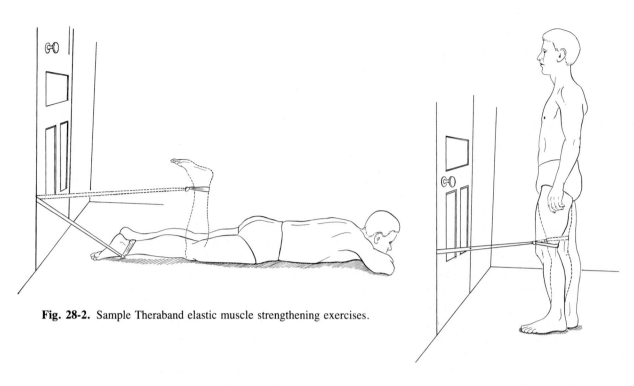

Fig. 28-2. Sample Theraband elastic muscle strengthening exercises.

of time on the job, stability of marriage, transportation to and from work, motivation, and the physical demands of the job. Because it is clearly more effective and economical to adapt the job to the individual rather than the other way around, job modification is the best way to overcome the difficulties individuals are having with their jobs. Although some efforts have been made in this direction, they are few and far between. The unwillingness of people to admit problems to their employers, strict union rules, insensitivity of management, and the lack of qualified expert consultants in the field make this problem almost insoluble. Although vocational rehabilitation services should be helpful in this respect, its counselors are more involved in retraining employees than in helping them stay at their current jobs. Also, their emphasis is more on the severely disabled than on those less impaired who could benefit more readily and at less expense. New legislation setting forth the rights of disabled people may create a climate in which needed reform may more readily occur.

RECREATION

As the length of the work week has declined during the past century, more time has become available for recreation, and recreational activities have come to represent a significant element in life. Many popular activities such as golf, hiking, tennis, water skiing, and even fishing require full use of the legs to be maximally enjoyable. For the older person who has given up an active life-style but now has more leisure time, travel has become an essential activity. However, travel, be it foreign or domestic, puts a heavy strain on the knees and must be limited or abandoned by those with arthritis. Some adaptations of present recreational

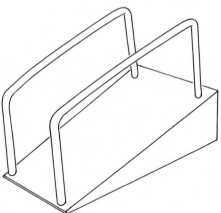

Fig. 28-3. The installation of rails and ramps around the home can facilitate daily life for chronically afflicted patients.

activities are certainly possible. Golf puts relatively little pressure on the knee, especially with the motorized golf carts generally in use today. By taking an extra acetaminophen or short-acting NSAID before a round, one can often successfully complete 9 or even 18 holes. By following well-groomed trails with gentle slopes, one can continue to hike in the woods. If the physician is willing to write a note to the airline affirming the degree of a patient's disability, a bulkhead seat can be made available that mitigates some of the discomfort of long-distance flights. If one can afford it, travel services can provide individual transportation service to ease the burdens of travel abroad. The most difficult but

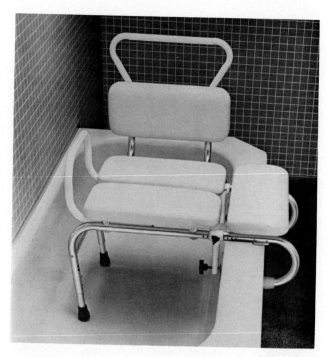

Fig. 28-4. Grab bars and a tub chair help to overcome obstacles to bathing and prevent falls. (Courtesy Fred Sammons Inc., Burr Ridge, Ill.)

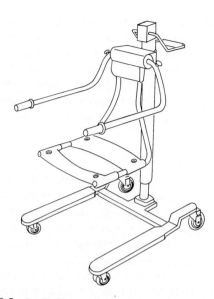

Fig. 28-5. A tub lift eases entry into whirlpools and baths.

perhaps most effective way of dealing with recreational blocks is to develop new interests that do not require total lower extremity integrity. If one lacks the imagination to find something attractive, an occupational therapist can administer a skills and interests inventory that can provide the basis for choosing new hobbies and recreational pursuits.

PSYCHOLOGICAL ASPECTS

Stress does not cause arthritis, but it certainly can aggravate it or precipitate it when present. Jacox,[27] comparing identical twins only one of whom had developed rheumatoid arthritis, found that the level of stress preceding onset was much higher in the affected than in the unaffected member of the pair. Most stresses, such as a disagreeable boss or a philandering son-in-law, cannot be eliminated, but people can be brought to see how stresses are affecting their symptoms and to modify their behavior. People cannot change their personalities but can gain insight into themselves that can help them deal more effectively with the way they react. Depression is a very common affliction in individuals with chronic arthritis.[28] For some it is a constitutive phenomenon that breaks out frequently at times of any major life change or stress. For others it is a more natural reaction to the necessity to endure pain and make major modifications in life. By being sensitive to such attitudes and emotional responses, the physician can provide support and insight that can be of great help and often inspire more gratitude than medications, exercises, or self-help devices. Medications such as fluoxetine (Prozac) for depression, cyclo-

benzaprine (Flexeril) to improve sleep pattern, or an occasional alprazolam (Xanax) for anxiety can be helpful if used appropriately. In our practice, a clinical psychologist provides essential help to patients needing counseling and psychological insight into the relationship between their symptoms and their emotional lives. If addiction to narcotics develops, the help of a psychiatrist with special interest and skill in this area needs to be sought.

TOTAL KNEE ARTHROPLASTY

A detailed discussion of this subject is beyond the scope of this chapter. For the individual with chronic arthritis of one or both knees, it is the ultimate solution, limited only by a few rare complications (dislocation, infection, thromboembolism, particulate synovitis) and eventual loosening in most, given sufficient time. The major indication for arthroplasty is pain that limits or prevents a person from doing what he or she most wants to do. The x-ray is most useful for making the diagnosis of chronic arthritis rather than defining the point in time when arthroplasty should be performed. However, individuals in whom severe worsening of symptoms coincides with rapid cartilage loss probably have a better outcome than those with minimal damage. In the latter case, one should pay special attention to the personality pattern of the individual. In particular, a person who complains of pain in other parts of the body for which no anatomic or physiologic explanation can be found may have a generalized pain syndrome that will not be much improved by surgery.

PSYCHOSOCIAL ASPECTS

Chronic arthritis affecting the knee, with or without involvement of other joints, can have profound effects on one's ability to maintain a life-style developed before the onset of arthritis. The most serious effect, of course, is on the ability to walk, climb stairs, or engage in such activities as tennis or heavy labor that require painless, normally functioning lower extremities. The limitations affecting any one individual go beyond the strictly mechanical impairments and are conditioned by personality, economic status, and ability to make satisfactory adjustments to a new way of life.

CONCLUSION

The management of the patient with chronic arthritis of the knee can be simple or complex, depending on the type of arthritis present, its severity, the presence of systemic disease of other joints or organs, and the psychosocial status of the affected individual. Although cure is seldom achievable, the physician who makes a proper diagnosis and takes the time to analyze all the factors involved in how this arthritis affects the life of his patient can do much to improve the well-being and functional status of the individual. Successful management often depends on a team effort involving rheumatologists, orthopedists, and physiatrists, as well as laboratory technicians, physical therapists, occupational therapists, and psychologists.

REFERENCES

1. Tapper EM, Hoover NW: Late results after meniscectomy, *J Bone Joint Surg [Am]* 51:517, 1969.
2. Lawrence RC, et al: Estimates of the prevalence of selected arthritic and musculoskeletal diseases in the United States, *J Rheumatol* 16:427, 1987.
3. Stecher RM: Heberden's nodes: a clinical description of osteoarthritis of the finger joints, *Ann Rheum Dis* 14:1, 1955.
4. Knowlton RG, et al: Genetic linkage of a polymorphism in the type II procollagen gene (COL2A1) to primary osteoarthritis associated with mild chondrodysplasia, *N Engl J Med* 322:526, 1990.
5. Felson DT, et al: Occupational physical demands, knee bending, and knee osteoarthritis: results from the Framingham study, *J Rheumatol* 19:1587, 1991.
6. Lawrence JS: Rheumatism in coal miners: III, occupational factor, *Br J Ind Med* 12:249, 1955.
7. Felson DT, et al: Obesity and knee osteoarthritis, the Framingham study, *Ann Intern Med* 107:18, 1988.
8. Pyron JG: *The epidemiology of osteoarthritis*. In Moskowitz RW, et al, editors: *Osteoarthritis, diagnosis and management*, Philadelphia, 1984, WB Saunders.
9. Neer CS, Craig EV, Fukuda H: Cuff tear arthropathy, *J Bone Joint Surg [Am]* 69:1232, 1983.
10. McCarty DJ, et al: Milwaukee shoulder: association of microspheroids containing hydroxyapatite crystals, active collagenose and neutral proteose with rotator cuff defects: I, clinical aspects, *Arthritis Rheum* 24:264, 1981.
11. Arnett FC: *HLA and the spondyloarthropathies*. In Calin A, editor: *Spondyloarthropathies*, Orlando, 1984, Grune & Stratton.
12. Dubost JJ, Sauvezie B: Late onset peripheral spondyloarthropathy, *J Rheumatol* 16:1214, 1989.
13. Miller TA, Jacobson ED: Gastrointestinal cytoprotection by prostaglandins, *Gut* 20:75, 1979.
14. Graham DY, Agraual NM, Roth SH: Prevention of NSAID-induced gastric ulcer with the synthetic prostaglandin, misoprostol: a multicenter, double-blind, placebo-controlled trial, *Lancet* 2:1277, 1988.
15. Kelley WN, Fox IH, Patella TD: *Gout and related disorders of purine metabolism*. In Kelley WN, et al, editors: *Textbook of rheumatology*, Philadelphia, 1989, WB Saunders.
16. Hollander JL, et al: Hydrocortisone and cortisone injected into arthritis joints, *JAMA* 147:1629, 1951.
17. Hollander JL: *Arthrocentesis technique and intrasynovial therapy*. In McCarty DJ, editor, *Arthritis and allied conditions, a textbook of rheumatology*, ed 10, Philadelphia, 1985, Lea & Febiger.
18. McCarty DJ: Treatment of rheumatoid joint inflammation with triamcinolone hexacetonide, *Arthritis Rheum* 15:157, 1972.
19. Ike RW, et al: Tidal irrigation versus conservative medication management in patients with osteoarthritis of the knee: a prospective randomized study, *J Rheumatol* 19:772, 1992.
20. Sledge CB, et al: Treatment of rheumatoid synovites of the knee with intraarticular injection of dyspropium 165–ferric hydroxide macroaggregates, *Arthritis Rheum* 29:153, 1986.
21. Harcom TM, et al: Therapeutic value of graded aerobic exercise training in rheumatoid arthritis, *Arthritis Rheum* 28:1, 1985.
22. Minor MA, et al: Efficacy of physical conditioning exercise in patients with rheumatoid arthritis and osteoarthritis, *Arthritis Rheum* 32:11, 1989.
23. Kovar PA, et al: Supervised fitness walking in patients with osteoarthritis of the knee, *Ann Intern Med* 116:7, 1992.
24. Fisher NM, et al: Muscle rehabilitation: its effect on muscular and functional performance of patients with knee osteoarthritis, *Arch Phys Med Rehabil* 72:6, 1991.
25. Mangine R, Heckmann TP, Eldridge VL: *Improving strength, endurance, and power*. In Scully RM, Barnes MR, editors: *Physical therapy*, Philadelphia, 1989, JB Lippincott.
26. Yelin EH, Henke CJ, Epstein WV: Work disability among persons with musculoskeletal conditions, *Arthritis Rheum* 29:1322, 1986.
27. Jacox RF: Personal communication.
28. Anderson KO, et al: Rheumatoid arthritis: review of psychological factors related to etiology, effects and treatment, *Psychol Bull* 98:358, 1985.

GENERAL INFORMATION AND REFERRAL SOURCES
Arthritis-related information resources

American Behçet's Foundation
421 21st Avenue SW
Rochester, MN 55902
(507) 282-9506

Services: Bestows grants for studies and research projects concerning Behçet's syndrome, gathers statistics on people with the disease, and educates the public and medical community on Behçet's syndrome.
Publications: Newsletter and brochures

American College of Rheumatology
17 Executive Park Drive, NE
Suite 480
Atlanta, GA 30329
(404) 633-3777

Services: Fosters development of rheumatology as a discipline. Composed of professionals devoted to the study of rheumatic diseases, education of physicians, and care of patients with these diseases.
Publications: Arthritis and Rheumatism, ARA Clinical Slide Collection on Rheumatic Diseases

The American Lupus Society
23751 Madison Street
Torrance, CA 90505
(213) 373-1335

Services: Engaged in the fight against lupus erythematosus. Assists lupus patients and their families in coping with the disease and involved in obtaining funds for lupus research. Chapters located throughout the country.

Publications: The Quarterly (newsletter), pamphlets, and other informational materials

Ankylosing Spondylitis Association
PO Box 5872
Sherman Oaks, CA 91413
(818) 990-3723

Services: Provides education information to patients, health professionals, and the general public on the disease and supports research.
Publications: Newsletter (quarterly), *Straight Talk on Ankylosing Spondylitis* (book), *Ankylosing Spondylitis–A Guidebook for Patients* (pamphlet), *Physical Therapy Exercises* (audiocassette with illustrated instructions)

Arthritis and Rheumatism Council
41 Eagle Street
London WCIR 4AR
England

Services: Finances research into the causes of and cures for the rheumatic diseases.
Publications: ARC (magazine) and *Reports on Rheumatic Diseases: A Guide to Arthritis* (series of handbooks to patients)

Arthritis Foundation
1314 Spring St. NE
Atlanta, GA 30309

Services: Over 70 chapters nationwide. Provides information and direct services such as self-help courses and pool exercise.
Publications: Bulletin of the Rheumatic Diseases and numerous pamphlets.

The Arthritis Society
250 Bloor Street East
Suite 401
Toronto, Ontario M4W 3PC
Canada
(416) 967-1414

Services: Devoted to funding and promoting arthritis research, patient care, and public education in the rheumatic diseases.
Publications: Arthritis News and various other publications

Lupus Foundation of America, Inc. (LFA)
1717 Massachusetts Avenue, NW
Suite 203
Washington, DC 20036
(202) 328-4500

Services: Clearinghouse for communications to and from the various LFA groups throughout the United States and Canada. Assists lupus patients with their problems, provides reference services and referrals, and works with other organizations on research.
Publications: Lupus News and various pamphlets

National Marfan Foundation
54 Irma Avenue
Port Washington, NY 11050
(516) 883-8712

Services: Disseminates accurate and timely information about Marfan syndrome and acts as a support network.
Publications: Connective Issues (newsletter) and *Marfan Syndrome* (pamphlet)

National Organization for Rare Diseases (NORD)
1182 Broadway
Suite 402
New York, NY 10001
(212) 686-1057

Services: Clearinghouse for information concerning rare disorders, monitors Orphan Drug Act, and stimulates research on rare diseases.
Publications: Orphan Disease Update

National Osteoporosis Foundation
1625 Eye Street, NW
Suite 1011
Washington, DC 20006
(202) 223-2226

Services: Supports a comprehensive education and research program designed to reduce the incidence of osteoporosis.
Publications: The Osteoporosis Report (Newsletter), *National Osteoporosis Foundation* (brochure), and *Osteoporosis: A Woman's Guide* (pamphlet)

National Psoriasis Foundation
6443 S.W. Beaverton Highway
Suite 210
Portland, OR 97221
(503) 297-1545

Services: Provides information and educational literature on psoriasis treatment and research.
Publications: National Psoriasis Foundation Bulletin, Annual Report, and patient education pamphlets

Osteogenesis Imperfecta Foundation
PO Box 838
Manchester, NH 03105
(516) 325-8992

Services: Supports medical research, educates the public about osteogenesis imperfecta, and disseminates information about the disease to patients and health professionals.
Publications: Breakthrough (newsletter), directories, and other literature

Paget's Disease Foundation, Inc.
PO Box 2772
Brooklyn, NY 11202
(718) 596-1043

Services: Dedicated to improving health care for people suffering from Paget's disease and allied disorders.
Publications: The PDF Update (newsletter) and pamphlets

Scleroderma Federation, Inc.
1377 K Street, NW
Suite 700
Washington, DC 20005
(703) 549-0666

Services: Coalition of various scleroderma organizations. Supports medical research and provides educational and support services to patients and their families.
Publications: Understanding and Managing Scleroderma (pamphlet)

Scleroderma International Foundation
704 Gardner Center Road
New Castle, PA 16101
(412) 652-3109

Services: Provides information to patients, physicians, and the general public on scleroderma.
Publications: The Connector (newsletter), *What is Scleroderma?* (pamphlet), and *From Isolation to Communication: An Anthology of Scleroderma Patients' Experiences* (booklet)

Scleroderma Research Foundation
Jobstown Road
PO Box 200
Columbus, NJ 08022
(609) 261-2200

Services: Provides information and support for patients and family members affected by scleroderma and funds medical research and awareness programs.
Publications: Informational pamphlets

Sjögren's Syndrome Foundation, Inc.
29 Gateway Drive
Great Neck, NY 11021
(516) 487-2243; (516) 364-8674

Services: Provides information to patients and their families about Sjögren's syndrome (chapters located throughout the country).
Publications: *The Moisture Seekers* (newsletter) and *A Handbook for Sjögren's Syndrome Patients*

United Scleroderma Foundation, Inc.
PO Box 350
Watsonville, CA 95077-0350
(408) 728-2202

Services: Provides information about scleroderma, maintains a physician referral and support network, and provides research grants.
Publications: Newsletter and pamphlets about scleroderma

Information resources

Clearinghouse on the Handicapped
Office of Special Education and Rehabilitative Services
US Department of Education
330 C Street, S.W., Room 3132
Washington, DC 20202-2319
(202) 732-1244; 732-1245

Services: Provides information and referral regarding federal and private services for the handicapped. Provides research information on recent developments bearing on handicapping conditions.
Publications: *Directory of National Information Sources on Handicapping Conditions and Related Services* (available from the Government Printing Office) and *Pocket Guide to Federal Help for the Disabled*

Consumer Information Center
Pueblo, CO 81009
(303) 948-3334

Services: Assists federal agencies in developing and releasing relevant and useful consumer information and helps increase public awareness of this information.
Publications: *Consumer Information Catalog* (lists more than 200 federal publications on topics such as careers, health, nutrition, education, and money management)

Information Center for Individuals with Disabilities
20 Park Place
Room 330
Boston, MA 02116
(617) 727-5540

Services: Assists disabled individuals in learning about the appropriate resources, agencies, and facts that promote a more independent life-style.
Publications: Monthly fact sheets and monthly newsletter

National Council on the Handicapped
800 Independence Avenue, SW
Suite 814
Washington, DC 20591
(202) 267-3846

Services: Establishes and implements policies concerning handicapped individuals.
Publications: Newsletter and other publications

National Easter Seal Society
2023 West Ogden Avenue
Chicago, IL 60612
(312) 243-8400

Services: Vary from state to state but may include physical and occupational therapy, vocational evaluation and training, camping and recreation, and psychological counseling. Contact local agencies for information.
Publications: List available

National Health Information Clearinghouse
PO Box 1133
Washington, DC 20013-1133
(202) 429-9091; (800) 336-4797

Services: Answers inquiries about disease prevention, clearing houses, professional associations, and voluntary organizations.
Publications: List available on request

National Highway Traffic Safety Administration
US Department of Transportation
400 Seventh Street, SW
Washington, DC 20590
(800) 424-9393; (202) 366-0123 in DC area

Services: Provides information and referral on effectiveness of occupant protection, such as the use of safety belts and child safety seats, and auto safety recalls.
Publications: "Consumer Information" briefs on various topics

Office of Disease Prevention and Health Promotion (ODHP)
PO Box 1133
Washington, DC 20013-1133
(800) 336-4797

Services: Information and referral for people with health questions. Database contains descriptions of health-related organizations and programs throughout the United States.
Publications: *Healthfinders* (series of resource lists on current health concerns) and *Health Information Resources in the Federal Government*

Local resources

The following local resources provide information on a variety of areas ranging from advocacy to transportation:

- Adult day care programs
- Area agencies on aging
- Churches, community, civic, and service groups
- Council or office on aging
- Departments of social services, human services, public assistance, or welfare
- Federal Information Centers. Provide information and referral regarding Federal and sometimes state and local governmental services. Look in phone directory under US Government, Federal Information Center, for listing.
- Geriatric Counselors or Care Managers. These individual or small group practices counsel older people and their families and help them find services to meet their particular needs. These practices operate on a fee-for-service basis and may be especially helpful to those whose incomes are too high to qualify for public programs.
- Independent Living Centers. Provide psychological counseling, transportation, vocational counseling, information on adaptive equipment, and other information to the physically disabled to aid them in a more independent life-style. For more information on centers, contact your local Rehabilita-

tion Services Division listed under the State Department of Human Resources.

- National Easter Seal Society
- Senior centers
- United States Government Printing Office. Provides information on all government printed materials. Call local US Government Information for telephone number in your area.

Publications

Consumer Resource Handbook. Published by the United States Office of Consumer Affairs. Contacts for available products and services in the marketplace. Order free copies from the Consumer Information Center, Pueblo, pecs CO 81009.

The Disability Bookshop. Prepared by The Disability Bookstore, PO Box 129, Vancouver, WA 98666, (206) 694-2462. Catalog includes books about cooking, computers, travel, sewing, gardening, education, etc. This is a shop-by-mail bookstore. Send $1.00 for postage and handling.

The Help Book. Prepared by city United Ways. Provides lists of people-serving agencies, describes the service and eligibility requirements of each, and gives the address, phone number, and contact at each agency.

Index

A

Acceptance, in grief process model, 90
Acetaminophen (Anacin 3; Tylenol), 52
Acetylsalicylic acid. *See* Aspirin
Achilles tendon, stretching of, 229
ACL. *See* Anterior cruciate ligament (ACL)
Acoustical streaming, 67
Active assisted flexion, 156
Active-assisted range of motion, for meniscal injury, 137
Activities of daily living, arthritis and, 321, 322-323
Adaptive phase, of injury, 90
Adductors, stretching of, 278
Adjustment problems, 96
Advil (ibuprofen), 49
Aerobic conditioning
    for dancers, 281
    for skiers, 289, 290
Aerobic dance, 274, 275, 279. *See also* Dance
Aesthetics, dance and, 274-275
Agility drills, 263
    for skiers, 291
Alternating current (AC), 55-56
Amenorrhea, 281
Anaerobic conditioning, for skiers, 289
Anaerobic power training, 260-261
Analgesic drugs, 45
Anaphylatoxin, 38
Anaprox (naproxen sodium), 49
Anger, in grief process model, 90
Anterior cruciate ligament (ACL)
    anatomy of, 12
    blood supply of, 12
    evaluation of
        diagnosis of injury and, 26-27
        Lachman's test for, 23
    female knee stability and, 299
    functions of, 23
    healing of. *See also* Ligaments, healing of
        negative factors in, 42-43
        positive factors in, 39-40
    injuries of
        boot-induced rupture, 284
        functional knee brace for, 109-110
        lateral capsular sign and, 29
        mechanisms of sprain in skiing, 284-285
        with meniscal tear, 136
        prophylactic lateral bracing for, 99-100, 103
        in skiers, 283
        tears, dancers and, 276
    mechanoreceptors of, 12-13
    reconstruction rehabilitation of, 153, 162-163
        electrical stimulation for, 59
        for gymnast, 234-239
        in hospital, 156-158
        office/therapy visits for, 158-159
        phase I of, 157-159
        phase II of, 159-161
        phase III of, 161-162
        postoperative bracing for, 111-112
        postoperative phase, 156-163
        postoperative strength assessment for, 162
        preoperative phase, 153-156
Anterior tibia, strengthening of, 232
Anterior tibial muscles, running and, 227
Anterior-posterior component
    control during taping, 131
    in patellar orientation, 130
Anterolateral instability tests, 23
Anti-inflammatory drugs, 45
Apley's test, positive, 135
Appetite suppressants, 319
Aquatic sports. *See also* Diving injuries; Swimming
    knee injuries in, 247

Arabesque, 235
Arachidonic acid, 46
Arc slides, 213
Arcuate ligament, 16
Arthritis
    activities of daily living and, 321, 322-323
    diagnosis of, 318
    injection therapy for, 320-321
    occupation and, 321-322
    pharmacologic management od, 319-320
    physical therapy for, 321
    psychological aspects, 323
    psychosocial aspects, 323-324
    recreation and, 322-323
    total knee arthroplasty for, 323
    types of, 318
    weight loss and, 319
Arthrography
    in clinical assessment, 29-30
    double-contrast, of meniscal injury, 135
Arthrometry, of functional knee brace, 107-108
Arthroscopy, limitations of, 31-32
Arthrotomy, postoperative muscle inhibition and, 58
Articular cartilage, healing of. *See also* Soft tissues, healing of
    negative factors in, 43
    positive factors in, 40, 42
Aspiration technique, for knee, 320
Aspirin
    adverse effects of
        gastrointestinal irritation and, 48
        prolonged bleeding time and, 48
        Reye's syndrome and, 48
        tinnitus and, 48
    for arthritis, 319
    effects of, 48-49
    historical background of, 48
    mechanism of action, 46
Assessment. *See* Clinical assessment
Associative focus, 95
Athletic training, electrical stimulation in, 60-61
Atrophy, electrical stimulation for, 59-60
Avulsion fracture, of tibial eminence, 285
Axes, for joint motion, 8

B

Baker's cyst, 171, 173
Balance, 74
Balance beam, 234, 235
Balance board, 212-213
Balance training, 74-75
    devices for, 74
Ballet, 274. *See also* Dance
    women and, 309-310
Ballottement, of patella, 320
BAPS board (Biomechanical Ankle Platform System), 74, 75
Bargaining, in grief process model, 90
Baseball
    importance of knee in, 219-221
    injuries
        rehabilitation exercise prescriptions for, 224-226
        statistics for, 220
    kinetic chains in, 221
    vs. tennis, rehabilitative differences in, 221-222
Basketball injuries
    agility exercises/drills, 213-215, 217
    conditioning for, 215, 217
    etiology of, 208
    in females, 208-209
    functional exercises, 212
    prevention of, 209
    proprioceptive exercises, 212
    rehabilitation program for, 209
        strengthening exercises, 209-211